Clinical Audiology

Clinical Audiology

Editor: Hannah Rivera

AMERICAN
MEDICAL PUBLISHERS
www.americanmedicalpublishers.com

AMERICAN
MEDICAL PUBLISHERS
www.americanmedicalpublishers.com

Cataloging-in-Publication Data

Clinical audiology / edited by Hannah Rivera.
p. cm.
Includes bibliographical references and index.
ISBN 978-1-63927-406-2
1. Audiology. 2. Hearing disorders--Treatment. 3. Hearing disorders--Diagnosis. 4. Audiometry.
5. Otolaryngology. I. Rivera, Hannah.
RF290 .C55 2022
617.8--dc23

American Medical Publishers,
41 Flatbush Avenue,
1st Floor, New York,
NY 11217, USA

ISBN 978-1-63927-406-2 (Hardback)

Contents

Preface

Clinical audiology is a field concerned with the treatment and prevention of hearing loss or damage. Besides vestibular and audiologic pathologies, the rehabilitation of various auditory disorders such as tinnitus, misophonia, hyperacusis and auditory processing disorders is under the scope of this field. Various testing strategies such as otoacoustic emission measurements, behavioural hearing tests and electrophysiologic tests are employed to determine a person's sensitivity to sounds. After diagnosis, assessing the degree or severity of hearing loss, determining the audio frequency range the ear is insensitive to and the location of the lesion that is causing the hearing loss, are vital to address the problem. Cochlear implants and hearing aids are some of the interventions of managing a hearing disorder. This book discusses the fundamentals as well as modern approaches of clinical audiology. It unfolds the innovative aspects of audiology and audiological health which will be crucial for the progress of this field in the future. The extensive content of this book provides the readers with a thorough understanding of the subject.

This book unites the global concepts and researches in an organized manner for a comprehensive understanding of the subject. It is a ripe text for all researchers, students, scientists or anyone else who is interested in acquiring a better knowledge of this dynamic field.

I extend my sincere thanks to the contributors for such eloquent research chapters. Finally, I thank my family for being a source of support and help.

Editor

1

Impaired Auditory-Vestibular Functions and Behavioral Abnormalities of *Slitrk6*-Deficient Mice

Yoshifumi Matsumoto[1], Kei-ichi Katayama[1], Takehito Okamoto[2], Kazuyuki Yamada[3], Noriko Takashima[1], Soichi Nagao[2], Jun Aruga[1]*

1 Laboratory for Behavioral and Developmental Disorders, RIKEN Brain Science Institute (BSI), Wako-shi, Japan, **2** Laboratory for Motor Learning Control, RIKEN Brain Science Institute (BSI), Wako-shi, Japan, **3** Support Unit for Animal Experiments, RIKEN Brain Science Institute (BSI), Wako-shi, Japan

Abstract

A recent study revealed that Slitrk6, a transmembrane protein containing a leucine-rich repeat domain, has a critical role in the development of the inner ear neural circuit. However, it is still unknown how the absence of *Slitrk6* affects auditory and vestibular functions. In addition, the role of *Slitrk6* in regions of the central nervous system, including the dorsal thalamus, has not been addressed. To understand the physiological role of Slitrk6, *Slitrk6*-knockout (KO) mice were subjected to systematic behavioral analyses including auditory and vestibular function tests. Compared to wild-type mice, the auditory brainstem response (ABR) of *Slitrk6*-KO mice indicated a mid-frequency range (8–16 kHz) hearing loss and reduction of the first ABR wave. The auditory startle response was also reduced. A vestibulo-ocular reflex (VOR) test showed decreased vertical (head movement–induced) VOR gains and normal horizontal VOR. In an open field test, locomotor activity was reduced; the tendency to be in the center region was increased, but only in the first 5 min of the test, indicating altered adaptive responses to a novel environment. Altered adaptive responses were also found in a hole-board test in which head-dip behavior was increased and advanced. Aside from these abnormalities, no clear abnormalities were noted in the mood, anxiety, learning, spatial memory, or fear memory–related behavioral tests. These results indicate that the *Slitrk6*-KO mouse can serve as a model of hereditary sensorineural deafness. Furthermore, the altered responses of *Slitrk6*-KO mice to the novel environment suggest a role of *Slitrk6* in some cognitive functions.

Editor: Fabien Tell, The Research Center of Neurobiology-Neurophysiology of Marseille, France

Funding: This study was funded by RIKEN Brain Science Institute (BSI) and supported by the Japan Society for the Promotion of Science. The funders had no role in study design, data collection and analysis, decision to publish, or preparation of the manuscript.

Competing Interests: The authors have declared that no competing interests exist.

* E-mail: jaruga@brain.riken.jp

Introduction

Slitrk6 belongs to the Slitrk family of transmembrane proteins with neurite outgrowth modulating activities [1,2]. Structurally, Slitrk members share two leucine-rich repeat domains located amino-terminal to the transmembrane domain. In the carboxy-terminus, there are conserved tyrosine residues flanked by amino acid sequences similar to those in the carboxy-terminal domain of the Ntrk neurotrophin receptor [3]. Among the six *Slitrk* family genes (*Slitrk1–6*) in mice, *Slitrk6* shows a unique expression pattern, with strong expression in the inner ear and modest expression in the dorsal thalamus at both embryonic and postnatal stages [1,4–6].

A recent study revealed that Slitrk6 promotes innervation and survival of inner ear sensory neurons in part by modulating neurotrophin–Ntrk signaling [5]. *Slitrk6*-knockout (KO) mice showed reduced cochlear innervation. In the vestibule, the innervation to the posterior crista was often lost, reduced, or sometimes misguided. These defects were accompanied by the loss of neurons in the spiral and vestibular ganglia. This study addressed only the embryonic to early postnatal morphological phenotype of *Slitrk6*-KO mice, and analyses of any functional deficits caused by the developmental defects of the inner ear remain to be conducted.

Previous studies reported Slitrk family members as candidate genes controlling several neuropsychiatric disorders [7–13]. Considering the expression of *Slitrk6* in the mature central nervous system [1,2] (http://www.brain-map.org/), it is possible that *Slitrk6* has a role in the expression of higher brain functions.

In the present study, we evaluated the neurological characteristics of the *Slitrk6*-KO mouse by performing systematic behavioral analyses and physiological tests related to inner ear functions. The results revealed deficits in the auditory, vestibular, and cognitive functions of *Slitrk6*-KO mice. We discussed the biological significance of *Slitrk6* and the similarities of deficits in the KO mice to the phenotypes of some neurological diseases.

Results

General features of the *Slitrk6*-KO mouse

The *Slitrk6* null allele (*Slitrk6*$^{-}$) was generated by replacing its entire protein-coding region by a loxP sequence [5]. Both male and female *Slitrk6*-KO (*Slitrk6*$^{-/-}$) mice grew without showing any external abnormalities and were fertile [5]. A slight, but significant reduction in body weight was observed in the adult male mice (wild type [WT]: $n = 10$, 26.5±0.57 g [mean ± SE]; KO: $n = 10$, 24.6±0.19 g at 12 weeks old). However, the reason for this weight reduction is not clear. We used adult male *Slitrk6*-KO mice and

WT (*Slitrk6*$^{+/+}$) littermates for the behavioral and inner ear function tests. The behavioral tests are listed in Table 1.

Auditory function defects in *Slitrk6*-KO mice

Auditory brain-stem response (ABR) is an electrical signal reflecting the neuronal activities related to auditory information processing. The ABR method has been shown to be effective for assessing auditory function in mice [14]. We recorded ABRs in anesthetized mice with ear and scalp electrodes. The responses were recorded upon delivering sound stimuli with certain ranges of frequencies (2–24 kHz) and strength (10–80 dB). Figure 1A presents the ABR waves from WT and *Slitrk6*-KO mice. To determine the hearing function of *Slitrk6*-KO mice, we first measured the thresholds for the appearance of a recognizable wave representing ABR (Fig. 1B). The results indicated significant increments (ca. 20 dB) of the sound intensity threshold for 8-kHz (WT = 48.5±2.6 [mean ± SE], KO = 62.2±2.22; $P<0.01$, Mann-Whitney's *U*-test) and 16-kHz (WT = 17.1±1.84, KO = 30±2.88; $P<0.05$) stimuli, but not for 2-, 4-, and 24-kHz stimuli at 4 weeks of age. When the amplitude and latency values of peaks I, II, and III with an 80-dB stimulus were compared between WT and *Slitrk6*-KO mice (Fig. 1C top), there was a significant decrement in the peak I absolute values of 16-kHz (WT = 5.42±0.43 [mean ± SE], KO = 3.55±0.31; $P=0.0031$), 8-kHz (WT = 2.51±0.15, KO = 1.36±0.16; $P=0.00020$), and 4-kHz (WT = 2.58±0.09, KO = 2.02±0.16; $P=0.012$) stimuli-induced

Table 1. Summary of Slitrk6 KO behavioral analyses.

Test	Parameter	Comparison to WT mice
Home cage activity	whole day	n.s.
	light phase	increment in KO mice (08:00–09:00, $P<0.05$)
	dark phase	decrement in KO mice (23:00–01:00, $P=0.68$)
Open field	total distance	decrement in KO mice (first 5 min, $P<0.01$)
	moving speed	decrement in KO mice ($P<0.01$)
	time in center area (%)	increment in KO mice (first 5 min, $P<0.01$)
Hole-board test	active time	n.s.
	total distance (cm)	n.s.
	head-dip latency (s)	decrement in KO mice ($P<0.05$)
	number of head dips	n.s.
	head dipping duration (s)	increment in KO mice ($P<0.05$)
	rearing duration (s)	n.s.
	number of rearing episodes	n.s.
Elevated plus maze	total distance (cm)	n.s.
	entry number	n.s.
	time in open arm (%)	n.s.
	number of entry to open arm (%)	n.s.
Light–dark box	total distance (cm)	n.s.
	number of transitions	n.s.
	latency to transition to dark box	n.s.
	distance travelled in light box (%)	n.s.
	time spent in light box (%)	n.s.
Morris water maze	total distance (cm)	n.s.
	movement time (s)	n.s.
	latency to platform (s)	n.s.
Fear conditioning	context test	n.s.
	cued test	n.s.
Hot plate test	lick	n.s.
Tail flick test	flinch	n.s.
	jump	n.s.
Rota- rod test	rotation	n.s.
Startle response	startle response	decrement in KO mice (95–120 dB, $P<0.01$)
	initial/final	n.s.
	prepulse inhibition	n.s.
Social interaction	number of contacts	n.s.
Tail suspension	immobility time (%)	decrement in KO mice ($P<0.01$)
Forced swimming	immobility time (%)	n.s.

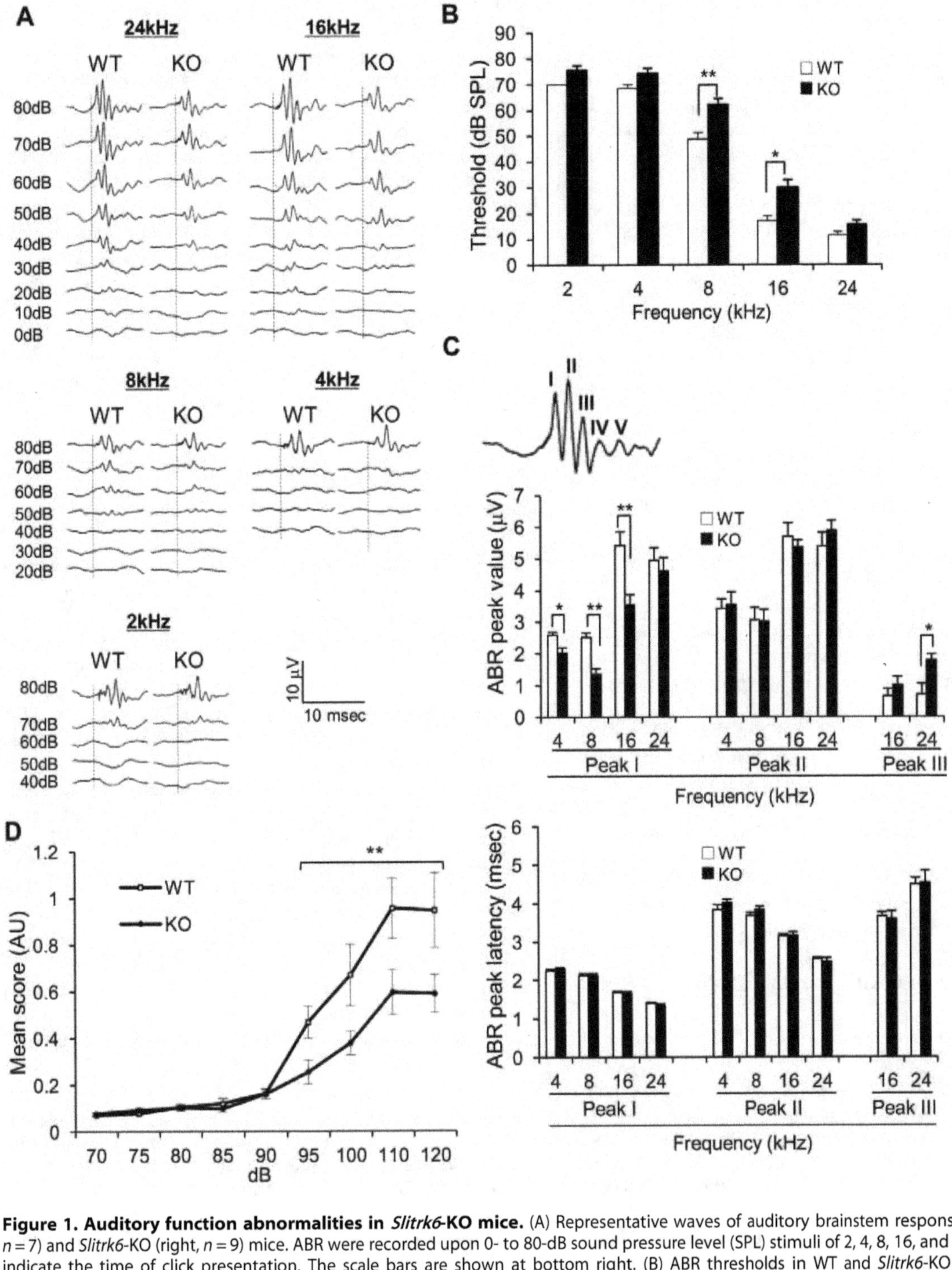

Figure 1. Auditory function abnormalities in *Slitrk6*-KO mice. (A) Representative waves of auditory brainstem response (ABR) from WT (left, $n=7$) and *Slitrk6*-KO (right, $n=9$) mice. ABR were recorded upon 0- to 80-dB sound pressure level (SPL) stimuli of 2, 4, 8, 16, and 24 kHz. The dash lines indicate the time of click presentation. The scale bars are shown at bottom right. (B) ABR thresholds in WT and *Slitrk6*-KO mice. *Slitrk6*-KO mice showed significantly higher thresholds to the 8- and 16-kHz stimuli than those of WT mice. (C) *Top:* Each peak number in a representative ABR wave. *Middle:* Comparison of the values of peaks I, II, and III between WT and *Slitrk6*-KO mice. Peak I of *Slitrk6*-KO mice was significantly reduced in the range of 8 to 16 kHz, and peak III was also significantly reduced at 24 kHz. *Bottom:* The latency to peaks I, II, and III. The latency did not show clear differences between WT and *Slitrk6*-KO mice. (D) Auditory startle response of WT ($n=10$) and *Slitrk6*-KO mice ($n=10$). *Slitrk6*-KO mice showed significantly lower startle responses to 95- to 120-dB sounds. $^{*}P<0.05$, $^{**}P<0.01$. All bars are mean ± standard error of the mean.

responses in *Slitrk6*-KO mice (Fig. 1C middle). There also was a significant increment in the peak III absolute values for the 24-kHz stimulus (Fig. 1C middle; WT $=0.69\pm0.34$, KO $=1.76\pm0.20$; $P=0.015$). However, the peak latency was not significantly different between the two genotypes (Fig. 1C bottom).

Auditory startle response (ASR) was included in the auditory function analysis. We measured the ASR following white noise stimulation with various sound intensities (Fig. 1D; 70–120 dB on 65-dB background noise). Compared with WT mice, *Slitrk6*-KO mice showed significant decrements of ASR toward the stronger sound stimuli (95–120 dB; $F_{1,18} = 9.7$, $P = 0.0059$, two-way ANOVA, main effect of genotype) but not toward the weaker ones (70–90 dB). While there was a clear difference in ASR between the genotypes, there were no significant differences in the prepulse (70, 75, and 80 dB) inhibition of ASR induced by a 120-dB stimulus (Table 1). Thus, both ABR and ASR results indicated that there was an auditory function deficit in the *Slitrk6*-KO mice.

Vertical vestibular function defects in *Slitrk6*-KO mice

A previous study revealed the frequent absence of vestibular nerve projection to the posterior crista in *Slitrk6*-KO mice [5]. Therefore, functions of the semicircular canal were investigated. We measured eye movements induced by rotation of the head on the plane of the horizontal semicircular canal, that is, the horizontal vestibulo-ocular reflex (hVOR), or on the plane perpendicular to the plane of the horizontal semicircular canal, the vertical vestibulo-ocular reflex (vVOR). The horizontal optokinetic response (hOKR), which shares the same neural circuit within the cerebellum as that of the hVOR, was measured as a reference. There were no clear differences in the hVOR or hOKR gains and phases between WT and *Slitrk6*-KO mice (Fig. 2A, B). For the vVOR, however, *Slitrk6*-KO mice showed significantly decreased gains at all four frequencies examined (Fig. 2C; $F_{1,12} = 11.7$, $P = 0.0051$, two-way ANOVA, main effect of genotype). There were no significant differences in the vVOR phases. These results indicated that there was a functional deficit in the semicircular canal of *Slitrk6*-KO mice.

We also performed behavioral tests related to vestibular functions, such as swimming, contact righting, and suspension [15]. In the suspension test, we did not see the trunk curling posture that is typically found in mice with impaired vestibular function [15] (data not shown). Swimming and contact righting did not show clear differences between the two genotypes (data not shown). In addition, *Slitrk6*-KO mice displayed a comparable performance to that of WT mice in the rota-rod test (Fig. 2D), which partly reflect vestibular function. These results suggested that the vestibular functional deficit in *Slitrk6*-KO mice is mild and selective for the posterior semicircular canal system.

Adaptive responses to environmental change are altered in *Slitrk6*-KO mice

In addition to inner ear–related abnormalities in *Slitrk6*-KO mice, novel phenotypes became clear based on their performance in a battery of behavioral tests (Table 1). First, we noticed altered activities of *Slitrk6*-KO mice in the home cage (Fig. 3). The activity level during the early dark phase tended to be lower (20:00–01:00, $P = 0.11$; 23:00–01:00, $P = 0.068$) and that during the beginning of the light phase was significantly higher (08:00–09:00, $P = 0.045$) than activity levels of the WT mice.

In an open field (OF) test with a 15-min observation period, the *Slitrk6*-KO mice showed less locomotor activity (Fig. 4A), although the difference was limited to the first 5 min (Fig. 4A; $P = 0.0023$). Furthermore, the percentage of time the *Slitrk6*-KO mice remained in the center area was significantly longer than the WT only in the first 5 min (Fig. 4B; $P = 0.0082$, Mann-Whitney's *U*-test). The abnormalities only in the early phase were thought to reflect some altered adaptive responses to the novel environment.

We also noted altered responses to a novel environment in the hole-board (HB) test, which was carried out for 5 min in a box that was the same size as the OF box. However, the HB box differed from the OF box in terms of color, brightness, and the presence of four holes on its floor. The total duration of head dipping into the holes by *Slitrk6*-KO mice was more than twice that of WT (Fig. 4D; $P = 0.046$). In addition, the latency to the first head dip was significantly shorter than that in the WT (Fig. 4E; $P = 0.028$).

Because *Slitrk6*-KO mice showed altered spontaneous activities in the three different contexts (home cage, OF box, and HB box), we evaluated whether these behavioral abnormalities were caused by elevated anxiety in a novel environment. We therefore performed the elevated plus maze test and light–dark box test, which are commonly used in neurobiological anxiety research. In these tests, however, we did not find any obvious differences between WT and *Slitrk6*-KO mice (Fig. 5). These results indicated that alterations of spontaneous activity in the home cage, OF, and HB tests are due to cognitive dysfunction in the *Slitrk6*-KO mice, rather than elevated anxiety.

The Morris water maze test, fear-conditioning test, forced swimming test, social interaction tests, tail flick test, and hot plate test did not show any abnormalities in the *Slitrk6*-KO mice as compared to the WT (Table 1).

Discussion

The *Slitrk6*-KO mouse is a novel animal model of sensorineural deafness

ABRs and ASRs indicated that there is an impaired auditory function in *Slitrk6*-KO mice. A mild (ca. 20-dB) elevation of the sound intensity threshold was observed for 8- and 16-kHz sound stimuli, resulting in a strong decrement of the ABR first wave (peak I). The results suggest that the reduction of peak I to the 80-dB stimulus is related to both the *Slitrk6* loss-of-function and the impaired auditory function. Although the precise origins of ABR waves are not yet well defined, it is generally agreed that the first wave represents activities of the auditory nerve and the late waves represent neural transmission within the central auditory circuit [16]. Our previous study revealed that during embryonic development of *Slitrk6*-KO mice the number of axon projection from the spiral ganglion to cochlear hair and the number of the spiral ganglion neurons were lower than seen in WT mice [5]. The total cell number in the spiral ganglion of *Slitrk6*-KO mice was one half that in WT, and the decreased number of the projection was clearly observed as late as 4 weeks after birth. Therefore, it is likely that the reduction of peak I may reflect these morphological differences in the inner ear neural circuit of *Slitrk6*-KO mice.

It is interesting that elevation of the sound intensity threshold was not observed for the 24-kHz sound stimulus. The frequency-selective sensitivity loss might not be fully explained by the innervation defects in the inner ear, considering that the projection impairment was generally observed from the basal to apical region of the cochlea. It is possible that some mechanism compensates for the desensitization to 24-kHz sounds. The enigmatic peak III increment might reflect such a process.

Many genes are associated with hearing impairment in mice [17,18], and 44 of them have been linked to human hereditary hearing loss [17]. Our findings indicate that *Slitrk6*-KO mice could be a novel model of sensorineural deafness. According to the current hereditary hearing loss database (http://hereditaryhearingloss.org), the nearest neighboring gene related to hearing impairment is an autosomal dominant nonsyndromic gene (DFNA 33, 13q34-qter) [19] approximately 27 Mb apart from *SLITRK6* (13q31.2). Thus, the involvement of functional deficits in *SLITRK6* in human hereditary hearing impairment awaits further investigation. Furthermore, *Slitrk6* inner ear abnormalities are known to involve altered neurotrophin-signaling [5]. NT-3 delivery has been attempted in model animals [20–22] with the aim of clinical treatment of hearing impairment, and it would be beneficial to

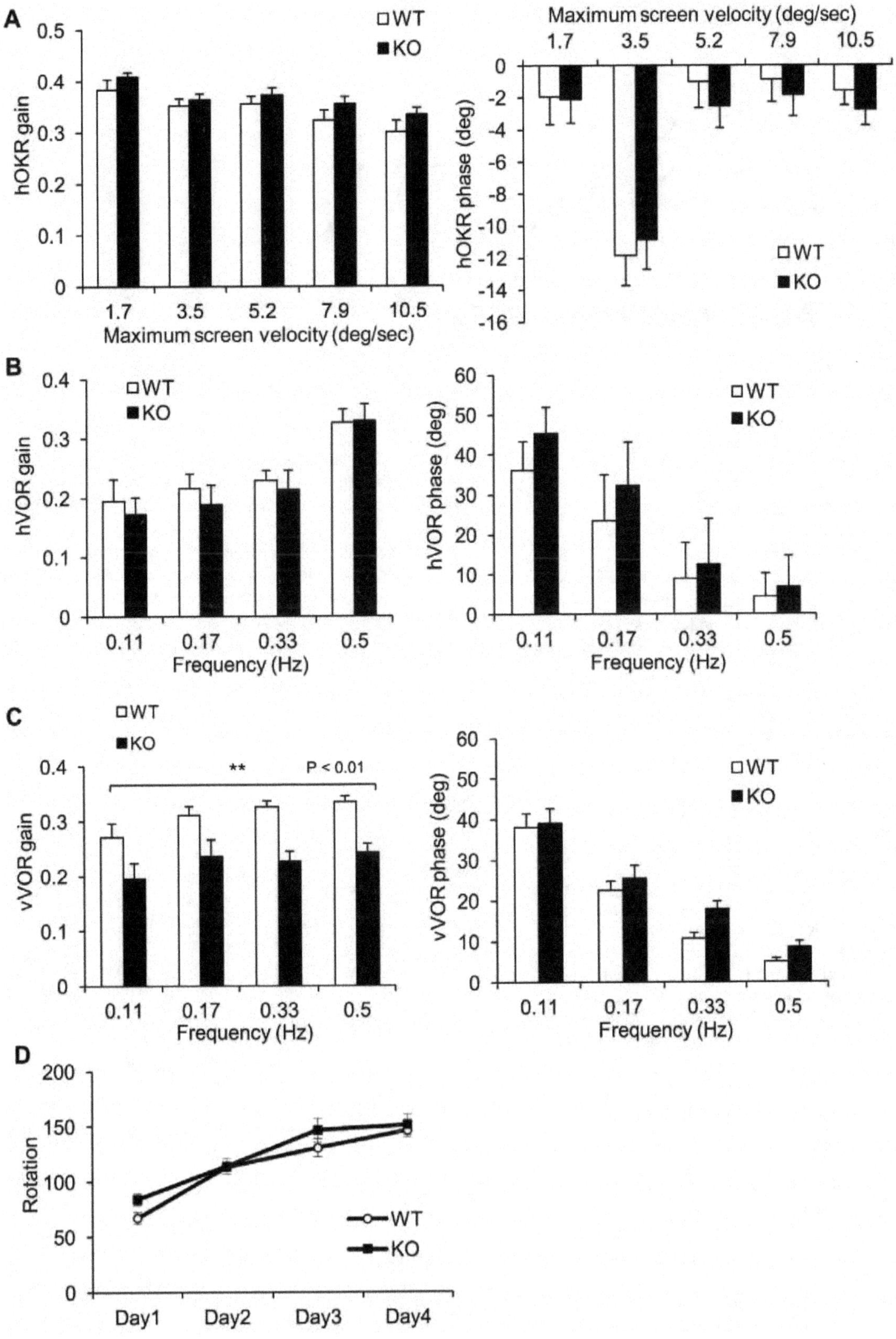

Figure 2. Vestibular function anomaly in *Slitrk6*-KO mice. (A) Dynamic characteristics of horizontal optokinetic response (hOKR) of WT ($n = 9$) and *Slitrk6*-KO ($n = 9$) mice. (B) Horizontal vestibulo-ocular reflex (hVOR). There were no differences in gains (left) or phases (right) between WT ($n = 9$) and KO ($n = 9$) in hVOR or hOKR. (C) Vertical vestibulo-ocular reflex (vVOR) of WT ($n = 8$) and *Slitrk6*-KO mice ($n = 6$). Gains of vVOR (left) of the *Slitrk6*-KO mice were significantly smaller than those of WT. (D) Rota- rod test. Rotation indicates the speed of rotation (rpm) at which the mice fell off or revolved around the rod. The values were comparable between WT ($n = 12$) and *Slitrk6*-KO ($n = 8$) mice, suggesting that there were no strong deficits of balancing function in *Slitrk6*-KO mice. Values are mean ± standard error of the mean.

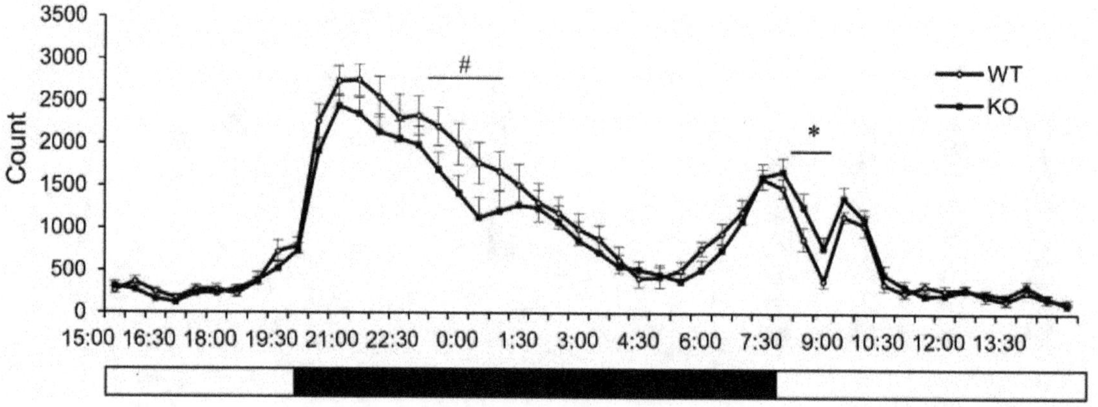

Figure 3. Spontaneous activity in home cage. Each vertical bar represents standard error of the mean. $^{\#}P = 0.068$; $^{*}P < 0.05$. WT, $n = 10$; KO, $n = 10$. Below the graph, open and black bars indicate light phase (08:00–20:00) and dark phase (20:00–08:00), respectively.

further clarify the mechanism of *Slitrk6* action in development of the inner ear and auditory signal processing.

Vestibular function abnormalities in *Slitrk6*-KO mice

Slitrk6-KO mice showed moderate deficit in the gain of vVOR, but not in hVOR. Based on the orientations of mouse semicircular canals [23], horizontal semicircular canals are selectively stimulated in the test of hVOR, whereas the anterior and posterior semicircular canals are equally stimulated in the test of vVOR in our assay system. The involvement of otolith in the head rotation used in our vVOR test was small, as the effect of gravity was minimal in the head rotation in nose-up position perpendicular to the earth axis. On the other hand, we previously showed that the neural projection to posterior crista, which develops to posterior semicircular canal, was often lost in *Slitrk6*-KO mice (78.3% at E13.5 [$n = 83$], 85.7% at E15.5 [$n = 28$], and 90.3% after P14 [$n = 62$]), but those to the anterior and horizontal canal cristae and otolith organs remained intact [5]. Thus, the defect of VOR (normal hVOR and impaired vVOR) is consistent with the anomaly of vestibular nerve projection (intact innervation of anterior and horizontal cristae and decreased innervation of posterior crista) in *Slitrk6*-KO mice. Concurrently, the VOR results suggest that function of *Slitrk6*-KO horizontal canal is not obviously impaired, indistinguishable from those of WT. However, the functional and structural properties of the remained inner ear neural circuits of *Slitrk6*-KO should be more carefully examined because embryonic *Slitrk6* expression broadly occurs in the inner ear sensory epithelia [5].

Many mutant mice with vestibular function abnormalities are listed in the current mouse genome informatics database (http://www.informatics.jax.org/). However, we did not find any mice with vertical-direction limited VOR abnormalities. In this regard, the vestibular dysfunction in *Slitrk6*-KO mice is unique. Together with the selective innervation defects to the posterior crista, *Slitrk6*-KO mice could serve as a useful model to study the role of the semicircular canal in vestibular function.

Although the vestibular function alteration was clear in the vVOR, it is unclear how the other behavioral phenotypes in *Slitrk6*-KO mice reflect the altered vestibular function. For example, *Slitrk6*-KO mice showed a significant decrement in the immobility time of the tail suspension test (Table 1). This alteration could indicate the absence of a normal vestibular response for vertical head movement. However, even if this is the case, the overall vestibular function deficit appears to be mild and selective. The vestibular innervation defects in the posterior canal may be partially compensated by the anterior semicircular canal and possibly the otolith organs, which also sense vertical head movements.

In humans, a posterior semicircular canal dysfunction is related to benign paroxysmal positional vertigo, in which displaced otoconia are thought to enter a semicircular canal, usually in the posterior one [24,25]. Although this is a disorder of late onset (mean onset 54 years old) [24], there are pediatric patients with balance and vestibular disorders [26,27]. Considering that significant associations exist between sensorineural hearing loss and balance disorders [26], it is possible that *SLITRK6* is involved in some pathophysiological processes of pediatric vestibular disorders.

Cognitive dysfunction of *Slitrk6*-KO mice

This study revealed novel behavioral phenotypes of *Slitrk6*-KO mice (Table 1). Among them, the abnormalities revealed by the OF and HB tests may reflect similar aspects of altered higher brain function in *Slitrk6*-KO mice. In both tests, the abnormalities appeared soon (within 5 min) after entry into the test boxes. Therefore, we assume that the novel environments induced the differential behaviors. Our findings clearly indicated a neurological basis for these behavioral abnormalities, which appeared to reflect increased attention to the environment and emotional responses similar to "restlessness" or "confusion."

It is tempting to correlate these behavioral abnormalities with the role of *Slirk6* in the thalamus, where its expression is clearly demarcated among regions of the central nervous system [1,4,6]. If we assume that the thalamic expression is significant, some sensory information processing during adaptive behaviors may be dysfunctional in *Slitrk6*-KO mice, considering the many roles played by the thalamus in relaying and modulating sensory signals [28–30]. Future studies should examine whether *Slitrk6* loss-of-function impairs the development or the function of the thalamic neural circuit. Clarification of the molecular function of *Slitrk6* will contribute to a better understanding of the higher function of the mammalian brain.

Materials and Methods

Animals

Animal experiments were approved by the Animal Experiment Committee of the RIKEN Brain Science Institute (approval no. H18-2B032), and the mice were maintained at the institute's

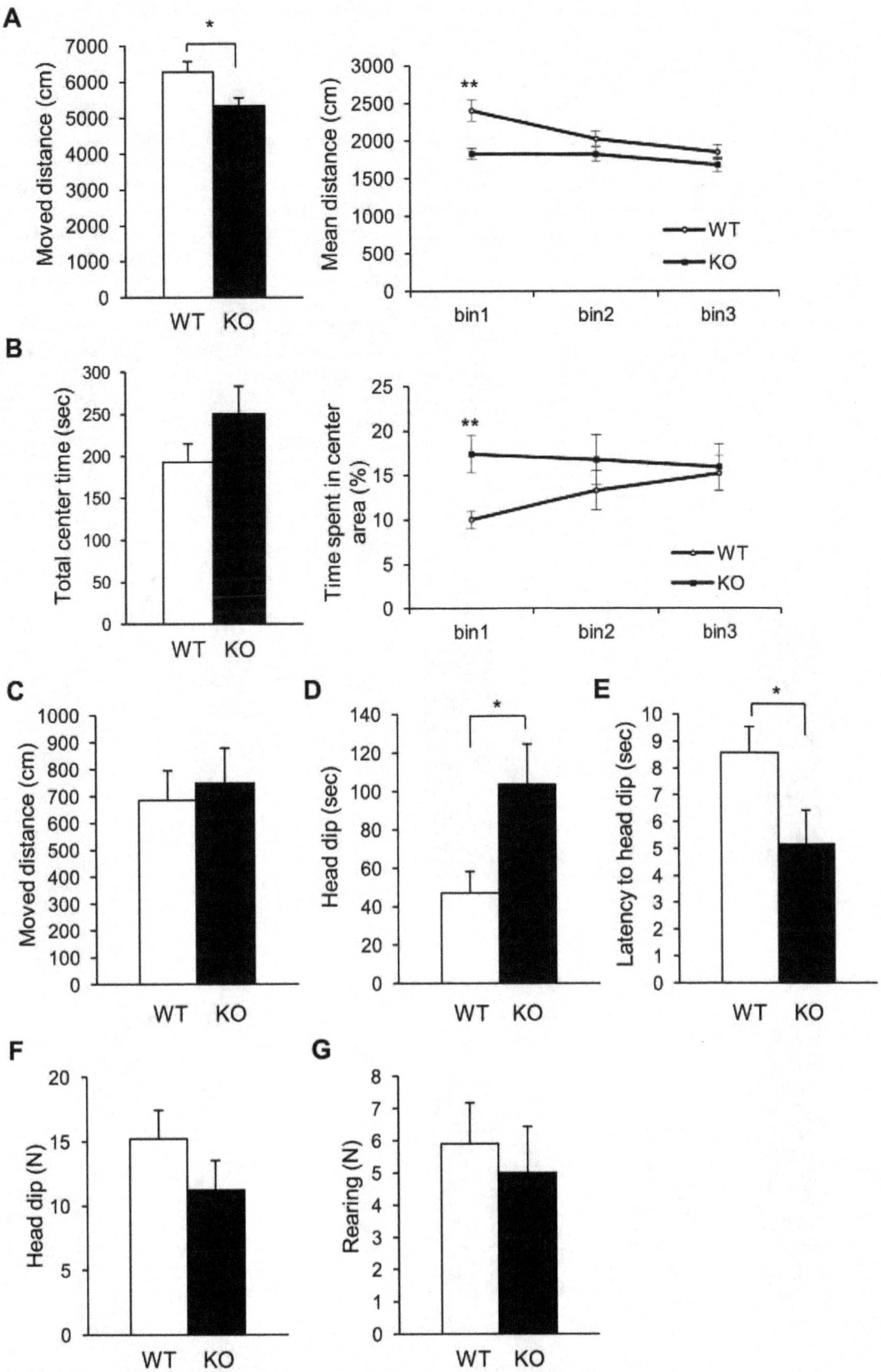

Figure 4. Altered adaptive responses to a novel environment in *Slitrk6*-KO mice. (A, B) Open field test. (A) The total distance moved was less in *Slitrk6*-KO than in WT mice (left). The distance moved in the first 5 min of the test was significantly lower in *Slitrk6*-KO mice (right). (B) In *Slitrk6*-KO mice, the total time spent in the center area was greater than that of the WT (left) and was significantly increased in the first 5 min of the test

(right). (C–G) Hole-board test. There were no significant differences in distance moved (C), number of rearing episodes (D), and number of head dips (E) between *Slitrk6*-KO and WT mice. Duration per head dip was significantly decreased in *Slitrk6*-KO mice (F). Latency time to head dip was significantly decreased in KO mice (G). Values are mean ± standard error of the mean. *$P<0.05$, **$P<0.01$ for Mann-Whitney's *U*-test (B, center area data) or Student's *t*-test (others). WT, $n=10$; KO, $n=10$.

Research Resource Center. The mice were kept on a 12-h light–dark cycle, with the dark cycle occurring from 20:00 to 08:00. All the testing described here was performed with adult male mice. The behavioral tests were started when the mice were 12 weeks old and completed before they reached the age of 16 weeks. In total, 45 pairs of WT and KO mice were used in this study.

Auditory brainstem response

For the measurement of ABRs, mice were anesthetized with an intraperitoneal injection of 60 mg/kg sodium pentobarbital (Nembutal, Dainippon Pharmaceutical Co., Ltd., Osaka, Japan), and needle electrodes were inserted at the vertex and pinna with a ground near the tail. ABRs were evoked with 4-ms tone pips at 40 per second with a 0.4-ms cosine squared rise–fall envelope and alternating in polarity to remove frequency-following responses. The voltage difference between the pinna and vertex was amplified (10,000×), filtered, digitized at 100 kHz, and averaged across 512 presentations. The sound level was decreased in 10-dB steps from an 80-dB sound pressure level. The threshold, amplitude, and latency of responses were defined by visual inspection of stacked waveforms.

Auditory startle response

In this test, each mouse was put into a small cage (30 or 35 mm diameter, 12 cm long) that was set on a sensor block within a sound-proof chamber (60×50×67 cm [height]). A dim light was equipped on the ceiling of the sound-proof chamber (10 lux at the center of the sensor block), and a 65-dB white noise was presented

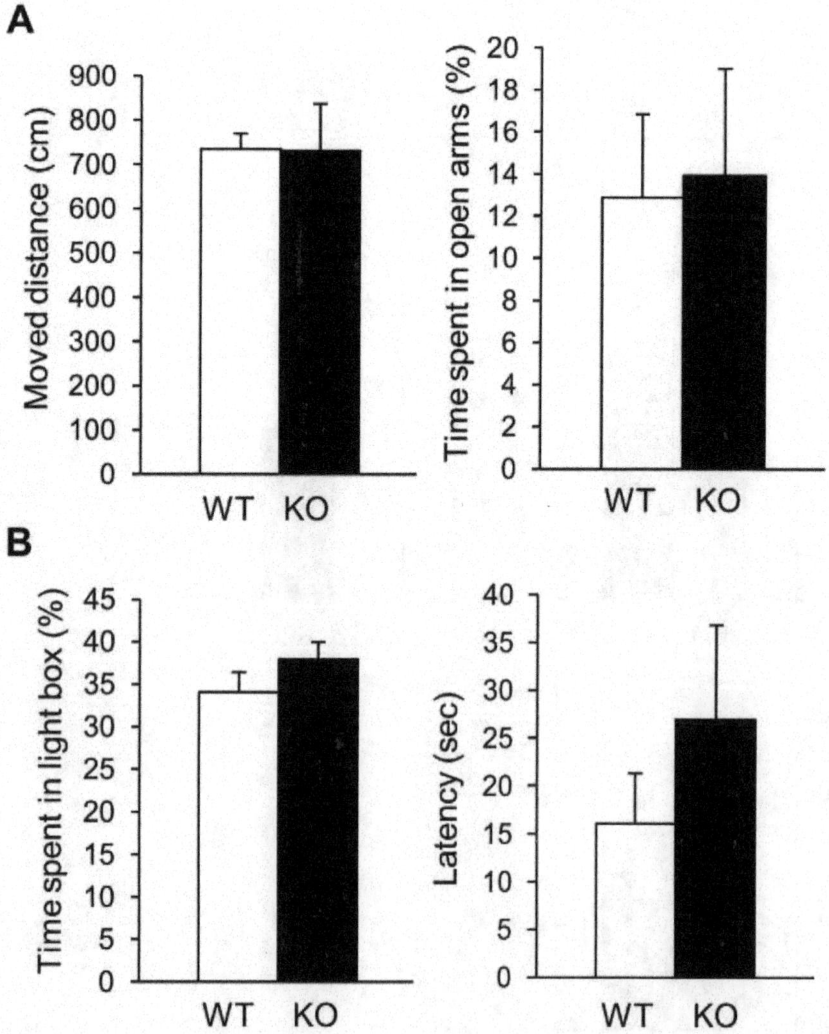

Figure 5. Normal anxiety level of *Slitrk6*-KO mice. (A) Elevated plus maze test. There was no difference between the genotypes in terms of distance traveled (left) or time spent in open arms (right). (B) Light–dark box test. Latency to the first entry into the dark box (left) and time spent in the light box (right) were not significantly different between WT and *Slitrk6*-KO mice. Values are mean ± standard error of the mean. WT, $n=10$; KO, $n=10$.

as background noise. In the ASR test, each mouse was acclimatized to the experimental condition for 5 min, then the experimental session began. In the first session, a 120-dB startle stimulus (40 ms) was presented to the mouse 10 times at random intertrial intervals (10–20 s). In the second session, the startle response to stimuli at various intensities was assessed. Five times of 70 to 120 dB (70, 75, 80, 85, 90, 95, 100, 110, 120 dB) white noise stimuli (40 ms) were presented in quasi-random order and random inter-trial intervals (10–20 sec). In the prepulse inhibition session, the mouse experienced five types of trials: (1) no stimulus; (2) startle stimulus (120 dB, 40 ms) only; (3) 70-dB prepulse (20 ms, lead time 100 ms) and 120-dB pulse; (4) 75-dB prepulse (20 ms, lead time 100 ms) and120-dB pulse; and (5) 80-dB prepulse (20 ms, lead time 100 ms) and 120-dB pulse. Each trial was repeated 10 times in quasi-random order at random intertrial intervals (10–20 s). In the final session, again a 120-dB startle stimulus (40 ms) was presented to the mouse 10 times at random intertrial intervals (10–20 s). The total duration of an ASR test was about 35 to 40 min. After each trial, holding chambers were washed with tap water, wiped with a paper towel, and dried. Apparatuses and software for data analysis used were commercially available ones (Mouse Startle, O'Hara, Tokyo, Japan).

Vestibulo-ocular reflex and optokinetic response eye movements

Eye movement was measured by the infrared TV method as described previously [31,32]. Under isofluorane (Escain, Mylan-Japan, Tokyo, Japan) anesthesia and aseptic conditions, a platform for head fixation was made on the mouse cranial bone using synthetic resin (Superbond C &B, Sun Medical, Tokyo, Japan) and one 15-mm stainless bolt. Two days after surgery, a mouse was mounted on the turntable surrounded by a checked-pattern (check size, 4°) screen (diameter, 60 cm; height, 60 cm), with the head fixed and the body loosely restrained in a plastic cylinder. The horizontal and vertical vestibulo-ocular reflexes (hVOR and vVOR, respectively) and horizontal optokinetic response (hOKR) eye movements were measured. The hVOR was tested in the dark by sinusoidal turntable oscillation at a frequency of 0.11–0.50 Hz and peak-to-peak amplitude of 10° on the plane parallel to the bilateral horizontal semicircular canals. The hOKR was tested in the light with sinusoidal screen oscillation at a frequency of 0.11–0.33 Hz and peak-to-peak amplitude of 10–20° (maximum screen velocity, 3.5–10.5°/s) on the same plane. The vVOR was tested in the dark with turntable oscillation at a frequency of 0.11–0.5 Hz and peak-to-peak amplitude of 10° on the plane perpendicular to the plane of the bilateral horizontal semicircular canals. During the test of vVOR, the mouse laid on its back in the plastic cylinder with the head-up position on the turntable [33]. More than 10 cycles of the evoked horizontal (hVOR and hOKR) or vertical (vVOR) eye movements free from artifacts due to blinks and saccades were averaged, and the mean amplitude and phase were calculated by a modified Fourier analysis [34]. A gain of the eye movement was defined as the ratio of the peak-to-peak amplitude of eye movements to that of the turntable or screen oscillation. The phase was defined as 0° when the peak of the eye movement was opposite to the peak of turntable oscillation in the hVOR and vVOR and when the peak of the eye movement matched the screen oscillation in the hOKR.

Rota-rod test

A mouse was placed on a rotating rod (O'Hara) and the time it was able to maintain its balance walking on top of the rod was measured. The speed of rotation was 4 rpm on day 1, and the speed was accelerated from 4 to 40 rpm over a 4-min period and then maintained at 40 rpm for another 1 min on days 2 to 5. Mice were tested in one trial for 2 min on day 1 and in four trials with a maximum time of 300 s (intertrial intervals were 20–30 s) on days 2 to 5. The time between placement and falling off or revolving around the rod was recorded manually.

Home cage activity

Spontaneous activity of each mouse in its home cage was measured using a 24-channel ABsystem 4.0 (Neuroscience, Tokyo, Japan). Cages were individually set into the stainless steel compartments of a negative breeding rack (JCL, Tokyo, Japan). An infrared sensor was equipped on the ceiling of each compartment and it detected movements of the mice. Home cage activity was measured for 1 week, starting from the afternoon of the day mice were transferred to the behavioral laboratory (day 1). Only data from days 2 to 8 were statistically analyzed. After termination of the home cage activity measurements, cages and bedding materials were changed and the mice were maintained in a micro-isolation rack (Allentown, PA, USA) throughout the behavioral screening.

Hole-board test

For this test, an OF system made of gray plastic (50×50×40 cm [height]) with four equally separated holes (3 cm diameter, each with an infrared sensor) on the floor was used (model ST-1/WII, Muromachi-kikai, Tokyo, Japan). The field was illuminated by fluorescent light (180 lux at the center of the field), and the level of background noise was approximately 50 dB. The behavior of each mouse was monitored by a CCD camera (placed about 1.5 m above the field). In the HB test, a mouse was introduced into the center of the field and allowed to explore freely for 5 min. Total moving time (s), distance traveled (cm), latency for head dipping (s), number of head dips, duration of head dipping (s), duration of rearing (s), and number of rearing episodes were measured as indices. Data were collected and analyzed using CompACT VAS system (Muromachi-kikai).

Open field, elevated plus maze, and light–dark box tests

Open field, elevated plus maze, and light–dark box tests were performed as described previously [35].

Statistical analyses

Statistical analyses were conducted using the SPSS statistical package (ver. 16.0, SPSS Japan Inc., Tokyo, Japan). Parametric data were analyzed by Student's *t*-test, and nonparametric data were analyzed by Mann-Whitney's *U*-test. Reported *P* values refer to Student's *t*-test unless otherwise noted. Effects of factors were analyzed by one-way ANOVA, two-way ANOVA with post hoc tests, and generalized linear model. Differences were defined as statistically significant when $P<0.05$.

Acknowledgments

We thank Hiromichi Goto (RIKEN Brain Science Institute) for teaching us how to perform the ABR measurement, and Azel Zine (University of Montpellier I) for valuable discussions.

Author Contributions

Conceived and designed the experiments: YM KK SN JA. Performed the experiments: YM KK TO KY NT SN. Analyzed the data: YM KK TO KY NT SN JA. Wrote the paper: YM KK KY SN JA.

References

1. Aruga J, Mikoshiba K (2003) Identification and characterization of Slitrk, a novel neuronal transmembrane protein family controlling neurite outgrowth. Mol Cell Neurosci 24: 117–129.
2. Aruga J, Yokota N, Mikoshiba K (2003) Human SLITRK family genes: genomic organization and expression profiling in normal brain and brain tumor tissue. Gene 315: 87–94.
3. Patapoutian A, Reichardt LF (2001) Trk receptors: mediators of neurotrophin action. Curr Opin Neurobiol 11: 272–280.
4. Aruga J (2003) Slitrk6 expression profile in the mouse embryo and its relationship to that of Nlrr3. Gene Expr Patterns 3: 727–733.
5. Katayama K, Zine A, Ota M, Matsumoto Y, Inoue T, et al. (2009) Disorganized innervation and neuronal loss in the inner ear of Slitrk6-deficient mice. PLoS One 4: e7786.
6. Stillman AA, Krsnik Z, Sun J, Rasin MR, State MW, et al. (2009) Developmentally regulated and evolutionarily conserved expression of SLITRK1 in brain circuits implicated in Tourette syndrome. J Comp Neurol 513: 21–37.
7. Abelson JF, Kwan KY, O'Roak BJ, Baek DY, Stillman AA, et al. (2005) Sequence variants in SLITRK1 are associated with Tourette's syndrome. Science 310: 317–320.
8. Shmelkov SV, Hormigo A, Jing D, Proenca CC, Bath KG, et al. (2010) Slitrk5 deficiency impairs corticostriatal circuitry and leads to obsessive-compulsive-like behaviors in mice. Nat Med 16: 598–602.
9. Piton A, Gauthier J, Hamdan FF, Lafreniere RG, Yang Y, et al. Systematic resequencing of X-chromosome synaptic genes in autism spectrum disorder and schizophrenia. Mol Psychiatry. In press.
10. Smith EN, Bloss CS, Badner JA, Barrett T, Belmonte PL, et al. (2009) Genome-wide association study of bipolar disorder in European American and African American individuals. Mol Psychiatry 14: 755–763.
11. Zuchner S, Cuccaro ML, Tran-Viet KN, Cope H, Krishnan RR, et al. (2006) SLITRK1 mutations in trichotillomania. Mol Psychiatry 11: 887–889.
12. Miranda DM, Wigg K, Kabia EM, Feng Y, Sandor P, et al. (2009) Association of SLITRK1 to Gilles de la Tourette syndrome. Am J Med Genet B Neuropsychiatr Genet 150B: 483–486.
13. Katayama K, Yamada K, Ornthanalai VG, Inoue T, Ota M, et al. (2010) Slitrk1-deficient mice display elevated anxiety-like behavior and noradrenergic abnormalities. Mol Psychiatry 15: 177–184.
14. Willott JF (2006) Overview of methods for assessing the mouse auditory system. Curr Protoc Neurosci Chapter 8: Unit8 21A.
15. Hardisty-Hughes RE, Parker A, Brown SD (2010) A hearing and vestibular phenotyping pipeline to identify mouse mutants with hearing impairment. Nat Protoc 5: 177–190.
16. Zhou X, Jen PH, Seburn KL, Frankel WN, Zheng QY (2006) Auditory brainstem responses in 10 inbred strains of mice. Brain Res 1091: 16–26.
17. Friedman LM, Dror AA, Avraham KB (2007) Mouse models to study inner ear development and hereditary hearing loss. Int J Dev Biol 51: 609–631.
18. Leibovici M, Safieddine S, Petit C (2008) Mouse models for human hereditary deafness. Curr Top Dev Biol 84: 385–429.
19. Bonsch D, Schmidt CM, Scheer P, Bohlender J, Neumann C, et al. (2009) A new gene locus for an autosomal-dominant non-syndromic hearing impairment (DFNA 33) is situated on chromosome 13q34-qter. (German) HNO 57: 371–376.
20. Carnicero E, Knipper M, Tan J, Alonso MT, Schimmang T (2002) Herpes simplex virus type 1-mediated transfer of neurotrophin-3 stimulates survival of chicken auditory sensory neurons. Neurosci Lett 321: 149–152.
21. Noushi F, Richardson RT, Hardman J, Clark G, O'Leary S (2005) Delivery of neurotrophin-3 to the cochlea using alginate beads. Otol Neurotol 26: 528–533.
22. Staecker H, Kopke R, Malgrange B, Lefebvre P, Van de Water TR (1996) NT-3 and/or BDNF therapy prevents loss of auditory neurons following loss of hair cells. Neuroreport 7: 889–894.
23. Calabrese DR, Hullar, TE (2006) Planar relationships of the semicircular canals in two strains of mice. J Assoc Res Otolaryngol 7: 151–159.
24. Salvinelli F, Firrisi L, Casale M, Trivelli M, D'Ascanio L, et al. (2004) Benign paroxysmal positional vertigo: diagnosis and treatment. Clin Ter 155: 395–400.
25. Korres SG, Balatsouras DG, Papouliakos S, Ferekidis E (2007) Benign paroxysmal positional vertigo and its management. Med Sci Monit 13: CR275–282.
26. O'Reilly RC, Morlet T, Nicholas BD, Josephson G, Horlbeck D, et al. Prevalence of vestibular and balance disorders in children. Otol Neurotol. In press.
27. Wiener-Vacher SR (2008) Vestibular disorders in children. Int J Audiol 47: 578–583.
28. Butler AB (1995) The dorsal thalamus of jawed vertebrates: a comparative viewpoint. Brain Behav Evol 46: 209–223.
29. Nunez A, Malmierca E (2007) Corticofugal modulation of sensory information. Adv Anat Embryol Cell Biol 187: 1–74.
30. Alitto HJ, Usrey WM (2003) Corticothalamic feedback and sensory processing. Curr Opin Neurobiol 13: 440–445.
31. Katoh A, Kitazawa H, Itohara S, Nagao S (1998) Dynamic characteristics and adaptability of mouse vestibulo-ocular and optokinetic response eye movements and the role of the flocculo-olivary system revealed by chemical lesions. Proc Natl Acad Sci USA 95: 7705–7710.
32. Shutoh F, Ohki M, Kitazawa H, Itohara S, Nagao S (2006) Memory trace of motor learning shifts transsynaptically from cerebellar cortex to nuclei for consolidation. Neuroscience 139: 767–777.
33. Harrod CG, Baker JF (2003) The vestibulo ocular reflex (VOR) in otoconia deficient head tilt (het) mutant mice versus wild type C57BL/6 mice. Brain Res 972: 75–83.
34. Jastreboff PW (1979) Evaluation and statistical judgment of neural responses to sinusoidal stimulation in cases with superimposed drift and noise. Biol Cybern 33: 113–120.
35. Sakatani S, Yamada K, Homma C, Munesue S, Yamamoto Y, et al. (2009) Deletion of RAGE causes hyperactivity and increased sensitivity to auditory stimuli in mice. PLoS One 4: e8309.

2

Pre-, Per- and Postoperative Factors Affecting Performance of Postlinguistically Deaf Adults using Cochlear Implants

Diane S. Lazard[1]*, Christophe Vincent[2], Frédéric Venail[3], Paul Van de Heyning[4], Eric Truy[5], Olivier Sterkers[6], Piotr H. Skarzynski[7,8], Henryk Skarzynski[7], Karen Schauwers[9], Stephen O'Leary[10], Deborah Mawman[11], Bert Maat[12], Andrea Kleine-Punte[4], Alexander M. Huber[13], Kevin Green[11], Paul J. Govaerts[9], Bernard Fraysse[14], Richard Dowell[10], Norbert Dillier[13], Elaine Burke[15], Andy Beynon[16], François Bergeron[17], Deniz Başkent[12,18], Françoise Artières[3,19], Peter J. Blamey[1,10]

1 Bionics Institute, Melbourne, Australia, **2** Service d'otologie et d'otoneurologie, Hôpital R.-Salengro, CHRU de Lille, Lille, France, **3** CHU Gui de Chauliac, Service d'ORL et Chirurgie Cervico-Faciale, Montpellier, France, **4** Department of Otorhinolaryngology and Head and Neck Surgery, Antwerp University Hospital, University of Antwerp, Antwerp, Belgium, **5** Hospices Civils de Lyon, Hôpital Edouard Herriot, Département d'ORL, de Chirurgie Cervico-Maxillo-Faciale et d'Audiophonologie, Lyon, France, **6** AP-HP, Hôpital Beaujon, Service d'ORL et Chirurgie Cervico-Faciale, Clichy, France, **7** Institute of Physiology and Pathology of Hearing, Warsaw, Poland, **8** Institute of Sensory Organs, Kajetany, Poland, **9** The Eargroup, Antwerp, Belgium, **10** Department of Otolaryngology, The University of Melbourne Cochlear Implant Clinic, The Royal Victorian Eye and Ear Hospital, Melbourne, Australia, **11** University of Manchester, Central Manchester University Hospitals NHS Foundation Trust, Manchester, United Kingdom, **12** University of Groningen, University Medical Center Groningen, Department of Otorhinolaryngology/Head and Neck Surgery, Cochlear Implant Center Northern Netherlands, Groningen, The Netherlands, **13** Department of Otorhinolaryngology, University Hospital of Zurich, Zurich, Switzerland, **14** Hôpital Universitaire Purpan, Service d'ORL et Chirurgie Cervico-Faciale, Toulouse, France, **15** St Thomas' Hospital, Auditory Implants Department, London, United Kingdom, **16** Otorhinolaryngology, Radboud University Nijmegen Medical Center, Mijmegen, The Netherlands, **17** Faculté de médecine, Université Laval, Québec City, Québec, Canada, **18** Graduate School of Medical Sciences (Research School of Behavioural and Cognitive Neurosciences), University of Groningen, Groningen, The Netherlands, **19** Institut Saint Pierre, Service d'Audiophonologie et ORL, Palavas les flots, France

Abstract

Objective: To test the influence of multiple factors on cochlear implant (CI) speech performance in quiet and in noise for postlinguistically deaf adults, and to design a model of predicted auditory performance with a CI as a function of the significant factors.

Study Design: Retrospective multi-centre study.

Methods: Data from 2251 patients implanted since 2003 in 15 international centres were collected. Speech scores in quiet and in noise were converted into percentile ranks to remove differences between centres. The influence of 15 pre-, per- and postoperative factors, such as the duration of moderate hearing loss (mHL), the surgical approach (cochleostomy or round window approach), the angle of insertion, the percentage of active electrodes, and the brand of device were tested. The usual factors, duration of profound HL (pHL), age, etiology, duration of CI experience, that are already known to have an influence, were included in the statistical analyses.

Results: The significant factors were: the pure tone average threshold of the better ear, the brand of device, the percentage of active electrodes, the use of hearing aids (HAs) during the period of pHL, and the duration of mHL.

Conclusions: A new model was designed showing a decrease of performance that started during the period of mHL, and became faster during the period of pHL. The use of bilateral HAs slowed down the related central reorganization that is the likely cause of the decreased performance.

Editor: Manuel S. Malmierca, University of Salamanca-Institute for Neuroscience of Castille and Leon and Medical School, Spain

Funding: DL was funded by Fondation Bettencourt-Schueller. The funders had no role in study design, data collection and analysis, decision to publish, or preparation of the manuscript. No additional external funding was received for this study.

Competing Interests: Most of the authors of this paper are involved in the purchase and application of cochlear implants from one or more of the four largest manufacturers (Advanced Bionics, Cochlear Limited, Med-El, and Neurelec). Peter Blamey is a co-inventor of technologies used in the device manufactured by Cochlear Limited and formerly received a share of royalties from the University of Melbourne. He is not a shareholder in Cochlear and no longer receives royalties. The hearing aid company, Blamey & Saunders Hearing Pty Ltd, regularly refers people with severe-to-profound hearing loss to cochlear implant clinics whenever it seems likely that a CI will provide a better clinical outcome than a HA. The Bionics Institute has a small shareholding in Cochlear Limited. DL received travel support from Cochlear in 2010/11. Neurelec partially funded her PhD work in 2009/10, but was not involved in the research project (fMRI). This dataset is a very rare resource enabling comparison of different devices from different manufacturers and from different cochlear implant clinics and the data analysts (Blamey and Lazard) designed the study and analysis in a way that treats data for these different devices equivalently to avoid any possibility of bias. Statistically significant differences between the device brands were found in the analysis, and the device brands have been de-identified in the manuscript to avoid use of the data for commercial advantage. This has been a difficult decision because de-identification of the brands is also withholding important information about clinical outcomes from potential patients and clinicians. The authors agree to share the (de-identified) data on request for academic, non-commercial purposes if the paper is published.

* E-mail: dianelazard@yahoo.fr

Introduction

In 1996, a three-stage model of auditory performance over time was described for 800 adult patients with severe to profound deafness who benefited from a cochlear implant (CI) [1]. The factors included in the model were (in order of relative importance) duration of severe to profound hearing loss (s/p HL), age at implantation, age at onset of s/p HL, duration of CI experience, and etiology. This study has been replicated with data from 2251 patients implanted in 15 different centres since 2002 (Blamey et al, in press). The new study used the same methods as in the 1996 study (general linear model) and confirmed the relevance of each factor. However, the relative effect of the factors has changed, including a relatively greater effect of duration of CI experience and age at onset of s/p HL, and relatively reduced importance of duration of s/p HL. These changes may have arisen from changes in the management of hearing loss, better and sustained use of hearing aids (HAs), different cochlear implant selection criteria, and improved CI devices. These changes were likely to have resulted in a higher average residual level of auditory processing and less reorganized cognitive functions in patients immediately prior to cochlear implantation, followed by a greater and more rapid post-operative improvement. Although the individual factors (duration of s/p HL, age at implantation, age at onset of s/p HL, duration of CI experience, and etiology) were all highly statistically significant in both studies, the proportion of the variance in the population accounted for by these factors was relatively small (21% in the 1996 study, and 10% in the more recent study, see Blamey et al, in press, for discussion of the variance difference). New factors (described below) are introduced in the present analysis to explain more of the variance and address additional hypotheses.

We speculated that central modifications might begin with the onset of moderate hearing loss (mHL), defined as the time from which subjects experienced a pure tone average (PTA) loss of more than 40 dB HL, and/or the time of the first use of HAs. It has been shown, in a functional magnetic resonance imaging (fMRI) study of a cohort of ten postlinguistically deaf subjects, that specific brain reorganizations associated with phonological processing in the right posterior superior temporal gyrus/supramarginal gyrus were influenced by the duration of s/p HL and/or the duration of mHL [2]. The hypothesis that mHL might also be an important factor in CI outcome required exploration in a larger group of subjects.

The relaxation of patient selection criteria since 1996 has resulted in a greater proportion of CI recipients with residual hearing [3–7]. At the same time, HA technology has improved [8–10] and a greater proportion of CI patients are using HAs pre- and post-operatively. Bimodal stimulation, combining electric and acoustic stimulation on the contralateral non-implanted ear, improves speech understanding in noise, sound localization, and music perception compared to the CI used alone [11,12]. HA use was included in the analyses to investigate the effects of these changes in clinical practice. Once deafness has become severe to profound, residual hearing and the use of HAs maintaining peripheral and central pathways might dampen a deleterious cerebral reorganization in favor of visual processing [13,14]. Thus we hypothesized that the negative effect of duration of s/p HL on CI outcome might be reduced by the use of HA(s).

The influence of several per- and postoperative factors, such as the surgical approach used (cochleostomy or round window approach) [15–18], the depth or angle of insertion of the electrode array [19–21], the number of active electrodes [21,22], have already been addressed. However the samples were small leading to controversial results. The large sample size of 2251 patients in the present study offered the opportunity to investigate the influence of these factors on CI speech performance with greater certainty.

The aim of the present study was to confirm the new model of auditory performance over time proposed in Figure 1 and to find a sensitive analysis that could test and control the effect of the factors previously outlined, on a large sample of CI recipients (2251). Apart from these factors, gender, level of education, PTA and unaided hearing threshold at 500 Hz of both ears, preoperative speech perception scores, date of surgery, ear chosen for implantation (better or worse ear), and CI brand were also included in the analysis.

Materials and Methods

Several new statistical analyses were conducted on the dataset described in Blamey et al (in press). The dataset consisted of retrospective information for 2251 CI recipients evaluated with various speech tests and conditions (quiet and noise) from 15 international centres. This project was approved by the Royal Victorian Eye and Ear Hospital Human Research Ethics Committee (Project 10/977H, Multicentre Study Of Cochlear Implant Performance In Adults). In a multicenter study, one of the

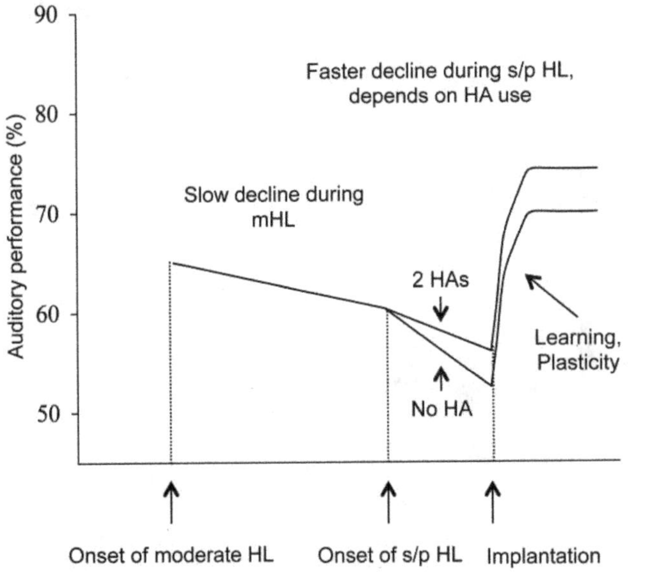

Figure 1. Three-stage model of mean expected auditory performance ranking over time for a hypothetical "average CI recipient". The detailed description of the Figure is in the Results section. mHL: moderate hearing loss; s/p HL: severe to profound hearing loss, HA: hearind aid.

challenges is to combine information in a useful manner despite the differences in evaluation methods and data recorded in the individual centres. All centres provided the core information on implant performance (on an open-set speech perception test in quiet and in noise without lipreading), duration of s/p HL, age at onset of s/p HL, etiology, and cochlear implant experience. Most centres provided additional information (such as use of HAs before surgery, duration of mHL, and amount of residual hearing) if it was available. The statistical analyses thus included additional factors beyond those used in Blamey et al. (in press) (duration of s/p HL, age at onset of s/p HL, duration of CI experience, and etiology). The number of data points included in each analysis varied because of missing data from some clinics on some factors.

Selection criteria for CI recipients included in the study were: Adult at the time of implantation (>18 years old); Onset of s/p HL after the age of 15 (time from which the patient could no longer use hearing alone to communicate even with the best-fitted hearing aids, and/or understand TV, and/or stopped using the telephone). Four brands of CIs were included (Advanced Bionics, Cochlear, Med-el, and Neurelec). Their proportions in the sample were 21%, 50%, 17%, and 7%, respectively (plus 5% missing data for this variable). Date of implantation was after 2002 for all recipients to include technically comparable improvements across brands.

Speech scores in quiet and in noise at two postoperative times for each recipient were requested from the clinics: one score collected early after activation of the CI (T1) and one score collected later on (T2). The choice of the date of the tests was free and varied between and within centres. The mean and standard deviation for T1 were 0.5 years and 0.8 years, respectively, and 2 years and 1.7 years for T2, respectively.

The four factors, used in the four-factor general linear model of Blamey et al (in press) were: *duration of s/p HL*, defined as the time in years between the onset of s/p HL and the date of implantation; mean and median *durations of s/p HL* were 7.4 years and 3.2 years, respectively (ranges: 0–60 years, standard deviation: 9.8); mean *age at onset of s/p HL* was 50 years (standard deviation: 17.3); *duration of implant experience* was defined as the time elapsed between the date of first activation and the dates of testing. It ranged from 2 months to 12 years; fifteen *etiologies* were defined. They are detailed in Figure 2 *Age at implantation* ranged from 17 years to 93 years (mean: 58, standard deviation: 15.8). It was not included in the four-factor general linear model of Blamey et al (in press) because it had less effect than *age at onset of s/p HL.*

In addition to duration of s/p HL, age at onset of s/p HL, duration of CI experience, and etiology, several pre-, per-, and post-operative factors were added to the statistical analyses.

The preoperative factors were:

- *gender.* There were 1017 females, 820 males, and 414 patients with missing gender data.
- *education level*, corresponding to the age at which the subject stopped studying. This factor was partitioned into ranges: stopping before the age of 12 years, before the age of 18 years, or continuing after 18 years old. These three ranges encompassed 21 subjects, 501 subjects, and 518 subjects, respectively, plus 1211 patients with missing data.
- *duration of moderate hearing loss (mHL)*, lasted from the onset of mHL to the onset of s/p HL. The ranges used for the analyses were: 0–4, 5–9, 10–14, 15–19, 20–24, 25–34, 35–44 and over 45 years. The mean duration of mHL was 17 years (range: 0 in case of sudden hearing loss to 74 years, standard deviation: 14.6 years).
- *preoperative HA use.* Centres reported whether the subject was using HAs, bilaterally, or monaurally, at the time of implantation. Four groups were defined: patients not using any HA, patients with a HA on the implanted side, patients with a HA on the ear contralateral to the implanted side, and patients wearing two HAs. These four ranges encompassed 429 subjects, 289 subjects, 386 subjects and 712 subjects, respectively (the rest had missing data).
- *pure tone average (PTA) of the implanted ear, and the better PTA of the two ears.* The latter will be called PTA of the better ear. PTAs represented the mean of unaided residual hearing levels in decibels (dB HL) at 500, 1000, 2000 Hz, for all centres. Four ranges were used: 40–49, 50–74, 75–99, and 100+dB HL.
- *hearing loss (HL) at 500 Hz.* This variable was included to test whether residual low frequencies were more relevant to maintaining functional auditory pathways. Similarly to PTA, HL at 500 Hz was considered for both the implanted ear and for the better ear. The ranges used were the same as for PTA.
- *preoperative speech scores in quiet.* These were aided speech scores before implantation. A percentile rank for each patient within each centre was calculated to allow for differences in test type (phonemes, monosyllabic words, dissyllabic words, sentences) in different languages and different levels of presentation (from 55 to 75 dB SPL). Using ranking removes differences in clinical practice without removing the relative differences between patients within each centre [1].
- *date at implantation.* Modifications of coding strategies since 2002 were tested indirectly through the date at implantation. Three ranges were used: 2002–2004, 2005–2007, 2008–2011. These three ranges encompassed 345 subjects, 822 subjects, and 1083 subjects, respectively (one date was missing).
- *implanted ear.* The implanted ear was classified as the better ear, the worse ear, or similar when both ears had the same amount of residual hearing. The better ear was implanted in 611 cases, the worse ear in 1142 cases, and the two ears had similar residual hearing in 294 cases (the rest had missing data).

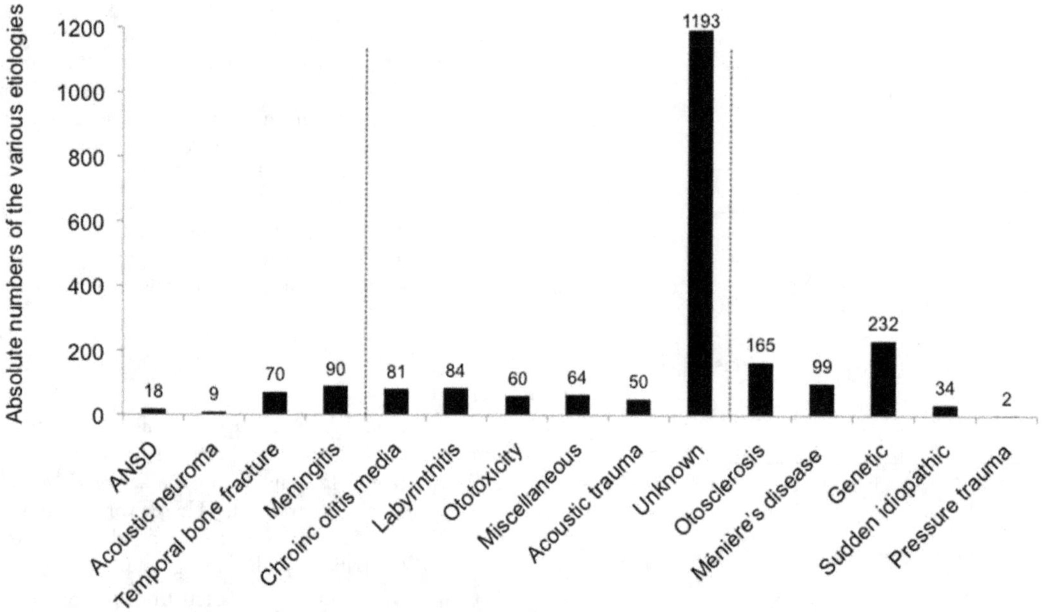

Figure 2. Absolute numbers of the various etiologies defined in the dataset. These etiologies are classified by poorest to best speech outcome in quiet with a CI. ANSD: Auditory neuropathy spectrum disorder. "Miscellaneous" included non-genetic congenital etiologies, cerebral ischemia, drepanocytosis, cephalic trauma without temporal bone fracture, etc. CI recipients presenting with the etiologies encompassed between the two vertical dotted lines showed performances around average, i.e. 50% of speech recognition (not statistically different from average). CI recipients presenting with etiologies on the left part of the dotted lines performed significantly below average. CI recipients presenting with etiologies on the right part of the dotted lines performed significantly better than average. Adapted from Blamey et al (in press).

Peroperatively, only one factor was studied:

- *surgical approach.* Cochleostomy and round window approaches were compared. They were performed in 1119 cases and 425 cases, respectively (information was missing in 707 cases).

The postoperative factors were:

- *CI brand.* CIs from four different manufacturers were represented in the dataset. Speech processors for Advanced Bionics were Auria and Harmony, for Cochlear processors included models from Esprit3G to CP810, for Med-el were Tempo+ and Opus 2, and for Neurelec the Digisonic SP processor.
- *angle of insertion of the electrode array*: Depth of electrode array insertion was expressed as an angle divided into three ranges: <370°, 370–539°, and ≥540°. It ranged from 135° to 730°.
- *percentage of active electrodes.* The number of active electrodes reported at the first testing was expressed relative to the total number of electrodes available on the electrode array, as the total number varies with the CI brand. The ranges used were: ≤70%, 71–85%, and >85%. The minimum percentage of active electrodes was 15%.

Statistical analyses of speech scores in quiet

Postoperative speech scores in quiet were transformed into percentile ranks for each patient within each centre. Using ranking removes differences in clinical practice without removing the relative differences between patients within each clinic. Indeed, for each clinic, the distribution varied uniformly from 0 to 100. The best performers from each centre had a percentile rank close to 100, and the poorest performers from each group had a percentile rank close to 0. The ranked data of the centres were combined for the global analysis. Preoperative and postoperative scores were ranked separately. Ranked postoperative scores were used as the dependent variables of the statistical analyses described below.

Each new factor that we wanted to test was added into the four-factor unbalanced analysis of variance using the General Linear Model (GLM; Minitab version 12), previously described in Blamey et al (in press) to create fifteen five-factor ANOVAs. Briefly, a GLM studies the influence of various independent factors on a dependant variable. The four-factor ANOVA described in Blamey et al (in press) was based on main well-established general factors (the independent factors), known to influence CI speech performance (the dependant variable). These four common factors were duration of s/p HL, age at onset of s/p HL, duration of CI experience, and etiology. In the present study, we wished to explore the influence of 15 other factors that have been less studied. Because entering 19 different independent factors was not possible with the software used (Minitab version 12) and because interpretation of the results would have been complicated, we entered into the former four-factor GLM a single new factor once at a time, leading to 15 different five-factor GLMs. From these 15 analyses, only factors with $p \leq 0.001$ were selected. These significant factors were further included in a single GLM analysis (a sixteenth analysis) to investigate the interrelations between them and produce a new model of auditory performance.

Statistical analyses of speech scores in noise

Postoperative speech scores in noise were ranked separately for each patient within each centre, and independently of scores in quiet. The noise used varied across centres from a cocktail party, to a pink noise, or a speech shaped noise, but was the same for all patients of the same center. Scores in noise at T1 and T2 were considered independent scores for the same patient, and used as dependent variables in the analysis used to explore the new model

Table 1. Results from the 15 five-factor GLM analyses.

Factor tested	F(df, dfe)	Significance p
Gender	(1, 2533) = 0.97	0.325
Education level	(2,1685) = 1.40	0.246
Duration of moderate HL	(7, 2155) = 7.44	0.000*
Hearing aid use	(3, 2833) = 6.99	0.000*
PTA of the implanted ear	(3, 2979) = 4.08	0.007
PTA of the better ear	(3, 3000) = 8.46	0.000*
HL at 500 Hz of the implanted ear	(3, 2860) = 3.98	0.008
HL at 500 Hz of the better ear	(3, 2881) = 7.43	0.000*
Ranked preoperative scores	(4, 2897) = 17.06	0.000*
Date at implantation	(2,3135) = 5.20	0.006
Implanted ear: better ear, worse ear	(2,2984) = 2.63	0.072
Surgical approach	(1, 2380) = 4.18	0.041
Brand	(3,2995) = 41.19	0.000*
Angle of insertion of the electrode array	(2,469) = 3.93	0.020
Percentage of active electrodes	(2,2273) = 35.77	0.000*

of auditory performance (the sixteenth analysis). This last analysis is detailed further in the Results section.

Results

Factors influencing CI outcome

The results from the 15 different five-factor GLM analyses are shown in Table 1. Only the results related to the new fifth factor are shown, the values for the four usual factors being stable across the 15 five-factor GLM analyses. The F ratio was used to test the significance of the fifth factor in each analysis. The number of degrees of freedom for the numerator is one less than the number of ranges for the factor. The number of degrees of freedom for the error term (dfe) differs from one analysis to another because some data were missing for some factors. The value of (dfe+32+df+1) is equal to the number of data points in each analysis (32 is the number of degrees of freedom used by the other factors in the analysis). Because of the large number of data points in the analyses, we considered $p<0.001$ as statistically significant. Factors with $0.05>p>0.001$ are referred to as "marginally significant" in the following discussion to provide the reader with some insight into the weaker trends in the data. Inclusion of the marginally significant factors in the new model of auditory performance would have complicated the model for a relatively small increase in its predictive power.

Gender, the implanted ear (worse, better, similar), and education level had no significant effect ($p>0.05$) and were not included in later analyses. The effects of PTA and HL at 500 Hz of the better ear produced p values lower than those of the implanted ear. We selected PTA in the better ear for the second analysis ahead of HL at 500 Hz, because the F factor was bigger (8.46 vs. 7.43). The effect of preoperative score was significant, but as demonstrated in Table 2, it was significantly influenced by other factors (age at onset of s/p HL, PTA of the better ear, HA use, $p<0.001$), and was therefore not included as an independent variable in the sixteenth analysis used to test the new model of auditory performance. Indeed, a fundamental assumption to perform a GLM analysis requires that the factors entered are independent. Date at implantation, the surgical approach, and the angle of insertion had marginally significant effects ($0.05>p>0.001$). The other new factors that had a significant influence ($p<0.001$) on CI outcomes were duration of mHL, HA use, CI brand, and percentage of active electrodes. Only these new relevant factors were consequently entered in the sixteenth analysis aiming to test the new model of performance over time (Figure 1).

A further multivariate GLM analysis (the sixteenth analysis), including all of the significant factors (9 in total), was conducted to determine the relative influence of these factors in the new model of performance over time shown graphically in Figure 1. Durations of s/p HL and mHL were treated as continuous covariates in the GLM analysis instead of categorical variables as they were in the previous analyses, to measure the rates of decrease (slopes) of auditory performance over time. Duration of s/p HL was nested within HA use to test the hypothesis that the negative effect of s/p HL might be affected by hearing aid use. The results of this analysis are provided in Table 3. All the factors studied still had a significant effect in the new analysis, except for the use of HA on its own and PTA of the better ear (marginally significant, and therefore not included in the final version of the model).

Effects of age at onset of s/p HL, etiology, duration of CI experience

The new analysis did not modify the relative importance of each of the main factors already studied in Blamey et al (in press), i.e. using a four-factor GLM analysis with categorical variables in Blamey et al (in press), or a nine-factor GLM analysis with two continuous variables (durations of s/p HL and of mHL) provided

Table 2. Results of a GLM analysis using ranked preoperative speech scores as dependent variable, and main preoperative factors (determined from Table 1).

Factor	Degree of freedom	Sum of squares	Mean squares	F	p
Age at onset of s/p HL	6	11221.1	2661.6	5.21	0.000
Duration of s/p HL	7	3112.3	416.2	0.81	0.575
Etiology	14	19822.6	1049.0	2.05	0.012
Duration of mHL	7	4001.1	571.6	1.12	0.349
PTA of the better ear	3	131808.3	30122.6	58.94	0.000
HA use	3	42184.3	13667.8	26.75	0.000
Error	1036	529436.7	511.0		
Total	1076	741586.5			

Table 3. Results of a GLM analysis testing the new model of auditory performance for speech in quiet.

Factor	Degree of freedom	Sum of squares	Mean squares	F	p
Age at onset of s/p HL	6	32144.8	5838.9	8.59	0.000
Etiology	14	14278.5	1382.3	2.03	0.013
Duration of CI experience	5	155534.2	33874.9	49.81	0.000
PTA of the better ear	3	12383.0	2804.4	4.12	0.006
HA use	3	8947.9	1196.2	1.76	0.153
Brand	3	53601.5	11313.2	16.63	0.000
Percentage of active electrodes	2	23669.7	12169.8	17.89	0.000
Duration of s/p HL(HA use)	4	40819.3	11120.1	16.35	0.000
Duration of mHL	1	17231.6	17231.6	25.34	0.000
Error	1894	1288090.5	680.1		
Total	1935	1646701.0			

Durations of severe to profound hearing loss and of moderate hearing loss were analysed as continuous (regression) variables. A separate regression coefficient was calculated for each hearing aid use category.

equivalent results for the F and p values of age at onset of s/p HL, etiology, and duration of CI experience. These values were $F = 35.31$, $p < 0.0001$ for CI experience in Blamey et al versus $F = 49.81$, $p < 0.0001$ in the new analysis. $F = 17.91$, $p < 0.0001$ for age at onset of s/p HL in Blamey et al versus $F = 8.59$, $p < 0.0001$ in the new analysis. $F = 2.46$, $p = 0.002$ for etiology in Blamey et al versus $F = 2.03$, $p = 0.013$ in the new analysis. Note that duration of s/p HL was treated as a continuous regression variable in the new analysis and as a categorical factor in the original analysis, so the F values for this factor were not comparable on theoretical grounds.

Effect of duration of s/p HL, influenced by the use of HAs

When nested with duration of s/p HL, each group of HA use had a significant effect. The regression analysis showed that wearing no HA before implantation induced a loss of CI speech performance of 0.83% per year of s/p HL ($p < 0.001$), using one HA on the future implanted ear induced a loss of CI speech performance of 0.64% per year of s/p HL ($p = 0.002$), using one HA on the ear contralateral to the implanted ear induced a loss of CI speech performance of 0.49% per year of s/p HL ($p = 0.017$), and using two HAs induced a loss of CI speech performance of 0.45% per year of s/p HL ($p = 0.003$). The slopes used in Figure 1 are the actual values derived from the nested GLM regression analysis.

Effect of duration of mHL

The GLM regression analysis for duration of mHL showed that CI speech performance reduced by 0.23% per year of mHL

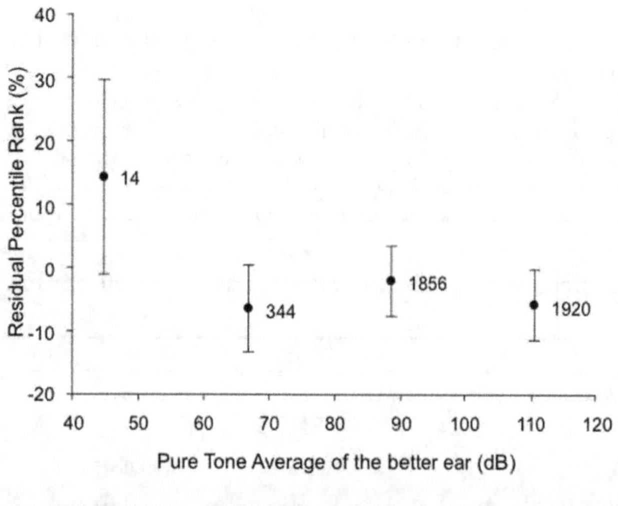

Figure 3. Significant effect of Pure Tone Average thresholds of the better ear on the residual percentile rank. Error bars indicate +/− two standard errors of the mean for each pure tone average range (approximately equivalent to the 95% confidence interval for each mean value shown on the graph; if two mean values fall within one error bar, then the means are not significantly different (p>0.05)). The numbers next to each symbol indicate the number of data points in that range.

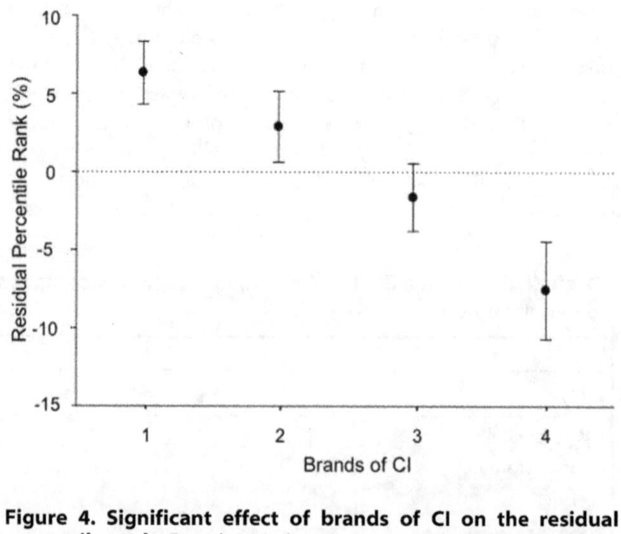

Figure 4. Significant effect of brands of CI on the residual percentile rank. Error bars indicate +/− two standard errors of the mean for each CI brand (approximately equivalent to the 95% confidence interval for each mean value shown on the graph; if two mean values fall within one error bar, then the means are not significantly different (p>0.05)). The numbers of data points for each brand were not indicated to avoid potential identification of the individual brands.

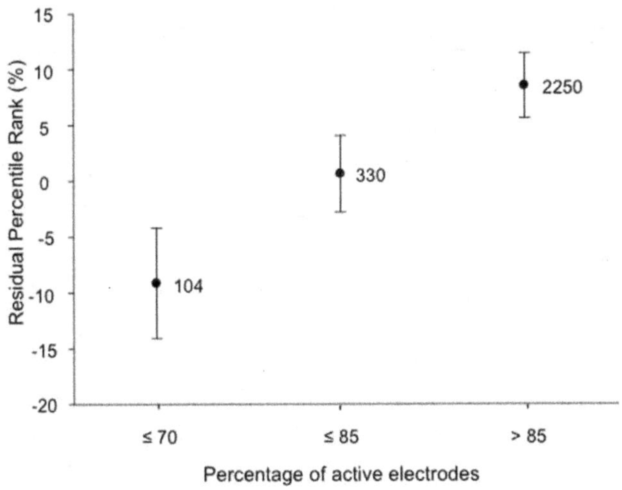

Figure 5. Significant effect of percentage of active electrodes on the residual percentile rank. Error bars indicate +/− two standard errors of the mean for each range (approximately equivalent to the 95% confidence interval for each mean value shown on the graph; if two mean values fall within one error bar, then the means are not significantly different ($p>0.05$)). The numbers next to each symbol indicate the number of data points in that range.

($p<0.001$). The slope used in Figure 1 is the actual value derived from the GLM regression.

Effect of PTA of the better ear

The effect of PTA of the better ear was marginal (Table 3, $F=4.12$, $p=0.006$). The results for the ranges used are represented in Figure 3. Patients with residual hearing better than 50 dB HL in the better ear had better CI speech scores. However, the variance of this group is large due to the small number of patients and possibly to the inclusion of patients presenting with auditory neuropathy spectrum disorder, who performed below the average outcome (Blamey et al, in press and Figure 2. Patients with severe HL and profound HL displayed similar CI performance.

Effect of CI brand

The effect of CI brand was significant (Table 3, $F=16.63$, $p<0.001$). The results are represented in Figure 4. The horizontal dotted line represents the average performance (50% of speech performance for the ranked scores in quiet). Although the difference between the mean percentile rankings of the highest and 2 lowest brands was significant, the mean scores of the highest and the lowest brand differed by only 14%.

Effect of percentage of active electrodes

The effect of percentage of active electrodes was significant (Table 3, $F=17.89$, $p<0.001$). Figure 5 shows the residual CI speech performance versus the percentage of active electrodes. A rise in performance was observed when the overall number of electrodes increased.

Defining a new model of auditory performance in quiet over time

The multivariate GLM analysis enabled a determination of the relative influence of the nine most relevant factors in a new model of performance. This model, proposed in Figure 1 for a hypothetical "average patient", starts at the beginning of mHL. It is important to note that "auditory performance" on the vertical axis of Figure 1 refers to the expected percentile rank with a CI if the hypothetical patient were to receive a CI. Mean expected auditory performance ranking with a CI for very short periods of mHL and s/p HL and no CI experience is about 65% relative to the mean ranking for all patients, which is always 50%. The percentages of performance lost per year of mHL or per year of s/p HL were derived from the regression analyses for these variables included in the GLM analysis. The slope of the relevant regression line has units of percentile rank change per year: during the period of mHL, mean expected CI auditory performance ranking slowly decreases by 0.23% per year. We have assumed about 20 years of mHL for the hypothetical patient in Figure 1, so auditory performance decreases down to 60%, where the hypothetical patient presents with a s/p HL. During the period of s/p HL, the decrease in mean expected ranking depends on HA use, at about 0.45% per year if 2 HAs are worn, and 0.89% if no HAs are worn. We have assumed about 10 years of s/p HL in Figure 1. The final stage represents the post-operative learning curve related to CI experience. The expected outcome for an individual patient will be influenced by the use or absence of HAs, the amount of residual hearing, the age of occurrence of the various events, the actual duration of mHL and s/p HL, the brand of CI, and the percentage of active electrodes postoperatively. Although explicit experimental measures, such as fMRI, are not routinely available, the effects of peripheral and central reorganization are partially taken into consideration by the factors tested. In total, the new model accounts for 22% of the variance in the data. The former model (four-factor GLM analysis) accounted for 10% of the variance in the present data set (Blamey et al in press).

Testing the new model of auditory performance in noise over time

The ranked speech perception scores in noise were subjected to the GLM analysis developed to test the new model of auditory performance to determine whether the nine most relevant factors had similar effects in quiet and in noise. After allowing for missing data, there were 1037 data points in the analysis of performance in noise. The results of this analysis are shown in Table 4. Duration of CI experience still had the greatest effect. The effect of CI brand in noise was this time marginally significant and much smaller than in quiet ($F(3,995)=3.80$, $p=0.01$ and $F(3,1894)=16.63$, $p<0.001$, respectively). The percentage of active electrodes had no significant effect in noise. The relative importance of duration of mHL was greater in noise, with a 50% steeper slope of decrease of auditory performance per year compared to the slope for auditory performance in quiet (−0.32% versus −0.23%). The slopes related to duration of s/p HL, ranging from −0.85% to −0.49%, were similar to those observed for auditory performance in quiet. In total, the percentage of variance accounted for by the new model in noise was the same as in quiet (22%).

Discussion

By including a large number of patients (2251) from 15 different centres, and removing the differences that may exist between clinical practices (speech material, level of presentation used) by using percentile ranking, the present study investigated the effects of variables that are routinely accessible from clinical files, to find those that have an effect on CI outcome.

Factors with little or no influence on CI outcome

Gender and level of education did not influence CI speech performance of postlinguistically deaf adults. The inclusion criteria

Table 4. Results of the new GLM analysis using ranked speech scores in noise with a CI as the dependent variable.

Factor	Degree of freedom	Sum of squares	Mean squares	F	p
Age at onset of s/p HL	6	27576.8	4499.3	6.56	0.000
Etiology	14	9395.5	697.0	1.02	0.434
Duration of CI experience	5	88794.2	18792.7	27.41	0.000
PTA of the better ear	3	8680.0	2893.3	4.22	0.006
HA use	3	6826.4	371.0	0.54	0.654
Brand	3	8887.2	2604.9	3.80	0.010
Percentage of active electrodes	2	1563.7	1838.3	2.68	0.069
Duration of s/p HL(HA use)	4	21207.3	5150.8	7.51	0.000
Duration of mHL	1	20823.8	16580.9	24.18	0.000
Error	995	682242.0	685.7		
Total	1036	875997.0			

of the present study paid particular attention to distinguish level of education and language acquisition. The age at beginning of s/p HL had to be later than 15 years old, in order to avoid bias related to potentially delayed development of speech processing in severely deaf children [23].

Implanting the better ear [24] or the worse ear [25], defined on PTA criteria only, had no effect [26]. In the sample studied, the clinical practice that was most frequently used was to implant the worse ear (56% of cases). The better ear was implanted in 30% of cases, and the 14% remaining concerned ears with symmetric PTA. It is likely that the actual choice of the side to implant was based on patients' reports rather than PTA. The ear with the better PTA is not always the ear with the more usable acoustic hearing, and the ear with the shortest duration of deafness is often preferred when aided performances are similar [27]. Preserving efficient residual hearing of the better ear (i.e. implanting the worse ear) is nowadays a general consensus, enabling the use of a HA contralateral to the CI [11,28,29]. The present study confirms that implantation of the poorer ear is unlikely to reduce the CI outcome significantly. The level of residual hearing of the better ear had a significant influence on CI outcome (Table 2), as discussed latter.

Surgical approach is a highly debated topic. Various publications defend one technique over the other one [15–18,30]. In this study, surgical approach had a marginally significant effect on outcomes ($p = 0.041$). Cochleostomy was practiced in 73% of cases, and the round window approach in 27%. Except for some electrode arrays for which a specified approach is recommended [17], the best approach may be the one that the surgeon controls best, depending on his/her surgical practice and habits, and on the local anatomy of the middle ear.

There were 504 data points from 4 different cochlear implant centers in the analysis for angle of insertion of the electrode array in Table 1. So far, the literature has been consistent in indicating the importance of studying electrode array placement, on postoperative CT scans, for CI outcome [19,20,31,32]. Predictors of good performance are: a greater number of electrodes within the scala tympani, an absence of translocation from the scala tympani to the scala vestibuli, a not excessively deep insertion, and a reduced distance to the modiolus. However, the present study found only a marginally significant effect of the angle of insertion ($p = 0.02$). It is noted that visibility of the electrode array and electrode contact positions may vary between scanners [33], that the angle of insertion may not correspond directly to the electrode array placement [32], and that the evaluation of the angle of insertion may require specific training of the radiologists involved.

The date at implantation was marginally significant ($p = 0.006$). However, Blamey et al (in press) and Zeng et al [34] suggest that the greater improvements in performance over time, compared with older studies [1], were related in part to improvements in coding strategies. Most of the major steps were taken before 2002, the beginning of the inclusions in the present study, and corresponded to a switch from F0F2, F0F1F2 and MPEAK strategies to Continuous Interleaved Sampling (CIS), and spectral-maxima (ACE or N of M) strategies [34,35]. Between 2002 and 2011, the coding strategies have remained much the same although other new sound processing features have been introduced, such as ADRO (Adaptive Dynamic Range Optimization) [8], and noise reduction algorithms [36,37], whose benefits are not explored by speech tests in quiet at conversational levels.

New factors with strong influence on CI outcome

Effects of age at onset of s/p HL, etiology, and duration of CI experience were similar to those found in Blamey et al (in press). They accounted for 10% of the variance in this previous study (four-factor GLM analysis) (Blamey et al in press).

Audiometric features, PTA of the implanted ear, PTA of the better ear, residual hearing at 500 Hz of the implanted ear, and residual hearing at 500 Hz of the better ear, had consistent significant effects (Table 1). The audiometric feature which had the bigger F value was PTA of the better ear ($F(3, 3000) = 8.46$, $p < 0.001$), compared with residual hearing at 500 Hz of the better ear ($F(3, 2881) = 7.43$, $p < 0.001$). These results suggest that using PTA, averaging the audiometric thresholds at 500, 1000 Hz and 2000 Hz, to define the severity of the hearing loss and the efficiency of the residual hearing, is a valuable practice, as audiometric thresholds at the low frequency studied (500 Hz) had a slightly smaller effect on the overall CI performances. The F values for the implanted ear, PTA and threshold at 500 Hz, were about half the corresponding values for the better ear. These results may indicate that speech performance with a CI does not rely more on the peripheral structures of the implanted ear, but more on the integrity of central processing. This possibility is consistent with the strong relationship between PTA in the better ear and pre-operative speech perception scores (Table 2). Whichever ear is implanted, what seems to matter is that the brain was not deprived of auditory inputs pre-operatively [26,38]. The redundant ascendant crossed auditory pathways seem to enable auditory processing independently of the side of the electric stimulation and of the asymmetric speech processing of the brain (see [39] and [40] for reviews of asymmetric speech processing). However, as shown in Figure 3, mean CI performances were similar for groups of recipients with unaided PTA of more than 65 dB. This result must be considered in the context of the other variables in the analysis that can modify the observed effects of the degree of residual hearing. For example, auditory processing and central preservation probably depend more on aided thresholds than unaided PTA, thus HA use may tend to reduce the observed effect of PTA. Durations of s/p HL and mHL are also included in the analysis as covariate factors which account for the effects of degree of hearing loss to a large extent. Thus inclusion of these interrelated variables in a single multivariate analysis may have acted to reduce the significance of the PTA factor in Table 3 relative to Table 1 where there were fewer interrelated variables.

Hearing aid use had a strong effect through its influence on the slope of the duration of s/p HL regression (Table 3 and Figure 1). As hypothesized, not using any HA accelerated the central and peripheral modifications induced by auditory deprivation. The amount of reduction of CI speech performance was 0.83% per year for the patients who used no HA during the period of s/p HL, while it was 0.45% per year for the patients who used two HAs during the period of s/p HL. These results confirm that inputs from HAs may slow down the pathological reorganization of auditory pathways induced by hearing loss [41,42]. Using only one HA on the future implanted ear was linked to a marginally greater reduction of CI speech performance than using only one HA on the ear contralateral to the implanted ear (0.64% per year of s/p HL vs 0.49%). Because general practice is to preserve the ear with the more efficient residual hearing [11,28,29], we may hypothesize that if the ear chosen to be implanted was the only one using a HA, the contralateral ear was profoundly deaf and probably presented with a much longer duration of s/p HL [27]. The central and peripheral auditory wiring might have been poorer in this case than when the HA was worn on the non-implanted ear. This may explain the greater negative effect of using one HA on the future implanted ear.

CI brand had a significant effect in the model of Figure 1 ($F(3, 1894) = 16.63$, $p<0.001$). It should be noted that these results are an average picture of the situation between 2002 and 2011. Some brands have already introduced new processors that were not included in this study. Technical improvements are continuing, and current performance may be different from this average over the last ten years. There was 14% difference between the best and poorest device in this analysis. This result may be considered rather small compared to the 0–100 range that exists in CI speech performance in quiet. An improvement to a particular device may easily change its positioning in the next decade. It is also important to note that other studies have found different results when comparing brands of CI [43]. The performance of each brand may vary depending on the characteristic tested (e.g. dynamic range, noise reduction strategy), the speech material used [43], and the test conditions as suggested by the present analysis of speech perception in noise. Another factor affecting these results may be the strategy used. In the present database, this item was not recorded, supposing that the default strategy of every brand was used in most of the cases. Other elements apart from performance, such as reliability, design of the electrode array and placement in the cochlea, may also be taken into consideration to evaluate a CI.

The percentage of active electrodes had a strong effect ($F(2, 1894) = 17.89$, $p<0.001$). Having more than 85% of active electrodes conferred a significant advantage in speech perception. A smaller percentage could reflect the number of electrodes inserted, and/or of deactivated electrodes (high impedance, facial stimulation, uncomfortable sensations) [22]. Reducing the percentage of active electrodes means that the actual number of intra-cochlear sites available for stimulation is reduced, indirectly reflecting the neural population stimulated [21]. It is important to note that the absolute number of electrodes was not studied here, because it is confounded with the other factors that differentiate the CI devices from different companies.

The negative effect of duration of mHL on auditory processing [2] was confirmed ($F(1, 1894) = 25.34$, $p<0.001$). The reduction of CI speech performance per year of mHL (0.23%) was smaller than the reduction during duration of s/p HL. Using HAs during the period of mHL may also slow this reduction (this information was not accessible in the present database). In Lazard et al [2], it was shown that non-speech sound processing (i.e. environmental sound processing) decreased with duration of mHL, releasing cognitive resources recycled to process phonology. A decline in phonological processing was also observed, but it was correlated with duration of s/p HL. It was proposed that cerebral plasticity prioritized reorganization in favor of oral communication. The delayed decline of phonological processing was related to a sustained reinforcement by lipreading.

Using the new model for speech perception in noise

The usual factors (duration of CI experience, age at onset of s/p HL) had the same importance in noise and in quiet. However, the results of the analysis in noise may be biased by the selection of only the best patients for testing in noisy conditions. Usually, poor performers are less likely to be tested in noise than the better performers, to avoid them having to face listening conditions that are too difficult. There were only about half as many data points in Table 4 as in Table 3, as indicated by the total degrees of freedom. The reduced significance of the percentage of active electrodes may come from this biased selection. It seems unlikely that in noise patients with a small number of active electrodes perform on average as well as patients with a greater number of active electrodes, although it is also possible that the noise obliterates some of the fine spectral detail that can be used with a larger number of electrodes. The modification of the importance of brand may also be explained by the selection of the best performers, or it may be that the differences across brands are dampened in difficult listening conditions, showing that speech understanding in noise with a CI remains challenging whatever the device. The increased effect of duration of mHL in noisy conditions may be related to cerebral reorganization of non-speech sound and environmental sound processing. Indeed, the cortical activation of some areas usually involved in non-speech sound and environmental sound processing starts to decrease during the period of mHL [2,41]. This last result may emphasize the importance of promoting the use of HAs to maintain the functional processing of both speech and environmental sounds in a noisy world.

Conclusions

Several questions were addressed in the present study. In particular, the model used did not find any significant effect of gender, level of education, or ear of implantation based on worse or better PTA. Surgical approach was marginally significant.

An older model including only 4 factors (duration of s/p HL, age at onset of s/p HL, etiology, and duration of CI experience) accounted for 10% of the variance in the same dataset as used in the present study (Blamey et al, in press). The new model described in the present study, and including the nine most significant factors among 15, accounted for 22% of the variance, and shed light on the roles of mHL, s/p HL and HA use. A part of the unexplained 78% of the variance is likely to be due to test/retest reliability of the speech perception measures used, some of which have only a relatively small number of test items. Indeed, the fewer items in a test, the greater the variability. The rest of the variance remains unexplained, but high order cognitive reorganization may be involved [42,44,45], as well as other variables not accessible from clinical information routinely collected.

Acknowledgments

Fifteen centres from Australia, Europe, and North America participated, the co-authors generously providing access to their own records. The authors want to highlight the fact that centers from USA were invited to participate, but they all declined the proposition.

Salomé Fontolliet (Faculté de médecine, Université Laval, Québec, Canada), Assia Terranti (Service d'otologie et d'otoneurologie, Hôpital R.-Salengro, CHRU de Lille, Lille, France), Alexandra Rousset (Department of Otolaryngology, The University of Melbourne Cochlear Implant Clinic, The Royal Victorian Eye and Ear Hospital, Melbourne, Australia), Isabelle Mosnier (AP-HP, Hôpital Beaujon, Service d'ORL et Chirurgie Cervico-Faciale, Clichy, France), Stéphane Gallégo (Hospices Civils de Lyon, Hôpital Edouard Herriot, Département d'ORL, de Chirurgie Cervico-Maxillo-Faciale et d'Audiophonologie, Lyon, France), Mathieu Marx (Hôpital Universitaire Purpan, Service d'ORL et Chirurgie Cervico-Faciale, Toulouse, France), Alec Fitzgerald O' Connor (St Thomas' Hospital, Auditory Implants Department, London, United Kingdom) are acknowledged for their contribution in collecting a great amount of data. The Bionics Institute acknowledges the support it receives from the Victorian Government through its Operational Infrastructure Support Program.

Author Contributions

Conceived and designed the experiments: DL CV FV PVdH ET OS PHS HS KS SO DM BM AKP AMH KG PJG BF RD ND EB AB FB DB FA PJB. Analyzed the data: DL PJB. Contributed reagents/materials/analysis tools: DL PJB. Wrote the paper: DL PJB. Critically revised the manuscript: DL CV FV PVdH ET OS PHS HS KS SO DM BM AKP AMH KG PJG BF RD ND EB AB FB DB FA PJB.

References

1. Blamey P, Arndt P, Bergeron F, Bredberg G, Brimacombe J, et al. (1996) Factors affecting auditory performance of postlinguistically deaf adults using cochlear implants. Audiol Neurootol 1: 293–306.
2. Lazard DS, Lee HJ, Truy E, Giraud AL (2012) Bilateral reorganization of posterior temporal cortices in post-lingual deafness and its relation to cochlear implant outcome. Hum Brain Mapp DOI: 10.1002/hbm.21504.
3. Cullen RD, Higgins C, Buss E, Clark M, Pillsbury HC 3rd, et al. (2004) Cochlear implantation in patients with substantial residual hearing. Laryngoscope 114: 2218–2223.
4. Rubinstein JT, Parkinson WS, Tyler RS, Gantz BJ (1999) Residual speech recognition and cochlear implant performance: effects of implantation criteria. Am J Otol 20: 445–452.
5. Kiefer J, von Ilberg C, Reimer B, Knecht R, Gall V, et al. (1998) Results of cochlear implantation in patients with severe to profound hearing loss–implications for patient selection. Audiology 37: 382–395.
6. Lenarz T (1998) Cochlear implants: selection criteria and shifting borders. Acta Otorhinolaryngol Belg 52: 183–199.
7. Dooley GJ, Blamey PJ, Seligman PM, Alcantara JI, Clark GM, et al. (1993) Combined electrical and acoustical stimulation using a bimodal prosthesis. Arch Otolaryngol Head Neck Surg 119: 55–60.
8. Blamey PJ (2005) Adaptive dynamic range optimization (ADRO): a digital amplification strategy for hearing aids and cochlear implants. Trends Amplif 9: 77–98.
9. Johnson JA, Cox RM, Alexander GC (2010) Development of APHAB norms for WDRC hearing aids and comparisons with original norms. Ear Hear 31: 47–55.
10. McDermott HJ (2011) A technical comparison of digital frequency-lowering algorithms available in two current hearing AIDS. PLoS One 6: e22358.
11. Potts LG, Skinner MW, Litovsky RA, Strube MJ, Kuk F (2009) Recognition and localization of speech by adult cochlear implant recipients wearing a digital hearing aid in the nonimplanted ear (bimodal hearing). J Am Acad Audiol 20: 353–373.
12. Sucher CM, McDermott HJ (2009) Bimodal stimulation: benefits for music perception and sound quality. Cochlear Implants Int 10 Suppl 1: 96–99.
13. Champoux F, Lepore F, Gagne JP, Theoret H (2009) Visual stimuli can impair auditory processing in cochlear implant users. Neuropsychologia 47: 17–22.
14. Lambertz N, Gizewski ER, de Greiff A, Forsting M (2005) Cross-modal plasticity in deaf subjects dependent on the extent of hearing loss. Brain Res Cogn Brain Res 25: 884–890.
15. Friedland DR, Runge-Samuelson C (2009) Soft cochlear implantation: rationale for the surgical approach. Trends Amplif 13: 124–138.
16. Addams-Williams J, Munaweera L, Coleman B, Shepherd R, Backhouse S (2011) Cochlear implant electrode insertion: in defence of cochleostomy and factors against the round window membrane approach. Cochlear Implants Int 12 Suppl 2: S36–39.
17. Souter MA, Briggs RJ, Wright CG, Roland PS (2011) Round window insertion of precurved perimodiolar electrode arrays: how successful is it? Otol Neurotol 32: 58–63.
18. Skarzynski H, Lorens A, Piotrowska A, Skarzynski PH (2010) Hearing preservation in partial deafness treatment. Med Sci Monit 16: CR555–562.
19. Finley CC, Holden TA, Holden LK, Whiting BR, Chole RA, et al. (2008) Role of electrode placement as a contributor to variability in cochlear implant outcomes. Otol Neurotol 29: 920–928.
20. Skinner MW, Ketten DR, Holden LK, Harding GW, Smith PG, et al. (2002) CT-derived estimation of cochlear morphology and electrode array position in relation to word recognition in Nucleus-22 recipients. J Assoc Res Otolaryngol 3: 332–350.
21. Yukawa K, Cohen L, Blamey P, Pyman B, Tungvachirakul V, et al. (2004) Effects of insertion depth of cochlear implant electrodes upon speech perception. Audiol Neurootol 9: 163–172.
22. Blamey PJ, Pyman BC, Gordon M, Clark GM, Brown AM, et al. (1992) Factors predicting postoperative sentence scores in postlinguistically deaf adult cochlear implant patients. Ann Otol Rhinol Laryngol 101: 342–348.
23. Pisoni DB, Kronenberger WG, Roman AS, Geers AE (2011) Measures of digit span and verbal rehearsal speed in deaf children after more than 10 years of cochlear implantation. Ear Hear 32: 60S–74S.
24. Group UCIS (2004) Criteria of candidacy for unilateral cochlear implantation in postlingually deafened adults I: theory and measures of effectiveness. Ear Hear 25: 310–335.
25. Chen JM, Shipp D, Al-Abidi A, Ng A, Nedzelski JM (2001) Does choosing the "worse" ear for cochlear implantation affect outcome? Otol Neurotol 22: 335–339.
26. Francis HW, Yeagle JD, Bowditch S, Niparko JK (2005) Cochlear implant outcome is not influenced by the choice of ear. Ear Hear 26: 7S–16S.
27. van den Broek E, Dunnebier EA (2009) Cochlear implantation in postlingually hearing-impaired adults: choosing the most appropriate ear. Int J Audiol 48: 618–624.
28. Firszt JB, Holden LK, Reeder RM, Skinner MW (2009) Speech recognition in cochlear implant recipients: comparison of standard HiRes and HiRes 120 sound processing. Otol Neurotol 30: 146–152.
29. Olson AD, Shinn JB (2008) A systematic review to determine the effectiveness of using amplification in conjunction with cochlear implantation. J Am Acad Audiol 19: 657–671; quiz 735.
30. O'Leary MJ, Fayad J, House WF, Linthicum FH Jr (1991) Electrode insertion trauma in cochlear implantation. Ann Otol Rhinol Laryngol 100: 695–699.
31. Skinner MW, Holden TA, Whiting BR, Voie AH, Brunsden B, et al. (2007) In vivo estimates of the position of advanced bionics electrode arrays in the human cochlea. Ann Otol Rhinol Laryngol Suppl 197: 2–24.
32. Radeloff A, Mack M, Baghi M, Gstoettner WK, Adunka OF (2008) Variance of angular insertion depths in free-fitting and perimodiolar cochlear implant electrodes. Otol Neurotol 29: 131–136.
33. Verbist BM, Joemai RM, Teeuwisse WM, Veldkamp WJ, Geleijns J, et al. (2008) Evaluation of 4 multisection CT systems in postoperative imaging of a cochlear implant: a human cadaver and phantom study. AJNR Am J Neuroradiol 29: 1382–1388.
34. Zeng F-G (2011) Advances in Auditory Prostheses. In: Zeng F, Popper A, Fay R, editors. Auditory Prostheses: New Horizons: Springer Handbook of Auditory Research 39. pp. 1–11.
35. Loizou PC (2006) Speech processing in vocoder-centric cochlear implants. Adv Otorhinolaryngol 64: 109–143.
36. Hamacher V, Doering WH, Mauer G, Fleischmann H, Hennecke J (1997) Evaluation of noise reduction systems for cochlear implant users in different acoustic environment. Am J Otol 18: S46–49.
37. Loizou PC, Lobo A, Hu Y (2005) Subspace algorithms for noise reduction in cochlear implants. J Acoust Soc Am 118: 2791–2793.

38. Friedland DR, Venick HS, Niparko JK (2003) Choice of ear for cochlear implantation: the effect of history and residual hearing on predicted postoperative performance. Otol Neurotol 24: 582–589.
39. Morris LG, Mallur PS, Roland JT Jr, Waltzman SB, Lalwani AK (2007) Implication of central asymmetry in speech processing on selecting the ear for cochlear implantation. Otol Neurotol 28: 25–30.
40. Lazard DS, Collette JL, Perrot X (2012) Speech processing: From peripheral to hemispheric asymmetry of the auditory system. Laryngoscope 122: 167–173.
41. Lazard DS, Giraud AL, Truy E, Lee HJ (2011) Evolution of non-speech sound memory in postlingual deafness: implications for cochlear implant rehabilitation. Neuropsychologia 49: 2475–2482.
42. Lazard DS, Lee HJ, Gaebler M, Kell CA, Truy E, et al. (2010) Phonological processing in post-lingual deafness and cochlear implant outcome. Neuroimage 49: 3443–3451.
43. Spahr AJ, Dorman MF, Loiselle LH (2007) Performance of patients using different cochlear implant systems: effects of input dynamic range. Ear Hear 28: 260–275.
44. Giraud AL, Lee HJ (2007) Predicting cochlear implant outcome from brain organisation in the deaf. Restor Neurol Neurosci 25: 381–390.
45. Strelnikov K, Rouger J, Demonet JF, Lagleyre S, Fraysse B, et al. (2010) Does brain activity at rest reflect adaptive strategies? Evidence from speech processing after cochlear implantation. Cereb Cortex 20: 1217–1222.

3

Audiovisual Segregation in Cochlear Implant Users

Simon Landry[1], Benoit A. Bacon[1,2], Jacqueline Leybaert[3], Jean-Pierre Gagné[4], François Champoux[1,4]*

1 Centre de Recherche en Neuropsychologie et Cognition (CERNEC), Montréal, Québec, Canada, **2** Department of Psychology, Bishop's University, Sherbrooke, Québec, Canada, **3** Université libre de Bruxelles, Bruxelles, Belgique, **4** Centre de recherche interdisciplinaire en réadaptation du Montréal métropolitain, Institut Raymond-Dewar, École d'orthophonie et d'audiologie, Université de Montréal, Montréal, Québec, Canada

Abstract

It has traditionally been assumed that cochlear implant users de facto perform atypically in audiovisual tasks. However, a recent study that combined an auditory task with visual distractors suggests that only those cochlear implant users that are not proficient at recognizing speech sounds might show abnormal audiovisual interactions. The present study aims at reinforcing this notion by investigating the audiovisual segregation abilities of cochlear implant users in a visual task with auditory distractors. Speechreading was assessed in two groups of cochlear implant users (proficient and non-proficient at sound recognition), as well as in normal controls. A visual speech recognition task (i.e. speechreading) was administered either in silence or in combination with three types of auditory distractors: i) noise ii) reverse speech sound and iii) non-altered speech sound. Cochlear implant users proficient at speech recognition performed like normal controls in all conditions, whereas non-proficient users showed significantly different audiovisual segregation patterns in both speech conditions. These results confirm that normal-like audiovisual segregation is possible in highly skilled cochlear implant users and, consequently, that proficient and non-proficient CI users cannot be lumped into a single group. This important feature must be taken into account in further studies of audiovisual interactions in cochlear implant users.

Editor: Claude Alain, Baycrest Hospital, Canada

Funding: This work was supported by the Natural Sciences and Engineering Research Council of Canada (NSERC). The funder had no role in study design, data collection and analysis, decision to publish, or preparation of the manuscript.

Competing Interests: The authors have declared that no competing interests exist.

* E-mail: francois.champoux@umontreal.ca

Introduction

It has been shown numerous times that when congruent visual and auditory cues are processed together perceptual accuracy is enhanced in both normally-hearing (NH) and in hearing-impaired individuals (e.g. [1–13]). In contrast, several investigations have demonstrated that when incongruent visual and auditory cues are processed together, audiovisual interactions seem to occur differently in hearing-impaired individuals, compared to NH. Specifically, audiovisual perception is dominated by auditory information in the NH, whereas it is dominated by vision in hearing-impaired individuals that are using a cochlear implant (CI). For example, a number of studies that used a McGurk effect paradigm [14] have shown that CI users are able to integrate auditory and visual information adequately [12,15,16] but that they essentially refer to the visual cues when incongruency makes integration difficult [11,17,18].

Tremblay et al. [19] recently suggested that when it came to audiovisual integration, not all CI users could be grouped together. In an audiovisual fusion task, only the CI users that were unable to recognize auditory speech sounds efficiently (yet showed normal sound detection performance) were referring primarily to visual cues to process speech information. Interestingly, the results of Tremblay et al. [19] also suggest that a number of CI users, namely those who are proficient in sound recognition, can show normal-like audiovisual interactions even in situations of incongruity. This notion is strongly supported by a recent study of audiovisual segregation; namely the ability to focus on the processing of one information stream while ignoring the irrelevant and incongruent information in an audiovisual task [20]. In an auditory task with visual distractors, proficient CI users performed in a normal-like manner, while non-proficient users did not; they were in fact much more disturbed by the visual distractors that involved movement (dots, lip movements) but not, however, by color changes. To our knowledge, this remains the only study of audiovisual segregation ability in CI users.

These two investigations [19,20] contrast with the general idea that all CI users rely more heavily on visual cues in conditions of incongruency [11,12,15–18]. More specifically, the results suggest that i) CI users can show normal-like performance in an audiovisual task, with the normal relative weight of visual and auditory cues, and ii) only the CI users that are non-proficient in highly demanding auditory tasks, such as speech identification, show abnormal, visual-oriented interactions.

Performance on audiovisual segregation tasks, however, has to be carefully assessed in order to fully confirm these conclusions. In particular, the question remains as to whether the reverse task, namely ignoring auditory distractors in a visual task, is performed differently in proficient and non-proficient CI users. The present study tackled this issue by comparing proficient CI users, non-proficient CI users and NH in a speechreading task with and without auditory distractors. In accordance with the results of Champoux et al. [20], it was hypothesized that only non-proficient users would differ from the NH. More precisely, it was hypothesized that speechreading would be affected by incongruent auditory information in NH and proficient CI, but not in non-proficient CI. The confirmation of these hypotheses would in effect also demonstrate that the results reported in Champoux et al. [20] were not due to the specificity of the task, the procedure or the stimuli used and confirm further the possibility of normal-like audiovisual interations in cochlear implant users.

Methods

Subjects

Twenty-four participants (seventeen CI users) were involved in the study. All CI users had received their implants at least one year prior to taking part in the study. The clinical profile of each participant has been described elsewhere (see [20]). All participants suffered from profound bilateral hearing loss (pure-tone detection thresholds at 80 dB HL or greater at octave frequencies ranging from 0.5 to 4 KHz) and were post-lingually deafened. The principal communication mode for all CI users was oral/lip-reading. In all participants, pure-tone detection thresholds with the CI, at octave frequencies ranging from 250 to 6000 Hz were within normal limits (30 dB HL or less). The Research Ethics Board of the Institut Raymond-Dewar approved the study and all the participants provided written informed consent. Figure 1 includes the picture of an audiologist. We confirm that this individual has seen this figure and the manuscript, and has provided written consent for publication.

Stimuli and design

A female speaker was filmed while she pronounced 120 consonant-vowel-consonant-vowel bi-syllabic words. The production of each stimulus began and ended in a neutral, closed mouth position and total duration of the stimuli was about 500 ms. Stimuli were presented in a baseline visual-only condition or in one of three incongruent audiovisual conditions (see Figure 1A). In the first audiovisual condition (AV-noise), visual stimuli were presented together with a comfortable level of white noise. The noise was generated with Cool Edit pro software (version 1.2: Syntrillium Software Corporation, San Jose, CA). This condition served as a second baseline and no difference was expected with the visual-only condition. In the second audiovisual condition (AV-reverse speech), visual stimuli were presented with reverse-speech sounds of the bisyllabic words. In the third audiovisual condition (AV-speech), visual stimuli were presented with non-altered speech sounds of the bisyllabic words. Temporal synchrony between the visual stimulus and the auditory utterance was

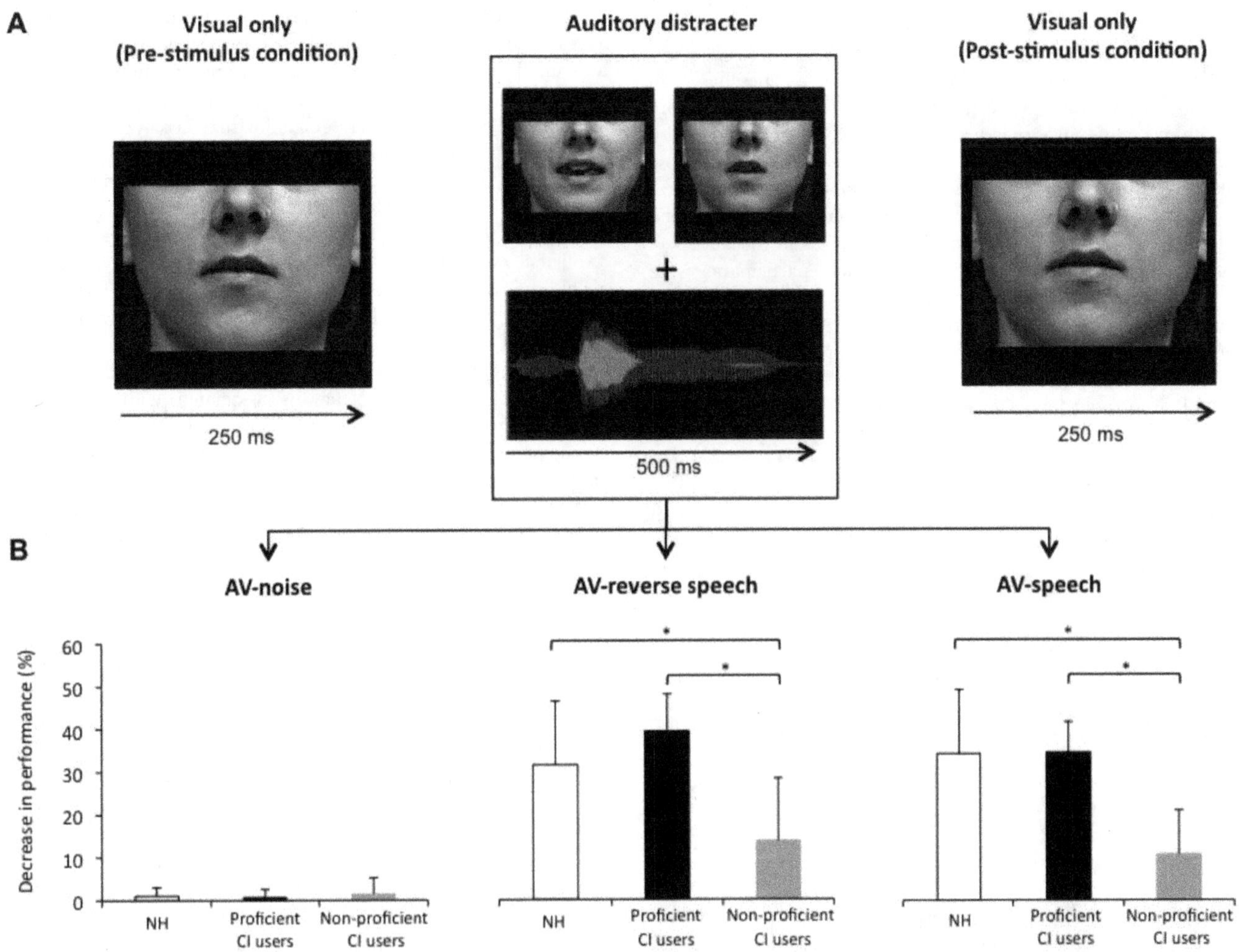

Figure 1. Experimental procedure and visual speech recognition performance in the three audiovisual conditions. (A) Illustration of the experimental procedure. Each visual stimulus began and ended in a static neutral position. Visual stimuli were either presented alone (baseline condition) or simultaneously with one of three types of auditory stimuli (white noise, reverse speech sounds and non-altered speech sounds). (B) Performance in the three audiovisual conditions is expressed as % decrease of performance compared to the baseline visual-only condition. In both the AV-reverse speech and AV-speech conditions, non-proficient CI users differ from both controls and proficient CI users. * : $p<.05$.

achieved by aligning the burst corresponding to the beginning of the test word in the auditory condition with the appearance of motion in the visual stimulus. An informal pre-evaluation confirmed that the reverse-speech and speech auditory stimuli were clearly detectable and identifiable as speech sounds by both proficient and non-proficient CI users.

Procedure

Forty stimuli from each of the three audiovisual conditions were presented in one block of 120 trials. The order of the stimuli was randomized with Presentation software (Neurobehavioral Systems Inc., San Pablo, CA). The visual stimuli were presented on a 17″ video monitor that was positioned at the participant's eye level at a viewing distance of 114 cm. The auditory stimuli were always presented at a comfortable listening level via two loudspeakers positioned at ear level and located on each side of the video monitor. The participants were asked to look at the screen, to completely ignore what they heard and to only report what they had read on the lips of the speaker. They were clearly informed that auditory input would always be incongruent with the visual stimulus and that their task was to report the visual stimulus. An experimenter was present throughout the procedure to ensure that the participants were looking at the screen before stimulus presentation and to monitor oculomotor behavior during stimulus presentation.

The procedure used to analyze segregation abilities has been described previously (see [20]). Prior to data collection, auditory speech recognition was measured in a counterbalanced order with a list of 40 bisyllabic words. These results confirmed those obtained with the same sample by Champoux et al. [20]. Most importantly, the proficient and non-proficient groups remained stable. The performance level of three CI users in the auditory-alone condition was extremely low, as these participants were barely able to differentiate speech from non-speech sounds. Hence, the results of these participants were not considered in the data analyses. Whereas the ability to accurately identify words presented auditorily varied considerably, all the other CI users ($n = 14$) were able to make the distinction between speech and non-speech sounds. These CI participants were divided in two groups: Proficient ($n = 7$) when their auditory speech recognition performance as measured with a list of 40 bisyllabic words was above 75% and non-proficient ($n = 7$), when auditory speech recognition performance was below 75%. The visual-alone baseline condition was used as a reference point from which to compute the percent decrement in performance in each of the three audiovisual conditions, i.e. decrease of performance = (% score in the visual-alone condition − % score in the audiovisual condition). A t-test found no significant difference ($p > .05$) between proficient and non-proficient CI users in the ability to discriminate bisyllabic words in a congruent audio-visual or visual-alone condition.

Results

Visual speech recognition performance in the three incongruent audiovisual conditions is shown in Figure 1B. To determine speechreading ability with or without irrelevant auditory distractors, a 3×3 mixed ANOVA with group (control, proficient CI users, non-proficient CI users) as a between-subjects factor and audiovisual condition (AV-noise, AV-reverse speech, AV-speech) as a within-subjects factor was conducted. There were main effects of condition ($F(2,36) = 114.537$, $p < .001$) and group ($F(2,18) = 9.901$, $p = .001$). The interaction between factors was also significant ($F(4,36) = 10.959$, $p = .001$). Post-hoc Tukey HSD tests revealed significant differences between the non-proficient group and the control group in the AV-reverse speech ($p = .049$) and AV-speech ($p = .005$) conditions. There were also significant differences between the non-proficient and the proficient group in the AV-reverse speech ($p = .005$) and AV-speech conditions ($p < .001$). Post-hoc analysis did not reveal any other differences between groups ($p > 0.05$) and as such the performance of proficient CI users was never statistically different from that of the NH controls. The performance level of every CI user was examined further in the three experimental conditions. There was a significant correlation between the decrease in speechreading performance and the proficiency to use the CI in the AV-reverse speech ($r = 0.686$, $p = .007$) and the AV-speech ($r = 0.824$, $p < .001$) conditions. There were however no significant relationships ($p > .05$) between visual recognition performance and the duration of deafness, the age at onset of hearing loss or the length of experience with CI.

Discussion

The present study aimed to investigate audiovisual segregation abilities in proficient and non-proficient CI users. Using a speechreading task and three types of auditory distractors, we showed that the presentation of auditory speech stimuli significantly impaired speechreading performance in proficient CI users, just like in NH participants, whereas speechreading performance was unaffected by auditory distractors in non-proficient CI users.

Traditionally, all CI users have been considered equal, and equally different from NH, in audiovisual tasks. In short, it is assumed that this population, although capable of normal integration, tends to rely more heavily on visual cues in conditions of incongruency (e.g. [11,12,15–18]. However, recent evidence from our laboratories [19,20] highlights the importance of CI proficiency in audiovisual interaction outcomes. We suggested that whereas CI users that were proficient at speech recognition could perform at normal-like levels, those that were not would favor visual cues and show anomalous audiovisual integration. The results presented here therefore support two notions: *i)* that CI speech recognition proficiency is associated with audiovisual interaction outcomes in this population and *ii)* that several CI users, namely the proficient ones, can show normal-like performance on an audiovisual task.

Cross-modal reorganization has been repeatedly shown to occur in the profoundly deaf (e.g. [21–24]). In fact, in CI users, there is an activation of the early auditory cortex in the presence of visual stimuli and this activation is greater for those who show poor speech recognition abilities [25]. In addition, CI users display atypical low-hierarchical visual activity during speech recognition tasks [26]. This activity in the visual cortex is less marked and less consistent in naive than in rehabilitated CI users, suggesting that these visual cortex activations are due not only to deafness-induced plasticity, but also to brain reorganizations related to the functional learning of associations between visual cues and oral speech [25]. Therefore, different levels of auditory-to-visual reorganization in cochlear implanted deaf subjects could explain the varying audiovisual segregation abilities reported in the present study: greater cross-modal reorganization would lead to the overuse of visual information and consequently to a greater capacity to ignore irrelevant auditory cues.

Some other issues, however, could also explain the pattern of results observed across tasks and groups. First, the three audiovisual tasks arguably did not require the exact same attentional resources. Indeed, speech stimuli were more salient and more complex than noise stimuli and consequently, were more likely to capture attention. Some studies, moreover, suggest that children with CI could perform poorly on attentional tasks [27,28], although performance might improve progressively with the use of a CI [29]. In our study, putative impairments of visual or auditory attentional processes have unfortunately not been evaluated. These capacities might need to be investigated further in those populations to better understand their implications in the present results.

In conclusion, our results strongly suggest that in terms of audiovisual interactions, proficient and non-proficient CI users should not be lumped into a single group. More specifically, we show that normal-like audiovisual interactions are possible in proficient users and we show that CI proficiency is associated with audiovisual interactions in CI users. CI proficiency must therefore be taken into account in further studies of audiovisual interactions in this population.

Author Contributions

Conceived and designed the experiments: FC JPG. Performed the experiments: FC SL. Analyzed the data: FC SL. Contributed reagents/materials/analysis tools: FC. Wrote the paper: FC BAB SL JL.

References

1. Perrott DR, Saberi K, Brown K, Strybel TZ (1990) Auditory psychomotor coordination and visual search performance. Percep Psychophys 48: 214–226.
2. Hughes HC, Reuter-Lorenz PA, Nozawa G, Fendrich R (1994) Visual-auditory interactions in sensorimotor processing: saccades versus manual responses. J Exp Psychol Hum Percept Perform 20: 131–153.
3. Frens MA, Van Opstal AJ, Van der Willigen RF (1995) Spacial and temporal factors determine auditory-visual interactions in human saccadic eye movements. Percep Psychophys 57: 802–816.
4. Grant KW, Walden BE, Seitz PF (1998) Auditory-visual speech recognition by hearing-impaired subjects: consonant recognition, sentence recognition, and auditory-visual integration. J Acoust Soc Am 103: 2677–2690.
5. McDonald JJ, Teder-Sälejärvi WA, Hillyard SA (2000) Involuntary orienting to sound improves visual perception. Nature 407: 906–908.
6. Teder-Sälejärvi WA, McDonald JJ, Di Russo F, Hillyard SA (2002) An analysis of audio-visual crossmodal integration by means of event-related potential (ERP) recordings. Brain Res Cogn Brain Res 14: 106–114.
7. Frassinetti F, Bolognini N, Làdavas E (2002) Enhancement of visual perception by crossmodal visuo-auditory interaction. Exp Brain Res 147: 332–343.
8. Sekiyama K, Kanno I, Miura S, Sugita Y (2003) Auditory-visual speech perception examined by fMRI and PET. Neurosci Res 47: 277–287.
9. Alegria J, Lechat J (2005) Phonological processing in deaf children: when lipreading and cues are incongruent. J Deaf Stud Deaf Educ 10: 122–133.
10. Bolognini N, Rasi F, Làdavas E (2005) Visual localization of sounds. Neuropsychologia 43: 1655–1661.
11. Van Wassenhove V, Grant KW, Poeppel D (2005) Visual speech speeds up the neural processing of auditory speech. Proc Natl Acad Sci U S A 102: 1181–1186.
12. Rouger J, Lagleyre S, Fraysse B, Deneve S, Deguine O, et al. (2007) Evidence that cochlear-implanted deaf patients are better multisensory integrators. Proc Natl Acad Sci U S A 104: 7295–7300.
13. Ross LA, Saint-Amour D, Leavitt VM, Molholm S, Javitt DC, et al. (2007) Impaired multisensory processing in schizophrenia: deficits in the visual enhancement of speech comprehension under noisy environmental conditions. Schizophr Res 97: 173–183.
14. McGurk H, McDonald J (1976) Hearing lips and seeing voices. Nature 264: 746–748.
15. Schorr EA, Fox NA, van Wassenhove V, Knudsen EI (2005) Auditory-visual fusion in speech perception in children with cochlear implants. Proc Natl Acad Sci U S A 102: 18748–18750.
16. Schwartz JL (2010) A reanalysis of McGurk data suggests that audiovisual fusion in speech perception is subject-dependent. J Acoust Soc Am 127: 1584–1594.
17. Rouger J, Fraysse B, Deguine O, Barone P (2008) McGurk effects in cochlear-implanted deaf subjects. Brain Res 1188: 87–99.
18. Desai S, Stickney G, Zeng FG (2008) Auditory-visual speech perception in normal-hearing and cochlear-implant listeners. J Acoust Soc Am 123: 428–440.
19. Tremblay C, Champoux F, Lepore F, Théoret H (2010) Audiovisual fusion and cochlear implant proficiency. Restor Neurol Neurosci 28: 283–291.
20. Champoux F, Lepore F, Gagné JP, Théoret H (2009) Visual stimuli can impair auditory processing in cochlear implant users. Neuropsychologia 47: 17–22.
21. Nishimura H, Hashikawa K, Doi K, Iwaki T, Watanabe Y, et al. (1999) Sign language "heard" in the auditory cortex. Nature 397: 116.
22. Finney EM, Fine I, Dobkins KR (2001) Visual stimuli activate auditory cortex in the deaf. Nat Neurosci 4: 1171–1173.
23. Sadato N, Okada T, Honda M, Matsuki K, Yoshida M, et al. (2005) Cross-modal integration and plastic changes revealed by lip movement, random-dot motion and sign languages in the hearing and deaf. Cereb Cortex 15: 1113–1122.
24. Bavelier D, Dye MW, Hauser PC (2006) Do Deaf individuals see better? Trends Cogn Sci 10: 512–518.
25. Doucet ME, Bergeron F, Lassonde M, Ferron P, Lepore F (2006) Cross-modal reorganization and speech perception in cochlear implant users. Brain 129: L3376–3383.
26. Giraud AL, Truy E, Frackowiak R (2001) Imaging plasticity in cochlear implant patients. Audiol Neurootol 6: 381–393.
27. Smith LB, Quittner AL, Osberger MJ, Miyamoto R (1998) Audition and visual attention: the developmental trajectory in deaf and hearing populations. Dev Psy 34: 840–850.
28. Yucel E, Derim D, Celik D (2008) The needs of hearing impaired children's parents who attend to auditory verbal therapy-counseling program. Int J Pediatr Otorhinolaryngol 72: 1097–1011.
29. Horn DL, Davis RA, Pisoni DB, Miyamoto RT (2005) Development of visual attention skills in prelingually deaf children who use cochlear implants. Ear Hear 26: 389–408.

4

Patterns of Retinal Damage Facilitate Differential Diagnosis between Susac Syndrome and MS

Alexander U. Brandt[1], Hanna Zimmermann[1], Falko Kaufhold[1], Julia Promesberger[2], Sven Schippling[3], David Finis[4], Orhan Aktas[5], Christian Geis[6], Marius Ringelstein[5], E. Bernd Ringelstein[7], Hans-Peter Hartung[5], Friedemann Paul[1,8,9], Ilka Kleffner[7], Jan Dörr[1,8]*

1 NeuroCure Clinical Research Center, Charité – Universitätsmedizin Berlin, Berlin, Germany, **2** Department of Ophthalmology, University of Münster, Münster, Germany, **3** Institute for Neuroimmunology and Clinical Multiple Sclerosis Research (inims), University Medical Center Hamburg Eppendorf, Hamburg, Germany, **4** Department of Ophthalmology, University Medical Center, Heinrich-Heine-University, Düsseldorf, Germany, **5** Department of Neurology, University Medical Center, Heinrich-Heine-University, Düsseldorf, Germany, **6** Department of Neurology, University of Würzburg, Würzburg, Germany, **7** Department of Neurology, University of Münster, Münster, Germany, **8** Clinical and Experimental Research Center for Multiple Sclerosis, Department of Neurology, Charité – Universitätsmedizin Berlin, Berlin, Germany, **9** Experimental and Clinical Research Center, Max Delbrück Center for Molecular Medicine and Charité – Universitätsmedizin Berlin, Berlin, Germany

Abstract

Susac syndrome, a rare but probably underdiagnosed combination of encephalopathy, hearing loss, and visual deficits due to branch retinal artery occlusion of unknown aetiology has to be considered as differential diagnosis in various conditions. Particularly, differentiation from multiple sclerosis is often challenging since both clinical presentation and diagnostic findings may overlap. Optical coherence tomography is a powerful and easy to perform diagnostic tool to analyse the morphological integrity of retinal structures and is increasingly established to depict characteristic patterns of retinal pathology in multiple sclerosis. Against this background we hypothesised that differential patterns of retinal pathology facilitate a reliable differentiation between Susac syndrome and multiple sclerosis. In this multicenter cross-sectional observational study optical coherence tomography was performed in nine patients with a definite diagnosis of Susac syndrome. Data were compared with age-, sex-, and disease duration-matched relapsing remitting multiple sclerosis patients with and without a history of optic neuritis, and with healthy controls. Using generalised estimating equation models, Susac patients showed a significant reduction in either or both retinal nerve fibre layer thickness and total macular volume in comparison to both healthy controls and relapsing remitting multiple sclerosis patients. However, in contrast to the multiple sclerosis patients this reduction was not distributed over the entire scanning area but showed a distinct sectorial loss especially in the macular measurements. We therefore conclude that patients with Susac syndrome show distinct abnormalities in optical coherence tomography in comparison to multiple sclerosis patients. These findings recommend optical coherence tomography as a promising tool for differentiating Susac syndrome from MS.

Editor: Markus Schuelke, Charité Universitätsmedizin Berlin, NeuroCure Clinical Research Center, Germany

Funding: This study was supported in part by Deutsche Forschungsgemeinschaft (DFG Exc. 257). The MS Center at the Department of Neurology, Heinrich-Heine-University Düsseldorf, is supported in part by the Walter-and-Ilse-Rose Stiftung. The Institute for Neuroimmunology and Clinical Multiple Sclerosis Research (inims), University Medical Center Hamburg Eppendorf, Hamburg, is supported in part by Hertie Stiftung. The funders had no role in study design, data collection and analysis, decision to publish, or preparation of the manuscript. No additional external funding was received for this study.

Competing Interests: The authors have declared that no competing interests exist.

* E-mail: jan-markus.doerr@charite.de

Introduction

Susac syndrome is a rare disease characterised by the clinical triad of encephalopathy, vision disturbances, namely visual field defects, and sensorineural hearing loss [1–3]. The exact prevalence of Susac syndrome is unknown, and its pathogenesis is still unclear; autoimmune processes that lead to an occlusion of small vessels in the brain, retina and inner ear are believed to play an important role [4,5]. The disease most often manifests in the third to fourth decade [6]. The prognosis mainly depends on the severity, the often self-limited and monophasic, sometimes fluctuating and rarely relapsing clinical course [7], and the appropriate treatment [8,9]. Retinal infarction presenting with scotoma is one of the clinical hallmarks, although often not predominant. Patients can present with episodic or permanent vision loss [6]. Fluorescein angiography (FAG) and funduscopy show branch retinal artery occlusions (BRAO), arterial wall hyperfluorescence and retinal arterial wall plaques, termed Gass plaques [10]. Retinal involvement can be missed in cases where patients do not complain about visual disturbances due to neuropsychological impairment, or when physicians are not familiar with the disease. In fact, in several reported cases BRAO was only detected after repeated FAG [6].

The diagnosis of Susac syndrome is straightforward, when the characteristic clinical triad is complete, when the physician is familiar with the clinical presentation, and when the crucial diagnostic procedures are carried out and show characteristic findings like BRAO in FAG. However, the diagnosis is often complicated by the fact that the characteristic signs usually do not occur concomitantly but rather develop successively with symptom-free intervals [3], which often enough results in a delayed or even completely missed diagnosis. Consensus criteria for the

Table 1. Demographic overview of Susac patients included in the study.

Subjects	n	9
Eyes	n	18
Gender	Male (%)	3 (33)
	Female (%)	6 (67)
Age (years)	Mean ± SD	33±11
	Min – Max	20–47
Time since diagnosis (months)	Mean ± SD	65±55
	Min – Max	3–173
Encephalopathy	No (%)	1 (11)
	Yes (%)	8 (89)
Hearing loss	No (%)	0 (0)
	Yes (%)	9 (100)
Visual impairment (eyes)	No (%)	3 (17)
	Yes (%)	15 (83)
	No (%)	3 (17)
	Yes (%)	15 (83)

Abbreviations: BRAO = branch retinal artery occlusion, SD = standard deviation.

diagnosis of Susac syndrome have not yet been established. In MRI, Susac syndrome usually presents with "punched-out" lesions, frequently in the corpus callosum and periventricular area [11]. A number of differential diagnoses, most of which occur more frequently than Susac syndrome, have to be taken into consideration [3]. In turn, Susac syndrome should be considered as differential diagnosis in various conditions. Due to some overlap in the clinical presentation and the patterns of MRI pathology multiple sclerosis (MS) is probably the most frequent misdiagnosis of Susac syndrome [2,8,11,12]. However, with respect to the different therapeutic approach, particularly the necessity of a first-line immunosuppressive treatment in Susac syndrome in contrast to primarily immunomodulatory approaches in MS, a prompt establishment of the diagnosis is essential. Additional diagnostic criteria allowing an early differential diagnosis are therefore highly warranted.

Optical coherence tomography (OCT) has recently become a valuable addition to the neurologist's diagnostic toolbox, proving its usefulness in a variety of disorders with neuro-ophthalmologic involvement [13–16]. OCT facilitates e.g. non-invasive quantification of both the thickness of the retinal nerve fibre layer (RNFLT), which represents unmyelinated axons of retinal ganglia converging to the optic disc to form the optic nerve and the macular volume which represents the volume of the central retina [13–16]. In a recently published case report we could demonstrate pathologic OCT findings in a patient with Susac syndrome [3]. Based on these findings we hypothesised that retinal changes (i) can be regularly detected by OCT in patients with Susac syndrome and (ii) differ from retinal pathology observed in MS. A different pattern of retinal pathology in Susac syndrome and MS would be of clinical value in terms of distinguishing patients with Susac syndrome from MS patients.

Methods

Objectives

To identify OCT changes in patients with Susac syndrome and to compare these changes with matched healthy controls and multiple sclerosis patients.

Table 2. Optical coherence tomography data of the nine patients with Susac syndrome.

Pat.	Sex	Age	Dur.	Eye	VS	BRAO	TMV [mm^3]	A [μm]	T [μm]	S [μm]	N [μm]	I [μm]
P1	m	20	26	OD	yes	yes	6.00	85	48	101	70	122
				OS	yes	yes	7.22	83	65	107	47	115
P2	m	32	58	OD	yes	yes	7.64	105	81	132	106	102
				OS	no	yes	7.66	108	77	141	98	115
P3	f	44	173	OD	yes	yes	5.67	61	51	54	51	88
				OS	yes	yes	6.11	61	49	64	53	77
P4	m	39	50	OD	yes	no	5.70	60	53	78	49	59
				OS	yes	yes	6.63	82	63	95	60	111
P5	f	22	41	OD	yes	yes	6.26	67	65	58	64	83
				OS	yes	yes	6.21	73	67	69	67	89
P6	f	30	128	OD	no	no	6.61	88	76	84	71	121
				OS	no	no	6.64	93	70	125	64	115
P7	f	20	66	OD	yes	yes	6.52	96	74	103	74	131
				OS	yes	yes	6.86	115	72	132	107	149
P8	f	45	69	OD	yes	yes	5.25	62	52	70	41	83
				OS	yes	yes	5.55	52	57	56	31	65
P9	f	47	3	OD	yes	yes	6.66	86	74	103	63	103
				OS	yes	yes	6.57	79	69	99	56	93

Abbreviations: Pat. = Patient No; Age = age of onset; Dur. = time since diagnosis at time of OCT measurement in months; OD = right eye; OS = left eye; VS = visual symptoms; BRAO = branch retinal artery occlusion; TMV = total macular volume in mm^3; A = average retinal nerve fibre layer thickness (RNFLT) in μm; T = temporal, S = superior, N = nasal, I = inferior quadrant's RNFLT in μm.

Study Design and Participants

This is a prospective, cross-sectional, multicentre observational study documenting OCT findings in Susac syndrome patients. Patients with definite diagnosis of Susac syndrome, aged ≥ 18 years were recruited from the neurologic outpatient clinics of five large university medical centres (Berlin, Münster, Düsseldorf, Hamburg, and Würzburg, Germany). Exclusion criteria were inability to provide informed consent. All included patients underwent complete neurological examination. Medical history, particularly with respect to encephalopathy, visual symptoms, and hearing loss was taken from all study participants. In cases where the classical clinical triad was not present, diagnosis was established on clinical presentation and MRI findings. Visual testing was performed with bedside visual field testing. Age and gender matched healthy controls (HC) and patients with relapsing remitting MS (RRMS) were randomly selected from the imaging research database of the NeuroCure Clinical Research Center (NCRC) at Charité – Universitätsmedizin Berlin by an investigator blinded to the OCT data.

Ethics

The study was approved by the local ethics committees and was conducted in accordance to the Declaration of Helsinki in its currently applicable version, the guidelines of the International Conference on Harmonisation of Good Clinical Practice (ICH-GCP), and the applicable German laws. All participants gave informed written consent.

Optical Coherence Tomography

RNFLT and TMV were measured with Stratus 3000 OCT (Carl Zeiss Meditec, California, USA) using "Fast RNFL 3.4" and "Fast Macula Thickness Map" protocols (software V4.0) by trained personnel. For RNFLT, a 3.4 mm diameter circular scan was acquired circumferentially to the optic disc, and for TMV six radial lines were taken, centred within the fovea. A good quality image was defined as having generalised signal distribution, a reflectance signal from either RNFL or retinal pigment epithelium strong enough to identify either layer, no missing parts caused by eye movements, and a signal strength of ≥7 of 10 [17]. Segmentation lines for upper and lower borders of RNFL were required to be on the internal limiting membrane and lower border of the RNFL. For the comparison of OCT measurements to normative data, the device's internal normative database, comprising of measurements of 170 eyes from HC was used as a reference. Percentile positions of measurements compared to these normative data are automatically given on the device's TMV and RNFLT report as below 1st percentile, between 1st and 5th percentile, between 5th and 95th percentile, and above 95th percentile.

Statistical methods

Differences in age and time since diagnosis between patients with Susac syndrome, HC and RRMS patients with and without a history of optic neuritis were analysed using Friedman's analysis for matched pairs. Differences between eyes from the groups were assessed using generalised estimating equation models (GEE) accounting for intra-patient/inter-eye dependencies. To further rule out possible age related effects or effects related to minor differences in time since diagnosis, GEE models were corrected for age and additionally with time since diagnosis for comparisons against RRMS patients. In all GEE, the diagnostic group was used as independent categorical variable. Mean values in text are given with standard deviation (SD) after a ± sign. All statistical tests were performed using SPSS 20 (IBM, Somers, NY, USA). For all calculations, statistical significance was established at $p<0.05$.

Results

Cohort description

Nine patients with Susac syndrome were prospectively recruited (six jointly from Berlin and Münster, one from each of the other

Table 3. Mean values from optical coherence tomography measurements of the macula (total macular volume and below) and the circular scan around the optic nerve head (RNFLT Average and below).

		Susac				**HC**				**MS-NON**				**MS-ON**			
		Mean	**SD**	**Min**	**Max**	**Mean**	**SD**	**Min**	**Max**	**Mean**	**SD**	**Min**	**Max**	**Mean**	**SD**	**Min**	**Max**
Total Macular Volume [mm³]		**6,43**	**0,67**	**5,25**	**7,66**	**7,14**	**0,35**	**6,65**	**7,84**	**7,09**	**0,36**	**6,51**	**7,75**	**6,73**	**0,49**	**6,04**	**7,68**
Inner Macula	**T [µm]**	240	33	172	284	269	18	238	296	269	13	237	286	253	20	220	294
	S [µm]	242	55	128	300	283	16	255	308	281	17	239	301	265	19	237	296
	N [µm]	271	26	207	306	282	17	256	312	279	16	243	302	266	19	241	302
	I [µm]	254	42	146	301	280	18	254	311	281	12	258	301	260	21	232	304
Outer Macula	**T [µm]**	205	27	160	243	229	11	213	252	229	11	211	251	219	18	193	252
	S [µm]	209	42	139	263	247	12	231	276	245	14	222	266	234	17	209	263
	N [µm]	246	18	211	267	264	14	248	291	262	16	232	291	248	18	214	281
	I [µm]	222	30	143	265	242	12	223	262	241	11	216	267	226	18	200	266
RNFLT Average [µm]		**81**	**18**	**52**	**115**	**107**	**9**	**91**	**120**	**102**	**14**	**87**	**137**	**95**	**11**	**74**	**118**
RNFLT	**T [µm]**	65	11	48	81	75	12	59	101	73	17	49	109	57	14	29	77
	S [µm]	93	28	54	141	133	14	104	158	123	17	104	164	113	16	87	150
	N [µm]	65	21	31	107	85	16	67	120	82	21	47	142	90	16	62	123
	I [µm]	101	24	59	149	132	14	109	150	128	17	105	163	120	16	89	139

Abbreviations: RRMS = relapsing-remitting multiple sclerosis; HC = healthy controls; SD = standard deviation; RNFLT = retinal nerve fibre layer thickness; t = temporal; S = superior; N = nasal; I = inferior.

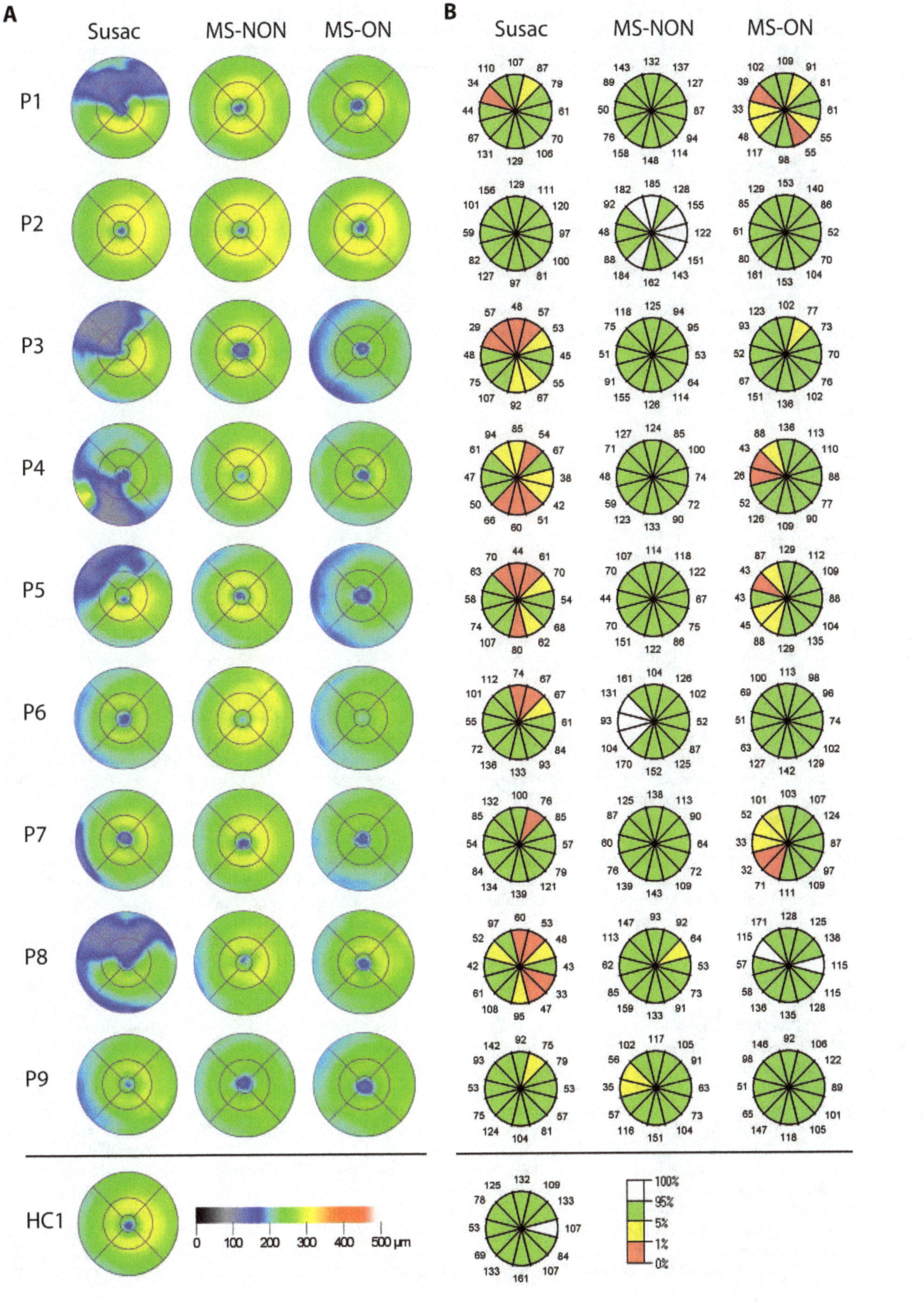
A
B
Susac
MS-NON
MS-ON
P1
P2
P3
P4
P5
P6
P7
P8
P9
HC1
0
100
200
300
400
500 µm
100%
95%
5%
1%
0%

Figure 1. Macular and ring scans from patients with Susac syndrome and matched RRMS patients. Shown are only the left eyes (randomly selected to save space) from each Susac patient (P1-9) and the corresponding left eyes from RRMS patients without history of optic neuritis (MS-NON) and RRMS patients with history of optic neuritis (MS-ON). On the bottom, a comparison of scans from one of the healthy controls is given. A) Colour coded is the calculated macular thickness from the device's segmentation algorithm with black to blue for reduced thickness and yellow to green for normal thickness (left legend on the bottom). The macular thickness map is calculated from six linear scans through the centre of the macula. Of note is the different distribution of the damage. B) For RNFLT scans, the thickness from 12 clock-hour segments of the circular scan is given. Colour coded is the thickness relative to the normative database with green and white meaning normal values above the 5th or 95th percentile and yellow and red meaning reduction of thickness below the 5th or 1st percentile (right legend on the bottom). Whereas some Susac patients' eyes show striking sectoral damage, eyes from RRMS patients show an even thinning with an accentuation in the outer temporal areas, that is further pronounced with a history of optic neuritis. Three Susac patients (P6, 7, 9) show a similar pattern.

three centres). A demographic overview is given in table 1, and a multiple case presentation is provided in table 2. The female to male ratio of 2:1 reflected that reported in the literature. All patients had a history of hearing loss, and all but one patient (P2) had symptoms of encephalopathy. All patients except one (P6) had a history of visual symptoms and provided accompanying reports of BRAO. Additionally, one patient (P2) had visual symptoms on the right eye. However, in this patient a report of BRAO did exist for both eyes. At the time of OCT investigation, no patient was in a clinically active phase of the disease.

Macular and retinal nerve fibre layer damage

Single case OCT measurements are given in table 2, and a synopsis is provided in table 3. In summary, compared to the normative database of the OCT device, most patients showed a reduction in either average RNFLT or macular measurements. All but one patient (P2) with a history of visual symptoms showed either reduced average RNFLT and/or diminished TMV in at least one eye. P2 showed a very mild clinical phenotype and TMV was above the 95th percentile when compared to the normative database of the device. Interestingly, one patient without visual symptoms and without documented BRAO (P6) did also present a pathological OCT with a strong RNFLT reduction in the superior quadrant of the right eye, although average RNFLT in this eye was normal (figures 1 and 2).

Importantly, TMV and RNFLT reduction were not evenly distributed over the entire scanning area but scattered over all sectors (figure 1 and figure 2). Patients with Susac syndrome showed a RNFLT below the 5th percentile in a mean 3.6±3.4 (range 0–10) of the twelve clock-hour sectors and a TMV below the 5th percentile in a mean 2.4±2.9 (range 0–7) of the nine macular sectors whereas the other sectors were within normal ranges. All but one patient (P2) showed this patchy retinal damage in at least one eye as indicated by the yellow and red areas in the RNFLT measurements and the dark blue areas in the TMV measurements (figure 1).

Comparison to matched healthy controls and multiple sclerosis patients

To compare OCT results from patients with Susac syndrome to results from HC and RRMS patients, either group of nine gender and age matched HC (mean age 33±11 years, 3/6 male/female), nine RRMS patients without any history of optic neuritis (mean age 32±10 years, 3/6 male/female, time since diagnosis 55±40 months) and nine RRMS patient with a previous bilateral optic neuritis (mean age 33±9 years, 3/6 male female, time since diagnosis 38±40 months) was considered. HC and RRMS patients were matched for gender, age and time since diagnosis. Gender was matched exactly 1:1. The differences in age were not significant (Friedman's analysis for matched pairs $p = 0.661$). Likewise, time since diagnosis of RRMS patients with and without previous optic neuritis was statistically not different from Susac patients (Friedman's analysis for matched pairs $p = 0.062$).

Average RNFLT was reduced in patients with Susac syndrome (average RNFLT 81±18 µm, table 3) in comparison to HC (average RNFLT 107±9 µm, coefficient $B = -25.5$, SE 6.2, $p < 0.001$, GEE), RRMS patients without previous optic neuritis (average RNFLT 102±14 µm, coefficient $B = -21.3$, SE 6.2, $p = 0.001$, GEE) and RRMS patients with a history of optic neuritis (average RNFLT 95±11 µm, coefficient $B = -13.5$, SE 5.8, $p = 0.019$, GEE) (figure 1B, 2 and 3). Accordingly, TMV was reduced in patients with Susac syndrome (TMV 6.43±0.67 mm^3, table 3) in comparison to HC (TMV 7.14±0.35 mm^3, coefficient $B = -0.71$, SE 0.22, $p = 0.001$, GEE), RRMS patients without history of optic neuritis (TMV 7.09±0.36 mm^3, coefficient $B = -0.67$, SE 0.20, $p = 0.001$, GEE) but not against RRMS patients with previous history of optic neuritis (TMV 6.73±0.49 mm^3, coefficient $B = -0.23$, SE 0.21, $p = 0.224$, GEE) (figure 1 and 3).

Discussion

In this cross-sectional, observational study we investigated nine patients with Susac syndrome using OCT and compared RNFLT and TMV data with nine gender and age matched HC and nine RRMS patients each with or without history of optic neuritis. Our main findings are (a) pathologic OCT measurements in most of the Susac patients with a history of visual symptoms when compared to the normative database of the OCT device; (b) reduced RNFLT and macular measurements when compared to gender and age matched HC; (c) a more severe retinal nerve fibre damage in patients with Susac syndrome as compared to RRMS patients irrespective the history of optic neuritis despite a similar disease duration, and most importantly (d) distinct patterns of retinal or retinal nerve fibre layer damage among patients with Susac syndrome compared to RRMS patients that can help to discriminate between both diseases.

Although a rare disease, Susac syndrome needs to be considered in the differential diagnosis of a variety of neurological disorders. Currently, its diagnosis is based primarily on the clinical presentation, the documentation of BRAO by FAG, and characteristic findings on cranial magnetic resonance imaging, including subtle changes such as fibre impairment detected by diffusion tensor imaging [18]. Recently, anti-endothelial antibodies in Susac syndrome were reported as a potential future diagnostic criterion and as a possible pathologic correlate [19,20].

The majority of patients with Susac syndrome in this study showed a characteristic and thus very distinct pattern of often severe and patchy retinal nerve fibre thinning in RNFLT and retinal damage in TMV. Compatible with the pathology of this retinal microangiopathy, retinal damage was usually scattered over distinct foci and not evenly distributed: whereas several sectors in RNFLT and/or TMV showed severe damage, other sectors remained completely normal. The notable exclusion from that rule was patient P2, who had a mostly normal RNFLT and TMV, despite visual symptoms and BRAO findings in FAG.

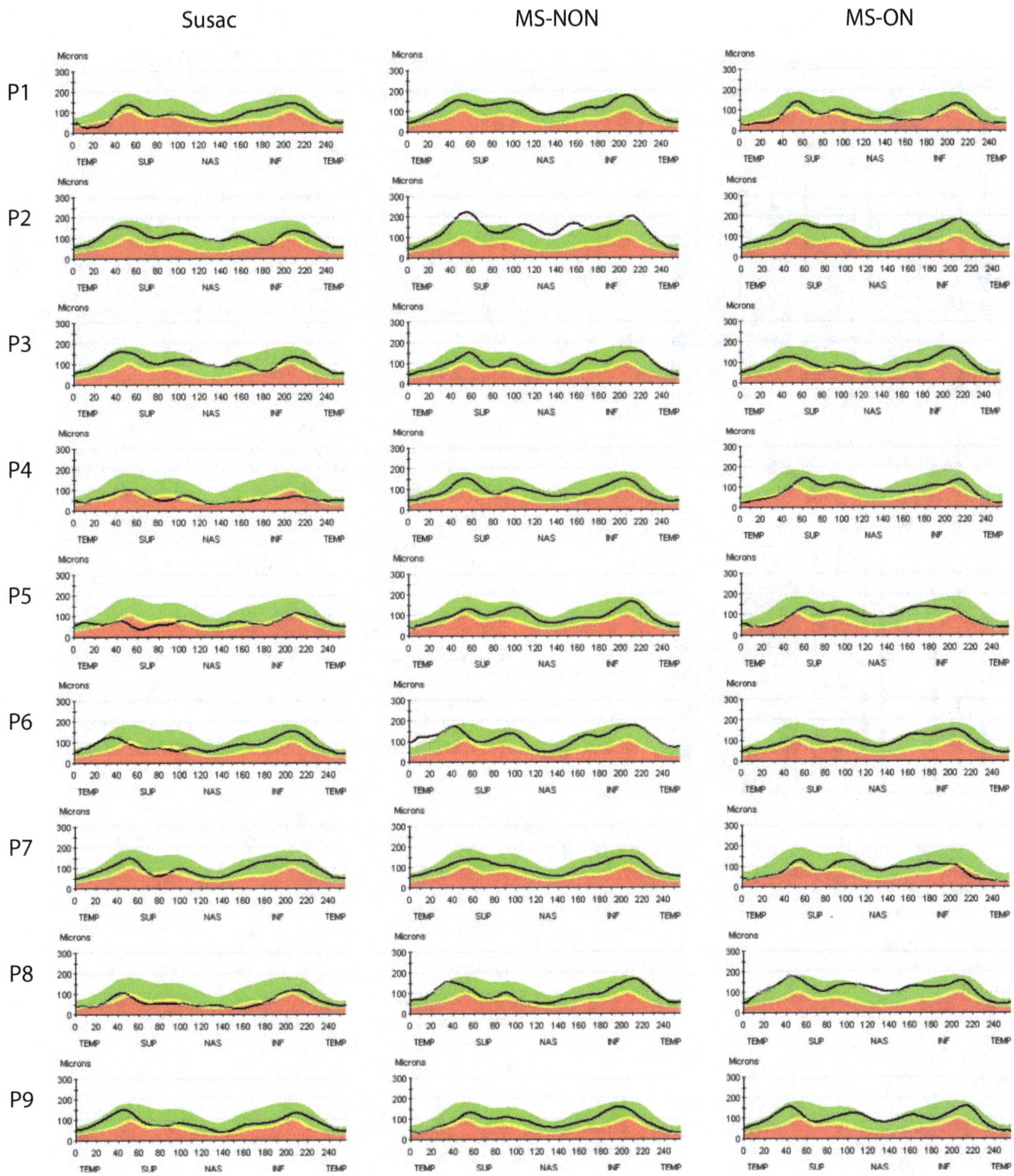

Figure 2. RNFLT from patients with Susac syndrome and matched RRMS patients. Shown are only the left eyes (randomly selected to save space) from each Susac patient (P1-9) and the corresponding left eyes from RRMS patients without history of optic neuritis (MS-NON) and RRMS patients with history of optic neuritis (MS-ON). Each graph represents the RNFLT from a peripapillary ring scan. Colour coded is the thickness relative to the normative database with green and white meaning normal values above the 5th or 95th percentile and yellow and red meaning reduction of thickness below the 5th or 1st percentile. Abbreviations: RNFLT = retinal nerve fibre layer thickness.

This presentation of Susac syndrome in OCT is in contrast to OCT findings in MS. Several publications that were recently reviewed in a meta-analysis [16], report an evenly distributed thinning of RNFL in MS that is slightly enhanced on the temporal quadrant after optic neuritis [21]. However, RNFL thinning in MS accumulates over time and becomes more severe especially in later stages of the disease. In early stages of MS and in clinically isolated syndrome (CIS), when differentiation of Susac syndrome is most important, RNFL thinning is barely detectable [22]. However, since Susac patients in this study's cohort had an

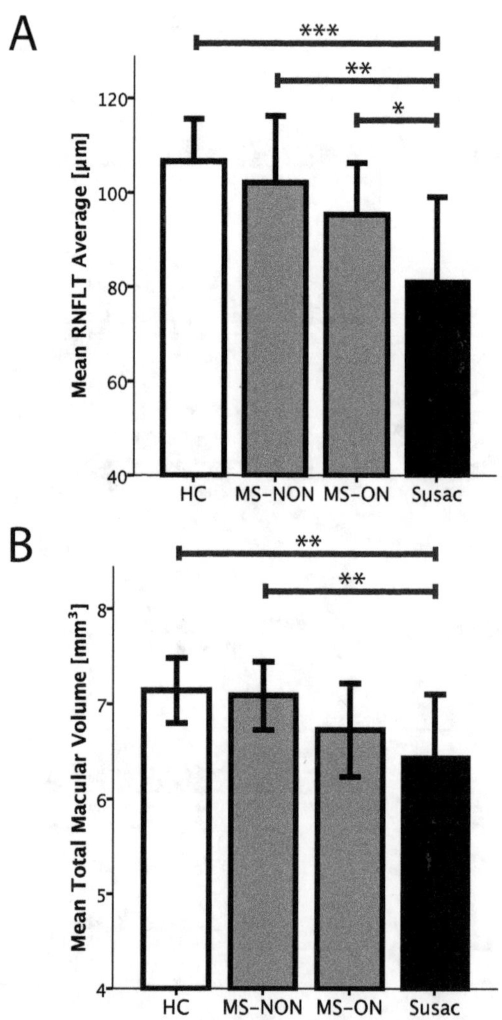

Figure 3. Comparison between healthy controls, RRMS patients and patients with Susac syndrome. Error bars indicate 1-fold standard deviation. Significance level from Generalised Estimating Equations are given as ***) $p<0.001$, **) $p<0.01$, and *) $p<0.05$. *Abbreviations*: HC = healthy control; RRMS = relapsing remitting multiple sclerosis; RNFLT = retinal nerve fibre layer thickness; MS-ON = RRMS patients with a previous, bilateral optic neuritis; MS-NON = RRMS patients without a history of optic neuritis.

established diagnosis already for several months or even years, it is not clear, how early Susac syndrome with acute visual impairment and BRAO translate into pathological OCT findings.

The crucial question in this context is at what time point OCT starts to show abnormal findings in patients with Susac syndrome. A few case reports and one study with nine BRAO patients without underlying Susac syndrome report an initial thickening of RNFL leading to final thinning after several months [23–25]. In general, one would suspect that structural retinal nerve fibre damage evolves some time after the underlying vessel pathology. One patient (P6) however showed an abnormal OCT even without BRAO in FAG pointing towards a potential usability of OCT in earlier stages of the disease when the diagnosis is yet not fully established. This issue should be addressed in a longitudinal study investigating the development of retinal lesions of newly diagnosed patients with Susac syndrome and BRAO over time including functional visual outcomes. Due to the design of our study, it was not possible to perform FAG and OCT at the same time, unfortunately limiting the possibility to make assertions on the co-occurrence of OCT and BRAO findings in this respect. Therefore, these questions are currently investigated in a follow up study.

Beyond differential diagnosis, the severe structural retinal damage in Susac syndrome especially in the macular scans detected by OCT supports an aggressive treatment regimen early after diagnosis [8]. This notion is further assisted by the fact that patient (P6) without visual symptoms showed a pathological OCT, suggesting early subclinical retinal damage. On the other hand, one patient (P2) with actual BRAO did not have pathological findings in OCT. Thus, BRAO does not always lead to pathological OCT findings. The dissociation of retinal damage and history of BRAO observed in P2 and P6 might suggest additional mechanisms independent of BRAO underlying retinal damage in this disease.

The reported study has important limitations that need to be considered. Due to the rarity of the disease, recruitment of a sufficient number of patients is challenging and prospective data on Susac syndrome derived from studies with more than five patients hardly exist. Although data on a limited number of nine patients obviously need to be interpreted cautiously, our study is among the largest prospective studies so far reported on Susac syndrome [26–28]. However, conclusions on the discriminatory ability of OCT between Susac syndrome and MS should be interpreted with care from this study with only small numbers.

Another important limitation of our study is the use of a time domain OCT device that measures macular volume using a six-line scan protocol instead of a volume/3D scan. A thickness map is generated via interpolating the measurements between the six line scans. The distinct and striking sectorial damage in the macular scans might therefore be under- or overestimated. Since the macular scan incorporates all retinal layers between the inner limiting membrane and the retinal pigment epithelium, it is not possible to determine via time domain OCT alone, which retinal layers are affected in Susac syndrome in comparison to optic neuritis. Because of the vascular nature of the disease, one might speculate though, that any damage would be more profound and affecting more retinal layers when compared to optic neuritis. Furthermore, the used time domain OCT device has known limitations in the reproducibility of sectoral RNFLT [29]. Next generation spectral domain OCT devices provide volume 3D scans and intra-retinal segmentation algorithms [30], possibly further enhancing the value of OCT in the differential diagnosis of Susac syndrome. However, in contrast to spectral domain OCT, time domain OCT is already widely available and patients with Susac syndrome show the reported distinct phenotype in comparison to MS even in time domain OCT, thus strengthening the importance of OCT application in differential diagnosis in routine or outpatient clinic settings.

In summary, we show that Susac patients regularly have distinct abnormalities in OCT scans. The sectorial pattern of retinal damage supports the hypothesis of a vascular origin with patchy lesions. Most importantly, our data recommends OCT as a tool in early primary and secondary diagnostics of Susac syndrome when differentiation from MS and other neuroimmunologic diseases can prove challenging.

Acknowledgments

We thank our study nurses Franziska Lipske and Katja Wolf for important logistical support.

Author Contributions

Conceived and designed the experiments: JD IK FP AUB. Performed the experiments: HZ FK JP SS DF MR OA CG IK JD. Analyzed the data: JD AUB FP. Wrote the paper: AUB IK JD. Provided important intellectual input into design and conduct of study: OA EBR HPH FP. Provided crucial logistic support: EBR CG OA MR HPH. Critically revised the manuscript for intellectual content: HZ FK JP SS DF OA CG MR EBR HPH FP.

References

1. Susac JO, Hardman JM, Selhorst JB (1979) Microangiopathy of the brain and retina. Neurology 29: 313–316.
2. Susac JO (1994) Susac's syndrome: the triad of microangiopathy of the brain and retina with hearing loss in young women. Neurology 44: 591–593.
3. Dörr J, Radbruch H, Bock M, Wuerfel J, Brüggemann A, et al. (2009) Encephalopathy, visual disturbance and hearing loss-recognizing the symptoms of Susac syndrome. Nat Rev Neurol 5: 683–688.
4. Petty GW, Engel AG, Younge BR, Duffy J, Yanagihara T, et al. (1998) Retinocochleocerebral vasculopathy. Medicine (Baltimore) 77: 12–40.
5. McLeod DS, Ying HS, McLeod CA, Grebe R, Lubow M, et al. (2011) Retinal and optic nerve head pathology in Susac's syndrome. Ophthalmology 118: 548–552.
6. Susac JO, Egan RA, Rennebohm RM, Lubow M (2007) Susac's syndrome: 1975–2005 microangiopathy/autoimmune endotheliopathy. J Neurol Sci 257: 270–272.
7. Petty GW, Matteson EL, Younge BR, McDonald TJ, Wood CP (2001) Recurrence of Susac syndrome (retinocochleocerebral vasculopathy) after remission of 18 years. Mayo Clin Proc 76: 958–960.
8. Rennebohm RM, Egan RA, Susac JO (2008) Treatment of Susac's Syndrome. Curr Treat Options Neurol 10: 67–74.
9. Rennebohm RM, Susac JO (2007) Treatment of Susac's syndrome. J Neurol Sci 257: 215–220.
10. Egan RA, Hills WL, Susac JO (2010) Gass plaques and fluorescein leakage in Susac Syndrome. J Neurol Sci 299: 97–100.
11. Rennebohm R, Susac JO, Egan RA, Daroff RB (2010) Susac's Syndrome – update. J Neurol Sci 299: 86–91.
12. O'Halloran HS, Pearson PA, Lee WB, Susac JO, Berger JR (1998) Microangiopathy of the brain, retina, and cochlea (Susac syndrome). A report of five cases and a review of the literature. Ophthalmology 105: 1038–1044.
13. Frohman EM, Costello F, Zivadinov R, Stuve O, Conger A, et al. (2006) Optical coherence tomography in multiple sclerosis. Lancet Neurol 5: 853–863.
14. Frohman EM, Fujimoto JG, Frohman TC, Calabresi PA, Cutter G, et al. (2008) Optical coherence tomography: a window into the mechanisms of multiple sclerosis. Nature Clinical Practice Neurology 4: 664–675.
15. Naismith RT, Tutlam NT, Xu J, Klawiter EC, Shepherd J, et al. (2009) Optical coherence tomography differs in neuromyelitis optica compared with multiple sclerosis. Neurology 72: 1077–1082.
16. Petzold A, de Boer JF, Schippling S, Vermersch P, Kardon R, et al. (2010) Optical coherence tomography in multiple sclerosis: a systematic review and meta-analysis. Lancet Neurol 9: 921–932.
17. Cheung CYL, Leung CKS, Lin D, Pang C-P, Lam DSC (2008) Relationship between retinal nerve fiber layer measurement and signal strength in optical coherence tomography. Ophthalmology 115: 1347–51, 1351.e1–2.
18. Kleffner I, Deppe M, Mohammadi S, Schiffbauer H, Stupp N, et al. (2008) Diffusion tensor imaging demonstrates fiber impairment in Susac syndrome. Neurology 70: 1867–1869.
19. Jarius S, Neumayer B, Wandinger KP, Hartmann M, Wildemann B (2009) Anti-endothelial serum antibodies in a patient with Susac's syndrome. J Neurol Sci 285: 259–261.
20. Magro CM, Poe JC, Lubow M, Susac JO (2011) Susac syndrome: an organ-specific autoimmune endotheliopathy syndrome associated with anti-endothelial cell antibodies. Am J Clin Pathol 136: 903–912.
21. Bock M, Brandt AU, Dörr J, Kraft H, Weinges-Evers N, et al. (2010) Patterns of retinal nerve fiber layer loss in multiple sclerosis patients with or without optic neuritis and glaucoma patients. Clin Neurol Neurosurg 112: 647–652.
22. Outteryck O, Zephir H, Defoort S, Bouyon M, Debruyne P, et al. (2009) Optical coherence tomography in clinically isolated syndrome: no evidence of subclinical retinal axonal loss. Arch Neurol 66: 1373–1377.
23. Asefzadeh B, Ninyo K (2008) Longitudinal analysis of retinal changes after branch retinal artery occlusion using optical coherence tomography. Optometry 79: 85–89.
24. Takahashi H, Iijima H (2009) Sectoral thinning of the retina after branch retinal artery occlusion. Jpn J Ophthalmol 53: 494–500.
25. Shah VA, Wallace B, Sabates NR (2010) Spectral domain optical coherence tomography findings of acute branch retinal artery occlusion from calcific embolus. Indian J Ophthalmol 58: 523–524.
26. Susac JO, Murtagh FR, Egan RA, Berger JR, Bakshi R, et al. (2003) MRI findings in Susac's syndrome. Neurology 61: 1783–1787.
27. Aubart-Cohen F, Klein I, Alexandra J-F, Bodaghi B, Doan S, et al. (2007) Long-term outcome in Susac syndrome. Medicine (Baltimore) 86: 93–102.
28. Kleffner I, Deppe M, Mohammadi S, Schwindt W, Sommer J, et al. (2010) Neuroimaging in Susac's syndrome: focus on DTI. J Neurol Sci 299: 92–96.
29. Cettomai D, Pulicken M, Gordon-Lipkin E, Salter A, Frohman TC, et al. (2008) Reproducibility of optical coherence tomography in multiple sclerosis. Arch Neurol 65: 1218–1222.
30. Saidha S, Syc SB, Ibrahim MA, Eckstein C, Warner CV, et al. (2011) Primary retinal pathology in multiple sclerosis as detected by optical coherence tomography. Brain 134: 518–533.

5

Screening of *MITF* and *SOX10* Regulatory Regions in Waardenburg Syndrome Type 2

Viviane Baral[1,2], Asma Chaoui[1,2], Yuli Watanabe[1,2], Michel Goossens[1,2,3], Tania Attie-Bitach[4], Sandrine Marlin[5], Veronique Pingault[1,2,3], Nadege Bondurand[1,2]*

1 INSERM, U955, equipe11, Créteil, France, **2** Université Paris Est, Faculté de Médecine, Créteil, France, **3** AP-HP, Hôpital H.Mondor-A. Chenevier, Service de biochimie et génétique, Créteil, France, **4** INSERM U781, Université Paris Descartes, Hôpital Necker-Enfants Malades, Paris, France, **5** Service de Génétique, Centre de référence «Surdités génétiques», INSERM U587, Hôpital Armand Trousseau, APHP, Paris, France

Abstract

Waardenburg syndrome (WS) is a rare auditory-pigmentary disorder that exhibits varying combinations of sensorineural hearing loss and pigmentation defects. Four subtypes are clinically defined based on the presence or absence of additional symptoms. WS type 2 (WS2) can result from mutations within the *MITF* or *SOX10* genes; however, 70% of WS2 cases remain unexplained at the molecular level, suggesting that other genes might be involved and/or that mutations within the known genes escaped previous screenings. The recent identification of a deletion encompassing three of the *SOX10* regulatory elements in a patient presenting with another WS subtype, WS4, defined by its association with Hirschsprung disease, led us to search for deletions and point mutations within the *MITF* and *SOX10* regulatory elements in 28 yet unexplained WS2 cases. Two nucleotide variations were identified: one in close proximity to the *MITF* distal enhancer (MDE) and one within the U1 *SOX10* enhancer. Functional analyses argued against a pathogenic effect of these variations, suggesting that mutations within regulatory elements of WS genes are not a major cause of this neurocristopathy.

Editor: Andreas R. Janecke, Innsbruck Medical University, Austria

Funding: This work was supported by Institut National de la Santé et de la Recherche Médicale (INSERM) and Agence Nationale de la Recherche (ANR-JCJC-2010). The funders had no role in study design, data collection and analysis, decision to publish, or preparation of the manuscript.

Competing Interests: The authors have declared that no competing interests exist.

* E-mail: nadege.bondurand@inserm.fr

Introduction

Waardenburg syndrome (WS) is characterised by the association of sensorineural hearing loss and pigmentation abnormalities, including depigmented patches of the skin and hair and vivid blue eyes or heterochromia iridis. Its prevalence is estimated to be 1 in 42,000 and it is responsible for 1–3% of all cases of congenital deafness [1,2]. Other features, such as dystopia canthorum, musculoskeletal abnormalities of the limbs, and Hirschsprung disease, are found in a subset of patients and used for the clinical classification of this syndrome into four subtypes (WS1-4). At the molecular level, WS is genetically heterogeneous, with six genes known to be involved: *PAX3* (encoding the paired box 3 transcription factor), *EDN3* (endothelin-3), *EDNRB* (endothelin receptor type B), *SOX10* (Sry bOX10 transcription factor), *MITF* (microphthalmia-associated transcription factor), and *SNAI2* (snail homolog 2) (for review, see [1]). WS2, which is defined by the absence of additional features, results from mutations occurring with different frequencies within the last three of these genes, *SOX10*, *MITF*, and *SNAI2*. Heterozygous *MITF* mutations have been reported in about 15% of cases [1,2], but homozygous deletions of the *SNAI2* gene, however, have been described in only two patients [3], arguing against a major involvement of this gene. Recently, we showed that another 15% of WS2 cases are due to heterozygous *SOX10* point mutations or deletions [1,4,5]. Some mutations are responsible for extended phenotypes, including peripheral and central neurological defects, and are referred to as PCW (Peripheral demyelinating neuropathy - Central dysmyelinating leucodystrophy - Waardenburg syndrome) [1,6]. Overall, 70% of WS2 remain unexplained at the molecular level, suggesting that other genes might be involved and/or that mutations within the known genes escaped previous screenings. It was therefore tempting to speculate that alteration of the expression level or sites of *MITF* or *SOX10*, which are tightly regulated during development, can lead to WS2.

Mitf/MITF, which encodes a member of the Myc supergene family of basic helix loop helix zipper (bHLH-Zip) transcription factors, is known as the key transcription factor in melanocyte development (for review, see [7,8,9]). This gene contains nine alternative promoters, producing multiple isoforms differing in their amino termini but sharing exons 2–9. Of all the different *Mitf* promoter elements, the melanocyte specific one (MITF-M) has generated the most interest because of its tissue specificity and function [8,9,10]. Various signalling molecules and transcription factors regulate expression from the MITF-M promoter, including Wnt, MSH, PAX3, SOX10, LEF-1, OC2, CREB, BRN2, and FoxD3 [9,10,11,12]. In humans, most of the responsive *MITF* promoter sequences lie within a region of 400 bp upstream of the MITF-M transcription initiation site. A distal regulatory region known as the MITF distal enhancer, or MDE, was characterised more recently [13]. This region of 298 bp, localised nearly 15 kb upstream of the human MITF-M transcription initiation site, is partially conserved in mouse and dog [13,14]. It contains at least two functional SOX10 binding sites and enhances M promoter activity in melanoma cells. In mouse, the importance of this element is consistent with the coat colour defects observed in the Mitf$^{mi\text{-}red\text{-}eyed\text{-}white}$ mutant, carrying a large deletion including this region [9].

The SOX10 transcription factor is an important pleiotropic regulator of neural crest development, regulating stem cell maintenance and cell lineage progression (for reviews, see [15,16,17]). Its function is well described, and recent studies shed light onto the complex regulation of its expression [18,19,20,21,22,23]. *In silico* analyses led to the identification of several enhancers of *SOX10*. We and others identified several of these regulatory elements, five upstream (U1–5) and one downstream (D6+7) of the human *SOX10* gene ([22,23,24]). The functional relevance of these elements was confirmed in different cell lines and in zebrafish, chicken and mouse models, where they drive expression in several neural crest derivatives [19,22]. Two of them, U1 and U3, which are localised 55 kb and 33 kb upstream of the *SOX10* gene respectively, drive *SOX10*/*Sox10* expression during melanocyte development in particular, at least in zebrafish and in melanoma cells ([18,19] and our unpublished results). These two sequences contain dimeric SOX consensus binding sites, which are essential for enhancer activity, as well as multiple binding sites for other factors known to play key roles in neural crest development [18,19,21].

Mutations within the *SOX10* gene are not only responsible for some WS2 cases but they also explain about 50% of WS4 cases, characterised by an association with Hirschsprung disease (HD, absence of enteric ganglia in the distal part of the intestine) [1,25]. Recently, we described the first characterisation of a large deletion encompassing several *SOX10* enhancers in a patient presenting with WS4 [24]. Taken together with previous results, this demonstrated that the disruption of highly conserved non-coding elements located within or at a long distance from the coding sequences of key genes can result in several neurocristopathies, particularly WS and HD ([24,26]). This led us to search for

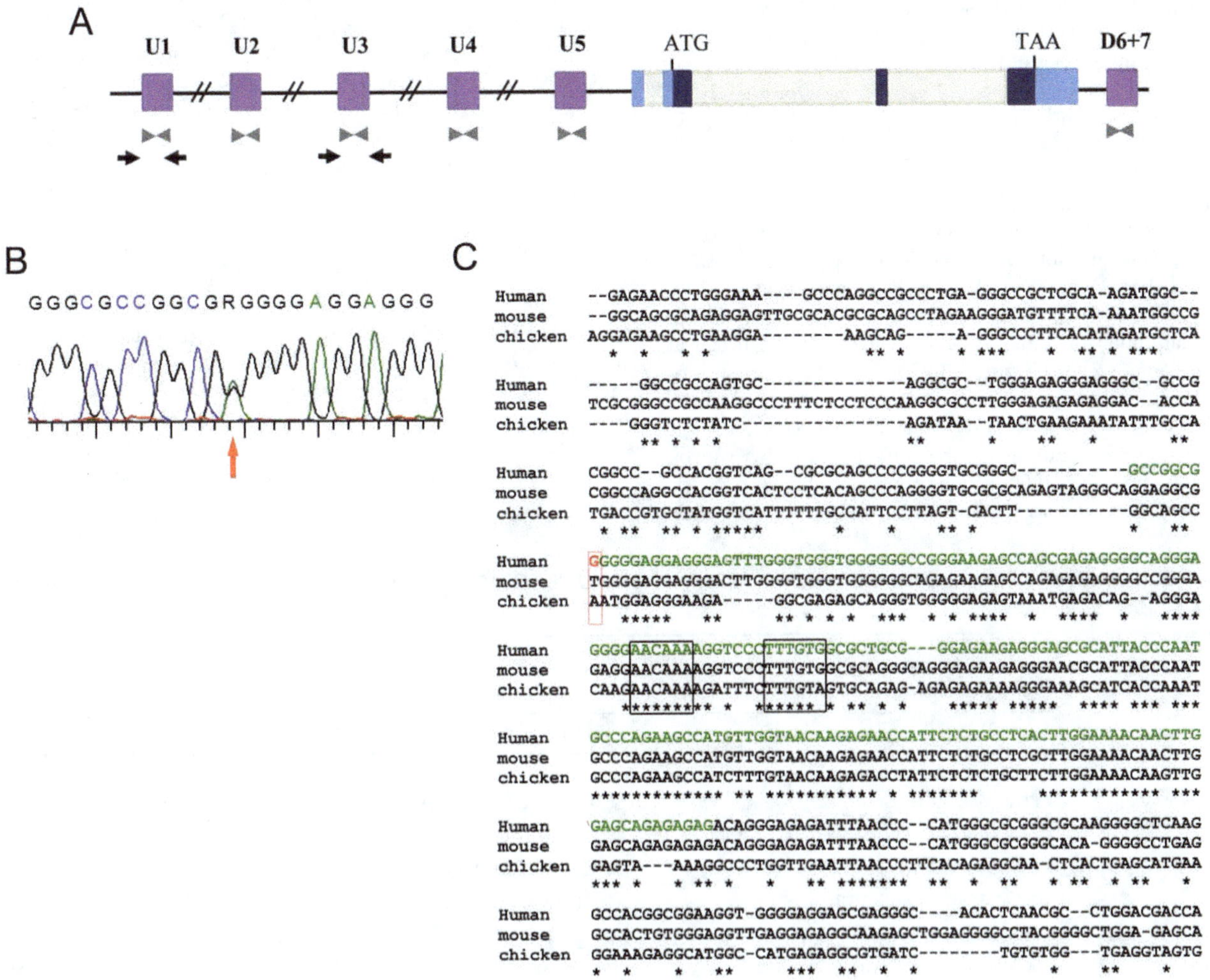

Figure 1. Variations identified in SOX10 regulatory regions. (A) Schematic view of the *SOX10* gene (start and stop codon are indicated) and putative enhancer regions located 100 kb around the human *SOX10* locus. SOX10-coding exons are in dark blue, noncoding exons in blue, intronic regions in grey and putative enhancers in purple. Grey arrowheads indicate the position of QMF-PCR primers. Black arrows indicate the position of primers used for PCR sequencing for screening. (B) Electropherogram showing the heterozygous variation identified. (C) Alignment of the nucleotide sequences of the human U1 region of *SOX10* (GenBank accession number NT_011520.12) and its corresponding *Mus musculus* (NT_039621.7) and *Gallus gallus* (NW_001471513.1) homologous regions. The asterisks indicate the nucleotides conserved between murine, chicken, and human sequences. The two previously described putative SOX10 binding sites are indicated by black open boxes. Nucleotides included in the region identified by DCODE analysis or previously published [22] are indicated in green. The location of the identified variation is indicated by a red open box.

deletions and point mutations within the *MITF* and *SOX10* regulatory elements in unexplained WS2 cases.

Materials and Methods

Patients

A total of 28 WS2 patients previously found to be negative for point mutations or deletions within the *MITF* and *SOX10* genes were investigated. *SNAI2* screening revealed an absence of anomalies in the two patients presenting with MDE and U1 variations. Genomic DNA was extracted from peripheral blood leukocytes using standard protocols. Written informed consent was obtained for all patients. The study has been validated by the ethical committee which waived requirement for a formal ethical approval in regards to the research performed.

Molecular analysis

Semi-quantitative fluorescent multiplex PCR (QMF-PCR) was used to amplify five of the regulatory regions located 5′ of the *SOX10* gene (U1-5) and one (D6+7) located 3′ of the gene in one fluorescently labelled multiplex reaction with two external controls, following previously described protocols ([24]). The same strategy allowed us to screen a 220 bp region of the *MITF* promoter using the following primers: 5′-TTAGATGATGTCTCCTCCAA-3′ and 5′-AAATGTTGATATCAATTTTTCC-3′.

In parallel, PCR amplification and direct sequencing of the U1, U3, MDE, and *MITF* promoter regions was performed using the primers described in Table 1. Thermo Scientific high fidelity DNA polymerase (Fermentas) was used for PCR amplification, with genomic DNA and 5% DMSO. The reaction started with an initial denaturation of 5 min at 95°C, followed by 35 cycles at 95°C for 1 min, 62°C (U1 and U3), 55°C (MITF promoter) or 58°C (MDE) for 1 min, and 72°C for 2 min. Then, 2 µl of the purified PCR products were used for direct sequencing.

Upon variation identification, the dbSNP (http://www.ncbi.nlm.nih.gov/snp) and 1000 genomes project (http://browser.1000genomes.org) databases were used to search for previously identified polymorphisms. In parallel, 50 controls (100 chromosomes) of matched geographical origins were confirmed negative for the variations identified in patients. The genomic location of the variations was given according to the international nomenclature based on the human chromosome 3 (NC_000003.11) and chromosome 22 (NC_000022.10) reference sequences. Analysis with the TFSEARCH program (Searching Transcription Factor Binding Sites, http://www.rwcp.or.jp/papia/) was used to seek putative transcription factor binding sites and their alteration upon variation identification.

Plasmid constructs, cell culture, transfection, and reporter assays

The MDE reporter construct (previously called pGL3-cis1) was kindly provided by Pr. Shigeki Shibahara [13]. The identified variation was inserted by site-directed mutagenesis using the QuikChange Site-Directed Mutagenesis Kit (Stratagene). The U1 enhancer region was amplified by PCR using control and patient DNA and the primers 5′- GAGCTCCCAGCCGCCCCCTACGACTGCCC-3′ and 5′-CTCGAGGCACAGGATGGGACGGGTTGAG-3′, containing SacI and XhoI restriction sites, respectively. After double digestion, the PCR products were cloned into the pTAL-luc vector (Clontech). The FoxD3 cDNA was amplified using the primers 5′-GGCACTCAAACCCTCTTCCCCTGAGCTCCG -3′ and 5′-GCAGCCTGGAGGTGCATTTGTTGCT -3′, and cloned into a TOPO-V5 expression vector (Invitrogen).

HeLa and SKMel5 cells (ATCC) were grown in Dulbecco's modified Eagle's medium (DMEM) supplemented with 10% foetal calf serum and transfected using Lipofectamine PLUS reagents (Invitrogen). Approximately 110,000 cells were plated on 12-well plates and transfected 1 day later with 0.5 µg of reporter plasmid and the FoxD3 expression plasmid. Twenty-four hours post-transfection, cells were washed twice with PBS and lysed, and the extracts were assayed for luciferase activity using the Luciferase Assay System (Promega) as previously described [4,5,27].

Table 1. Sequences of primers used for PCR and sequencing of U1 and U3 SOX10 enhancers regions as well as *MDE* and promoter regions of *MITF* sequences.

	Primer sequence (5′→3′)		
Primer	**Forward**	**Reverse**	**PCR size (bp)**
SOX10			
U1 PCR	CCAGCCGCCCCCTACGACTGCCC	GCACAGGATGGGACGGGTTGAG	476
U1 SEQ	CCAGCCGCCCCCTACGACTGCCC	GTCGTCCAGGCGTTGAGTGT	
U3 PCR	CTCAGGAGGGCTGGAGAGTGGTG	GGGGCATCAGCGAATCTGTTTTG	902
U3 SEQ	TGCCAGGCAGCAGAGGCTGG	AGCAGAGCAAGGGCCTGGTG	
	TTCCAACATGTCATTACAGT	CGACGTTGACATTGTTCCCA	
	TGGGAACAATGTCAACGTCG		
***MITF* promoter**			
PCR and SEQ	GCCCGGTCTTCCTGATGTGAGGTCA	GACTTATCCCTCCCTCTACTTTCTA	636
SEQ	TGATCTGACAGTGAGTTTGA	AGGCCAATTCACTATTCATC	
***MITF*-MDE**			
PCR	CCTGGGTTCAGGTGATTCTCCTG	AGCCCCTCAAGCCAGCAACGGG	652
SEQ	CAGGCATATGCCACCACACC	CGGAGAAAGTCAATATGGACATTTGTTC	

Expected PCR product size are reported. SEQ indicates the primers used for sequencing. pb: base pais.

Results

Analysis of *SOX10* regulatory sequences

Based on the recent identification of a WS4 patient presenting with a large deletion encompassing three SOX10 enhancers, we first screened for deletions of SOX enhancers using the previously described QMF-PCR strategy ([24]). Analysis of the U1–5 and D6+7 regions (Fig. 1A, grey arrowheads indicate the position of the primers) revealed an absence of deletions or detectable rearrangement within the 28 WS2 cases included in our study. The high enhancer activity of U1 and U3 sequences observed in melanoma cells ([19] and our unpublished results), along with their crucial function during zebrafish melanocyte development, led us to analyse these regions in more detail. We searched for point variations within these two regulatory elements (see Fig. 1A, black arrows, and Table 1 for primer sequences) by a direct PCR sequencing strategy. No variations were found within U3, but one was identified within U1: g.38434799C>T on chromosome 22 (G>A on the reverse sequence, Fig. 1B), which has not been reported in polymorphism databases. This nucleotide, which lies 5′ of the most conserved sequence, is not evolutionarily conserved (Fig. 1C). The patient was born of a healthy non consanguineous couple. He presented with a white frontal forelock and bilateral profound hearing loss revealed by neonatal hearing screening. Temporal bones CT scan showed no malformation and a cochlear implantation has been performed. His older sister presented with isolated, bilateral profound hearing loss diagnosed at the age of 6 months. No sign of skin, hair or irides depigmentation was observed. *GJB2* mutations screening was found negative. The parents and sister testing revealed the variation was inherited from the mother and was not carried by the sister.

TFSEARCH analysis indicated that the concerned variation may alter putative ADR1 (alcohol dehydrogenase (ADH) II synthesis regulator) and/or AP-2 (activator protein-2) binding sites (Fig. 2A).

The effect of this variation on the ability of U1 to direct reporter gene expression was tested *in vitro*. To this end, wild-type or mutated versions of U1 were cloned upstream of a minimal promoter directing basal luciferase expression, and constructs were transfected into SKMel5 and HeLa cell lines, and their enhancer activity was tested 24 hours later. The wild-type U1 sequence conferred a 107.8±24.2-fold and a 79.9±16.6-fold increase in activation in SKMel5 and HeLa cells, respectively (Fig. 2B), confirming the ubiquitous enhancer activity of this element [19,23]. Under our experimental conditions, the identified variation did not significantly alter U1 enhancer activity. Indeed, a 94.8±22.1-fold and an 86.1±8.8-fold increase in activation were observed in SKMel5 and HeLa cells, respectively. Altogether, our results argued that the variation identified in this patient did not confer any significant functional consequences.

Analysis of *MITF* regulatory sequences

We used similar strategies to search for deletions and point mutations within the known *MITF* regulatory sequences. First, we used QMF-PCR to screen for deletions within the well known MITF-M promoter region (Fig. 3A, grey arrows indicate the positions of the primers). No deletion or rearrangement were identified. In parallel, we used direct PCR sequencing strategies to analyse i) the 400 bp promoter region and 100 bp downstream of the M transcription initiation site (Fig. 3A and Table 1); and ii) the MDE region and around 150 bp of flanking regions (Fig. 3A,

A

```
GCCCCGGGGT GCGGGCGCCG GCGGGGGGAG GAGGGAGTTT GGGTGGGTGG entry  score
    ----->                                            ADR1   98.5
                      ----->                          ADR1   96.9
                 <------------                        AP-2   94.0
<-----                                                ADR1   93.8
                  ----->                              ADR1   92.3
                 ------->                             MZF1   92.2
                   <------------                      AP-2   90.0
                          ---------------->           p300   89.1
                         ------>                      ADR1   87.7
                             ----->                   ADR1   87.7
                                ---------->           Lyf-1  87.0
                                 -------------->      NGFI-C 86.8
                       ------>                        ADR1   86.2

GCCCCGGGGT GCGGGCGCCG GCGAGGGGAG GAGGGAGTTT GGGTGGGTGG entry  score
    ----->                                            ADR1   98.5
<-----                                                ADR1   93.8
                 ------->                             MZF1   90.4
                  ----->                              ADR1   89.2
                          ---------------->           p300   89.1
                         ------>                      ADR1   87.7
                             ----->                   ADR1   87.7
                                ---------->           Lyf-1  87.0
                                 -------------->      NGFI-C 86.8
                       ------>                        ADR1   86.2
```

B

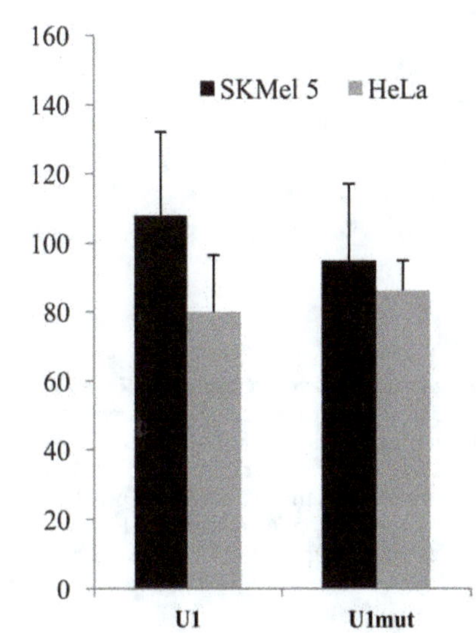

Figure 2. Functional analysis of the variation identified within U1. (A) TFSEARCH results obtained upon analysis of 50 bp around the variation. The top panel corresponds to the wild-type sequence, whereas the bottom panel corresponds to the mutated sequence. Variation and affected binding sites are indicated in red. (B) Functional consequences of the variation. Wild-type and mutated versions of the U1 sequences were cloned upstream of a minimal promoter driving basal luciferase expression and assayed for enhancer activity in SKMel5 and HeLa cells. Reporter gene activation is presented as fold-induction relative to the empty vector. Results represent the mean ± standard error of three to five different experiments, each performed in duplicate.

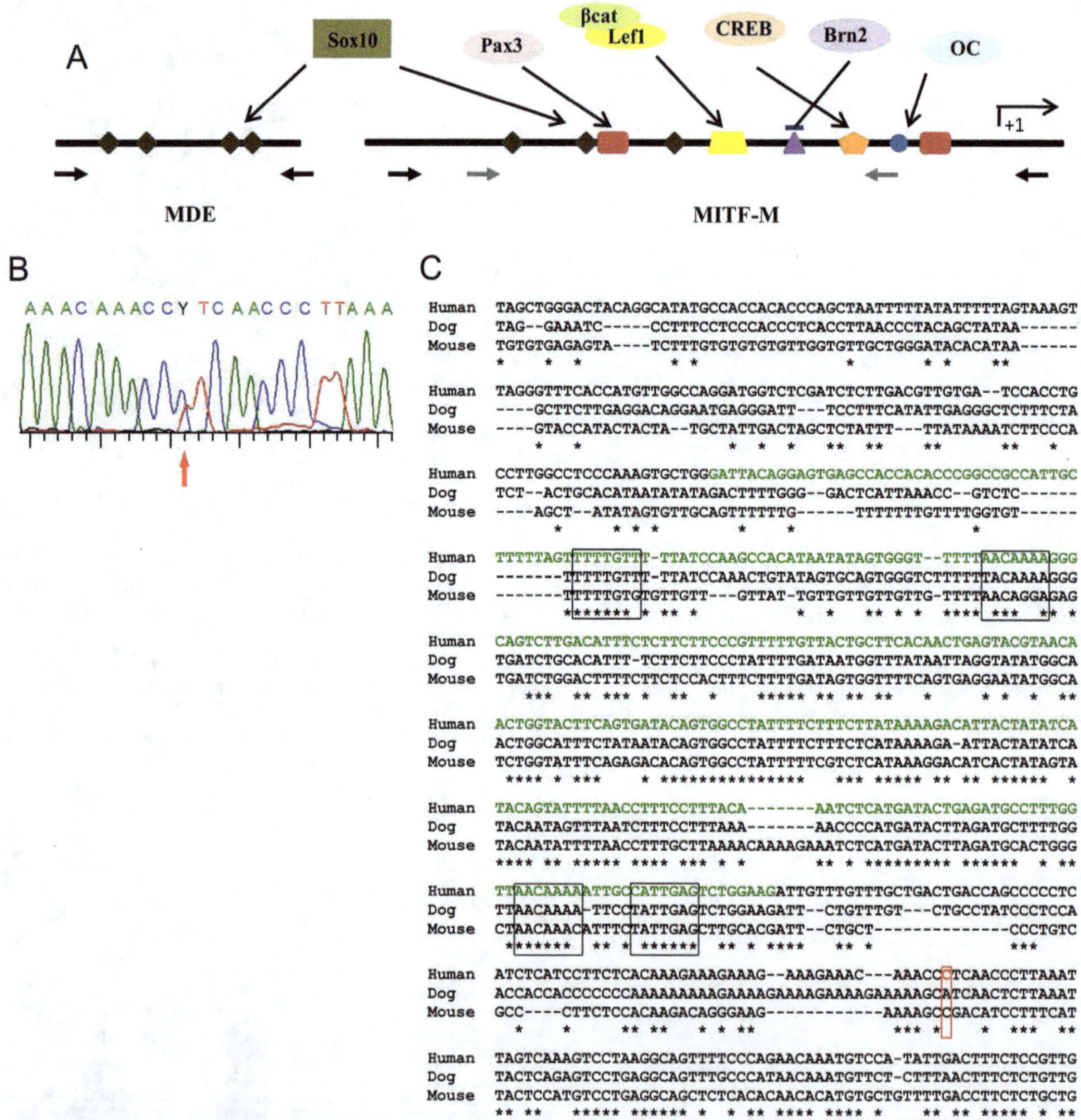

Figure 3. Variations identified in *MITF* regulatory regions. (A) Schematic view of the MITF-M promoter and MDE enhancer regions showing binding sites for transcription factors known to regulate *MITF/Mitf* expression in melanocytes. Note the presence of several SOX10 binding sites in both promoter and enhancer regions. Grey arrows indicate the position of QMF-PCR primers. Black arrows indicate the position of primers used for PCR and sequencing screening. (B) Electropherogram showing the heterozygous variation identified. (C) Alignment of the nucleotide sequences of human MDE (GenBank accession number NT_022459) and its corresponding *Mus musculus* (NT_039353) and canine (AC191512.6) homologous regions. The asterisks indicate the identical nucleotides between murine, canine, and human sequences. The four putative SOX10 binding sites are indicated by black boxes. The previously described human MDE 298 bp region [13] is indicated in green. The location of the identified variation is indicated by a red open box. Note that it affects a nucleotide conserved between humans and mice, but not dogs.

black arrows, and Table 1 for primer sequences). No variation was identified within the promoter region, but one nucleotidic substitution, not reported in polymorphism databases, was found within the 3′ flanking region of the previously defined MDE region: g.69972010C>T on chromosome 3 (Fig. 3B). The affected nucleotide is conserved in mouse but not in dog (Fig. 3C). This variation was identified in a WS2 patient who is the unique child of a non consanguineous couple. He presented with bilateral profound sensorineural hearing impairment diagnosed at 8 months of age. The temporal bones CT scan and fundus oculi were normal. At 16 months, he presented with a synophrys without any other dymorphism. His mother was born with a white frontal forelock and her hair has begun greying at 16 years. Several cases of premature hair greying have been noted in the maternal lineage. The molecular result was confirmed on a second sample but the parents were not available for testing.

The region containing the identified variation was described as able to reduce the enhancer activity of MDE, but no transcription factor binding sites were reported [13]. TFSEARCH analysis revealed that the region contained a putative HFH-2 (HNF-3 Forkhead homolog 2; FoxD3) binding site. The variation lies within a CAP (cAMP receptor protein) binding site and could create an additional FoxD3 putative binding site (Fig. 4A).

To test its functional relevance, the consequences of this variation on the ability of MDE to direct reporter gene expression was analysed in melanoma cells as previously described [13]. Briefly, wild-type or mutated versions of MDE (MDE or MDEmut) constructs were transfected into SKMel5 cells and their enhancer activity was tested 24 hours later. A 99.4±17.4-fold and a 104.3±22.4-fold increase in activation was observed in the wild-type and mutated versions of MDE, respectively (Fig. 4B). The presence of putative FoxD3 binding sites within the wild-type MDE sequence as well as the presence of an additional site within the patient's sequence led us to test the role of FoxD3 on MDE regulation. Co-transfection with FoxD3 reduced the fold-activation to 27±7.8, suggesting a repressive role for this transcription factor on MITF promoter activity [27,28,29] and on MDE (Fig. 4C). Nevertheless, no further repression was observed upon transfection with the mutated construct. Indeed, the same repressive effect was observed for the mutated MDE sequence (Fig. 4C), arguing against any pathogenic effect caused by the variation.

Discussion

In this study, we report the screening of *SOX10* and *MITF* regulatory elements in WS2 patients that had not been previously characterised at the molecular level. No deletion was identified

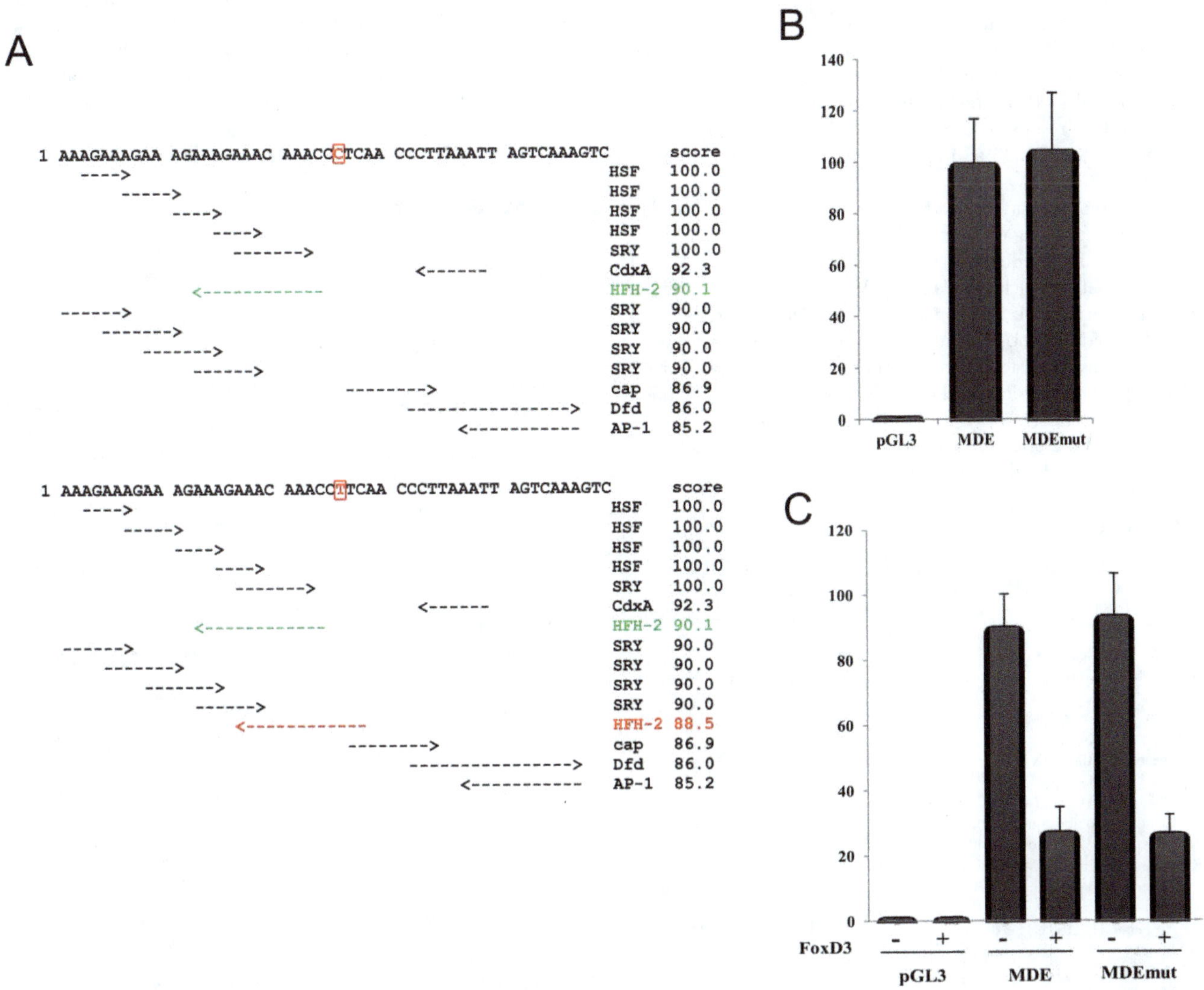

Figure 4. Functional consequences of the variation identified within MDE. (A) TFSEARCH results obtained upon analysis of 50 bp around the variation. The top panel corresponds to the wild-type sequence, whereas the bottom panel corresponds to the mutated sequence. The HFH2 additional binding site is indicated in red; the one present in both wild-type and mutated sequences is indicated in green. (B) Wild-type and mutated versions of the MDE reporter construct were assayed for enhancer activity in SKMel5 melanoma cell lines. Reporter gene activation is presented as fold-induction relative to the empty vector. Results represent the mean ± standard error of seven different experiments, each performed in duplicate. (C) Wild-type and mutated versions of the MDE reporter construct were co-transfected with a FoxD3 expression vector. Reporter gene activation is presented as the fold-induction relative to the empty vector. Results represent the mean ± standard error of three different experiments, each performed in duplicate.

upon QMF-PCR analysis of the *MITF* promoter and the *SOX10* regulatory regions. Sequencing of U1 and U3 SOX10 enhancers, as well as the *MITF* promoter and enhancer regions, led to the identification of two new variations: one in close proximity to the *MITF* enhancer sequence MDE, and one within the U1 enhancer. Each of these variations could potentially create or alter transcription factor binding sites: creation of an HFH2/FOXD3 site in the case of MDE, and alteration of ADR1 and AP2 binding sites in the case of U1. However, combined functional analyses and familial segregation suggested an absence of deleterious effects for these two variations.

For MITF, TFSEARCH analysis revealed that the 298 bp MDE region contained at least two putative HFH2/FOXD3 binding sites. One of these, described in Figure 4, is very close to the variation identified. Interestingly, recent reports shed light on the involvement of FOXD3 in the regulation of *Mitf* expression *in vivo* and *in vitro*. Several groups working in mouse or zebrafish showed that this transcription factor represses *MITF* expression through promoter regulation [28,29,30,31]. However, direct binding of FOXD3 to the *MITF* promoter region has been proposed by some and refuted by others. Thomas *et al.* suggested that functional FoxD3 binding sites might exist elsewhere in the gene [31]. Our results are in agreement with this last observation and suggest that FoxD3 also represses *MITF* expression through MDE regulation.

Recent reports have found that the disruption of highly conserved non-coding elements, both within or at a long distance from the coding sequences of key genes, resulted in several neurocristopathies, including HD and WS type 4 ([24,26]). These findings serve to open new routes to the molecular description of these disorders. The *MITF* and *SOX10* regulatory sequences were therefore considered to be good candidates for yet unexplained WS2 cases. The very low level of sequence variation we identified here argues against a major implication of these regulatory sequences in WS2 and leaves about 70% of WS2 still unexplained at the molecular level. Future studies will aim at screening the noncoding regions of these genes, but priority should be given to the discovery of new WS2 genes.

The recent identification of a deletion encompassing the *SOX10* regulatory elements U1 and U3 in a patient with WS4 [24], as well as their functional importance during enteric nervous system development ([22] and our unpublished observations), opens the possibility that variations within regulatory sequences could be at the origin of other phenotypes, or play a role in phenotypic variability. This paradigm parallels another *SOX* gene close to *SOX10*, *SOX9*. The involvement of the latter in campomelic dysplasia (CD) was demonstrated 17 years ago [32,33], but long distance genomic alterations at this locus have been recently associated with isolated disorders of sex development as well as isolated Pierre Robin sequence (PRS), both typical features of CD [34,35,36,37]. In addition to enlarging the list of diseases associated with *SOX9* mutations in human, these results clearly demonstrate that endophenotypes of CD can result from tissue-restricted alterations of *SOX9* expression due to disruption of tissue-specific, long-distance regulatory regions [26,37]. The increasing number of *SOX10* regulatory elements identified and the tissue-specific expression patterns of some of them lead us to speculate that endophenotypes of WS4, such as isolated HD, might also be linked to mutations within regulatory sequences of *SOX10*, hypothesis that will be tested in the near future.

Acknowledgments

Authors would like to thank Bruno Costes and Natacha Martin for sequencing and Alexandre Torgomian for technical assistance in figure drawing.

Author Contributions

Conceived and designed the experiments: NB. Performed the experiments: VB AC YW NB VP. Analyzed the data: NB VP. Contributed reagents/materials/analysis tools: TAB SM VP MG. Wrote the paper: NB VP. Approved final version of the manuscript: VB AC YW MG TAB SM VP NB.

References

1. Pingault V, Ente D, Dastot-Le Moal F, Goossens M, Marlin S, et al. (2010) Review and update of mutations causing Waardenburg syndrome. Hum Mutat 31: 391–406.
2. Read AP, Newton VE (1997) Waardenburg syndrome. J Med Genet 34: 656–665.
3. Sanchez-Martin M, Rodriguez-Garcia A, Perez-Losada J, Sagrera A, Read AP, et al. (2002) SLUG (SNAI2) deletions in patients with Waardenburg disease. Hum Mol Genet 11: 3231–3236.
4. Bondurand N, Dastot-Le Moal F, Stanchina L, Collot N, Baral V, et al. (2007) Deletions at the SOX10 gene locus cause Waardenburg syndrome types 2 and 4. Am J Hum Genet 81: 1169–1185.
5. Chaoui A, Watanabe Y, Touraine R, Baral V, Goossens M, et al. (2011) Identification and functional analysis of SOX10 missense mutations in different subtypes of waardenburg syndrome. Hum Mutat 32: 1436–1449.
6. Inoue K, Khajavi M, Ohyama T, Hirabayashi S, Wilson J, et al. (2004) Molecular mechanism for distinct neurological phenotypes conveyed by allelic truncating mutations. Nat Genet 36: 361–369.
7. Arnheiter H (2011) The discovery of the microphthalmia locus and its gene, Mitf. Pigment Cell Melanoma Res 23: 729–735.
8. Shibahara S, Takeda K, Yasumoto K, Udono T, Watanabe K, et al. (2001) Microphthalmia-associated transcription factor (MITF): multiplicity in structure, function, and regulation. J Investig Dermatol Symp Proc 6: 99–104.
9. Steingrimsson E, Copeland NG, Jenkins NA (2004) Melanocytes and the microphthalmia transcription factor network. Annu Rev Genet 38: 365–411.
10. Hou L, Pavan WJ (2008) Transcriptional and signaling regulation in neural crest stem cell-derived melanocyte development: do all roads lead to Mitf? Cell Res 18: 1163–1176.
11. Sommer L (2010) Generation of melanocytes from neural crest cells. Pigment Cell Melanoma Res 24: 411–421.
12. Vance KW, Goding CR (2004) The transcription network regulating melanocyte development and melanoma. Pigment Cell Res 17: 318–325.
13. Watanabe K, Takeda K, Yasumoto K, Udono T, Saito H, et al. (2002) Identification of a distal enhancer for the melanocyte-specific promoter of the MITF gene. Pigment Cell Res 15: 201–211.
14. Tsuchida S, Takizawa T, Abe K, Okamoto M, Tagawa M (2009) Identification of microphthalmia-associated transcription factor isoforms in dogs. Vet J 182: 283–293.
15. Harris ML, Baxter LL, Loftus SK, Pavan WJ (2010) Sox proteins in melanocyte development and melanoma. Pigment Cell Melanoma Res 23: 496–513.
16. Mollaaghababa R, Pavan WJ (2003) The importance of having your SOX on: role of SOX10 in the development of neural crest-derived melanocytes and glia. Oncogene 22: 3024–3034.
17. Wegner M (2005) Secrets to a healthy Sox life: lessons for melanocytes. Pigment Cell Res 18: 74–85.
18. Antonellis A, Bennett WR, Menheniott TR, Prasad AB, Lee-Lin SQ, et al. (2006) Deletion of long-range sequences at Sox10 compromises developmental expression in a mouse model of Waardenburg-Shah (WS4) syndrome. Hum Mol Genet 15: 259–271.
19. Antonellis A, Huynh JL, Lee-Lin SQ, Vinton RM, Renaud G, et al. (2008) Identification of neural crest and glial enhancers at the mouse Sox10 locus through transgenesis in zebrafish. PLoS Genet 4: e1000174.
20. Betancur P, Bronner-Fraser M, Sauka-Spengler T (2010) Genomic code for Sox10 activation reveals a key regulatory enhancer for cranial neural crest. Proc Natl Acad Sci U S A 107: 3570–3575.
21. Wahlbuhl M, Reiprich S, Vogl MR, Bosl MR, Wegner M (2011) Transcription factor Sox10 orchestrates activity of a neural crest-specific enhancer in the vicinity of its gene. Nucleic Acids Res.
22. Werner T, Hammer A, Wahlbuhl M, Bosl MR, Wegner M (2007) Multiple conserved regulatory elements with overlapping functions determine Sox10 expression in mouse embryogenesis. Nucleic Acids Res 35: 6526–6538.
23. Yokota Y, Saito D, Tadokoro R, Takahashi Y (2011) Genomically integrated transgenes are stably and conditionally expressed in neural crest cell-specific lineages. Dev Biol 353: 382–395.

24. Bondurand N, Fouquet V, Baral V, Lecerf L, Loundon N, et al. (2012) Alu-mediated deletion of SOX10 regulatory elements in Waardenburg syndrome type 4. Euro J Human Genetics In press.
25. Amiel J, Sproat-Emison E, Garcia-Barcelo M, Lantieri F, Burzynski G, et al. (2008) Hirschsprung disease, associated syndromes and genetics: a review. J Med Genet 45: 1–14.
26. Amiel J, Benko S, Gordon CT, Lyonnet S (2010) Disruption of long-distance highly conserved noncoding elements in neurocristopathies. Ann N Y Acad Sci 1214: 34–46.
27. Bondurand N, Pingault V, Goerich DE, Lemort N, Sock E, et al. (2000) Interaction among SOX10, PAX3 and MITF, three genes altered in Waardenburg syndrome. Hum Mol Genet 9: 1907–1917.
28. Curran K, Lister JA, Kunkel GR, Prendergast A, Parichy DM, et al. (2010) Interplay between Foxd3 and Mitf regulates cell fate plasticity in the zebrafish neural crest. Dev Biol 344: 107–118.
29. Curran K, Raible DW, Lister JA (2009) Foxd3 controls melanophore specification in the zebrafish neural crest by regulation of Mitf. Dev Biol 332: 408–417.
30. Ignatius MS, Moose HE, El-Hodiri HM, Henion PD (2008) colgate/hdac1 Repression of foxd3 expression is required to permit mitfa-dependent melanogenesis. Dev Biol 313: 568–583.
31. Thomas AJ, Erickson CA (2009) FOXD3 regulates the lineage switch between neural crest-derived glial cells and pigment cells by repressing MITF through a non-canonical mechanism. Development 136: 1849–1858.
32. Foster JW, Dominguez-Steglich MA, Guioli S, Kwok C, Weller PA, et al. (1994) Campomelic dysplasia and autosomal sex reversal caused by mutations in an SRY-related gene. Nature 372: 525–530.
33. Wagner T, Wirth J, Meyer J, Zabel B, Held M, et al. (1994) Autosomal sex reversal and campomelic dysplasia are caused by mutations in and around the SRY-related gene SOX9. Cell 79: 1111–1120.
34. Benko S, Fantes JA, Amiel J, Kleinjan DJ, Thomas S, et al. (2009) Highly conserved non-coding elements on either side of SOX9 associated with Pierre Robin sequence. Nat Genet 41: 359–364.
35. Benko S, Gordon CT, Mallet D, Sreenivasan R, Thauvin-Robinet C, et al. (2011) Disruption of a long distance regulatory region upstream of SOX9 in isolated disorders of sex development. J Med Genet 48: 825–830.
36. Georg I, Bagheri-Fam S, Knower KC, Wieacker P, Scherer G, et al. (2010) Mutations of the SRY-responsive enhancer of SOX9 are uncommon in XY gonadal dysgenesis. Sex Dev 4: 321–325.
37. Gordon CT, Tan TY, Benko S, Fitzpatrick D, Lyonnet S, et al. (2009) Long-range regulation at the SOX9 locus in development and disease. J Med Genet 46: 649–656.

6

Discrimination Task Reveals Differences in Neural Bases of Tinnitus and Hearing Impairment

Fatima T. Husain[1,2]*, Nathan M. Pajor[2], Jason F. Smith[2], H. Jeff Kim[3], Susan Rudy[3], Christopher Zalewski[3], Carmen Brewer[3], Barry Horwitz[2]

1 Department of Speech and Hearing Science, University of Illinois at Urbana-Champaign, Champaign, Illinois, United States of America, **2** Brain Imaging and Modeling Section, National Institute on Deafness and Other Communication Disorders, National Institutes of Health, Bethesda, Maryland, United States of America, **3** Otolaryngology Branch, National Institute on Deafness and Other Communication Disorders, National Institutes of Health, Bethesda, Maryland, United States of America

Abstract

We investigated auditory perception and cognitive processing in individuals with chronic tinnitus or hearing loss using functional magnetic resonance imaging (fMRI). Our participants belonged to one of three groups: bilateral hearing loss and tinnitus (TIN), bilateral hearing loss without tinnitus (HL), and normal hearing without tinnitus (NH). We employed pure tones and frequency-modulated sweeps as stimuli in two tasks: passive listening and active discrimination. All subjects had normal hearing through 2 kHz and all stimuli were low-pass filtered at 2 kHz so that all participants could hear them equally well. Performance was similar among all three groups for the discrimination task. In all participants, a distributed set of brain regions including the primary and non-primary auditory cortices showed greater response for both tasks compared to rest. Comparing the groups directly, we found decreased activation in the parietal and frontal lobes in the participants with tinnitus compared to the HL group and decreased response in the frontal lobes relative to the NH group. Additionally, the HL subjects exhibited increased response in the anterior cingulate relative to the NH group. Our results suggest that a differential engagement of a putative auditory attention and short-term memory network, comprising regions in the frontal, parietal and temporal cortices and the anterior cingulate, may represent a key difference in the neural bases of chronic tinnitus accompanied by hearing loss relative to hearing loss alone.

Editor: Ed X. Wu, The University of Hong Kong, Hong Kong

Funding: The research was supported by the National Institutes of Health-National Institute on Deafness and Other Communication Disorders Intramural Research Program and a grant from the Tinnitus Research Consortium to FTH. The funders had no role in study design, data collection and analysis, decision to publish, or preparation of the manuscript.

Competing Interests: The authors have declared that no competing interests exist.

* E-mail: husainf@illinois.edu

Introduction

Subjective tinnitus is the phantom perception of sound in the absence of an external source. The annoyance and distress associated with tinnitus range from mild to severe, with the latter type having a major impact on a person's life, making sleep difficult and intellectual work challenging [1]. The incidence of tinnitus is higher above the age of 50, consistent with the increased incidence of hearing loss with age. As per the National Center for Health Statistics survey (1999) of non-institutionalized Americans reported in [2], approximately 200 men and 100 women per 1000 persons suffer from hearing loss in the 45–64 year range and approximately 70 men and 40 women per 1000 persons suffer from tinnitus in the same 45–64 year age range. Hearing loss causes reorganization of the central auditory processing pathways and associated areas in the brain, possibly leading to tinnitus. However, not everyone with hearing loss has tinnitus and about 10% of those with tinnitus have normal hearing [2,3]. One of the challenges in studying the neural bases of chronic tinnitus is dissociating the effects and mechanisms of tinnitus from those of hearing loss alone. The nature of the interaction between hearing loss and tinnitus has long been noted. Hearing loss is the most common risk factor for developing tinnitus and the most correlated condition with tinnitus [1,4,5]. Few studies, however, have taken hearing loss into account when investigating the neural correlates of tinnitus. Most studies have either compared patients with tinnitus and hearing loss with normal hearing controls [6], compared participants with normal hearing and tinnitus with normal hearing controls [7,8,9], or used specific paradigms that allowed participants to serve as their own controls [10,11,12]. In the present study, we chose to use two control groups against which to compare the group with tinnitus and hearing loss: those with normal hearing and those with similar hearing loss. The inherent assumption was that comparing participants with tinnitus and hearing loss against participants with hearing loss alone would allow us to better identify the neural correlates of tinnitus. This, of course, may be a simplification in that it is possible that the underlying pathophysiology of tinnitus with hearing loss differs from that with tinnitus and normal hearing. Increasing evidence from brain imaging studies suggests that large-scale networks subserving attention, emotion, and cognition are affected in chronic tinnitus [10,11,12,13,14,15]. However, the engagement of these networks has been implicated indirectly rather than through explicit tasks targeting attention, cognition or emotional processing. At the same time, animal studies have noted the involvement of multimodal networks in tinnitus [16,17]. The current study was therefore designed to identify differences in the sensory and cognitive networks across chronic tinnitus and hearing loss conditions, possibly related to short-term memory and auditory processing. Short-term memory tasks have been successfully used to investigate influences of aging and hearing loss on cognitive behavior [18,19,20,21,22]. Depending on the task being used, brain imaging studies have investigated neural bases of attention, working memory, and cognitive and sensory effort in older adults with normal hearing or hearing loss. Our study was motivated in part by recent behavioral studies [23,24,25] that corroborate anecdotal evidence of the distracting effect of tinnitus on real-world tasks involving sounds. In the behavioral studies, deficits ascribed to tinnitus in cognitive and other demanding tasks typically take the form of slower responses rather than lower accuracy. This would suggest that subjects with tinnitus in our study would exhibit longer reaction time than those without tinnitus in completing an active discrimination task. Further, in the present study we account for hearing loss that often accompanies tinnitus and may contribute to the severity and annoyance of tinnitus [1,26] and may result in structural changes [27,28].

We used two tasks to investigate the neural bases of short-term memory and auditory processing in individuals with hearing loss without tinnitus, participants with hearing loss accompanied by tinnitus and normal hearing control subjects without tinnitus. Both tasks used identical non-speech stimuli; they differed only in the tasks: passive listening or active discrimination. We had previously used similar tasks and stimuli to investigate short-term memory and auditory processing in young normal-hearing adults [29]. The stimuli included pure tones and frequency-modulated sweeps that were employed in separate scanning (echo-planar imaging) runs [29]. Relative to rest, a distributed network involving the temporal, frontal and parietal cortices was preferentially activated for the discrimination task. In a recent pitch discrimination fMRI study of individuals with tinnitus [30], participants discriminated a series of tonal pips with three different frequencies. Activations in the middle frontal gyrus, putamen and left-hemispheric insula were observed in six tinnitus patients and in the right hemispheric anterior insula for the six controls in addition to auditory cortices, for the task relative to the rest. They also found the caudate nucleus, superior frontal gyrus and anterior cingulate to be more responsive in the tinnitus patients compared to the controls. The two studies [29,30] suggest that discrimination task using simple non-speech sounds is a valid method to differentiate some of the neural correlates of tinnitus from those of normal hearing or hearing loss. However, note that in the Wunderlich study, the participants in the tinnitus group had various degrees of hearing loss, ranging from none to mild, especially at higher frequencies. The small number of subjects and the lack of controls with hearing loss limit the usefulness of the study.

We wanted to test differences in behavior and neural response of those with hearing loss with and without tinnitus, for sounds they could hear and discriminate well. Both of these groups would be compared to a control group of normal hearing participants without tinnitus. We ensured that all participants could hear the sounds equally well by (a) recruiting only those with either normal hearing for octave frequencies 0.25–8 kHz (control group) or normal hearing through 2 kHz (i.e. they have bilateral high-frequency sensorineural hearing loss) and (b) creating stimuli that included frequencies only up to 2 kHz. Our prediction was that the response of a distributed set of regions in the frontal, parietal and temporal cortices would be enhanced for those with hearing loss and would be increased further for those with hearing loss and tinnitus compared to normal hearing controls during these tasks. Such increased response would be more apparent for the discrimination task relative to the passive listening task because of the greater engagement of a distributed cortical network in the former, possibly due to attentional and short-term memory processing. The prediction was based on our previous fMRI study of young normal hearing adults using similar stimuli and a discrimination task. However, because all participants could hear the sounds and if their behavior did not differ significantly, the null hypothesis would be that there would be no appreciable difference in the response of the auditory processing network between the normal hearing and hearing impaired group without tinnitus; the group with tinnitus would differ due to the additional distracting factor of chronic tinnitus.

Methods

Subjects

Three groups of participants were recruited in the study from the greater Washington, D.C. metropolitan area. All participants gave written informed consent. The National Institutes of Health/National Institute of Neurological Disorders and Stroke-National Institute on Deafness and Other Communication Disorders Institutional Review Board approved the study (protocol 06-DC-0218) and all participants were suitably compensated.

The tinnitus group (TIN) consisted of 8 male volunteers (age range = 42–64 yr, mean = 56.13 yr, SD = 7.04 yr) with bilateral, mild to moderately-severe high-frequency sensorineural hearing loss and chronic subjective tinnitus that had persisted for between 3–38 years at the time of their scan (Table 1). The tinnitus percept was most frequently described as a buzzing, ringing, hissing or a whistle sound. Others described a hum, clear tone or pulsating percept (all subjects denied changes in time with heartbeat or respiration). One subject perceived the sound of cicadas. Five subjects described more than one of the above sounds. Tinnitus severity was evaluated by the Tinnitus Handicap Inventory and all subjects were either grade 1 – slight or grade 2 – mild (range = 10–26, mean = 17.25, SD = 5.01) [31,32]. We assessed laterality of the tinnitus percept via questionnaires. We excluded potential participants if they did not have symmetrical (bilateral) hearing loss or non-lateralized tinnitus percept. Six subjects experienced their tinnitus bilaterally or in the "middle of the head." Two subjects described their tinnitus as more left lateralized but still central. Of the 28 (6 female) individuals with tinnitus screened for this study, only 8 male patients met our criteria for symmetrical high-frequency sensorineural hearing loss and chronic tinnitus. The others were not included in the study due to our stringent exclusionary criteria of the type of hearing loss, type of tinnitus, and other physical or mental health issues.

The second group (HL) (n = 7) was matched in age (age range = 31–64 yr, mean = 51.38 yr, SD = 11.45 yr), gender and hearing loss and had bilateral, mild to moderately-severe hearing loss but did not have tinnitus. The third group (NH) (n = 11) was age (age range = 32–63 yr, mean = 48.09 yr, SD = 10.42 yr) and gender-matched and had normal hearing with no tinnitus. All subjects scored in the minimal depression range on the Beck Depression Inventory (BDI-II) [33,34] (range = 0–10, mean for TIN = 1.45, mean for HL = 0.57, mean for NH = 0.75) (Table 1). After initial screening, all potential participants were evaluated by a licensed medical practitioner and were excluded if they had current, or a history of, temporomandibular joint problems, hyperacusis, Meniere's disease, benign positional vertigo or any other health issues that may have presented complications or contraindications with MRI. We explicitly excluded for hyperacusis not only because of possible noise-exposure in the MRI scanner but also because of studies showing elevated auditory activity due to this factor [35].

Table 1. Demographic and clinical characteristics of the participants in the study.

Variables	Normal Hearing N = 11	Hearing Loss N = 7	Tinnitus N = 8
Age (M/SD)	48.09/10.42	51.38/11.45	56.13/7.04
Sex N (M/F)	11/0	7/0	8/0
BDI-II (M/SD)	0.75/2.81	0.57/0.73	1.45/1.49
THI (M/SD)	n/a	n/a	17.25/5.01
Duration of tinnitus (M/SD) in years	n/a	n/a	14.43/12.56

BDI = Beck Depression Inventory, THI = Tinnitus Handicap Inventory.

Audiometric evaluation

All participants underwent full audiologic evaluation before and after the scanning session at the NIH Clinical Center. The audiologic examination, including speech recognition and pure-tone air- and bone-conduction thresholds (0.25–8 kHz), was conducted in a double-walled audiometric test suite using ER-3A transducers in accordance with American National Standards Institute standards (American National Standards Institute, S3.1-1999 American National Standard Maximum Permissible Ambient Noise Levels for Audiometric Test Rooms (Standard S3.1), New York, NY: American National Standards Institute, 2003, and S3.1-1996 American National Standard Specification for Audiometers (Standard S3.6). New York, NY: American National Standards Institute; 2004). Additional audiometric measures, including distortion product otoacoustic emissions, tympanometry, and acoustic reflex thresholds and decay, were conducted to ensure that there were no audiometric signs of conductive or retrocochlear pathology. Loudness tolerance evaluation using recorded samples of scanner noise was also conducted to ensure that each participant's loudness discomfort levels were sufficiently high to permit scanning without loudness discomfort. We excluded potential participants who exhibited symptoms of hyperacusis, either via loudness tolerance evaluation or subjective questionnaire. All participants in the NH group had pure-tone thresholds of 25 dB HL or less for all of the test frequencies. Participants in the TIN and HL groups had pure-tone thresholds of 25 dB HL or less for 0.25–2 kHz, and sensorineural hearing loss in the mild to moderately-severe range (no greater than 70 dB as defined by [36] and noted at http://www.asha.org/public/hearing/disorders/types.htm) for 3–8 kHz. There were no statistically significant differences in the pure-tone average hearing loss (across all testing frequencies) ($p = 0.89$ using Wilcoxon Rank Sum test) or at the higher frequencies (4, 6, 8 kHz) ($p = 0.69$ using Wilcoxon Rank Sum test) for the TIN and HL groups. Using the method described in [37], we calculated maximum steepness of the audiogram for the TIN and HL groups. There were no statistically significant differences in maximum steepness ($p = 0.19$ using Wilcoxon Rank Sum test) between the two groups. The hearing loss of all groups is depicted in Figure 1.

Stimuli and Tasks

Stimuli used in the study consisted of pure tones and frequency modulated sweeps. There were three pure tones: 3 low frequency tones (0.5, 0.6, 0.7 kHz) and 3 high frequency tones (1.5, 1.7, 1.9 kHz). There were two types of frequency modulated sweep stimuli: "down-up" and "up-down". The up-down stimuli consisted of a 200 ms up sweep, a 100 ms pure tone and a 200 ms down sweep. The three segments were concatenated such that each complete stimulus was continuous and the total duration was 500 ms. For both the up-down and the down-up stimuli, the 100 ms pure tone frequency was 1 kHz. There were 3 up-down stimuli with varying frequencies. The starting frequencies of the up-down stimuli were 0.65, 0.55, 0.45 kHz. The initial 200 ms up sweep always ended at 1 kHz (the frequency of the pure tone) regardless of the starting frequency. The down sweep then started at a frequency of 1 kHz and dropped in frequency to 0.65, 0.55 and 0.45 kHz to match each beginning frequency. The down-up stimuli were identical to the up-down in duration and segmentation but consisted of a concatenated down sweep, pure tone (with frequency at 1 kHz) and up sweep. There were 3 down-up stimuli with starting and ending frequencies of 2.0, 1.8, 1.6 kHz. Each stimulus-pair (either 'same' or 'different') was presented 5 times in pseudo-random order with 10 silent (rest) trials mixed amongst the listening trials. Thus, there were 30 trials with pure tones and 30 trials with the sweeps, with equal distribution of same and different trials. The tones and sweeps were generated using Audition 2.0 (Adobe Systems Inc., San Jose, CA). None of the stimuli overlapped the hearing loss range of the listeners who had normal hearing at frequencies less than 2 kHz. The sounds were further low-pass filtered with a cut-off point at 2 kHz and were normalized to have the same root-mean-square amplitude. Sounds were played at most comfortable level for the participants, during the 'silent' portion of the sparse sampling acquisition. Post-hoc measurements revealed that this was between 70–80 dB SPL.

Subjects performed (a) a passive listening task (PL) where they listened to pairs of stimuli without responding and (b) a discrimination task (DT) in which they responded whether a pair of tones or a pair of sweeps was 'same' or 'different'. Responses were collected via button-presses. Subjects performed a brief training session for 5–10 minutes to familiarize them with the tasks and stimuli. The training sounds were similar to but not identical to the stimuli used in the experiment. Subjects began the actual experiment once they achieved a threshold of 85% accuracy on the task.

Data Acquisition

Participants were scanned in a 3 Tesla GE Excite scanner using an eight-channel receive-only coil. Subjects were scanned using an Echo Planar Imaging (EPI) sparse sampling technique (shown in Figure 2) so that the stimuli were presented in silence. Three different types of stimuli were used: pure tones, frequency modulated sweeps and music samples. Thirty-two T2*-weighted axial slices ($TR = 2000$ ms, $TE = 30$ ms) were collected for each volume in an interleaved order with a 2.6 mm slice thickness, 1.2 mm slice gap, and a 2.5 mm by 2.5 mm within plane resolution (96 by 96 Matrix, 240 mm FOV). We obtained 70 image volumes for each EPI run, including 60 image volumes for the task and 10 for the resting condition. Because of the timing of

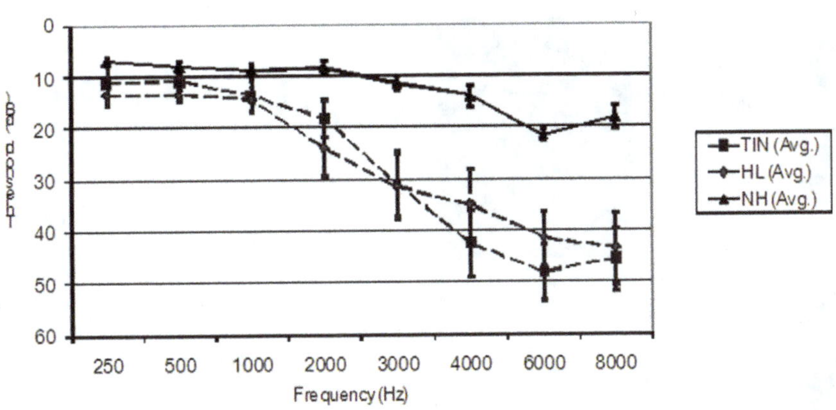

Figure 1. Average audiograms of the participants including error bars that depict standard error of the mean.

sparse sampling and BOLD delay, the image volume targeted neural activity related to the delay, the second stimulus and beginning of the response period. Subject behavior was recorded using button presses.

Data Processing

Statistical parametric software (SPM5, Wellcome Trust Centre for Neuroimaging, http://www.fil.ion.ucl.ac.uk/spm/software/spm5/) was used to analyze the data. The fMRI data were pre-processed: images were realigned, co-registered to a high resolution template, normalized to MNI space, and finally smoothed with an 8-mm full-width-half-maximum filter. The smoothed data from individual subjects was entered into a fixed-effects analysis for purposes of statistical analyses at group level. A design matrix of all three groups was defined comprising contrasts testing for significant effects of various task components from each group. The contrasts were Task (either DT or PL)>Rest or Rest>Task. Because the PL and DT tasks were in separate EPI runs, they were analyzed separately. To analyze commonalities across the two hearing loss groups (TIN, HL), we performed a conjunction analysis [38]. Voxel clusters were considered to be statistically significant if they were $p<0.05$ corrected for multiple comparisons using family-wise error (FWE) either at the voxel or cluster-level, unless otherwise stated.

Results

Behavioral Results

There were no statistically significant differences between the three groups for the discrimination task, either in accuracy or response times. Behavioral responses of two normal hearing participants were excluded in the analysis: the button responses of one were inadvertently not recorded for all trials and the other only performed at 55% accuracy. We had set the inclusion criterion at 75% accuracy. All included participants, regardless of group, performed at or near ceiling; the lowest individual score was 87% accuracy. The group scores were as follows: normal hearing (N = 9, mean = 92, standard deviation = 5.75), hearing loss (N = 7, mean = 91.8, standard deviation = 4.65), tinnitus (N = 8, mean = 91.0, standard deviation = 4.25).

fMRI Results

Passive Listening task. As shown in Figure 3 and Table 2, all three groups, on average, showed greater response of the bilateral superior temporal cortex, including regions in the superior and middle temporal gyri and superior temporal sulcus, when listening to the stimuli compared to rest. We also observed greater response of some loci in bilateral inferior and middle frontal gyri for the normal hearing control group. When we

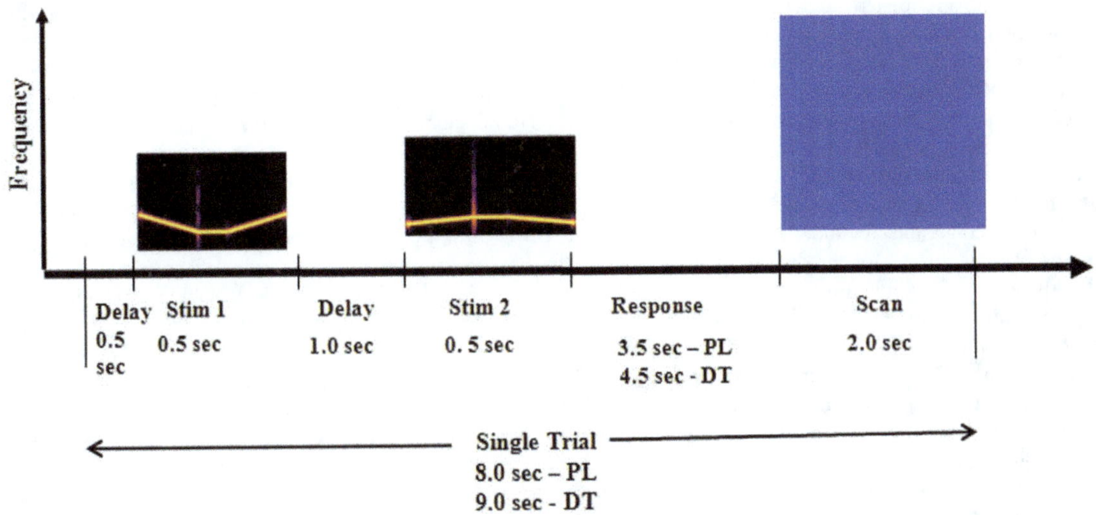

Figure 2. Timeline of a trial using sparse imaging technique. PL = passive listening, DT = discrimination task.

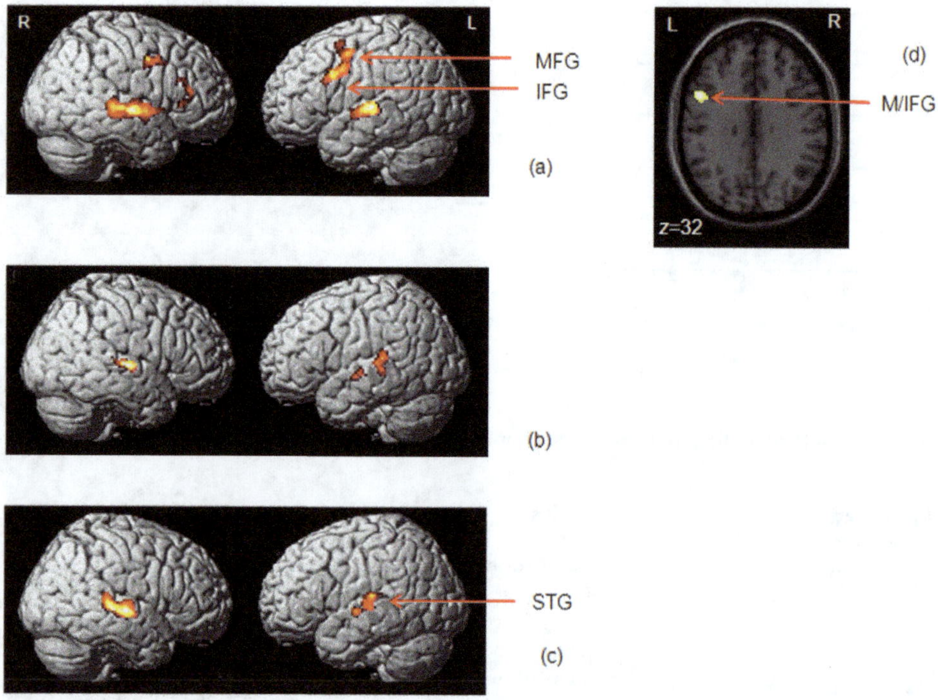

Figure 3. Statistical parametric maps of the passive listening task. Statistical parametric maps of the passive listening task (PL>Rest) rendered on a template brain for (a) normal hearing, (b) hearing loss and (c) tinnitus with hearing loss groups. Results of the NH>TIN comparison showed greater response in the left middle/inferior frontal gyri are depicted in (d). All reported clusters are $p<0.05$ FWE corrected for multiple comparisons at the voxel or cluster-level. Some clusters are highlighted in the figure - MFG: middle frontal gyrus, IFG: inferior frontal gyrus, STG: superior temporal gyrus.

performed pair-wise comparisons of the groups, the only statistically significant region of difference was in the left inferior and middle frontal gyri for the NH>TIN contrast (Figure 3D).

Discrimination task. All three groups, on average, showed greater response of the bilateral superior and middle temporal cortex when discriminating sounds compared to rest (see Figure 4 and Table 3). In addition, there was widespread activation of other regions that varied with subject group. Recall that all participants, regardless of the group, could hear the sounds and task performance across the groups was similarly at or near ceiling. On average, the normal hearing group activated the bilateral middle frontal gyrus, inferior parietal lobule, thalamus and putamen, central posterior cingulate, left cerebellum, and hippocampus and right superior frontal gyrus and anterior cingulate to a greater extent for the discrimination task relative to test. The HL group preferentially activated most of the same regions as the NH group, but to a greater extent, and additionally activated the left postcentral gyrus, right cerebellum and right caudate. The TIN group, on average, did not show wide-spread response in the frontal and parietal cortices for the discrimination task compared to rest, although, they exhibited activations in the anterior cingulate and dorsomedial frontal gyrus and in the bilateral precentral and postcentral gyri. We also conducted Rest>DT comparisons. If the Rest>DT contrast yielded extensive clusters of activation, a likely interpretation would be that there is higher activity in the rest condition rather than the task conditionfor those regions. Melcher et al. [9] have noted greater activity in the inferior colliculus in participants with tinnitus relative to those without tinnitus, suggesting increased baseline activity due to tinnitus. However, except for one suprathreshold cluster for the HL group in the left parahippocampal gyrus (MNI coordinates: −28, −44, −12), we did not find any activation clusters for the other groups for Rest>DT contrast. To investigate the effect of hearing loss and tinnitus we performed group-wise comparisons, the results of which are described next.

Effect of Hearing Loss. Conjunction analysis, which was used to identify commonalities between HL and TIN groups, revealed widespread activations in the bilateral superior temporal cortex and in the central regions of anterior cingulate and in the medial frontal gyri (Figure 5A, left and right, respectively).

We next determined the effect of hearing loss alone without the confounding factor of tinnitus, by comparing HL and NH groups (Table 4). The following regions showed increased response for the HL group compared to the NH control group during discrimination: bilateral superior temporal gyrus, right postcentral gyrus, right inferior parietal lobule, left precentral gyrus, left superior frontal gyrus and left transverse temporal gyrus (Figure 5B, left) and central dorsomedial frontal gyrus, central anterior cingulate (Figure 5B, right). For the reverse contrast of NH>HL, the suprathreshold voxel clusters were in the left posterior cingulate (Figure 5C, right), left inferior parietal lobule, including the supramarginal gyrus (Figure 5C, left) and the left parahippocampal gyrus (Figure 5C, center).

Effect of Tinnitus. We contrasted the activation patterns for the TIN group separately against the NH and HL groups (Figure 6, Table 4). We observed increased response for the TIN group relative to the NH group in left transverse and superior temporal gyri, right superior frontal gyrus, and right superior and middle temporal gyri (Figure 6A). We did not find any suprathreshold clusters of voxels for the TIN>HL contrast. We observed an extensive network of regions showing decreased response for the

Table 2. Local maxima for the individual groups and the inter-group contrasts for the passive listening task compared to rest.

Contrast	MNI coordinates			Z score	Cluster size	Gyrus(Brodmann Area)
	x	*y*	*z*			
NH group PL>Rest	−50	−20	2	6.09 *#	597	L superior temporal gyrus (21/22)
	66	−16	−2	5.69*#	888	R superior and middle temporal gyri, superior temporal sulcus (21/22)
	−50	10	32	4.87*#	634	L inferior and middle frontal gyri (44/6)
	40	26	4	4.08*	150	R inferior and middle frontal gyri (45/46)
	44	0	40	3.84*	173	R middle frontal gyrus (9)
HL group PL>Rest	−46	−32	12	5.62*#	455	L transverse and superior temporal gyri, superior temporal sulcus (41/42/22)
	46	−20	2	4.41*	293	R superior temporal gyrus (22)
TIN group PL>Rest	60	−28	2	5.13*#	623	R superior and middle temporal gyri, superior temporal sulcus (42/22/21)
	−52	−12	−2	4.23*	358	L superior and middle temporal gyrus, superior temporal sulcus (42/22/21)
NH>TIN	−50	10	32	4.17*	300	L inferior and middle frontal gyri (44,6,9)

All reported clusters are p<0.05 FWE corrected for multiple comparisons at the voxel (indicated by * next to the Z-score) or cluster-level (indicated by #), cluster extent is 50 voxels.

TIN group in the HL>TIN contrast in the left superior and middle temporal gyri, bilateral inferior frontal gyri, left inferior parietal lobule, left superior and middle frontal gyri and right cerebellum (Figure 6B). We did not find any suprathreshold clusters of voxels for the NH>TIN contrast, although there was a trend ($p = 0.16$ FWE corrected) at right superior frontal gyrus.

Discussion

Our study employed passive listening and active discrimination tasks to investigate differences in the neural bases of hearing loss and chronic tinnitus. We found bilateral superior temporal cortex response for passive listening of sounds across all three groups (hearing loss, hearing loss with tinnitus, and normal hearing without tinnitus). There were no regions of significant difference for the passive listening task between the three groups, except participants in the NH group activated the left inferior/middle frontal gyrus to a greater extent relative to those in the hearing loss groups with and without tinnitus (TIN and HL). The patterns of response across the three groups varied more for the discrimination task compared to the passive listening task. In the discrimination task compared to rest, we found an elevated response in the frontal and parietal cortices in addition to the temporal cortex for the normal hearing and hearing impaired without tinnitus participants. This is not surprising because the discrimination task is a short-term memory task. The activation patterns seen in the normal hearing control group are similar to those seen in our previous study of young normal hearing adults [29]. However, we observed an increased response of the frontal and parietal cortices for the HL group relative to the NH and TIN groups. The TIN group demonstrated heightened response in bilateral temporal and left frontal cortices when compared with the NH group and decreased response in the temporal, frontal and parietal cortices with respect to the HL group.

One of the surprising results of our study was that high-frequency hearing loss affected perception and discrimination of low-frequency sounds, not in terms of behavior, but in terms of the response of the auditory, frontal and parietal cortices. Because the sounds were low-pass filtered at 2 kHz to be within the normal hearing range of all participants, the null hypothesis was that there would be no difference in the response of brain for the participants regardless of their hearing status (disregarding tinnitus). This was mostly true for the passive listening task; however, we observed differential involvement of a distributed set of brain regions in the three groups for the discrimination task, varying both on hearing and tinnitus status.

The distributed set of regions (prefrontal cortex, inferior parietal cortex, anterior cingular cortex) highlighted in our results have been proposed previously to play an important role in auditory attention and working memory. Although our study did not employ tasks that require attention explicitly, the short-term memory task uses attention implicitly. Studies investigating attention in the auditory modality have reported on the involvement of the following cortical and subcortical structures: prefrontal cortex, parietal cortex, superior temporal gyrus, temporoparietal junction, anterior cingulate gyrus, basal ganglia, thalamus and inferior colliculus (for reviews, see [39,40,41,42,43]). Whereas the putative attention and working memory network can be large and distributed [43,44], for the purposes of the present study and to simplify terminology, we will use the term auditory attention and short-term memory (AASM) network and restrict its definition to include frontal cortex, parietal cortex, superior temporal gyrus and anterior cingulate cortex.

Cognitive scientists and neuroscientists have suggested that cognitive function may be affected by sensory difficulties in older adults [45]. The incoming signal, the receiver (ear, cochlea) and the perception/cognition system may all contribute to imperfect cognitive performance. Several cognitive theories have been forwarded that relate the interaction of these agencies. One such theory, the 'effortfulness hypothesis' [46], holds that either with degraded sensory abilities [47] or in noisy conditions [48] individuals tend to increase effort to achieve successful perception. Increased effort in initial stages of processing drains cognitive resources from speech processing and other higher-level cognitive processes [45,49,50]. Treisman's 'levels of analysis' model of

Table 3. Local maxima for the individual groups (cluster extent = 50 voxels) for the discrimination task compared to rest.

Contrast	MNI coordinates			Z score	Cluster size	Gyrus (Brodmann Area)
	x	*y*	*z*			
NH group DT>Rest	58	−12	2	Inf*#	681	R superior and middle temporal gyrus (22,21)
	−44	−42	24	8.62*#	898	L transverse and superior temporal gyrus, inferior parietal lobule (42,22,40)
	54	4	−8	7.6*#	249	R superior and middle temporal gyrus (22,21)
	−40	−20	−12	6.5*#	112	L hippocampus
	12	−10	10	6.44*#	528	R thalamus, putamen
	−52	2	30	6.39*#	123	L inferior and middle frontal gyrus (44, 6)
	−52	−20	2	6.34*#	274	L superior and middle temporal gyrus (22,21)
	36	−48	38	6.25*#	128	L inferior parietal lobule (40)
	0	−34	26	6.16*#	110	posterior cingulate (23)
	−34	−10	62	6.12*#	86	L precentral gyrus, middle frontal gyrus (4,6)
	−26	−66	−36	5.99*#	51	L cerebellum
	−22	14	−2	5.82*#	88	L putamen
	48	−54	52	5.79*#	92	R inferior parietal lobule (40)
	8	26	40	5.46*#	54	R anterior cingulate, dorsomedial frontal gyrus (32, 8)
	36	44	26	5.32*#	60	R middle and superior frontal gyrus (10)
	44	−24	58	5.23*#	36	L thalamus, putamen
HL group DT>Rest	60	−28	8	Inf*#	2804	R superior temporal gyrus (42, 22)
	−54	−44	22	Inf*#	4318	L postcentral gyrus, inferior parietal lobule (1, 2, 3, 40)
	0	10	58	Inf	1039	Dorsomedial frontal gyrus, anterior cingulate (6, 8, 32)
	−36	50	10	6.89*#	232	L middle frontal gyrus (10,44)
	−54	−40	−4	6.5*#	129	L superior and middle temporal gyrus (22, 21)
	2	−62	−10	6.5*#	98	R cerebellum
	34	52	14	6.49*#	345	R middle and inferior frontal gyrus (10, 46)
	8	−76	−24	6.15*#	104	R cerebellum
	24	14	0	6.11*#	389	R putamen
	16	−2	10	6.11*#	129	R putamen, caudate
	−6	34	28	5.97*#	54	L anterior cingulate, dorsomedial frontal gyrus (32, 9)
	−18	−58	−32	5.91*#	65	L cerebellum
	54	4	36	5.87*#	56	R inferior frontal gyrus (44)
	−10	−20	4	5.86*#	76	L thalamus
	−30	−60	46	5.4*#	56	L inferior parietal lobule (40)
TIN group DT>Rest	−58	−22	4	Inf*#	2372	L superior temporal gyrus (22)
	54	−26	10	Inf*#	2806	R superior temporal gyrus (42, 22)
	36	−22	70	Inf*#	260	R precentral gyrus, superior frontal gyrus (4, 6)
	−2	12	44	6.69*#	846	L dorsomedial frontal gyrus, anterior cingulate (6, 32)
	−22	6	6	6*#	356	L putamen
	−40	−14	64	5.97*#	133	Left precentral and postcentral gyri (4, 1, 2, 3)
	60	4	16	5.86*#	91	R inferior frontal gyrus (44, 6)
	34	−52	64	5.74*#	56	R postcentral gyrus, superior parietal lobule (5, 7)
	24	6	4	5.63*#	164	R putamen
	56	−30	44	5.55*#	57	R postcentral gyrus (1, 2, 3)
	−38	−58	56	5.38*#	56	L inferior and superior parietal lobule (40, 5, 7)

All reported clusters are p≤0.05 FWE corrected for multiple comparisons at the voxel (indicated by * next to the Z-score) or cluster-level (indicated by #).

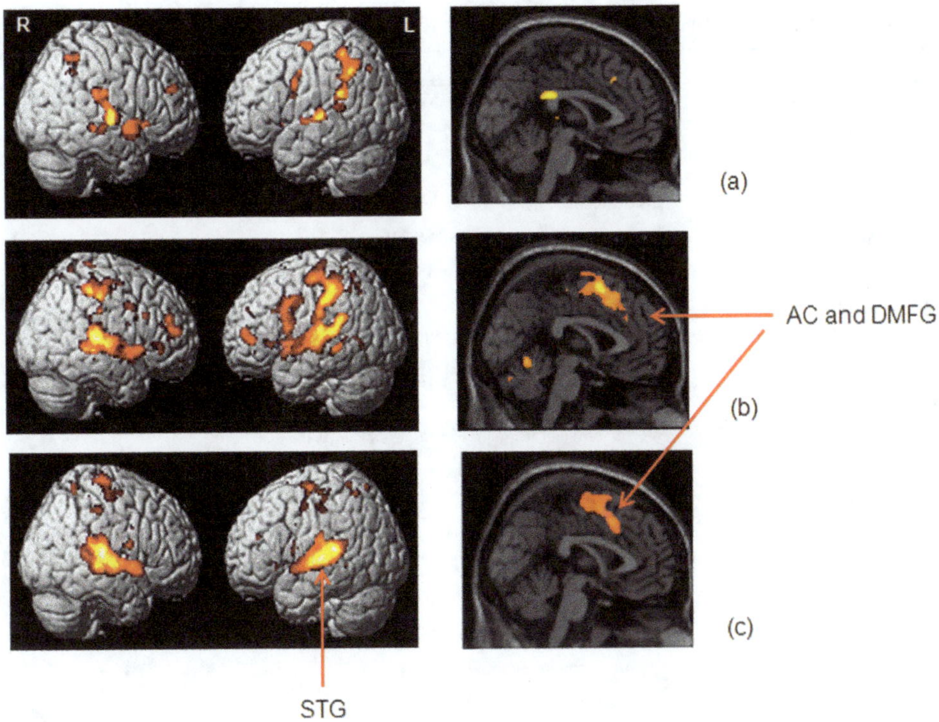

Figure 4. Statistical parametric maps of the discrimination task. Statistical parametric maps of the discrimination task (DT>Rest) rendered on a template brain for (a) normal hearing, (b) hearing loss and (c) tinnitus with hearing loss groups are shown on the left. The sagittal sections shown are located at $x = 0$ for all groups are shown on the right. All reported clusters are $p<0.05$ FWE corrected for multiple comparisons at the voxel or cluster-level. Some clusters are highlighted in the figure - AC: anterior cingulate, DMFG: dorsomedial frontal gyrus, STG: superior temporal gyrus.

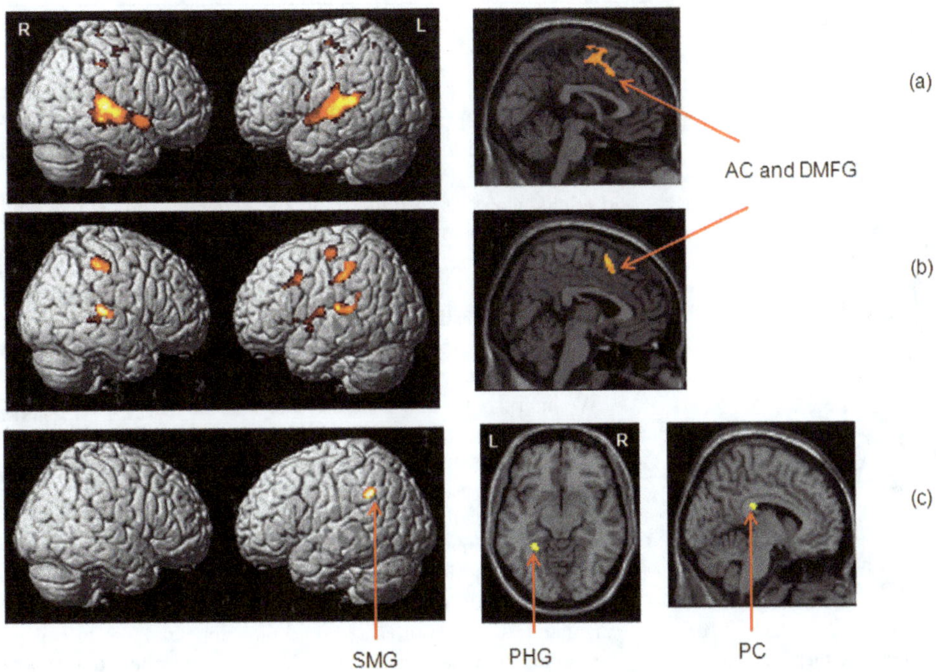

Figure 5. Effect of hearing loss. Statistical parametric maps for (a) conjunction of HL and TIN rendered on a template brain and sagittal slice at $x = 0$, (b) contrast HL>NH rendered on a template brain and sagittal slice at $x = 4$, and (c) contrast NH>HL rendered on a template brain, axial slice at $z = -12$, and sagittal slice at $x = -6$. All reported clusters are $p<0.05$ FWE corrected for multiple comparisons at the voxel or cluster-level. Some clusters are highlighted in the figure - AC: anterior cingulate, DMFG: dorsomedial frontal gyrus, SMG: supramarginal gyrus, PHG: parahippocampal gyrus, PC: posterior cingulate.

Table 4. Local maxima for the inter-group contrasts (cluster extent = 20 voxels) for the discrimination task compared to rest.

Contrast	MNI coordinates			Z score	Cluster size	Gyrus (Brodmann Area)
	x	*y*	*z*			
HL>NH	58	−26	48	6.37*#	203	R postcentral gyrus (1,2)
	60	−28	8	5.66*#	286	R superior temporal gyrus (42, 22)
	−56	−30	38	5.64*#	276	R postcentral gyrus, inferior parietal lobule (1, 2, 40)
	−46	−18	60	5.15#	106	L precentral gyrus (4)
	−44	−28	12	5.02*#	312	L transverse and superior temporal gyrus (42, 22)
	−32	−26	72	4.79#	29	L superior frontal gyrus (6)
	−50	−22	−4	4.75#	68	L superior and middle temporal gyri (21)
	−2	10	56	4.61*#	203	R dorsomedial frontal gyrus, anterior cingulate (8, 6,32)
NH>HL	−28	−44	−12	4.7#	54	L parahippocampal gyrus (37, 36)
	−4	−28	24	4.69#	113	L posterior cingulate (23)
	−52	−48	36	4.67#	86	L inferior parietal lobule, supramarginal gyrus (40)
HL>TIN	−54	−44	22	6.07#	88	L superior temporal gyrus (42, 22)
	−36	52	10	5.03#	163	L superior and middle frontal gyri (10)
	54	22	26	4.71#	73	R inferior frontal gyrus (44, 46)
	−50	−34	42	4.52#	152	L inferior parietal lobule (40)
	−50	10	36	4.2*	150	L inferior frontal gyrus (44)
	6	−78	−24	4.14*	182	R cerebellum
	−42	−68	4	4.09*	164	L middle temporal gyrus (22, 37)
TIN>HL	No significant differences					
TIN>NH	−50	−38	8	5.62*#	979	L transverse and superior temporal gyrus (41, 42, 22)
	54	−26	8	5.26*#	451	R superior and middle temporal gyrus (42, 22, 21)
	36	−22	70	5.04#	34	R superior frontal gyrus (6)
NH>TIN	No significant differences					

All reported clusters are $p \leq 0.05$ FWE corrected for multiple comparisons at the voxel (indicated by * next to the Z-score) or cluster-level (indicated by #).

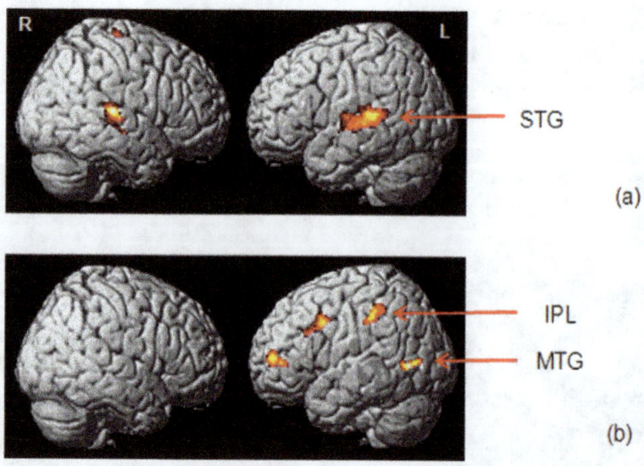

Figure 6. Effect of tinnitus. Statistical parametric maps rendered on a template brain for the contrasts (a) TIN>NH and (b) HL>TIN, showing increased and decreased response, respectively, due to tinnitus. The contrasts NH>TIN and TIN>HL did not result in any suprathreshold voxels. All reported clusters are $p<0.05$ FWE corrected for multiple comparisons at the voxel or cluster-level. Some clusters are highlighted in the figure – STG: superior temporal gyrus, IPL: inferior parietal lobule, MTG: middle temporal gyrus.

attention [51,52] provides a framework for investigating bottom-up auditory and top-down cognitive interactions [53] due to both hearing loss and tinnitus. Using such a framework to study hearing in adults allows us to understand the dynamic, competitive, and 'mutually compensatory' activity [53] between auditory and cognitive factors, and where attentional resources may be allocated. Attentional resources apply to working memory [54] by limiting processing of unattended inputs and facilitating that of attended inputs [55] and may be used to index effort due to hearing loss or tinnitus.

We interpret the differential response of the AASM network as follows. The hearing loss group likely engages attentional resources to a greater extent compared to normal hearing participants in order to compensate for their hearing impairment. The hearing loss group activates superior temporal, superior frontal, inferior parietal, and anterior cingular cortices significantly more than the normal hearing group (Table 4). Note that normal hearing participants exhibited marginal involvement of the anterior cingulate (just above threshold) and they appeared also to engage the frontal and parietal cortices (Table 3). Further, our results suggest that those who, in addition to having hearing loss, perceive tinnitus use their attentional resources in a different manner. We speculate that attention needs to be diverted to a phantom sound while at the same time actively processing external, relevant stimuli. In order to attend to external stimuli, subjects with tinnitus (similar to other groups) activated superior and middle temporal cortex and anterior cingulate to a greater extent for the discrimination task when contrasted to rest. However, compared to the hearing loss group, there was less widespread response of the superior and middle frontal gyri and inferior parietal cortices by the tinnitus group for the discrimination task relative to rest (Table 4). This implies that the compensatory mechanisms differ for tinnitus and hearing loss and may result in differing functional neural response. Nevertheless, studies explicitly targeting the attentional network in the two hearing loss groups, with and without tinnitus, are needed to confirm the role of the AASM in hearing loss and chronic tinnitus.

The role of the attentional network in mediating chronic tinnitus has been inferred from a number of whole-brain imaging studies. Use of lidocaine allowed [13] to temporarily suppress tinnitus in their participants; subtracting the tinnitus-suppressed blood flow pattern from that during the tinnitus perception state led to the visualization of a broad temporal-parietal network possibly related to attention and a paralimbic network possibly related to emotion. By employing aversive stimuli to simulate tinnitus-like conditions in normal hearing volunteers without tinnitus, [56] also found dorsolateral prefrontal and paralimbic structures to be responsive to the aversive sounds. Mirz et al. contrasted tinnitus perception with tinnitus suppression to identify a frontal-temporal network as associated with chronic tinnitus sensation [11]. All these studies found auditory and attention processing regions in the cortex to be involved in mediating tinnitus perception. However, few imaging studies have investigated involvement of the attentional network using behavioral tasks.

Neurophysiological studies employing electroencephalography (EEG) have also implicated the involvement of the attentional network in tinnitus perception; however, for the most part they have not taken into account the effect of hearing loss and have reported disparate findings. Jacobson and colleagues [6] observed that an electrophysiological index of early selective auditory attention ('negative difference wave') was greater and the N100 component occurred later in tinnitus patients relative to controls, suggesting there are differences in early selective attention between patients with bothersome tinnitus and controls. The negative difference wave was obtained by subtracting the event-related potential (ERP) component of an ignore-frequent-stimulus from the ERP component of an attend-frequent-stimulus. The participants in the study had high-frequency hearing loss (not affecting thresholds at 0.5 and 1 kHz) whereas the controls had normal hearing. A later study by [57] however, did not find any group differences in latency of N100 across passive and selective listening conditions. In a recent event-related potentials study [58], high distress related to tinnitus was associated with smaller changes in the event-related potentials between attended and unattended auditory task conditions. Both controls and those with mild tinnitus exhibited greater changes in N100 amplitude and phase locking between the attended and unattended task conditions. Tinnitus patients may have had some high-frequency hearing loss; the criterion for inclusion was normal hearing up to 2 kHz. Although our results suggest differential involvement of the attentional network, the study was not explicitly designed to test attentional load. There remains a need to conduct a brain imaging study explicitly investigating the role of the attentional network in tinnitus perception and delineate it from the response of the attentional network in hearing loss alone.

Although we found brain activation pattern differences between the groups, we did not find any statistically significant behavioral differences. Behavioral studies have noted attentional deficits in selective and divided attention in chronic tinnitus sufferers, specifically in the form of slower response times. In one such study [25], investigators found slower reaction times in individuals with severe tinnitus relative to controls in visual Stroop tasks with color and word naming components and in a demanding dual task involving word reading or category naming. Dornhoffer et al. [23] found no significant differences between individuals with tinnitus and controls in terms of arousal to a repetitive sensory stimulation as measured by a brainstem-thalamus P50 potential or by habituation as measured by the ability to suppress a second stimulus. They did, however, find statistically significant slower reaction times in the tinnitus group compared to the control group. This is in contrast to our study, where we found cortical-level activation differences between tinnitus and non-tinnitus groups but no reaction-time differences at the behavioral level. Hallam et al. [24] have posited that tinnitus impairs cognitive efficiency because of the self-reported concentration problems by tinnitus sufferers. In their study, Hallam et al. [24] tested tinnitus and non-tinnitus sufferers on five cognitive tasks that probed sustained attention, reaction time, verbal fluency and immediate and delayed memory. The tinnitus group was slower than the hearing-impaired and normal hearing control groups in reaction time tasks, but had similar behavior on the verbal fluency task as the hearing impaired group, and both groups performed worse than the normal hearing group. The other tasks showed similar performances between the groups. Hallam et al. interpreted these results as suggesting that 'cognitive inefficiency in tinnitus participants is related to the control of attentional processes' (page 218, [24]). With regards to the present study, it is possible that the discrimination task used did not engage the attentional system to the extent that resulted in differences in behavior. Nevertheless, even without overt behavioral differences our results showed that there were differences in the attentional network among the three groups for the same task.

We compared TIN and HL groups in order to understand better the neural correlates of tinnitus, however, the interaction between hearing loss and tinnitus may not be linear. The TIN and HL comparison gave us greater understanding of the brain regions most affected by hearing loss and those that may be most influenced by tinnitus, within the context of simple listening tasks. The relation between hearing loss and tinnitus is complex and includes other cortical and subcortical networks such as those subserving emotion or somatosensory processing [14,17]. Whereas peripheral hearing loss may be the most prominent trigger for tinnitus, pathophysiology resulting in tinnitus may be quite different than in hearing loss without tinnitus [59,60]. Further, the compensatory effects in the two conditions (hearing loss with tinnitus and hearing loss without tinnitus) may be different and not necessarily become evident by direct comparisons. In order to control for some aspects of hearing loss, we carefully matched the hearing loss profiles for the HL and TIN groups. However, it is possible that other peripheral hearing factors such as cochlear dead regions, differences in hearing loss slopes, differences in etiology of hearing loss between the two groups may be responsible for some of the variations seen in the fMRI results. As is true of almost any patient population and particularly so of tinnitus, the tinnitus patient population is heterogeneous [4]. The type of tinnitus, laterality, duration of tinnitus, pitch and loudness of the percept, presence of hyperacusis, concomitant disorders such as depression and anxiety may influence the neural correlates of tinnitus.

We collected structural MR and diffusion tensor imaging (DTI) data on the same group of participants in the current study [27]. We observed that the hearing loss group without tinnitus had the most profound changes in both white and gray matter relative to the other groups, those with normal hearing and those with hearing loss accompanied by tinnitus. This is in contrast to our fMRI findings that showed large scale changes in both the tinnitus and hearing loss without tinnitus groups. The gray matter decreases seen in the HL group relative to TIN and NH groups were in the anterior cingulate, putamen and the middle frontal gyrus. These changes are in the same regions as the reductions seen in the hearing loss group and the tinnitus group for the discrimination task compared to rest contrast in the fMRI study. Impaired sustained attention may have an impact on gray matter, as has been observed in studies of schizophrenia [61]. This suggests that functional compensation due to sensory deprivation may result in long-term structural changes. There was no significant alteration of the gray or white matter in the TIN group compared to the NH group.

We chose to perform a fixed-effects analysis because of the limited number of participants in our study and additionally, the patients belonged to a subset (bilateral hearing loss with mild tinnitus) of a complex heterogeneous population. Fixed-effects analysis also lends itself to conjunction analysis [38] as we have demonstrated in Figure 5. Conjunction analysis allows us to identify common activation patterns across groups. In the study, we used conjunction analysis to characterize shared neural correlates of the two hearing loss groups. Regardless of the analytical method, generalization of the study results to the larger patient group of those with tinnitus is limited beyond a systems-level interpretation. For instance, individuals with unilateral tinnitus and normal hearing may exhibit different responses compared to the patients in the present study, at a lower sensory or subcortical level, although they may exhibit commonalities at a higher, non-sensory level. It is also likely that those with severe tinnitus may exhibit different responses of the AASM network compared to the participants with mild tinnitus in our study. Meta-analysis of a series of brain imaging studies employing short-term working memory tasks with differing attentional demands in individuals with different types of tinnitus may allow us to draw more robust conclusions about the role of the attentional network in hearing loss or tinnitus.

In conclusion, our study suggests the differential involvement of a putative AASM network in hearing loss with and without tinnitus. This network consisted of regions in the frontal, parietal and temporal cortices and the anterior cingulate. In participants with hearing loss without tinnitus, the attentional network response was enhanced relative to normal hearing controls. In individuals with tinnitus and hearing loss, the response of some nodes of the attentional network was diminished with respect to hearing loss only group, whereas response of other nodes was enhanced. This suggests a complex role for the attentional network in those with chronic tinnitus and studies are needed that will elaborate on the functioning of this network.

Acknowledgments

We are grateful to Dr. Allen Braun of the Language Section, NIDCD, NIH, for his assistance with patient evaluation.

Author Contributions

Conceived and designed the experiments: FTH NMP BH. Performed the experiments: FTH NMP JFS HJK SR CZ CB. Analyzed the data: FTH NMP JFS. Wrote the paper: FTH NMP BH. Screening and detailed audiological testing: CZ CB. Otolaryngological consulting and screening: HJK. Medical, general health consulting, testing, and screening: SR.

References

1. Davis A, Rafaie EA (2000) Epidemiology of tinnitus. In: Tyler RS, ed. Tinnitus Handbook. San Diego, CA: Singular.
2. Lockwood AH, Salvi RJ, Burkard RF (2002) Tinnitus. N Engl J Med 347: 904–910.
3. Vernon JA, ed. (1997) Tinnitus: treatment and relief. Boston, MA: Allyn and Bacon.
4. Moller AR (2007) Tinnitus: presence and future. Prog Brain Res 166: 3–16.
5. Sindhusake D, Golding M, Newall P, Rubin G, Jakobsen K, et al. (2003) Risk factors for tinnitus in a population of older adults: the blue mountains hearing study. Ear Hear 24: 501–507.
6. Jacobson GP, Calder JA, Newman CW, Peterson EL, Wharton JA, et al. (1996) Electrophysiological indices of selective auditory attention in subjects with and without tinnitus. Hear Res 97: 66–74.
7. Landgrebe M, Langguth B, Rosengarth K, Braun S, Koch A, et al. (2009) Structural brain changes in tinnitus: grey matter decrease in auditory and non-auditory brain areas. Neuroimage 46: 213–218.
8. Muhlau M, Rauschecker JP, Oestreicher E, Gaser C, Rottinger M, et al. (2006) Structural brain changes in tinnitus. Cereb Cortex 16: 1283–1288.
9. Melcher JR, Sigalovsky IS, Guinan JJ, Jr., Levine RA (2000) Lateralized tinnitus studied with functional magnetic resonance imaging: abnormal inferior colliculus activation. J Neurophysiol 83: 1058–1072.
10. Lockwood AH, Salvi RJ, Coad ML, Towsley ML, Wack DS, et al. (1998) The functional neuroanatomy of tinnitus: evidence for limbic system links and neural plasticity. Neurology 50: 114–120.
11. Mirz F, Gjedde A, Ishizu K, Pedersen CB (2000) Cortical networks subserving the perception of tinnitus–a PET study. Acta Otolaryngol Suppl 543: 241–243.
12. Mirz F, Pedersen B, Ishizu K, Johannsen P, Ovesen T, et al. (1999) Positron emission tomography of cortical centers of tinnitus. Hear Res 134: 133–144.
13. Andersson G, Lyttkens L, Hirvela C, Furmark T, Tillfors M, et al. (2000) Regional cerebral blood flow during tinnitus: a PET case study with lidocaine and auditory stimulation. Acta Otolaryngol 120: 967–972.
14. Cacace AT (2003) Expanding the biological basis of tinnitus: crossmodal origins and the role of neuroplasticity. Hear Res 175: 112–132.
15. Giraud AL, Chery-Croze S, Fischer G, Fischer C, Vighetto A, et al. (1999) A selective imaging of tinnitus. Neuroreport 10: 1–5.
16. Kaltenbach JA (2006) The dorsal cochlear nucleus as a participant in the auditory, attentional and emotional components of tinnitus. Hear Res 216–217: 224–234.
17. Bauer CA (2004) Mechanisms of tinnitus generation. Curr Opin Otolaryngol Head Neck Surg 12: 413–417.
18. Tun PA, McCoy S, Wingfield A (2009) Aging, hearing acuity, and the attentional costs of effortful listening. Psychol Aging 24: 761–766.
19. Parbery-Clark A, Strait DL, Anderson S, Hittner E, Kraus N (2011) Musical experience and the aging auditory system: implications for cognitive abilities and hearing speech in noise. PLoS One 6: e18082.
20. Stewart R, Wingfield A (2009) Hearing loss and cognitive effort in older adults' report accuracy for verbal materials. J Am Acad Audiol 20: 147–154.
21. Craik FI, Byrd M (1982) Aging and cognitive deficits: the role of attentional resources. In: Craik FI, Trehub S, eds. Aging and Cognitive Processes. New York, NY: Plenum. pp 191–211.
22. Salthouse TA (1994) The aging of working memory. Neuropsychology 8: 535–543.
23. Dornhoffer J, Danner C, Mennemeier M, Blake D, Garcia-Rill E (2006) Arousal and attention deficits in patients with tinnitus. Int Tinnitus J 12: 9–16.
24. Hallam RS, McKenna L, Shurlock L (2004) Tinnitus impairs cognitive efficiency. Int J Audiol 43: 218–226.
25. Stevens C, Walker G, Boyer M, Gallagher M (2007) Severe tinnitus and its effect on selective and divided attention. Int J Audiol 46: 208–216.
26. Brown SC (1990) Older Americans and tinnitus: A demographic study and chartbook. In: Johnson RC, Hotto SA, eds. GRI monograph series A, No 2: Gallaudet Research Institute, Gallaudet University.
27. Husain FT, Medina RE, Davis CW, Szymko-Bennett Y, Simonyan K, et al. (2011) Neuroanatomical changes due to hearing loss and chronic tinnitus: a combined VBM and DTI study. Brain Res 1369: 74–88.
28. Wong PC, Ettlinger M, Sheppard JP, Gunasekera GM, Dhar S (2010) Neuroanatomical characteristics and speech perception in noise in older adults. Ear Hear 31: 471–479.
29. Husain FT, Fromm SJ, Pursley RH, Hosey LA, Braun AR, et al. (2006) Neural bases of categorization of simple speech and nonspeech sounds. Hum Brain Mapp 27: 636–651.
30. Wunderlich AP, Schonfeldt-Lecuona C, Wolf RC, Dorn K, Bachor E, et al. (2009) Cortical Activation during a Pitch Discrimination Task in Tinnitus Patients and Controls - An fMRI Study. Audiol Neurootol 15: 137–148.
31. McCombe A, Baguley D, Coles R, McKenna L, McKinney C, et al. (2001) Guidelines for the grading of tinnitus severity: the results of a working group commissioned by the British Association of Otolaryngologists, Head and Neck Surgeons, 1999. Clin Otolaryngol Allied Sci 26: 388–393.
32. Newman CW, Jacobson GP, Spitzer JB (1996) Development of the Tinnitus Handicap Inventory. Arch Otolaryngol Head Neck Surg 122: 143–148.

33. Beck AT, Steer RA (1984) Internal consistencies of the original and revised Beck Depression Inventory. J Clin Psychol 40: 1365–1367.
34. Steer RA, Clark DA, Beck AT, Ranieri WF (1999) Common and specific dimensions of self-reported anxiety and depression: the BDI-II versus the BDI-IA. Behav Res Ther 37: 183–190.
35. Gu JW, Halpin CF, Nam EC, Levine RA, Melcher JR (2010) Tinnitus, diminished sound-level tolerance, and elevated auditory activity in humans with clinically normal hearing sensitivity. J Neurophysiol 104: 3361–3370.
36. Clark JG (1981) Uses and abuses of hearing loss classification. ASHA 23: 493–500.
37. Konig O, Schaette R, Kempter R, Gross M (2006) Course of hearing loss and occurrence of tinnitus. Hear Res 221: 59–64.
38. Friston KJ, Holmes AP, Price CJ, Buchel C, Worsley KJ (1999) Multisubject fMRI studies and conjunction analyses. Neuroimage 10: 385–396.
39. Hugdahl K, Westerhausen R, Alho K, Medvedev S, Laine M, et al. (2009) Attention and cognitive control: unfolding the dichotic listening story. Scand J Psychol 50: 11–22.
40. Janata P (2005) Brain networks that track musical structure. Ann N Y Acad Sci 1060: 111–124.
41. Palmer AR, Hall DA, Sumner C, Barrett DJ, Jones S, et al. (2007) Some investigations into non-passive listening. Hear Res 229: 148–157.
42. Shinn-Cunningham BG, Best V (2008) Selective attention in normal and impaired hearing. Trends Amplif 12: 283–299.
43. Fritz JB, Elhilali M, David SV, Shamma SA (2007) Auditory attention–focusing the searchlight on sound. Curr Opin Neurobiol 17: 437–455.
44. Deco G, Corbetta M (2011) The Dynamical Balance of the Brain at Rest. Neuroscientist. In press.
45. Lindenberger U, Baltes PB (1994) Sensory functioning and intelligence in old age: a strong connection. Psychol Aging 9: 339–355.
46. Rabbitt PM (1968) Channel-capacity, intelligibility and immediate memory. Q J Exp Psychol 20: 241–248.
47. McCoy SL, Tun PA, Cox LC, Colangelo M, Stewart RA, et al. (2005) Hearing loss and perceptual effort: downstream effects on older adults' memory for speech. Q J Exp Psychol A 58: 22–33.
48. Gao X, Stine-Morrow EA, Noh SR, Eskew RT, Jr. (2010) Visual noise disrupts conceptual integration in reading. Psychon Bull Rev 18: 83–88.
49. Li KZ, Lindenberger U (2002) Relations between aging sensory/sensorimotor and cognitive functions. Neurosci Biobehav Rev 26: 777–783.
50. Pichora-Fuller MK, Souza PE (2003) Effects of aging on auditory processing of speech. Int J Audiol 42 Suppl 2: 2S11–16.
51. Treisman AM (1964) Selective Attention in Man. Br Med Bull 20: 12–16.
52. Treisman AM (1969) Strategies and models of selective attention. Psychol Rev 76: 282–299.
53. Craik FI (2007) The role of cognition in age-related hearing loss. J Am Acad Audiol 18: 539–547.
54. Baddeley A (1992) Working memory. Science 255: 556–559.
55. Sussman ES, Bregman AS, Wang WJ, Khan FJ (2005) Attentional modulation of electrophysiological activity in auditory cortex for unattended sounds within multistream auditory environments. Cogn Affect Behav Neurosci 5: 93–110.
56. Mirz F, Gjedde A, Sodkilde-Jrgensen H, Pedersen CB (2000) Functional brain imaging of tinnitus-like perception induced by aversive auditory stimuli. Neuroreport 11: 633–637.
57. Jacobson GP, McCaslin DL (2003) A reexamination of the long latency N1 response in patients with tinnitus. J Am Acad Audiol 14: 393–400.
58. Delb W, Strauss DJ, Low YF, Seidler H, Rheinschmitt A, et al. (2008) Alterations in Event Related Potentials (ERP) associated with tinnitus distress and attention. Appl Psychophysiol Biofeedback 33: 211–221.
59. Moller AR (2003) Pathophysiology of tinnitus. Otolaryngol Clin North Am 36: 249–266, v–vi.
60. Syka J (2002) Plastic changes in the central auditory system after hearing loss, restoration of function, and during learning. Physiol Rev 82: 601–636.
61. Salgado-Pineda P, Baeza I, Perez-Gomez M, Vendrell P, Junque C, et al. (2003) Sustained attention impairment correlates to gray matter decreases in first episode neuroleptic-naive schizophrenic patients. Neuroimage 19: 365–375.

Increased p66Shc in the Inner Ear of D-Galactose-Induced Aging Mice with Accumulation of Mitochondrial DNA 3873-bp Deletion: p66Shc and mtDNA Damage in the Inner Ear during Aging

Lisa Wu[1,2]⁹, Yu Sun[1]⁹, Yu-Juan Hu[1], Yang Yang[1], Ling-Li Yao[1], Xing-Xing Zhou[1], Hao Wang[1], Rui Zhang[1], Xiang Huang[3], Wei-Jia Kong[1,3,4]*

1 Department of Otorhinolaryngology, Union Hospital, Tongji Medical College, Huazhong University of Science and Technology, Wuhan, People's Republic of China, **2** Department of Otolaryngology-Head and Neck Surgery, Xiangya Hospital, Central South University, Changsha, People's Republic of China, **3** Institute of Otorhinolaryngology, Union Hospital, Tongji Medical College, Huazhong University of Science and Technology, Wuhan, People's Republic of China, **4** Key laboratory of Neurological Disease, Ministry of Education, Wuhan, People's Republic of China

Abstract

Aging has been associated with mitochondrial DNA damage. P66Shc is an age-related adaptor protein that has a substantial impact on mitochondrial metabolism through regulation of the cellular response to oxidative stress. Our study aimed to establish a D-galactose (D-gal)-induced inner ear aging mouse model and to investigate the potential role of p66Shc and its serine 36-phosphorylated form in the inner ear during aging by using this model. Real-time PCR was performed to detect the mtDNA 3873-bp deletion and the level of p66Shc mRNA in the cochlear lateral wall. Western blot analysis was performed to analyze the total and mitochondrial protein levels of p66Shc and the level of Ser36-P-p66Shc in the cochlear lateral wall. Immunofluoresence was performed to detect the location of the Ser36-P-p66Shc expression in the cochlear lateral wall. The results showed that the accumulation of the mtDNA 3873-bp deletion, total and mitochondrial protein levels of p66Shc and level of Ser36-P-p66Shc were significantly increased in the cochlear lateral wall of the D-gal-treated group when compared to the control group and that Ser36-P-p66Shc was mainly localized in the cytoplasm of the cells in the stria vascularis. During aging, the oxidative stress-related increase of p66Shc and Ser36-P-p66Shc might be associated with the accumulation of the mtDNA 3873-bp deletion in the inner ear.

Editor: Yidong Bai, University of Texas Health Science Center at San Antonio, United States of America

Funding: This work was supported by grants from the Major State Basic Research Development Program of China (973 Program) (2011CB504504) and the National Nature Science Foundation of China (30730094 and 81000408). The funders had no role in study design, data collection and analysis, decision to publish, or preparation of the manuscript.

Competing Interests: The authors have declared that no competing interests exist.

* E-mail: entwjkong@yahoo.com.cn

⁹ These authors contributed equally to this work.

Introduction

Age-related hearing loss (ARHL) or presbycusis is the most common sensory deficit in the elderly, and it has become a severe social and health problem. Although many theories underlying presbycusis have been proposed, the overall mechanisms remain speculative. Among these theories, many studies support the idea that a mitochondrial malfunction plays an important role in presbycusis [1–3]. The mitochondrion is the organelle that generates the high energy intermediate ATP and is also a major source and major target of reactive oxygen species (ROS) [4,5]. ROS that originates from the mitochondrial respiratory chain can damage macromolecules, especially mitochondrial DNA (mtDNA) [6]. Mammalian mtDNA is a closed circular molecule of approximately 16 kb and encodes many critical components of the oxidative phosphorylation pathway, which is responsible for generating ATP for the cell. Thus, a deletion in the mtDNA would lead to a mitochondrial malfunction. The 3867-bp deletion in mice that corresponds to the mtDNA 4977-bp deletion in humans and the mtDNA 4834-bp deletion in rats, which are also called common deletions (CD), is the most common mtDNA damage associated with aging [7–9]. According to the NCBI reference sequence for mtDNA (NC_005089.1), there are 6 bp added to the mtDNA 3867-bp deletion. Thus, it is more accurately a mtDNA 3873-bp deletion. The mtDNA 3873-bp deletion occurs within nt9089– nt12961 or nt9104– nt12976, which are flanked by a 15-bp direct-repeat sequence (AGCCCTACTAATTAC), and results in a partial to complete loss of the following mtDNA genes coding for components of oxidative phosphorylation (OXPHOS): COX3, ND3, ND4L, ND4, ND5 and 5 tRNAs (tRNA-Gly, tRNA-Arg, tRNA-His, tRNA-Ser and tRNA-Leu). Previous studies have suggested that the mtDNA deletion is associated with pathological disorders of presbycusis in human beings, rats and mice [10–13]. We have previously utilized overdoses of D-galactose (D-gal) to induce an aging model of rats, which harbor increased amounts of the mtDNA 4834-bp deletion in the central and peripheral auditory system [14–19]. Moreover, we found that below a certain level, the mtDNA 4834-bp deletion might not directly lead to a hearing impairment but rather act as a predisposing factor that can greatly enhance the sensitivity of the inner ear to aminoglycoside antibiotics [17]. These findings suggest that the mtDNA deletion plays an important role in presbycusis. As the inner ear tissue of live humans is inaccessible and the genetic and environmental background of individuals with hearing loss is nonhomogeneous, studies on presbycusis are limited. The mouse is one of the mammals, after humans, whose genome has been sequenced. Additionally, approximately 99% of human genes have homologs in the mouse [20]. Thus, compared to the D-gal-induced aging rat, the D-gal-induced aging mouse would provide a more ideal model to explore the potential mechanisms involved in inner ear aging.

The p66Shc protein is a Src homologue and collagen homologue (Shc) adaptor protein, which has the ability to interact with other proteins that mediate cell signaling [21]. It is encoded by the mammalian shcA gene, which also encodes the two other ShcA adaptor proteins p46Shc and p52Shc that are named for their molecular masses [22]. However, only the p66Shc isoform participates in mitochondrial ROS generation and acts as an oxidative signal regulator, which translates oxidative signals to the mitochondria [23,24]. P66shc-null mice display an increased lifespan and enhanced resistance to oxidative stress [25]. Upon oxidative stress, p66Shc is phosphorylated at a serine residue (Ser36), and the phosphorylation of Ser36 is necessary for the cellular response to oxidative stress [25]. A portion of p66Shc partially localizes within the membrane space of the mitochondria where it oxidizes cytochrome c (Cytc), thus producing ROS [23]. Since the publication by Migliaccio, the p66Shc protein has been recognized as an important element of the free radical theory of aging [24], and many age-related diseases were suggested to associate with p66Shc [26–29]. However, no study of p66Shc in presbycusis has previously been reported.

As the stria vascularis is an essential structure of the inner ear that contains abundant mitochondria and has the highest rate of aerobic oxidation in the inner ear [30,31], we focused on the cochlear lateral wall as the major subject of our study. We established a D-gal-induced aging mouse model that harbored increased levels of the mtDNA 3873-bp deletion in the cochlear lateral walls and investigated the total and mitochondrial levels of p66Shc and the Ser36-phosphorylated form of p66Shc (Ser36-P-p66Shc) in this aging model. Our results suggested that p66Shc and Ser36-P-p66Shc might play a critical role in inner ear aging and the formation and accumulation of mtDNA damage in the inner ear.

Table 1. The ABR threshold (dB SPL).

Frequency	NS group (n = 10)	LD group (n = 10)	HD group (n = 10)
4 kHz	39.0±3.94	38.5±5.80	38.0±6.75
8 kHz	30.0±4.83	30.5±5.50	27.5±4.86
16 kHz	23.0±4.22	23.0±4.83	22.5±4.25
32 kHz	34.5±4.38	37.0±4.25	36.0±3.16

The data are expressed as mean±standard deviation. (NS, the group treated with normal saline; LD, the group treated with 800 mg/kg D-gal; HD, the group treated with 1000 mg/kg D-gal. $p>0.05$ when compared to the NS group.).

Table 2. The plasma SOD activity and MDA levels.

	NS group (n = 6)	LD group (n = 6)	HD group (n = 6)
T-SOD (U/ml)	198.62±10.35	170.67±19.11**	146.52±13.42**#
MDA (μmol/ml)	1.22±0.20	2.52±0.49**	3.25±0.47**^

The data are expressed as the mean±standard deviation. (NS, the group treated with normal saline; LD, the group treated with 800 mg/kg D-gal; HD, the group treated with 1000 mg/kg D-gal. **, $p<0.01$ when compared to the NS group; #, $p<0.05$ when compared to the LD group; ^, $p<0.01$ when compared to the LD group.).

Materials and Methods

Animals and Treatment

One hundred and two male Kunming mice (median body weight of 22 g; 7–8 weeks old) with normal hearing were purchased from the Laboratory Animal Center of Tongji Medical College of Huazhong University of Science and Technology. The Kunming mouse strain is an outbred strain of the Swiss mouse strain, which came to Kunming, China in 1944 from the Indian Haffkine Institute, and was widely used for the D-galactose-induced aging mice [32–36]. The mice were acclimated to the new environment (23°C; 12-h light/dark cycle) for at least one week before the start of the experiments. All the animals had free access to water and food. The animals were randomly assigned to three groups (n = 34 for each group) depending on the dose of D-gal (Sigma Chemical, St. Louis, MO), as follows: a low dose (LD) group, high dose (HD) group and control group. Mice were treated with a daily subcutaneous injection of the D-gal solutions (LD group, 800 mg/kg of D-gal; HD group, 1000 mg/kg of D-gal) or an equal volume of normal saline (NS) (for control group) in the neck for 10 weeks. The animal studies were performed in accordance with the guidelines for the care and use of laboratory animals that were prepared by the Institution of Laboratory Animals of Huazhong University of Science and Technology. The protocol was approved by the Committee on the Ethics of Animal Experiments of Huazhong University of Science and Technology (Permit Number: S244). All surgeries were performed under a mixture of ketamine and chlorpromazine anesthesia, and all efforts were made to minimize suffering.

Auditory Brainstem Response

At the beginning and at the end of the treatment, the hearing functions of the mice were tested by auditory brainstem responses (ABR). Mice (n = 10 for each group) were anaesthetized with a mixture of ketamine (120 mg/kg) and chlorpromazine (20 mg/kg) and placed on a heated mat in an audiometric chamber. The sound delivery tube of the insert earphone was tightly fitted into the external auditory canal. Electrodes were placed subdermally over the vertex (active), right mastoid (reference) and left mastoid (ground). The ABR responses were measured with a tone burst stimulus at 4, 8, 16 and 32 kHz using a computer-based signal averaging system (Tucker-Davis Technology, Alachua, FL, USA), as Yu described previously [37]. The threshold was verified by two unblinded investigators.

Tissue Sample Preparation

Mice were killed after the last subcutaneous injections. All animals were euthanized under deep anesthesia with chlorpromazine and ketamine hydrochloride, and the temporal bones and plasma were collected. For immunofluorescence experiments, the

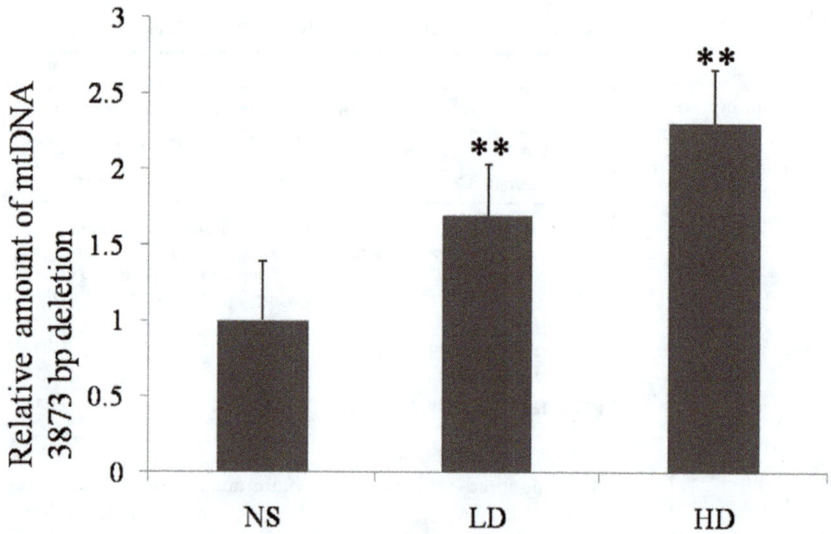

Figure 1. The effect of D-gal on the amount of mtDNA 3873-bp deletion in the cochlear lateral wall of the experimental groups. The accumulation of the mtDNA 3873-bp deletion in the D-gal-treated groups was significantly higher when compared to the control group. (NS, the group treated with normal saline; LD, the group treated with 800 mg/kg D-gal; HD, the group treated with 1000 mg/kg D-gal. **, p<0.01 when compared to the NS group.).

cochleae from 12 animals (n = 4 from each group) were perfused slowly with cold 4% paraformaldehyde in phosphate-buffered saline (PBS) and then kept in the same fixative at 4°C overnight. Following fixation, the cochleae were decalcified with disodium EDTA. Then, the decalcified cochleae were paraffin embedded, and 5-μm sections were cut and mounted on glass slides for analysis of immunofluorescent labeling. For experiments involving DNA, total RNA and total or mitochondrial protein detection, the cochlear lateral wall, which included the stria vascularis and spiral ligament, was isolated under a stereomicroscope (Zeiss, Germany). Then, the DNA and total RNA from 18 animals (n = 6 from each group) were extracted with a genomic DNA Kit (Tiangen, China) and RNAiso Plus reagent (TaKaRa, Japan), respectively. cDNA was reverse transcribed using a PrimeScript® RT reagent kit (Perfect Real Time; TaKaRa, Japan). The total protein from 18 animals (n = 6 from each group) was isolated with RIPA lysis buffer (Beyotime, China). The mitochondrial proteins from 36 animals (n = 12 from each group) were isolated with the Tissue Mitochondria Isolation Kit (Beyotime, China). Protein concentrations were determined with the BCA Protein Assay Kit (Beyotime, China), with BSA as the standard.

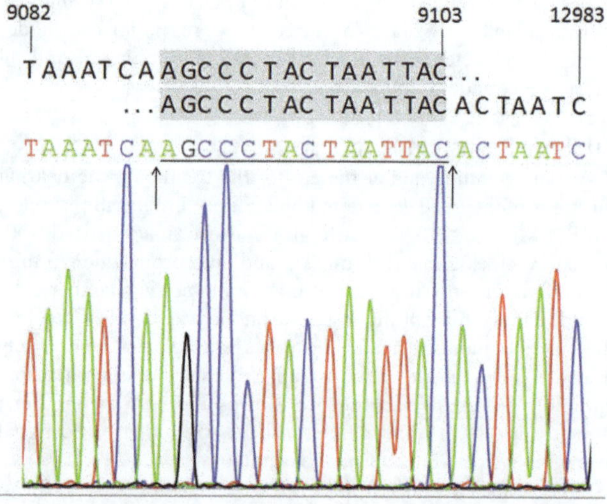

Figure 2. Schematic diagram and sequences of the mtDNA 3873-bp deletion (nt9089–nt12961 or nt9104–nt12976). Bold black letters indicate the nucleotide sequences flanking the breakpoints of the deleted mtDNA, and shaded letters indicate the direct repeats. The sequences of the PCR products are shown below the schematic diagram. The arrowheads point to the possible breakpoints.

SOD Activity and MDA Assay of Plasma

The SOD (Superoxide Dismutase) activity and MDA (Malondialdehyde) levels in the plasma were quantified with colorimetric kits (Jiancheng, China) according to the manufacturer's instructions [17].

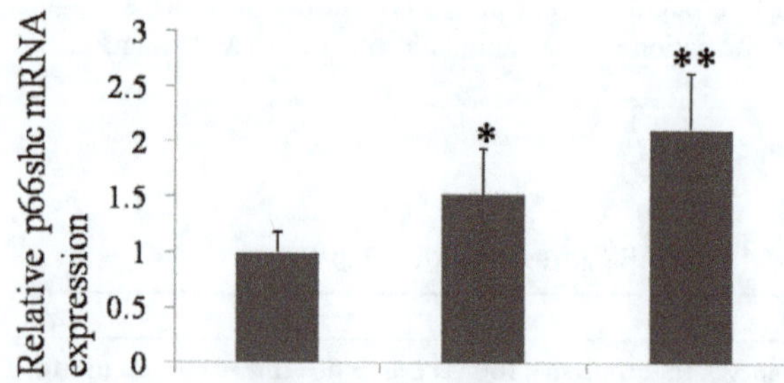

Figure 3. The effect of D-gal on the mRNA levels of p66Shc in the cochlear lateral wall of the experimental groups. With the increasing doses of D-gal, the mRNA levels of p66Shc were increased. (NS, the group treated with normal saline; LD, the group treated with 800 mg/kg D-gal; HD, the group treated with 1000 mg/kg D-gal. *, p<0.05 when compared to the NS group. **, p<0.01 when compared to the NS group.).

Real-time PCR

To evaluate the mtDNA damage induced by D-gal, a sequence designed according to the description of Brossas et al. [38], which represented the new fusion sequence (NFS) that is present in only the deleted mtDNA, was used as a measurement of the mtDNA 3873-bp deletion. Because the D-loop region of mtDNA is rarely deleted, it can represent the conserved segment and be used to determine the copy number of mtDNA. All gene-specific primers used in this study were designed and synthesized at TaKaRa Biotechnology (Dalian) Co. Ltd. and were previously tested for optimal efficiency. The primer pairs for the mtDNA 3873-bp deletion and D-loop were as follows: NFS forward, 5′-CGAAAC-CACATAAATCAAGCCCTAC-3′; NFS reverse, 5′-AAT-GATTCGTATGCTGTACATAGCTGTT-3′; D-loop forward, 5′-GGGCTGATTAGACCCGATACCAT-3′; and D-loop reverse, 5′-TACCATCCTCCGTGAAACCAACA-3′. The primer pairs for p66Shc and the internal standard (β-actin) were as follows: p66Shc forward, 5′-CCGAC-TACCTGTGTTCCTTCTT-3′; p66Shc reverse, 5′-CCCATCTTCAGCAGCCTTTCC-3′; β-actin forward, 5′-CATCCGTAAAGACCTCTATGCCAAC-3′; and β-actin reverse, 5′-ATGGAGCCACCGATCCACA-3′. The DNA and cDNA products were subjected to real-time PCR with the ABI StepOnePlus^{TM} instrument equipped with StepOne software (ABI) for 40 cycles (95°C for 30 s, 95°C for 5 s and 60°C for 5 s) by using the SYBR® Premix Ex Taq^{TM} (Tli RNaseH Plus) kit (TaKaRa, Japan). Each reaction was performed in duplicate and analyzed by melting curves at the end to confirm specificity. The products obtained with primers for detection of the mtDNA 3873-bp deletion were excised from a gel. Then, the products were gel purified, cloned and analyzed using an ABI Prism 377 DNA sequencer (Applied Biosystems, Foster City, CA). The ΔCt method ($Ct_{deletion}$-$Ct_{D\text{-}loop}$) was used to calculate the abundance of the mtDNA deletion. The relative amount of the mtDNA 3873-bp deletion and the mRNA levels of p66Shc were calculated with the $2^{-\Delta\Delta Ct}$ method.

Western Blot

We detected the total protein level of p66Shc, p52Shc and p46Shc by using an antibody against SHC (Abcam, USA), which detects the three isoforms simultaneously by binding to a similar domain in all three proteins. The total protein level of SHC and the level of Ser36-P-p66Shc (p66Shc phosphorylated at serine 36) were measured with the corresponding antibodies and normalized to the level of glyceraldehyde-3-phosphate dehydrogenase (GADPH). The mitochondrial p66Shc levels were measured with the SHC antibody and normalized to the voltage-dependent anion channel (VDAC1). For this analysis, 20 μg of protein was separated by 10% or 12% SDS-PAGE and then transferred to nitrocellulose membranes. The SHC and Ser36-P-p66Shc levels were detected after incubation with primary antibodies (SHC, Ser36-P-p66Shc and VDAC1, 1:1000, Abcam, USA; GAPDH, 1:5000, Kangchen, China), which was followed by an incubation with a horseradish peroxidase (HRP)-conjugated goat anti-rabbit (1:5000, Santa Cruz, USA) or goat anti-mouse (1:2000, Santa Cruz, USA) immunoglobulin, as appropriate. The immunoreactivity was determined using the ECL reaction kit (Beyotime, China) according to the manufacturer's instructions by exposure on medical film. The band density was quantified with the Image-Pro Plus 6.0 software (Media Cybernetics, Inc., USA).

Immunofluorescent Labeling

After deparaffinization, rehydration, antigen retrieval and nonspecific antigen site blocking, immunofluorescence was performed on the sections overnight at 4°C with the monoclonal anti-Ser36-P-p66Shc antibody (1:40, Abcam, USA), which were then incubated for 1 h with the fluorescently tagged secondary antibody. Control staining was performed without the primary antibody. Images were taken with a laser scanning confocal microscope (Nikon, Japan).

Statistical Analysis

All data are presented as the mean±standard deviation (Mean±S.D.). Statistical analyses were performed with the SPSS 13.0 software (IBM, Armonk, NY, USA). One-way analysis of variance (ANOVA) was used for comparisons of the relative expression levels for the different groups. The least significant difference (LSD) post-hoc test was used to compare differences between two of the groups. Differences with a p-value<0.05 were considered to be statistically significant.

Results

D-gal did not Induce Hearing Loss

To determine the effect of the mtDNA 3873-bp deletion on hearing, the auditory status was evaluated with ABR after the last D-gal administration. There was no significant difference in the ABR threshold (Table 1) among the three experimental groups ($p>0.05$).

Decreased SOD Activity and Increased MDA Levels in Plasma Induced by D-gal

The SOD activity in the plasma of mice treated with the low and high doses of D-gal was 170.67±19.11 U/ml and 146.52±13.42 U/ml, respectively, which was significantly lower than that of the control group (198.62±10.35 U/ml) ($p<0.01$). The MDA levels in the plasma of mice treated with the low and high doses of D-gal were 2.52±0.49 μmol/ml and 3.25±0.47 μmol/ml, respectively, which were significantly higher than that of the control group (1.22±0.20 μmol/ml) ($p<0.01$) (Table 2).

Accumulation of the Mitochondrial DNA 3873-bp Deletion Induced by D-gal

The amount of mtDNA 3873-bp deletion was significantly increased in the cochlear lateral wall of the D-gal-treated groups. Compared to the control group, the accumulation of the mtDNA 3873-bp deletion in the low and high dose D-gal groups was increased by approximately 1.70-fold and 2.30-fold, respectively (Fig. 1). The products obtained with the primers for the mtDNA 3873-bp deletion were sequenced to prove the presence of the mtDNA 3873-bp deletion (Fig. 2).

Increased mRNA Levels of p66Shc Induced by D-gal

The mRNA levels were significantly increased in the cochlear lateral wall of the D-gal-treated groups (Fig. 3). Compared to the control group, the relative expression levels in the low and high dose D-gal-treated groups were increased approximately 1.53-fold and 2.12-fold, respectively.

Increased Total Protein Levels of p66Shc and Ser36-P-p66Shc Induced by D-gal

The result showed that the total protein level of p66Shc was increased in the cochlear lateral wall of the D-gal-treated groups. However, the relative changes of the total protein levels of p52Shc and p46Shc between the groups were not statistically significant ($p>0.05$). The levels of Ser36-P-p66Shc were increased in the

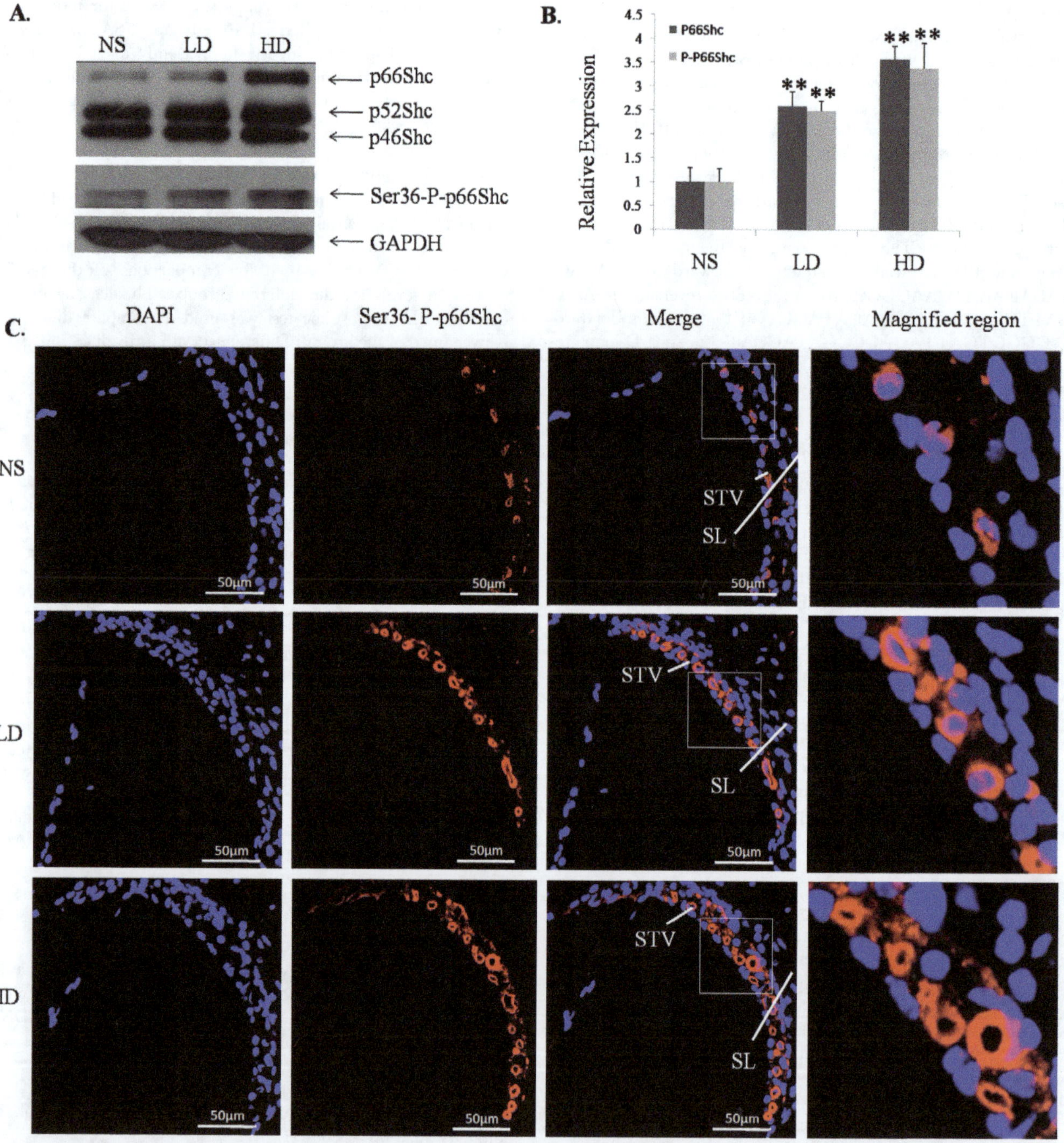

Figure 4. The expression of total SHC protein and Ser36-P-p66Shc in the cochlear lateral wall of the experimental groups. A, Western blot assessment of the protein expression of SHC and Ser36-P-p66Shc in the NS, LD and HD groups. B, Semiquantitative representation of the total protein levels of p66Shc and Ser36-P-p66Shc compared to the control group. C, Cochlea sections were subjected to immunofluorescent labeling of Ser36-P-p66Shc; Ser36-P-p66Shc was mainly expressed in the cytoplasm of cells in the stria vascularis. (NS, the group treated with normal saline; LD, the group treated with 800 mg/kg D-gal; HD, the group treated with 1000 mg/kg D-gal. STV, stria vascularis; SL, spiral ligament. **, $p<0.01$ when compared to the NS group.).

cochlear lateral wall of the D-gal-treated groups (Fig. 4A and B). Compared to the control group, the total protein levels of p66Shc in the low and high dose groups were increased approximately 2.59-fold and 3.58-fold, respectively, and the levels of Ser-P-p66Shc were increased approximately 2.48- and 3.39-fold, respectively.

In addition, we analyzed the location of the Ser36-P-p66Shc expression by using immunofluorescent labeling. We found that Ser36-P-p66Shc was mainly expressed in the cytoplasm of the cells in the stria vascularis, and it was increased with the increasing doses of D-gal (Fig. 4C).

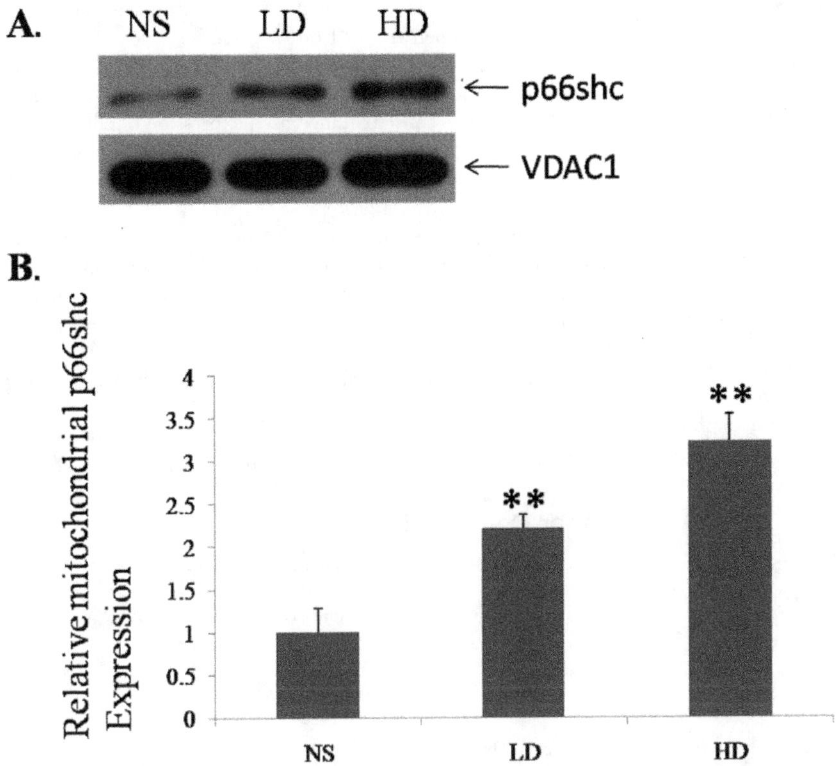

Figure 5. The mitochondrial protein expression of p66Shc in the cochlear lateral wall of the experimental groups. A, Western blot assessment of the protein expression of p66Shc in the NS, LD and HD groups. B, Semiquantitative representation of the relative abundance of the mitochondrial protein levels of p66Shc in D-gal-treated groups compared to the control group. (NS, the group treated with normal saline; LD, the group treated with 800 mg/kg D-gal; HD, the group treated with 1000 mg/kg D-gal. **, $p<0.01$ when compared to the NS group.).

Increased Mitochondrial Protein Level of p66Shc Induced by D-gal

To detect the protein levels of p66Shc in the mitochondria, we utilized western blot analysis. The mitochondrial protein levels of p66Shc were significantly increased in the cochlear lateral wall of the D-gal-treated mice (Fig. 5A). Compared to the control group, the mitochondrial protein levels of p66Shc in the D-gal-treated groups were increased approximately 2.21-fold and 3.22-fold in the low and high dose groups, respectively (Fig. 5B).

Discussion

According to the oxidative stress theory by Denham Harman, the age-related loss of physiological function is due to the progressive accumulation of oxidative damage, which ultimately determines the lifespan of an organism [39]. In this study, we used an overdose of D-gal that was thought to result in the generation of superoxide anions and oxygen-derived free radicals and the formation of advanced glycation end products (AGEs) [40–42], which triggers excess ROS and abnormally high oxidative stress, to accelerate the aging of mice. We demonstrated that the plasma SOD activity was decreased and the MDA level in plasma was increased in the D-gal-treated mice. The changes of these two age-related biochemical markers were similar to those that occur during the natural aging process in humans and other animals [43–45]. The CD is an important biomarker of aging [46–48]. Our previous study on the D-gal-induced rats that mimic aging reported that the amount of CD in the inner ear of the high dose D-gal group was increased 3.69-fold compared to the control group [18]. Zhang et al. [13] reported that the level of the CD in the inner ear of 17- to 19-month-old mice was increased 3.32 fold compared to 7- to 10-month-old mice. In this study, we demonstrated that the amount of CD in the cochlear lateral wall of the high dose D-gal group was increased 2.30-fold compared to the control group. These data indicated that we established a mouse model of aging in the inner ear by using D-gal, which was similar to the D-gal-induced inner ear aging rat model. Corresponding to our previous study in rats [16,17,19], there was no significant difference in the ABR threshold among the three experimental groups. The result of the mouse aging model further confirmed the result from the rat aging model that, below a certain level, the mtDNA deletion does not directly lead to a hearing impairment [16,17,19].

Most of the p66Shc protein is distributed throughout the cytosol, while a fraction of p66Shc localizes within the inner membrane and intermembrane space of the mitochondria; additionally, oxidative stress stimulates an increase in the mitochondrial p66Shc level [23,49–51]. Protein kinase C β (PKCβ) is activated by oxidative stress and phosphorylates p66Shc on the Ser36 residue, which triggers its translocation to the mitochondria [52,53]. Our data showed that the mRNA and total protein levels of p66Shc and levels Ser36-P-p66Shc were significantly increased in the cochlear lateral wall of the D-gal-induced aging mice. High amounts of Ser36-P-p66Shc indicate a high activation of the PKCβ pathway and higher oxidative stress in a tissue [54,55]. Thus, the increased levels of Ser36-P-p66Shc indicated higher oxidative stress in the cochlea lateral wall of the D-gal-induced aging mice. Furthermore, we analyzed the location of the Ser36-P-p66Shc expression in the cochlear lateral wall by using immunofluorescent labeling. The results showed that Ser36-P-p66Shc was mainly expressed in the cytoplasm of the cells in the stria vascularis, which also indicates that there is higher oxidative stress in the stria vascularis. Migliaccio et al. [25] reported that their study of mouse embryo fibroblasts showed that p66Shc was activated upon exposure to agents that induce oxidative stress. Our results further established a positive correlation between the levels of oxidative stress and the amount of p66Shc in the cochlear lateral wall of mice. Consistent with the Ser36-P-p66Shc level, which was increased in the D-gal-induced aging mice, the mitochondrial protein levels of p66Shc were also increased. This result indicates that p66Shc was translocated to the mitochondria in the D-gal-induced aging mice. Pinton et al. [56] reported that phosphorylation of p66Shc at Ser36 triggers a mitochondrial accumulation of p66Shc. It was reported that before Ser36-P-p66Shc is translocated to the mitochondria, it is isomerized by the peptidyl-prolyl isomerase Pin1 and then recognized and dephosphorylated by the phosphatase PP2A [56,57]. Thus, mitochondrial p66Shc is unphosphorylated.

In the intermembrane space of the mitochondria, p66Shc oxidizes Cytc, resulting in the generation of H_2O_2 via the transfer of electrons from the reduced Cytc to oxygen and, thus, increasing the intracellular ROS level [23], which has been suggested to lead to the accumulation of the mtDNA 3873-bp deletion [58]. Trinei et al. [59] reported that the mtDNA 3873-bp deletion was detected in liver samples of wildtype mice, while it was barely detectable in matched tissues from p66Shc$^{-/-}$ mice. This result indicates that the p66Shc expression was correlated with the level of the mtDNA 3873-bp deletion. Therefore, our data indicating that oxidative stress caused an increased expression of p66Shc and Ser36-P-p66Shc and the translocation of p66Shc to the mitochondria may be associated with the accumulation of the mtDNA 3873-bp deletion in the inner ear.

In conclusion, we established a D-gal-induced inner ear aging mouse model in this study and demonstrated the accumulation of the mtDNA 3873-bp deletion in the lateral wall of the D-gal-treated mice, which may be associated with an oxidative stress-related increase in the expression of p66Shc and Ser36-P-p66Shc and the translocation of p66Shc to the mitochondria. Considering that oxidative stress has been associated with numerous human aging processes in addition to presbycusis, the role of p66Shc as a signaling agent may have important therapeutic implications.

Author Contributions

Conceived and designed the experiments: LW YS YJH YY. Performed the experiments: LW XXZ HW RZ. Analyzed the data: LW YS LLY. Contributed reagents/materials/analysis tools: LW YS XH. Wrote the paper: LW YS WJK.

References

1. Someya S, Prolla TA (2010) Mitochondrial oxidative damage and apoptosis in age-related hearing loss. Mech Ageing Dev 131: 480–486.
2. Yamasoba T, Someya S, Yamada C, Weindruch R, Prolla TA, et al. (2007) Role of mitochondrial dysfunction and mitochondrial DNA mutations in age-related hearing loss. Hear Res 226: 185–193.
3. Seidman MD, Khan MJ, Bai U, Shirwany N, Quirk WS (2000) Biologic activity of mitochondrial metabolites on aging and age-related hearing loss. Am J Otol 21: 161–167.
4. Finkel T, Holbrook NJ (2000) Oxidants, oxidative stress and the biology of ageing. Nature 408: 239–247.
5. Beckman KB, Ames BN (1998) The free radical theory of aging matures. Physiol Rev 78: 547–581.
6. Jang YC, Remmen VH (2009) The mitochondrial theory of aging: insight from transgenic and knockout mouse models. Exp Gerontol 44: 256–260.
7. Mohamed SA, Hanke T, Erasmi AW, Bechtel MJ, Scharfschwerdt M, et al. (2006) Mitochondrial DNA deletions and the aging heart. Exp Gerontol 41: 508–517.
8. Nicklas JA, Brooks EM, Hunter TC, Single R, Branda RF (2004) Development of a quantitative PCR (TaqMan) assay for relative mitochondrial DNA copy number and the common mitochondrial DNA deletion in the rat. Environ Mol Mutagen 44: 313–320.
9. Zeng Z, Zhang Z, Yu H, Corbley MJ, Tang Z, et al. (1999) Mitochondrial DNA deletions are associated with ischemia and aging in Balb/c mouse brain. J Cell Biochem 73: 545–553.
10. Seidman MD, Bai U, Khan MJ, Murphy MJ, Quirk WS, et al. (1996) Association of mitochondrial DNA deletions and cochlear pathology: a molecular biologic tool. Laryngoscope 106: 777–783.
11. Seidman MD, Bai U, Khan MJ, Quirk WS (1997) Mitochondrial DNA deletions associated with aging and presbyacusis. Arch Otolaryngol Head Neck Surg 123: 1039–1045.
12. Zhang X, Han D, Ding D, Dai P, Yang W, et al. (2002) Deletions are easy detectable in cochlear mitochondrial DNA of Cu/Zn superoxide dismutase gene knockout mice. Chin Med J (Engl) 115: 258–263.
13. Zhang X, Han D, Ding D, Dai P, Yang W, et al. (2002) Cochlear mitochondrial DNA3867bp deletion in aged mice. Chin Med J (Engl) 115: 1390–1393.
14. Chen B, Zhong Y, Peng W, Sun Y, Kong WJ (2010) Age-related changes in the central auditory system: comparison of D-galactose-induced aging rats and naturally aging rats. Brain Res 1344: 43–53.
15. Chen B, Zhong Y, Peng W, Sun Y, Hu YJ, et al. (2011) Increased mitochondrial DNA damage and decreased base excision repair in the auditory cortex of D-galactose-induced aging rats. Mol Biol Rep 38: 3635–3642.
16. Kong WJ, Wang Y, Wang Q, Hu YJ, Han YC, et al. (2006) The relation between D-galactose injection and mitochondrial DNA 4834 bp deletion mutation. Exp Gerontol 41: 628–634.
17. Kong WJ, Hu YJ, Wang Q, Wang Y, Han YC, et al. (2006) The effect of the mtDNA4834 deletion on hearing. Biochem Biophys Res Commun 344: 425–430.
18. Zhong Y, Hu YJ, Chen B, Peng W, Sun Y, et al. (2011) Mitochondrial transcription factor A overexpression and base excision repair deficiency in the inner ear of rats with D-galactose-induced aging. FEBS J 278: 2500–2510.
19. Zhong Y, Hu YJ, Yang Y, Peng W, Sun Y, et al. (2011) Contribution of common deletion to total deletion burden in mitochondrial DNA from inner ear of d-galactose-induced aging rats. Mutat Res 712: 11–19.
20. Boguski MS (2002) Comparative genomics: the mouse that roared. Nature 420: 515–516.
21. Rajendran M, Thomes P, Zhang L, Veeramani S, Lin MF (2010) p66Shc–a longevity redox protein in human prostate cancer progression and metastasis: p66Shc in cancer progression and metastasis. Cancer Metastasis Rev 29: 207–222.
22. Pelicci G, Lanfrancone L, Grignani F, McGlade J, Cavallo F, et al. (1992) A novel transforming protein (SHC) with an SH2 domain is implicated in mitogenic signal transduction. Cell 70: 93–104.
23. Giorgio M, Migliaccio E, Orsini F, Paolucci D, Moroni M, et al. (2005) Electron transfer between cytochrome c and p66Shc generates reactive oxygen species that trigger mitochondrial apoptosis. Cell 122: 221–233.
24. Migliaccio E, Mele S, Salcini AE, Pelicci G, Lai KM, et al. (1997) Opposite effects of the p52shc/p46shc and p66shc splicing isoforms on the EGF receptor-MAP kinase-fos signalling pathway. EMBO J 16: 706–716.
25. Migliaccio E, Giorgio M, Mele S, Pelicci G, Reboldi P, et al. (1999) The p66shc adaptor protein controls oxidative stress response and life span in mammals. Nature 402: 309–313.
26. Berry A, Capone F, Giorgio M, Pelicci PG, de Kloet ER, et al. (2007) Deletion of the life span determinant p66Shc prevents age-dependent increases in emotionality and pain sensitivity in mice. Exp Gerontol 42: 37–45.
27. Percy CJ, Brown L, Power DA, Johnson DW, Gobe GC (2009) Obesity and hypertension have differing oxidant handling molecular pathways in age-related chronic kidney disease. Mech Ageing Dev 130: 129–138.
28. Rota M, LeCapitaine N, Hosoda T, Boni A, De Angelis A, et al. (2006) Diabetes promotes cardiac stem cell aging and heart failure, which are prevented by deletion of the p66shc gene. Circ Res 99: 42–52.
29. Ljubicic V, Menzies KJ, Hood DA (2010) Mitochondrial dysfunction is associated with a pro-apoptotic cellular environment in senescent cardiac muscle. Mech Ageing Dev 131: 79–88.
30. Yao X, Rarey KE (1996) Detection and regulation of Cu/Zn-SOD and Mn-SOD in rat cochlear tissues. Hear Res 96: 199–203.
31. VOSTEEN KH (1960) The histochemistry of the enzymes of oxygen metabolism in the inner ear. Trans Southeast Sect Am Urol Assoc 1960: 230–241.
32. Lu J, Wu DM, Hu B, Zheng YL, Zhang ZF, et al. (2010) NGF-Dependent activation of TrkA pathway: A mechanism for the neuroprotective effect of troxerutin in D-galactose-treated mice. Brain Pathol 20: 952–965.
33. Lu J, Wu DM, Zheng YL, Hu B, Zhang ZF, et al. (2010) Ursolic acid attenuates D-galactose-induced inflammatory response in mouse prefrontal cortex through inhibiting AGEs/RAGE/NF-kappaB pathway activation. Cereb Cortex 20: 2540–2548.

34. Zhang ZF, Lu J, Zheng YL, Hu B, Fan SH, et al. (2010) Purple sweet potato color protects mouse liver against d-galactose-induced apoptosis via inhibiting caspase-3 activation and enhancing PI3K/Akt pathway. Food Chem Toxicol 48: 2500–2507.
35. Shan Q, Lu J, Zheng Y, Li J, Zhou Z, et al. (2009) Purple sweet potato color ameliorates cognition deficits and attenuates oxidative damage and inflammation in aging mouse brain induced by d-galactose. J Biomed Biotechnol 2009: 564737.
36. Liu CM, Ma JQ, Lou Y (2010) Chronic administration of troxerutin protects mouse kidney against D-galactose-induced oxidative DNA damage. Food Chem Toxicol 48: 2809–2817.
37. Sun Y, Tang W, Chang Q, Wang Y, Kong W, et al. (2009) Connexin30 null and conditional connexin26 null mice display distinct pattern and time course of cellular degeneration in the cochlea. J Comp Neurol 516: 569–579.
38. Brossas JY, Barreau E, Courtois Y, Treton J (1994) Multiple deletions in mitochondrial DNA are present in senescent mouse brain. Biochem Biophys Res Commun 202: 654–659.
39. HARMAN D (1956) Aging: a theory based on free radical and radiation chemistry. J Gerontol 11: 298–300.
40. Gong Y, Liu L, Xie B, Liao Y, Yang E, et al. (2008) Ameliorative effects of lotus seedpod proanthocyanidins on cognitive deficits and oxidative damage in senescence-accelerated mice. Behav Brain Res 194: 100–107.
41. Lu J, Wu DM, Hu B, Cheng W, Zheng YL, et al. (2010) Chronic administration of troxerutin protects mouse brain against D-galactose-induced impairment of cholinergic system. Neurobiol Learn Mem 93: 157–164.
42. Wu DM, Lu J, Zheng YL, Zhou Z, Shan Q, et al. (2008) Purple sweet potato color repairs d-galactose-induced spatial learning and memory impairment by regulating the expression of synaptic proteins. Neurobiol Learn Mem 90: 19–27.
43. Ho SC, Liu JH, Wu RY (2003) Establishment of the mimetic aging effect in mice caused by D-galactose. Biogerontology 4: 15–18.
44. Song X, Bao M, Li D, Li YM (1999) Advanced glycation in D-galactose induced mouse aging model. Mech Ageing Dev 108: 239–251.
45. Inal ME, Kanbak G, Sunal E (2001) Antioxidant enzyme activities and malondialdehyde levels related to aging. Clin Chim Acta 305: 75–80.
46. Eshaghian A, Vleugels RA, Canter JA, McDonald MA, Stasko T, et al. (2006) Mitochondrial DNA deletions serve as biomarkers of aging in the skin, but are typically absent in nonmelanoma skin cancers. J Invest Dermatol 126: 336–344.
47. Meissner C, Bruse P, Mohamed SA, Schulz A, Warnk H, et al. (2008) The 4977 bp deletion of mitochondrial DNA in human skeletal muscle, heart and different areas of the brain: a useful biomarker or more? Exp Gerontol 43: 645–652.
48. Dumont P, Burton M, Chen QM, Gonos ES, Frippiat C, et al. (2000) Induction of replicative senescence biomarkers by sublethal oxidative stresses in normal human fibroblast. Free Radic Biol Med 28: 361–373.
49. Ventura A, Maccarana M, Raker VA, Pelicci PG (2004) A cryptic targeting signal induces isoform-specific localization of p46Shc to mitochondria. J Biol Chem 279: 2299–2306.
50. Orsini F, Migliaccio E, Moroni M, Contursi C, Raker VA, et al. (2004) The life span determinant p66Shc localizes to mitochondria where it associates with mitochondrial heat shock protein 70 and regulates trans-membrane potential. J Biol Chem 279: 25689–25695.
51. Nemoto S, Combs CA, French S, Ahn BH, Fergusson MM, et al. (2006) The mammalian longevity-associated gene product p66shc regulates mitochondrial metabolism. J Biol Chem 281: 10555–10560.
52. Gopalakrishna R, Jaken S (2000) Protein kinase C signaling and oxidative stress. Free Radic Biol Med 28: 1349–1361.
53. Pinton P, Rimessi A, Marchi S, Orsini F, Migliaccio E, et al. (2007) Protein kinase C beta and prolyl isomerase 1 regulate mitochondrial effects of the life-span determinant p66Shc. Science 315: 659–663.
54. Le S, Connors TJ, Maroney AC (2001) c-Jun N-terminal kinase specifically phosphorylates p66ShcA at serine 36 in response to ultraviolet irradiation. J Biol Chem 276: 48332–48336.
55. Lebiedzinska M, Duszynski J, Rizzuto R, Pinton P, Wieckowski MR (2009) Age-related changes in levels of p66Shc and serine 36-phosphorylated p66Shc in organs and mouse tissues. Arch Biochem Biophys 486: 73–80.
56. Pinton P, Rimessi A, Marchi S, Orsini F, Migliaccio E, et al. (2007) Protein kinase C beta and prolyl isomerase 1 regulate mitochondrial effects of the life-span determinant p66Shc. Science 315: 659–663.
57. Wulf G, Finn G, Suizu F, Lu KP (2005) Phosphorylation-specific prolyl isomerization: is there an underlying theme? Nat Cell Biol 7: 435–441.
58. Zhang W, Liu Y, An Z, Huang D, Qi Y, et al. (2011) Mediating effect of ROS on mtDNA damage and low ATP content induced by arsenic trioxide in mouse oocytes. Toxicol In Vitro 25: 979–984.
59. Trinei M, Giorgio M, Cicalese A, Barozzi S, Ventura A, et al. (2002) A p53-p66Shc signalling pathway controls intracellular redox status, levels of oxidation-damaged DNA and oxidative stress-induced apoptosis. Oncogene 21: 3872–3878.

8

Effect of Hearing Aids on Auditory Function in Infants with Perinatal Brain Injury and Severe Hearing Loss

Alma Janeth Moreno-Aguirre, Efraín Santiago-Rodríguez*, Thalía Harmony, Antonio Fernández-Bouzas

Unidad de Investigación en Neurodesarrollo "Dr. Augusto Fernández Guardiola", Instituto de Neurobiología, Universidad Nacional Autónoma de México (UNAM), Campus Juriquilla, Querétaro, México

Abstract

Background: Approximately 2–4% of newborns with perinatal risk factors present with hearing loss. Our aim was to analyze the effect of hearing aid use on auditory function evaluated based on otoacoustic emissions (OAEs), auditory brain responses (ABRs) and auditory steady state responses (ASSRs) in infants with perinatal brain injury and profound hearing loss.

Methodology/Principal Findings: A prospective, longitudinal study of auditory function in infants with profound hearing loss. Right side hearing before and after hearing aid use was compared with left side hearing (not stimulated and used as control). All infants were subjected to OAE, ABR and ASSR evaluations before and after hearing aid use. The average ABR threshold decreased from 90.0 to 80.0 dB ($p = 0.003$) after six months of hearing aid use. In the left ear, which was used as a control, the ABR threshold decreased from 94.6 to 87.6 dB, which was not significant ($p > 0.05$). In addition, the ASSR threshold in the 4000-Hz frequency decreased from 89 dB to 72 dB ($p = 0.013$) after six months of right ear hearing aid use; the other frequencies in the right ear and all frequencies in the left ear did not show significant differences in any of the measured parameters ($p > 0.05$). OAEs were absent in the baseline test and showed no changes after hearing aid use in the right ear ($p > 0.05$).

Conclusions/Significance: This study provides evidence that early hearing aid use decreases the hearing threshold in ABR and ASSR assessments with no functional modifications in the auditory receptor, as evaluated by OAEs.

Editor: Olivier Baud, Hôpital Robert Debré, France

Funding: This work was sponsored by Programa de Apoyo a Proyectos de Investigación e Innovación Tecnológica (PAPIIT))IN205006-17,Universidad Nacional Autónoma de México (UNAM),México. The funders had no role in study design, data collection and analysis, decision to publish, or preparation of the manuscript.

Competing Interests: The authors have declared that no competing interests exist.

* E-mail: santiagorode@unam.mx

Introduction

Perinatal brain injury (PBI) consists of a large group of conditions that produce mild to severe impairments in motor, visual, auditory and cognitive functions [1,2]. Hearing loss affects 1 to 3 per 1000 normal newborns and 2 to 4 per 100 of infants who require neonatal intensive care [3,4]. Early hearing loss detection can only be achieved with sensitive diagnostic techniques. Ideally, hearing loss screening should be performed before 3 months of age, and an appropriate intervention should be implemented no later than 6 months of age [5].

Currently, the most useful techniques for early hearing loss detection are auditory brainstem responses (ABRs) and otoacoustic emissions (OAEs); however, new techniques such as auditory steady state responses (ASSRs) have been developed. These techniques show high sensitivity for detecting hearing loss in healthy and PBI infants [6–10].

The three techniques mentioned above measure different aspects of auditory function. OAEs evaluate the activity of the cochlear outer hair cells (OHCs) [6]. ABRs assess the conduction properties of pathways from the auditory nerve to the inferior colliculus and can determine auditory threshold. On the other hand, it has been demonstrated that ABRs can only detect frequencies in a narrow range, perhaps between 2000–4000 Hz [11–13].

More recently, auditory steady-state responses (ASSR) have been reported as a reliable and objective technique for evaluating hearing thresholds, with the advantage that several frequency-specific thresholds can be assessed simultaneously, and one frequency-specific audiometry can be obtained [9,14–17].

One treatment for hearing loss is the use of hearing aids (HA), and cochlear implants are employed in selected cases. However, severe and moderate hearing loss may not be identified until the second year of life, and mild hearing loss is usually not detected until the child begins school [18]. After the first year of life, the sensible epochs for language acquisition have elapsed. As a result, the prescription of auditory aids is most useful during the first year of life [19].

Therefore, our aim was to analyze the effects of HA use on auditory function as evaluated by modifications in OAEs, ABRs and ASSRs in a group of infants with PBI and severe, profound hearing loss.

Methods

Infants with PBI attending a specialized neurodevelopment research unit were included in this study. PBI was suspected when an injury that occurred between the 28th week of gestation and 28 days after birth gave rise to abnormal neurological examination and abnormal magnetic resonance image (MRI) findings. All infants underwent a neurological examination in addition to the following evaluations: otoscopy, tympanometry, acoustic stapedial ipsilateral reflex (ASIR), OAEs, ABR, ASSRs and MRI. A total of 13 infants with severe or profound bilateral sensorineural hearing loss were included in this study. The parents of all infants provided written informed consent, and the study was approved by the institutional review board of the Institute of Neurobiology, National Autonomous University of México.

The tympanometry test was carried out using MT10 equipment (Interacocustics, Denmark), with a base frequency of 1000 Hz (high frequency tympanometry), maximum pressure of 200 daPa, minimum pressure of −200 daPa, maximum compliance of 2.00 ml, minimum compliance of 0.00 ml, and a unit gradient in ml. The results were considered normal when the output values were as follows: a compliance of 0.3 to 1.3 ml, a pressure of ±50 daPa, and a unit gradient of 1 to 2 ml. The results were classified according to Jerger's curves as follows: type 'A' (normal compliance and pressure), type 'B' (without compliance peak and abnormal negative pressure), and type 'C' (normal compliance and abnormal negative pressure) [20]. The ASIR test was carried out using MT10 equipment (Interacoustics, Denmark). The ASIR was measured with trains of tone bursts between 70 and 110 dB HL. Frequencies of 500, 1000, 2000, and 4000 Hz were used. The ASIR response was biphasic, with an initial positive plateau followed by a longer negative one. For stimuli below 80 dB HL, the pattern of the reflex was monophasic, with a single positive peak. The presence of this peak was considered as a response, whereas its absence was classified as a lack of a response.

OAEs were elicited with ILO-V6 Otodynamics equipment (Otodynamic Limited, United Kingdom). The test was performed using a probe with two transducers and one microphone. Transient OAEs (TEOAEs) were produced by a brief click (80 μs) with a peak intensity of 80±5 dB SPL at frequencies of 1000, 2000, 3000, 4000, 6000 and 8000 Hz. The stability and sensitivity of this test is between 90 and 100%. In the distortion product OAEs (DPOAEs), the stimuli consisted of two pure tones (F1–F2) of frequencies ranging from 1000 to 8000 Hz, at an intensity of 70 dB SPL. The stimulus, signal to noise ratio, and emission reproducibility were recorded. A response was considered satisfactory when the signal was 5 dB above noise level with a maximum 60 s response time gate.

ABRs and ASSRs were studied in sleeping infants in a soundproof room using the AUDIX system (Neuronic Mexicana, S.A, México City). The ABR test was performed 100 μs monaural rarefaction clicks with intensities between 20 and 100 dB HL (hearing level), with a repetition rate of 11.2 Hz. An average of 2000 stimuli and a sweep time of 15 ms were used. The signal was recorded with an Ag/AgCl electrode disk in Cz with mastoids M1 and M2 as reference; impedance was kept under 5 kOhms in all electrodes. Two channels for ipsi- and contralateral registers were used. Amplifier gain was 100,000, with low-bandpass filters at 100 Hz and high-bandpass filters at 3000 Hz. The latency and amplitude of waves I to V and interpeak latencies I–III, III–V and I–V were obtained. A test was considered normal when the threshold for wave V was 30 dB HL; mild alterations were considered between 40 and 50 dB HL, moderate between 60 and 70 dB HL and severe when the threshold was higher than 80 dB HL.

The ASSR study was carried out with intensities between 20 and 100 dB HL in 5 to 10 dB steps. Stimuli were a combination of five carrier tones: 500, 1000, 2000, 4000 and 8000 Hz modulated in amplitude at rates: 95, 98, 101 and 105 Hz. Electrodes were placed in the mastoids (M1 or M2) as an active channel, and Cz was used as reference. Impedance was kept under 5 kOhms in all electrodes. Amplifier gain was 100,000 with low-cut filters at 10 Hz and high-cut filters at 300 Hz; the analysis period was 1.37 ms, and approximately 24 epochs were averaged. The frequency spectrum was obtained with the Fast Fourier Transform. Each spectral peak was considered as a vector in an X–Y coordinate system, where its length represented the amplitude of the spectral peak. The level of significance between the signal and noise spectral components was determined with Hotelling's T2-test [21]. The significance level for the statistical detection of a signal was $p<0.05$. The ASSR thresholds were analyzed and classified as normal or abnormal by comparison with normal threshold values during the first year of life [22].

Hearing loss severity was evaluated based on calculated with the pure tone average (PTA) [14,23], and was modified for pediatric age [24]. Hearing loss was classified as mild when the PTA threshold increased between 10 and 15 dB HL; moderate when PTA increased between >15 and 40 dB HL; severe when PTA increased between >40 and 60 dB HL, and profound when PTA increased >60 dB HL. When only mild abnormalities were found in one or two frequencies, hearing loss was classified as minimally altered.

Infants with profound hearing loss used a behind the ear (BTE) hearing aid with digital technology in the right ear; the left ear was not stimulated and was used as a control. The digital BTE hearing aid was adjusted with software (Aventa Standalone 2.2 version 2002–2006 GN Resound, U.S.) in 6 frequency bands (250, 500, 100, 2000, 4000 and 6000 Hz), and the maximum gain was established according to the threshold. To adjust the BTE hearing aids to each particular infant, an instant mold was made for the right ear. Indications for the use of BTE hearing aids were 4 to 6 hours a day in comfort program and volume set to 4 (maximum volume). Statistical analyses of the differences between auditory thresholds at the first and second evaluations of the two ears were carried out using Student's t-test for paired samples.

Results

Of the 378 infants evaluated, only 13 (3.4%) presented bilateral sensorineural severe to profound hearing loss. The study group consisted of 7 females and 6 males; 6 premature infants and 7 full-term infants. Premature infants had a gestational age of 35±1.6 weeks and full-term infants 39.2±1.2 weeks. At the first evaluation, the premature mean age was of 4.4±1.4 months, and the full-term mean age was 4.9±1.7 months. Tympanometry tests were carried out in all infants in the study group, and all results were normal (curve type A). The ASIR was absent in all frequencies evaluated.

Otoacoustic Emissions

The TEOAE and DPOAE tests were carried out in all 13 infants. In the basal test, all infants exhibited no response in any of the frequencies. In the second evaluation, after six months of right ear HA use, OAEs showed no significant differences ($p>0.05$) (Figure 1).

Auditory Brain Responses

a) Latencies. In the first evaluation, nine infants (69.2%) exhibited ABRs with mean latency in the right ear as follows: for wave I, 2.66±0.54 ms; wave II, 3.67±1.24 ms; wave III, 5.13±0.98 ms; wave IV, 6.87±0.89 ms; and wave V, 7.36±1.59 ms. Only 4 infants (30.8%) showed an absence of

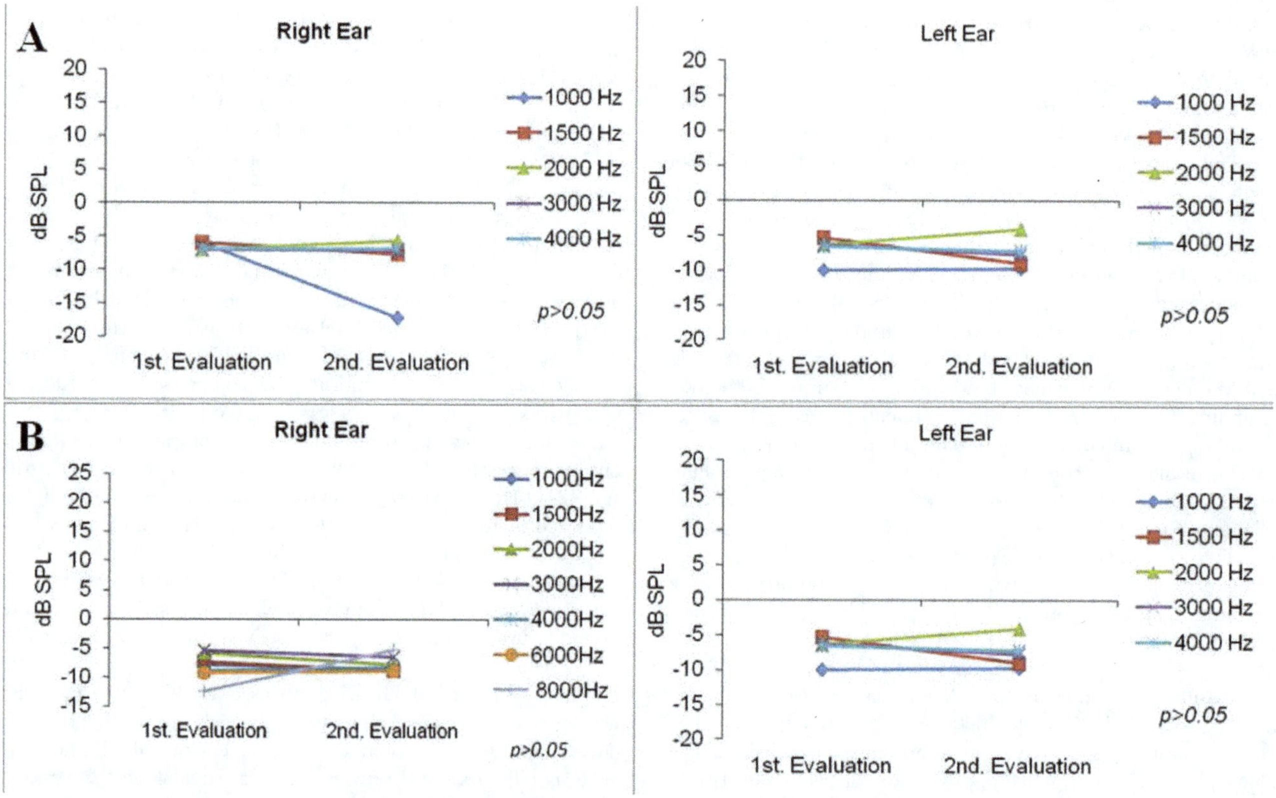

Figure 1. Otoacoustic emissions. (A) Transient otoacoustic emissions values were obtained in both ears at the following frequencies: 1000, 1500, 2000 and 4000 Hz in the first and second evaluations (after using a hearing aid in the right ear). (B) Distortion product otoacoustic emissions values were obtained in both ears at the following frequencies: 1000, 1500, 2000, 3000, 4000, 6000 and 8000 Hz in the first and second evaluations. No significant differences were found ($p>0.05$).

waves I to V when maximum stimulation (100 dB) was applied. In the second evaluation (after right ear HA use), all ABR waves were present in 9 infants (69.2%), and other infants (7.7%) presented waves IV and V; ABRs elicited no response in 3 infants (23.1%). The mean latencies in the right and left ears are shown in Table 1. No significant differences were observed between the right and left sides and between the first and second evaluations in either ear ($p>0.05$).

b) Inter-wave latencies. In the first evaluation, only 9 infants (69.2%) presented waves I, III and V that allowed the assessment of inter-wave latencies. The mean values for the right and left ears are shown in Table 1. There were no significant differences between the first and second evaluations after right ear HA use in any of the control left ears ($p>0.05$).

c) Thresholds. In the first right ear evaluation, wave V was present in 9 infants (69.2%). To calculate the mean threshold, a numerical value of 110 dB was given to the infants with no response at 100 dB. The mean hearing threshold was 90.0±15.8 dB. In the second evaluation after right ear HA use, a significant decrease to 80.0±19.1 dB ($p=0.003$) was observed. In the left ear, 7 infants (53.9%) presented wave V. The mean hearing threshold was 94.6±17.1 dB. In the second evaluation, the threshold decreased to 87.7±17.8 dB ($p=0.069$). However, in the first evaluation of the right side, the ratio of wave V absence in preterm/term infants was one:three. On the left side, the no-

Table 1. Auditory Brain Responses (Latencies).

Ear	Evaluation	Waves					Inter-wave latencies		
		I	II	III	IV	V	I–III	III–V	I–V
Right	First	2.66 (0.54)	3.67 (1.23)	5.13 (0.98)	6.87 (0.89)	7.36 (0.76)	2.25 (0.47)	2.23 (0.63)	4.48 (0.52)
	Second	2.57 (0.34)	3.26 (0.38)	4.87 (0.73)	6.43 (0.61)	7.08 (0.61)	2.30 (0.65)	2.21 (0.71)	4.51 (0.52)
Left	First	2.43 (0.30)	3.15 (0.16)	4.71 (0.61)	6.35 (0.70)	7.15 (0.72)	2.28 (0.74)	2.43 (0.63)	4.71 (0.84)
	Second	2.43 (0.27)	3.02 (0.33)	4.40 (0.32)	6.11 (0.48)	6.80 (0.58)	1.97 (0.74)	2.43 (0.70)	4.40 (0.71)

Mean latencies in milliseconds (standard deviation).
Second evaluation after six months of right ear hearing aid use.
No significant difference between two evaluations and right and left side $p>0.05$.

Table 2. Auditory Brain Responses (Hearing Thresholds).

Subject	GA	First Evaluation		Second Evaluation	
		Right ear	Left ear	Right ear	Left ear
1	31	90	NR 100	70	100
2	36	NR 100	NR 100	80	100
3	36	90	90	80	90
4	40	70	70	70	80
5	31	90	80	80	80
6	42	80	100	80	80
7	39	NR 100	NR 100	NR 100	NR 100
8	38	80	90	70	90
9	38	90	70	70	60
10	41	NR 100	NR 100	NR 100	NR 100
11	33	70	70	50	60
12	32	70	NR 100	60	70
13	38	NR 100	NR 100	NR 100	NR 100
Mean (SD)	36.5(3.7)	90.0* (15.8)	94.6 (17.3)	80.0* (19.1)	87.6 (17.8)

GA = gestational age in weeks.
NR = No Response.
Hearing thresholds in decibels Hearing Level (dB HL).
Second evaluation after six months of hearing aid use (Right Ear).
Right ear, significant difference between two evaluations *$p = 0.003$.
Left ear; no significant differences between two evaluations $p = 0.07$.

response ratio observed was three:three. All infants without a response in the initial evaluation had a response in the second evaluation (Table 2).

Auditory Steady State Responses

In the first evaluation, the mean hearing thresholds for the right ear in the frequencies tested were as follows : 500 Hz, 85.0±16.3 dB; 1000 Hz, 83.5±19.1 dB; 2000 Hz, 84.0±16.1 dB; 4000 Hz, 89.2±17.1 dB; and 8000 Hz, 90.4±15.9 dB. After right ear HA use, the mean thresholds of all frequencies decreased to 75.7±26.9 dB, 77.3±17.9 dB, 75.4±21.6 dB, 72.3±27.1 dB, and 79.6±19.6 dB, respectively. Only one significant decrease in the mean hearing threshold in the 4000 Hz frequency ($p = 0.013$) was found (Table 3). There were no significant differences between the first and second evaluation in any of the measured frequencies ($p > 0.05$) in the left ear (Table 3).

Discussion

The aim of this study was to analyze the effects of early HA use (before six months of age) on auditory function in a group of infants. Main finding of our study is that in infants with PBI and severe to profound hearing loss, the use of a HA decreased the hearing threshold evaluated based on ABR and ASSR tests, with no modifications in auditory receptor function, as assessed based on OAEs.

All the infants in our study presented with severe to profound sensorineural hearing loss without OAEs in the basal evaluation. The causes of hearing loss in our group of infants with PBI were similar to those found in other studies, and included hyperbilirrubinemia, ototoxic antibiotics, and hypoxic-ischemic encephalopathy [25–27]. All these factors affect the cochlear OHCs with mild alterations to inner hair cells (IHCs) [28]. It is known that the absence of OAEs is indicative of OHC damage with mild and moderate hearing loss (30 to 60 dB), but does not indicate hearing threshold alterations. Therefore, it is possible that infants in our study with severe to profound hearing loss presented both OHC and IHC dysfunction, but with enough IHC functionality to maintain residual hearing. This is important because OHC damage characteristically produces increases in hearing threshold and decreases in frequency selectivity [6].

We propose that the preserved function of those IHCs may be sufficient for environmental sounds (with the amplification of the HA) to stimulate the receptor, auditory pathways and auditory cortex. This may also explain why infants with severe to profound hearing loss with total damage to the OHCs and partial damage to the IHCs presented no OAEs, and yet IHC and auditory pathway activation were enough to produce action potentials that allowed ABR and ASSR evaluations. In agreement with this concept, Kempt proposes two types of sensory hearing loss, transmissive and transduction types, depending on the alteration of the OHCs or IHCs, respectively [28].

Auditory pathway properties were evaluated based on ABRs. These responses were present in nine of 13 infants in the initial evaluation; after six months of right ear HA use, the number of infants with ABR responses was the same. However, in the first evaluation of the right side, the proportion of wave V absence in preterm/term infants was one/three, while it was three/three on the left side. Independent of side or prematurity, all infants without a response in the initial evaluation had a response in the second evaluation. This can be explained as an effect of age, which allows for maturation and better myelination of the auditory pathways with the appearance of ABR in the second evaluation.

When the hearing thresholds were compared, the right side decreased 10 dB with no significant changes in the latencies or amplitudes of Waves I to V. In the left ear, no significant decrease in the hearing threshold was observed between the two evaluations. Therefore, we postulated that the effect observed on the right side was due to the six months of HA use. It is possible that hearing pathway maturation has some contribution to this effect, as was observed in the analysis of the proportion of ABR absence.

Although many studies have been carried out to analyze plastic reorganization of auditory cortex after experimental and human hearing loss and subsequent correction with cochlear implants; only a few studies have analyzed the plastic changes of auditory pathways after HA [29–31].

The decrease in hearing threshold observed with ABRs was also found for ASSRs, where the hearing threshold in the 4000 Hz frequency decreased from 89 dB to 72 dB after right ear HA use. This finding is relevant because it is known that the hearing threshold obtained with ABRs only evaluates a narrow frequency spectrum, between 2000 and 4000 Hz. In addition, it has been reported that ABR generators of Wave V are located in the mesencephalic region at the level of the inferior colliculus. Previously published, inconclusive results indicated that ASSR electrical sources might be localized in the brain stem and cortex at the level of left and right supratemporal plane [32].

The decrease in hearing threshold found in both tests but only on the right side after HA use suggests an increase in ABR and ASSR amplitude to the same intensity of the stimulus; the increase in amplitude may be due to an increase in the number of auditory pathway fibers synchronically activated or to an increase in synaptic efficacy in some nuclei of this pathway [18,30].

Experimental models of hearing loss have shown decreases in the number or size of neurons in cochlear nucleus and trapezoid

Table 3. Auditory Steady State Responses (Hearing Thresholds).

	500 Hz				1000 Hz				2000 Hz				4000 Hz				8000 Hz			
	First evaluation		Second evaluation		First evaluation		Second evaluation		First evaluation		Second evaluation		First evaluation		Second evaluation		First evaluation		Second evaluation	
Subject	RE	LE	RE	LE	RE	LE	RE	LE	RE	LE	RE	LE	RE	LE	RE	LE	RE	LE	RE	LE
1	80	100	100	70	100	100	100	90	90	100	80	70	100	100	50	60	100	100	80	100
2	100	100	100	100	70	100	70	50	80	50	100	50	100	100	100	100	100	100	100	100
3	100	100	100	100	90	90	90	90	100	80	100	80	100	50	100	50	100	90	100	90
4	100	100	80	70	100	80	80	90	70	100	70	90	100	90	100	100	60	100	80	100
5	80	100	40	100	60	100	80	85	100	60	50	70	90	90	100	100	100	80	60	100
6	50	90	30	70	90	70	70	30	80	80	90	50	80	50	30	100	60	60	100	100
7	NR	NR	100	100	NR	NR	90	NR	NR	NR	100	100	NR	NR	NR	NR	NR	NR	80	NR
8	75	70	75	70	75	100	75	100	50	80	50	80	60	60	60	60	75	70	75	70
9	70	60	70	40	40	40	80	50	70	70	80	60	50	80	40	50	100	80	100	60
10	NR	NR	100	100	NR	NR	100	90	80	80	100	80	NR	NR	90	90	100	NR	100	NR
11	80	30	30	35	90	80	30	30	70	70	30	40	80	70	30	30	80	70	30	30
12	70	60	80	90	70	60	70	80	100	40	80	100	100	50	80	90	100	60	80	90
13	NR	NR	90	100	NR	NR	70	NR	NR	NR	70	100	NR	NR	80	NR	NR	NR	70	NR
Mean (SD)	85 (16.3)	85.4 (23)	76.5 (26.9)	80.4 (23.3)	83.5 (19.1)	86.2 (19.4)	77.3 (17.9)	75.8 (26.1)	83.8 (16.1)	77.7 (19.6)	76.9 (22.5)	74.6 (20.3)	89.2* (17.1)	80 (21.2)	73.8* (28.1)	79.2 (25.3)	90.4 (15.9)	85.4 (16.1)	81.2 (20.4)	87.7 (21.7)

Hz = Hertz.
RE = Right Ear.
LE = Left Ear.
NR = No Response.
Significant difference between two evaluations $^{*}p = 0.013$.

body [33,34]. Some changes in neuronal morphology have been reported in the superior olivary complex and lateral lemniscus [35]. In other auditory pathway structures, bilateral deafness is required to induce synaptic density changes in the inferior colliculus [36]. Conversely, functional changes have been observed even in unilateral deafness. These changes are relevant to explain the decrease in threshold in our group of infants. In normal hearing animals, cochlear stimulation activates nearly 30% of neurons in the inferior colliculus; this percentage increases to 70% in unilateral deaf adult animals, and 90%, when the cochlear lesion is produced during the neonatal period [37]. In addition, a reduction in temporal neuronal resolution has been observed in neonatal bilateral deafened animals in relation to normal or unilateral deaf animals used as controls.

On the other hand, the maturation pattern of electrically evoked auditory brainstem responses in deaf infants during the first two years after cochlear implant has been compared with the ABR maturation pattern of normal hearing infants [30]. These authors reported a decrease in wave V latency and auditory threshold only when the cochlear implant was adapted to infants with early-onset deafness; infants with late-onset deafness showed no modifications in latencies. They concluded that the modifications in latency and wave V threshold are due to plastic changes in auditory pathways that may include increased myelination or synaptic efficiency. These plastic changes may be similar to those found in our study, where a decrease in wave V threshold in the ABR assessment was present after right ear HA use.

The present study included a small sample size. As a result, the conclusions should be considered with caution. Additionally, compliance with HA use could only be measured indirectly with mothers' self-reports of the duration of HA use.

In conclusion, auditory function in infants is modified after early stimulation with HA before 6 months of age, causing a decrease in the hearing threshold determined based on ABR and ASSR evaluations, with no modifications in auditory receptor function as evaluated based on OAEs.

Acknowledgments

We appreciate the technical assistance and support of David Avila Acosta, Engineers Héctor Belmont Tamayo and Paulina Alvarez García.

Author Contributions

Conceived and designed the experiments: AJM-A ES-R. Performed the experiments: AJM-A ES-R. Analyzed the data: AJM-A ES-R TH AF-B. Contributed reagents/materials/analysis tools: AJM-A AF-B. Wrote the paper: AJM-A ES-R.

References

1. Volpe JJ (1997) Brain injury in the premature infant. Neuropathology, clinical aspects, pathogenesis, and prevention. Clin Perinatol 24: 567–587.
2. du Plessis AJ, Volpe JJ (2002) Perinatal brain injury in the preterm and term newborn. Curr Opin Neurol 15: 151–157.
3. Borg E (1997) Perinatal asphyxia, hypoxia, ischemia and hearing loss. An overview. Scand Audiol 26: 77–91.
4. Davidson J, Hyde ML, Alberti PW (1989) Epidemiologic patterns in childhood hearing loss: a review. Int J Pediatr Otorhinolaryngol 17: 239–266.
5. American Academy of Pediatrics Joint Committee on Infant Hearing (2007) Year 2007 Position Statement: Principles and Guidelines for Early Hearing Detection and Intervention Programs. Pediatrics 120: 898–921.
6. Kemp DT, Ryan S (1991) Otoacoustic emission tests in neonatal screening programmes. Acta Otolaryngol 482: 73–84.
7. Erenberg A, Lemons J, Sia C, Trunkel D, Ziring P (1999) Newborn and infant hearing loss: detection and intervention. American Academy of Pediatrics. Task Force on Newborn and Infant Hearing. Pediatrics 103: 527–530.
8. Norton SJ, Gorga MP, Widen JE, Folsom RC, Sininger Y, et al. (2000) Identification of neonatal hearing impairment: summary and recommendations. Ear Hear 21: 529–535.
9. Pérez-Abalo MC, Savio G, Torres A, Martin V, Rodríguez E, et al. (2001) Steady state responses to multiple amplitude-modulated tones: an optimized method to test frequency-specific thresholds in hearing-impaired children and normal hearing subjects. Ear Hear 22: 200–211.
10. Santiago-Rodríguez E, Harmony T, Bernardino M, Porras-Kattz E, Fernández-Bouzas A, et al. (2005) Auditory steady-state responses in infants with perinatal brain injury. Pediatr Neurol 32: 236–240.
11. Jewett DL, Romano MN, Williston JS (1970) Human auditor y evoked potentials: possible brain stem components detected on the scalp. Science 167: 1517–1518.
12. Picton TW, Hillyard SA, Krausz HI, Galambos R (1974) Human auditory evoked potentials. I. Evaluation of components. Electroencephalogr Clin Neurophysiol 36: 179–190.
13. Hyde ML, Riko K, Malizia K (1990) Audiometric accuracy of the click ABR in infants at risk for hearing loss. J Am Acad Audiol 1: 59–66.
14. Picton TW, Durieux-Smith A, Champagne S, Whittingham J, Moran L, et al. (1998) Objective evaluation of aided thresholds using auditory steady-state responses. J Am Acad Audiol 9: 315–331.
15. Cone-Wesson B, Parker J, Swiderski N, Rickards F (2002) The auditor y steady-state response: full-term and premature neonates. J Am Acad Audiol 13: 260–269.
16. Johns MS, Purcell DW, Dimitrijevic A, Picton TW (2002) Advantages and caveats when recording steady-state responses to multiple simultaneous stimuli. J Am Acad Audiol 13: 246–259.
17. Savio G, Pérez-Abalo MC, Gaya J, Hernández O, Mijares E (2006) Test accuracy and prognostic validity of multiple auditory steady state responses for targeted hearing screening. Int J Audiol 45: 109–120.
18. Eggermont JJ, Ponton CW (2003) Auditory-evoked potential studies of cortical maturation in normal hearing and implanted children: correlations with changes in structure and speech perception. Acta Otolaryngol 123: 249–252.
19. Yoshinaga-Itano C (2003) Early intervention after universal neonatal hearing screening: impact on outcomes. Ment Retard Dev Disabil Res Rev 9: 252–266.
20. Margolis RH, Bass-Ringdahl S, Hanks WD, Holte L, Zapala DA (2003) Tympanometry in newborns infants:1 kHz norms. J Am Acad Audiol 14: 383–392.
21. Valdés JL, Pérez-Abalo MC, Martín V (1997) Comparison of statistical indicators for the automatic detection of 80 Hz auditory steady state responses. Ear Hear 18: 420–429.
22. Savio G, Cárdenas J, Pérez-Abalo M, González A, Valdés J (2001) The low and high frequency auditory steady state responses mature at different rates. Audiol Neurootol 6: 279–287.
23. Ozdek A, Karacay M, Saylam G, Tatar E, Aygener N, Korkmaz MH (2010) Comparison of pure tone audiometry and auditory steady-state responses in subjects with normal hearing and hearing loss. Arch Otorhinolaryngol 267: 43–49
24. Moreno-Aguirre AJ, Santiago-Rodríguez E, Harmony T, Fernández-Bouzas A, Porras-Kattz E (2010) Analysis of auditory function using brainstem auditory evoked potentials and auditory steady state responses in infants with perinatal brain injury. Int J Audiol 49: 110–5.
25. Meyer C, Witte J, Hildmann A, Hennecke KH, Schunck KU, et al. (1999) Neonatal screening for hearing disorders in infants at risk: Incidence, risk factors and follow-up. Pediatrics 104: 900–4.
26. Poblano A, Belmont A, Sosa J, Vargas AM, Limón G, et al. (2003) Amikacin alters auditory brainstem conduction time in newborns. J Perinat Med 31: 237–241.
27. Martínez-Cruz CF, Poblano A, Fernández-Carrocera LA (2008). Risk factors associated with sensorineural hearing loss in infants at the neonatal intensive care unit: 15- year experience at the National Institute of Perinatology (Mexico City). Arch Med Res 39: 686–94.
28. Kemp DT (2002) Otoacoustic emissions, their origin in cochlear function, and use. Br Med Bull 63: 223–241.
29. Pantev C, Dinnesen A, Ross B, Wollbrink A, Knief A (2006) Dynamics of auditory plasticity after cochlear implantation: a longitudinal study. Cereb Cortex 16: 31–36.
30. Thai-Van H, Cozma S, Boutitie F, Disant F, Truy E, et al. (2007) The pattern of auditory brainstem response wave V maturation in cochlear-implanted children. Clin Neurophysiol 118: 676–689.
31. de Villers-Sidani E, Chang EF, Bao S, Merzenich MM (2007) Critical period window for spectral tuning defined in the primary auditory cortex (A1) in the rat. J Neurosci Res 27: 180–189.
32. Herdman AT, Lins O, Van Roon P, Stapells DR, Scherg M, et al. (2002) Intracerebral sources of human auditory steady-state responses. Brain Topogr 15: 69–86.
33. Tierney TS, Rusell FA, Moore DR (1997) Susceptibility of developing cochlear nucleus neurons to deafferentation-induced death abruptly ends just before onset of hearing. J Comp Neurol 378: 295–306.
34. Pasic TR, Moore DR, Rubel EW (1994) Effect of altered neuronal activity on cell size in the medial nucleus of the trapezoid body and ventral cochlear nucleus of the gerbil. J Comp Neurol 348: 111–120.

35. Powell TPS, Erulkar SD (1962) Transneuronal cell degeneration in the auditory relay nuclei of the cat. J Anat 96: 249–268.
36. Hardie NA, Martsi-McClintock A, Aitkin LM, Shepherd RK (1998) Neonatal sensorineural hearing loss affects synaptic density in the auditory midbrain. Neuroreport 9: 2019–22.
37. McAlpine D, Martin RL, Mossop JE, Moore DR (1997) Response properties of neurons in the inferior colliculus of the monaurally deafened ferret to acoustic stimulation of the intact ear. J Neurophysiol 78: 767–79.

9

Categories of Auditory Performance and Speech Intelligibility Ratings of Early-Implanted Children without Speech Training

Huiqun Zhou[1,2], Zhengnong Chen[1,2]*, Haibo Shi[1,2], Yaqin Wu[1,2], Shankai Yin[1,2]*

1 Department of Otolaryngology, Affiliated Sixth People's Hospital to Shanghai Jiao Tong University, Shanghai, China, 2 Otolaryngology Institute, Shanghai Jiao Tong University, Shanghai, China

Abstract

Objective: To assess whether speech therapy can lead to better results for early cochlear implantation (CI) children.

Patients: A cohort of thirty-four congenitally profoundly deaf children who underwent CI before the age of 18 months at the Sixth Hospital affiliated with Shanghai Jiaotong University from January 2005 to July 2008 were included. Nineteen children received speech therapy in rehabilitation centers (ST), whereas the remaining fifteen cases did not (NST), but were exposed to the real world, as are normal hearing children.

Methods: All children were assessed before surgery and at 6, 12, and 24 months after surgery with the Categories of Auditory Performance test (CAP) and the Speech Intelligibility Rating (SIR). Each assessment was given by the same therapist who was blind to the situation of the child at each observation interval. CAP and SIR scores of the groups were compared at each time point.

Results: Our study showed that the auditory performance and speech intelligibility of trained children were almost the same as to those of untrained children with early implantation. The CAP and SIR scores of both groups increased with increased time of implant use during the follow-up period, and at each time point, the median scores of the two groups were about equal.

Conclusions: These results indicate that great communication benefits are achieved by early implantation (<18 months) without routine speech therapy. The results exemplify the importance of enhanced social environments provided by everyday life experience for human brain development and reassure parents considering cochlear implants where speech training is unavailable.

Editor: Joel Snyder, UNLV, United States of America

Funding: This work was supported by the Ministry of Health Sector Fund (grant no. 201202001) and the joint research projects of Shanghai municipal hospitals (grant no. SHDC12010119). The funders had no role in study design, data collection and analysis, decision to publish, or preparation of the manuscript.

Competing Interests: The authors have declared that no competing interests exist.

* E-mail: jassey@126.com (ZC); yinshankai@china.com (SY)

Introduction

Cochlear implantation (CI) already has an established role as a treatment for profound hearing impairment. Candidacy for CI has changed gradually but significantly since the first multichannel devices were implanted in the late 1970s. Increasing experience with CI has resulted in children of younger ages being considered as CI candidates [1,2]. The earliest age of approved cochlear implantation was reduced by the US Food and Drug Administration from 24 months in 1990 to 18 months in 1998 and to 12 months in 2000.

Many factors have been found to affect the outcome of implantation, such as duration of deafness [3], age at onset of deafness and age at implantation [4,5], duration of implant use, length of daily device use [6], and preoperative level of residual hearing [7]. Although not all reports are in agreement on the effects of these variables [8], all appear to agree that earlier implantation produces better outcomes [9]. Most children implanted before the age of 2 years are able to develop speech and language at a rate equal to similarly aged children with normal hearing [10]. More and more children have received cochlear implants before 2 and even at 1 year of age to obtain better results.

Although the overall outcome for patients with cochlear implants has steadily improved with advances in cochlear implant technology, some patients receive little benefit from the latest cochlear implant technology even after many years of daily use of the device. Speech therapy is thought to be important in improving speech-recognition performance. Previous studies had demonstrated the benefits of training in speech-recognition skills of CI users and have shown promising results in adult, postlingually deafened CI recipients. However, access to rehabilitation provided by hospitals and hearing clinics is limited for many hearing-impaired patients due to time constraints, expense, and the proximity of patients to the rehabilitation site [11], which is even more serious for children under 2 years old. Many families considering CI for their children are concerned that the non-availability of speech training or other rehabilitation might make CI ineffective. To assess how important speech therapy in the rehabilitation centers is in children with early implantation, in this study, we compared CAP and SIR results between patients with speech therapy and those without.

Methods

The protocol was approved by ethics committees of Shanghai Jiaotong University. Written informed consent was obtained from parents. The supporting Strobe Checklist is available as supporting information (Table S1).

Thirty-four congenitally profoundly deaf children who underwent CI before the age of 18 months at the Sixth Hospital affiliated with Shanghai Jiaotong University from January, 2005 to July, 2008 were included. These children were totally or almost totally deaf, and did not wear a hearing aid before or after surgery. Children with significant cognitive delay determined by Griffiths' mental development scales (<86) or with cochlear malformations presented by CT scan were excluded. 19 children received routine speech therapy in rehabilitation centers after the surgery (ST), and the remaining 15 cases did not (NST), but were exposed to the real world, as are normal hearing children. Usually, speech therapy begins with an emphasis on auditory training (detection, recognition, discrimination, and perception), followed by speech orthodontic treatment, articulation training, and language training according to the child's performance. Training took place two or three times per week and lasted 6–12 months. All children received the MED-EL COMBI 40+ cochlear implant, and the speech processing strategy during the follow-up period was continuous interleaved sampling.

For the 34 patients, the age at the time of CI ranged from 7 to 18 months (mean = 14.2 months, SD = 2.63). The ages of the children in the ST group ranged from 8 to 18 months (mean = 14.8 months, SD = 2.86), and the ages of the children in the NST group ranged from 7 to 18 months (mean = 13.95 months, SD = 2.98). The difference in age between the two groups was not significant (Student's *t*-test, $P = 0.22$).

The CAP (Table S2) was used to measure the speech perception performance of the implanted children. It measures supraliminal performance, which reflects everyday auditory performance in a more realistic way. The CAP comprises a hierarchical scale of auditory perceptive ability ranging from 0 "displays no awareness of environmental sounds" to 7 "can use the telephone with a familiar talker" [12].

The SIR (Table S3) was used to measure the speech intelligibility of the implanted children by quantifying their everyday spontaneous speech. It is a time-effective global outcome measure of speech intelligibility in real-life situations. SIR consists of five performance categories ranging from "prerecognizable words in spoken language" to "connected speech is intelligible to all listeners" [13].

All children were assessed before surgery and 6, 12, and 24 months after surgery using CAP and SIR. To eliminate test bias, the children enrolled in this study were mixed with other children who were not enrolled, and each child was rated by the same speech and language therapist who was blind to the child's situation and was not allowed to ask for information such as the duration of cochlear implant use and whether the child received speech therapy prior to scoring. The CAP and SIR scores of the groups at each time point were compared using Mann-Whitney rank-sum test, while the percentage of children at level 3 or higher at the four time points between the two groups were compared using Fisher Exact Test.

Results

Comparison of CAP scores of the two groups

The median CAP scores for the two groups are shown in Figure 1. CAP scores in both groups increased with increasing time of implant use during the follow-up period after implantation, and at each time point, the median CAP score of the two groups were comparable. Before implantation, the median CAP score for the ST group was 0, and it increased to 4 at 6 months, 5 at 12 months, and 7 at 24 months after cochlear implantation. An identical change was noted for the median CAP score in the NST group. The median CAP score for that group showed that values increased from 0 at implantation to 3 at 6 months, 5 at 12 months, and 7 at 24 months. The median CAP values of the two groups were not significantly different at any point during the follow-up (Mann-Whitney rank-sum test, $P>0.05$).

The numbers and percentages of children with scores at each CAP level before, at 6 months after, and at 1 and 2 years after CI were calculated. The percentage of children at level 3 or higher increased from 0 before surgery to 73.7%, 89.5%, and 100% at 6, 12, and 24 months after implantation in the ST group, respectively; the percentages were 0 before surgery and 73.3%, 86.7%, and 100% at 6, 12, and 24 months after implantation in the NST group (Table 1). There was no significant difference in scores at the four time points between the ST and NST groups (Fisher Exact Test, P>0.05).

Comparison of SIR scores between the two groups

The median SIR values increased in a manner similar to CAP values in the two groups (Fig. 2). Before CI, the median SIR value of the ST group was 1, and it increased to 2 at 6 months, 3 at 12 months, and 5 at 24 months. For the NST group, the median SIR value was 1 before implantation and it increased to 2 at 6 months, 3 at 12 months, and 5 at 24 months. No significant difference

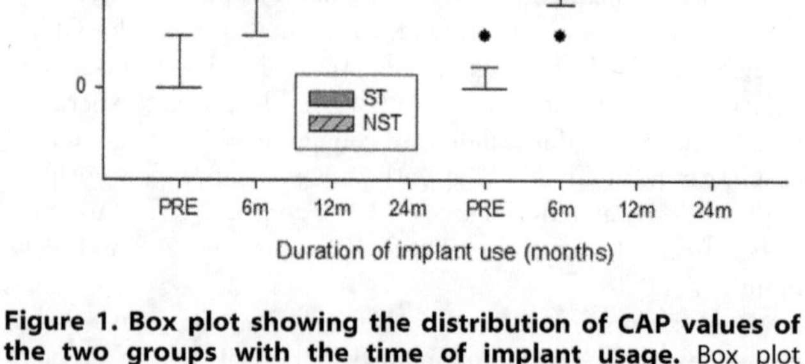

Figure 1. Box plot showing the distribution of CAP values of the two groups with the time of implant usage. Box plot explanation: upper horizontal line of box, 75th percentile; lower horizontal line of box, 25th percentile; horizontal bar within box, median; upper horizontal bar outside box, 90th percentile; lower horizontal bar outside box, 10th percentile. Circles represent outliers.

Table 1. Numbers of patients in each CAP category before implantation, 6, 12, 24 months after implantation.

CAP	Before		6 months		12 months		24 months	
Category	**ST**	**NST**	**ST**	**NST**	**ST**	**NST**	**ST**	**NST**
0	17 (89.5%)	14 (93.3%)	0 (0%)	0 (0%)	0 (0%)	0 (0%)	0 (0%)	0
1	2 (10.5%)	1 (6.7)	2 (10.5%)	1 (6.6%)	0 (0%)	0 (0%)	0 (0%)	0
2	0 (0%)	0 (0%)	3 (15.8%)	3 (20.0%)	2 (10.5%)	2 (13.3%)	0 (0%)	0
3	0 (0%)	0 (0%)	4 (21.1%)	4 (26.7%)	1 (5.3%)	1 (6.7%)	0 (0%)	0
4	0 (0%)	0 (0%)	7 (36.8%)	4 (26.7%)	3 (15.8%)	1 (6.7%)	2 (10.5%)	1 (6.7%)
5	0 (0%)	0 (0%)	3 (15.8%)	3 (20.0%)	5 (26.3%)	6 (40.0%)	2 (10.5%)	2 (13.3%)
6	0 (0%)	0 (0%)	0 (0%)	0 (0%)	6 (31.6%)	4 (26.6%)	5 (26.3%)	4 (26.7%)
7	0 (0%)	0 (0%)	0 (0%)	0 (0%)	2 (10.5%)	1 (6.7%)	10 (52.7%)	8 (53.3%)
Total	19	15	19	15	19	15	19	15

between the groups in median SIR values was observed at any time point during the follow-up period (Mann-Whitney rank-sum test, $P>0.05$).

The numbers and percentages of children with scores at each level of SIR before, at 6 months after, and at 1 and 2 years after CI were calculated (Table 2). In this study, categories 3, 4, and 5 were all defined as intelligible, following a previous study [14]. The percentage increased from 0 before surgery to 47.4% at 6 months, 73.7% at 12 months, and 100% at 24 months after CI in the ST group, whereas in NST group, the percentages were 0 before surgery, 40% at 6 months, 73.3% at 12 months, and 100% at 24 months after CI. There was no significant difference at the four time points between the ST and NST groups (Fisher Exact Test, $P>0.05$).

Discussion

In this study, our results showed that the auditory performance and speech intelligibility of trained children in the rehabilitation centers were almost the same as those of untrained children with early implantation. After implantation, the CAP and SIR scores of both groups increased with increasing time of implant use during the follow-up period, and at each time point, the median scores of the two groups were comparable.

Speech therapy has been shown to be effective in the rehabilitation of patients with cochlear implantation in previous

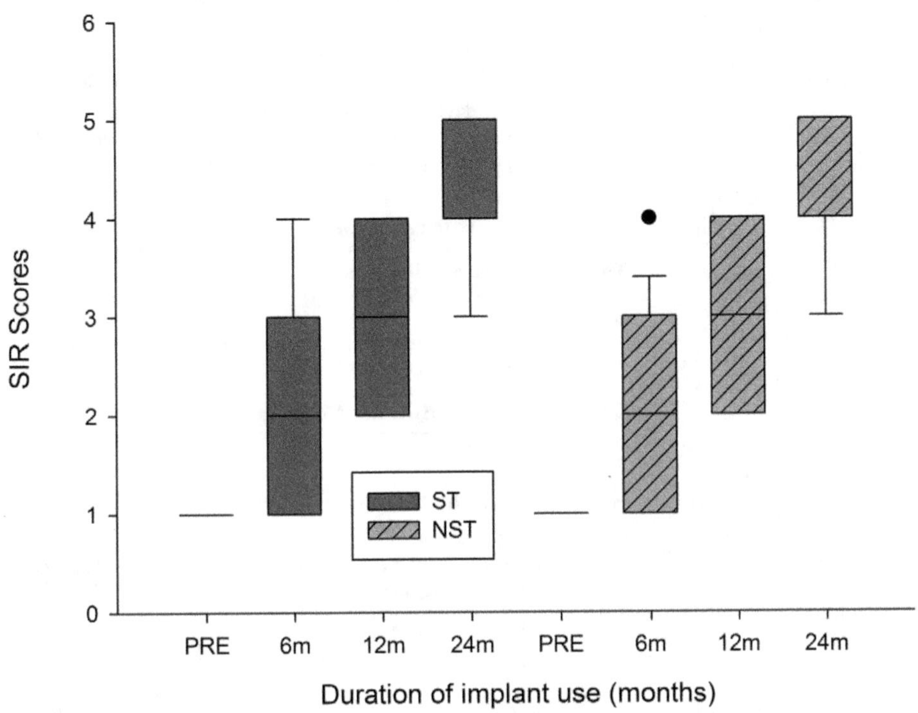

Figure 2. Box plot showing the distribution of SIR values of the two groups with the time of implant usage. Box plot explanation: upper horizontal line of box, 75th percentile; lower horizontal line of box, 25th percentile; horizontal bar within box, median; upper horizontal bar outside box, 90th percentile; lower horizontal bar outside box, 10th percentile. Circles represent outliers.

Table 2. Numbers of patients in each SIR category before implantation, 6, 12, 24 months after implantation.

SIR	Before		6 months		12 months		24 months	
Category	ST	NST	ST	NST	ST	NST	ST	NST
1	19 (100%)	15 (100%)	5 (26.3%)	4 (26.7%)	0 (0%)	0 (0%)	0 (0%)	0 (0%)
2	0 (0%)	0 (0%)	5 (26.3%)	5 (33.3%)	5 (26.3%)	4 (26.7%)	0 (0%)	0 (0%)
3	0 (0%)	0 (0%)	7 (36.9%)	5 (33.3%)	6 (31.6%)	5 (33.3%)	4 (21.1%)	3 (20%)
4	0 (0%)	0 (0%)	2 (10.5%)	1 (6.7%)	8 (42.1%)	6 (40%)	2 (10.5%)	3 (20%)
5	0 (0%)	0 (0%)	0 (0%)	0 (0%)	0 (0%)	0 (0%)	13 (68.4%)	9 (60%)
Total	19	15	19	15	19	15	19	15

studies [15,16]. It has been thought to be one of the methods that can accelerate the learning process because postlingually deafened cochlear implant patients must adapt to both spectrally reduced and spectrally shifted speech due to the limited number of electrodes and the limited length of the electrode array after implantation. Several studies have revealed better auditory resolution, speech perception, and music perception after receiving training [15,16], suggesting great promise as part of the aural rehabilitation of adult, postlingually deafened cochlear implant recipients.

Our results may seem inconsistent with previous studies. However, our negative result was not the only one demonstrating no efficacy in CI patients receiving speech training. Mixed and generally poor outcomes have been revealed from previous CI speech-training studies [17,18]. For example, Dawson and Clark (1997) found that three of five patients showed minimal or no improvement in vowel perception after training [18]. Most authors believe these results were due to training protocols, training materials, and training frequencies used. However, none of these factors has been confirmed, and the exact reason remains unknown.

Some studies have found that earlier implantation leads to better language outcomes, suggesting that there may be sensitive periods for central auditory and spoken language development at a younger age [19,20]. There is considerable evidence for a developmentally sensitive period during which the auditory cortex is highly plastic, although it has not been defined clearly [10,21]. If the auditory system is deprived of sensory input during this sensitive period, then the central auditory system is susceptible to large-scale reorganization. Very early implantation may be necessary to allow at least relatively normal organization of auditory pathways in congenitally deaf children. This might be a potential factor explaining why earlier implantation leads to good results in children even without speech training.

The length of the speech therapy for the children in this study might be insufficient to see results. A previous study reported that the generally poor outcomes of CI speech training patients might well be due to the amount and type of training used [22]. We cannot exclude this possibility. However, many studies that reported marked benefits used training protocols of less than 6 months' duration. Since they focused on adult, postlingually deafened cochlear implant recipients, comparison of these studies and ours was not proper.

The CAP and SIR are non-linear, hierarchical scales, with poor accuracy and little detail [23], and therefore they may not reveal the real conditions in these children. This may be the main limitation of the present study. However, the very young children have not established spoken language skills or the level of behavior and cooperation necessary for a more formal assessment [14]. Therefore, indirect measures may have to be used [23]. Further investigations should be undertaken using more accurate and detailed parameters and should also be conducted over a longer term with more cases. On the other hand, the benefits of ST for the early implantation children were so subtle that they could not be distinguished using real-life situation-based measures, and so might be of little clinical significance.

Conclusions

These results indicate that great communication benefits achieved by early implantation (<18 months) without routine speech therapy, the results exemplify the importance of enhanced social environments provided by everyday life experience for human brain development and reassure parents considering cochlear implants where speech training is unavailable. Further studies should be conducted to confirm our results.

Supporting Information

Table S1 Strobe checklist.

Table S2 Categories of auditory performance.

Table S3 Speech intelligibility ratings.

Author Contributions

Conceived and designed the experiments: CZN YSK. Performed the experiments: ZHQ CZN SHB WYQ YSK. Analyzed the data: ZHQ CZN. Contributed reagents/materials/analysis tools: CZN. Wrote the paper: ZHQ.

References

1. Geers AE (2004) Speech, language, and reading skills after early cochlear implantation. Arch Otolaryngol Head Neck Surg 130: 634–638.
2. Dettman SJ, Pinder D, Briggs RJ, Dowell RC, Leigh JR (2007) Communication development in children who receive the cochlear implant younger than 12 months: risks versus benefits. Ear Hear 28: 11S–18S.
3. Hiraumi H, Tsuji J, Kanemaru S, Fujino K, Ito J (2007) Cochlear implants in post-lingually deafened patients. Acta Otolaryngol Suppl: 17–21.
4. O'Neill C, O'Donoghue GM, Archbold SM, Nikolopoulos TP, Sach T (2002) Variations in gains in auditory performance from pediatric cochlear implantation. Otol Neurotol 23: 44–48.

5. Snik AF, Makhdoum MJ, Vermeulen AM, Brokx JP, van den Broek P (1997) The relation between age at the time of cochlear implantation and long-term speech perception abilities in congenitally deaf subjects. Int J Pediatr Otorhinolaryngol 41: 121–131.
6. Fryauf-Bertschy H, Tyler RS, Kelsay DM, Gantz BJ, Woodworth GG (1997) Cochlear implant use by prelingually deafened children: the influences of age at implant and length of device use. J Speech Lang Hear Res 40: 183–199.
7. Pyman B, Blamey P, Lacy P, Clark G, Dowell R (2000) The development of speech perception in children using cochlear implants: effects of etiologic factors and delayed milestones. Am J Otol 21: 57–61.
8. Geers AE, Nicholas JG, Moog JS (2007) Estimating the Influence of Cochlear Implantation on Language Development in Children. Audiol Med 5: 262–273.
9. Svirsky MA, Robbins AM, Kirk KI, Pisoni DB, Miyamoto RT (2000) Language development in profoundly deaf children with cochlear implants. Psychol Sci 11: 153–158.
10. Moore DR, Shannon RV (2009) Beyond cochlear implants: awakening the deafened brain. Nat Neurosci 12: 686–691.
11. Wu JL, Yang HM, Lin YH, Fu QJ (2007) Effects of computer-assisted speech training on Mandarin-speaking hearing-impaired children. Audiol Neurootol 12: 307–312.
12. Archbold S, Lutman ME, Marshall DH (1995) Categories of Auditory Performance. Ann Otol Rhinol Laryngol Suppl 166: 312–314.
13. Allen MC, Nikolopoulos TP, O'Donoghue GM (1998) Speech intelligibility in children after cochlear implantation. Am J Otol 19: 742–746.
14. Allen C, Nikolopoulos TP, Dyar D, O'Donoghue GM (2001) Reliability of a rating scale for measuring speech intelligibility after pediatric cochlear implantation. Otol Neurotol 22: 631–633.
15. Fu QJ, Galvin JJ III (2008) Maximizing cochlear implant patients' performance with advanced speech training procedures. Hear Res 242: 198–208.
16. Yucel E, Sennaroglu G, Belgin E (2009) The family oriented musical training for children with cochlear implants: speech and musical perception results of two year follow-up. Int J Pediatr Otorhinolaryngol 73: 1043–1052.
17. Busby PA, Roberts SA, Tong YC, Clark GM (1991) Results of speech perception and speech production training for three prelingually deaf patients using a multiple-electrode cochlear implant. Br J Audiol 25: 291–302.
18. Dawson PW, Clark GM (1997) Changes in synthetic and natural vowel perception after specific training for congenitally deafened patients using a multichannel cochlear implant. Ear Hear 18: 488–501.
19. Sharma A, Dorman MF, Kral A (2005) The influence of a sensitive period on central auditory development in children with unilateral and bilateral cochlear implants. Hear Res 203: 134–143.
20. Houston DM, Miyamoto RT (2010) Effects of early auditory experience on word learning and speech perception in deaf children with cochlear implants: implications for sensitive periods of language development. Otol Neurotol 31: 1248–1253.
21. Gilley PM, Sharma A, Dorman MF (2008) Cortical reorganization in children with cochlear implants. Brain Res 1239: 56–65.
22. Fu QJ, Nogaki G, Galvin JJ III (2005) Auditory training with spectrally shifted speech: implications for cochlear implant patient auditory rehabilitation. J Assoc Res Otolaryngol 6: 180–189.
23. Govaerts PJ, De Beukelaer C, Daemers K, De Ceulaer G, Yperman M, et al. (2002) Outcome of cochlear implantation at different ages from 0 to 6 years. Otol Neurotol 23: 885–890.

10

Otitis Media in a New Mouse Model for CHARGE Syndrome with a Deletion in the *Chd7* Gene

Cong Tian[1,2,4], Heping Yu[1,4], Bin Yang[4], Fengchan Han[1,4], Ye Zheng[1], Cynthia F. Bartels[2], Deborah Schelling[2], James E. Arnold[1], Peter C. Scacheri[2], Qing Yin Zheng[1,2,3,4]*

1 Department of Otolaryngology-Head and Neck Surgery, University Hospitals of Cleveland, Case Western Reserve University School of Medicine, Cleveland, Ohio, United States of America, **2** Department of Genetics and Genome Sciences, Case Western Reserve University School of Medicine, Cleveland, Ohio, United States of America, **3** Case Comprehensive Cancer Center, Cleveland, Ohio, United States of America, **4** The Transformative Otology and Neuroscience Center, Binzhou Medical University, Yantai, Shandong Province, China

Abstract

Otitis media is a middle ear disease common in children under three years old. Otitis media can occur in normal individuals with no other symptoms or syndromes, but it is often seen in individuals clinically diagnosed with genetic diseases such as CHARGE syndrome, a complex genetic disease caused by mutation in the *Chd7* gene and characterized by multiple birth defects. Although otitis media is common in human CHARGE syndrome patients, it has not been reported in mouse models of CHARGE syndrome. In this study, we report a mouse model with a spontaneous deletion mutation in the *Chd7* gene and with chronic otitis media of early onset age accompanied by hearing loss. These mice also exhibit morphological alteration in the Eustachian tubes, dysregulation of epithelial proliferation, and decreased density of middle ear cilia. Gene expression profiling revealed up-regulation of *Muc5ac*, *Muc5b* and *Tgf-β1* transcripts, the products of which are involved in mucin production and TGF pathway regulation. This is the first mouse model of CHARGE syndrome reported to show otitis media with effusion and it will be valuable for studying the etiology of otitis media and other symptoms in CHARGE syndrome.

Editor: Xin Zhang, Indiana University School of Medicine, United States of America

Funding: This work was supported by the National Institute of Child Health and Development (R01HD056369 to PCS), the National Human Genome Research Institute (R01HG004722 to PCS) and the National Institute on Deafness and Other Communication Disorders (R01DC009246, R01DC007392, R21DC005846 and Taishan Scholar to QYZ). The funders had no role in study design, data collection and analysis, decision to publish, or preparation of the manuscript.

Competing Interests: The authors have declared that no competing interests exist.

* E-mail: qing.zheng@case.edu

Introduction

Otitis media (OM), inflammation of the middle ear, is the most prevalent disease in children [1]. OM leads to 24 million pediatric office visits and $4 billion in health care costs annually in the United States [2]. The pathogenesis of otitis media is influenced by multiple factors such as exposure to infectious pathogens, Eustachian tube anatomy, immunologic status, genetic predisposition, and innate mucosal defense [3]. The observations of a higher incidence of OM in white infants than in black and Asian infants and of the high incidence of OM in patients with genetic disease, such as CHARGE syndrome studied in this paper, indicate that genetic factors play an important role in development of otitis media [4].

CHARGE syndrome, a multiple congenital anomaly syndrome, has an incidence of approximately 1 in 10,000 individuals globally [5]. CHARGE syndrome is characterized by retarded growth and development as well as abnormalities of the eye, heart, choana, genitalia, and middle and inner ear. [6]. Virtually all individuals with CHARGE syndrome have recurrent otitis media with effusion in their first year of life. Approximately two-thirds of individuals clinically diagnosed with CHARGE syndrome have a mutation in the *Chd7* gene [7], encoding the chromodomain helicase DNA-binding protein 7 (CHD7). Recent evidence suggests that *Chd7* functions as a regulator of genes which play a role in cell-lineage specification in the nucleus and as a positive regulator of rRNA biogenesis in the nucleolus [8,9,10].

Here we present a novel mouse model for CHARGE syndrome with a spontaneous deletion mutation in the *Chd7* gene. This mouse model exhibits a high incidence of otitis media and associated hearing loss together with several other features that are commonly observed in CHARGE patients such as eye abnormality, growth retardation, and balance defects. Otitis media was not reported in any of the previously described animal models for CHARGE syndrome and to date, there are no published studies that have examined the pathogenesis of otitis media in human CHARGE syndrome patients [11]. By further study, we found that Eustachian tube dysfunction, dysregulated epithelial proliferation, and decreased middle ear cilia density can explain the incidence of OM in *Chd7* mutant mice. This mouse model facilitates the study of serous otitis media etiology in CHARGE syndrome patients and helps establish a common pathway for development of otitis media in humans in general.

Results

Circling mice have a deletion mutation in the *Chd7* gene

We identified a spontaneous mouse mutant exhibiting head bobbing and circling behavior transmitted in an autosomal dominant fashion. To determine the chromosomal location of the *Ome* mutation, heterozygous *Ome* mice on the BALB/cByJ background were mated with inbred C57BL/6J mice to generate F1 mice. Those F1 mice that exhibited circling behavior were backcrossed to BALB/cByJ inbred mice to produce N2 mice. Ninety of 180 total N2 progeny were affected. From these 90, genomic DNA was prepared as previously described [12] and genotyped by polymorphic microsatellite marker analysis via agarose electrophoresis, utilizing standard conditions and protocols. The initial genome scan was carried out on pooled DNA samples. After detection of linkage on Chr 4, microsatellite markers *D4Mit149*, *D4Mit235*, *D4Mit181*, *D4Mit18*, *D4Mit1*, *D4Mit292*, and *D4Mit193* were scored on individual DNA samples. Candidate genes localized to the critical region between markers *D4Mit181* (4.23 cM, NCBI Build 37, 9501070–9501202) and *D4Mit18* (6.01 cM, NCBI Build 37, 13937604–13937829) were identified by scanning the Ensembl genome database (Release 62).

Based on these mapping studies, and given that these mice show a remarkably similar phenotype to other mouse models with known mutations in *Chd7*, we hypothesized that these mice harbored a mutation in the *Chd7* gene, and set out to identify the causative mutation. Because most reported *Chd7* mutations are of the nonsense and frameshift type, we first sequenced the mouse *Chd7* gene by conventional Sanger sequencing to identify such a mutation. Several DNA variants were detected between *Ome* and mouse sequence NCBIM37; however, all were predicted to be benign polymorphisms (data not shown) and no difference between *Ome*/+ and littermate +/+. We then tested whether the mice harbored a heterozygous deletion or duplication mutation within the *Chd7* gene, which would have evaded detection by conventional DNA sequencing. To do this, we quantified *Chd7* exon copy number by quantitative PCR (qPCR) of genomic DNA isolated from mutant and wild-type mice. Relatively similar levels of *Chd7* exons 1, 4, 6, 18, and 38 were detected between wild-type and mutant mice (Figure 1A). However, *Chd7* exons 2 and 3 were amplified to levels approximately one-half of those in wild-type mice, consistent with a heterozygous deletion of these two exons. Genomic deletion of *Chd7* exons 2 and 3 resulted in an mRNA transcript with exon 1 aberrantly spliced to exon 4 (Figure 1B, C). The translation initiation codon is located in exon 2, and in silico translation of the aberrant *Chd7* transcript predicts a protein containing a premature stop codon. We therefore conclude that the deletion of *Chd7* exons 2–3 is the causative mutation in these mice, likely resulting in haploinsufficiency of *Chd7*.

Ocular anomalies, growth retardation, and circling behavior in mutant mice

Keratoconjunctivitis sicca was observed in about 60% of the mutant mice (Table 1). Though mutant mice have smaller body size and weight at weaning age (Table 1), their life span is comparable to that of wild-type mice. Mutant breeder males can live at least 12 months until retired from breeding (data not shown). $Chd7^{Ome/+}$ male mice were slightly less fecund than wild type, but most breeding pairs succeeded to generate offspring. $Chd7^{Ome/+}$ mice also showed circling behavior (Video S1) and poor swimming ability (Video S2), which directly indicates a balance defect, compared to a normal swimmer (Video S3).

Hearing deficiency was detected in *Chd7* mutant mice

A time-course observation of the ABR thresholds of $Chd7^{Ome/+}$ and wild-type mice is shown in Figure 2. The results showed that the mean ABR thresholds of $Chd7^{Ome/+}$ mice in each age-group from P21 to P120 (n≥3 at each time point) were significantly higher than those of wild-type mice at all the frequencies tested (Figure 2A). We also performed DPOAE tests over a similar time course and the results showed that mutant mice have amplitudes below zero at every frequency tested from P21 to P120 (n≥3 at each time point), substantially lower than those in wild-type mice (Figure 2B). Tympanometry measurement showed lower compliance values in the mutant mice (Figure 2C), which indicate abnormal middle ear function in the mutant mice. Though the mutant mice with otitis media tended to show cochlear microphonics (CM) responses at higher sound pressure levels compared to responses at lower sound pressure levels in littermate control mice, all the mutant mice (n = 5) did successfully generate CM peaks (Figure 2D).

Otitis media was observed in a majority of $Chd7^{Ome/+}$ mice

To evaluate the incidence rate of otitis media in $Chd7^{Ome/+}$ mice, 12 mice ranging in age from 21 to 77 days were randomly selected for otitis media screening by otoscopic and histological analysis. Of the 12 $Chd7^{Ome/+}$ mice examined, all 12 had effusion in the middle ear space of one or both ears, although the effusion volume varied (Table 2). Figure 3 shows representative images of the histology of $Chd7^{Ome/+}$ mouse ears. Effusion (Figure 3B, E, K), thickened epithelia (Figure 3E, K), a dilated periosteum (Figure 3K), and inflammatory cells (Figure 3L, M) were observed in most of the mutant mice. Effusion with inflammatory cells was also observed in the Eustachian tube opening in the middle ear cavity of most of the mutant mice (Figure 3I). The effusion content was quite variable with respect to quantity of inflammatory cells, which consisted mainly of polymorphonuclear cells (Figure 3L, M). Additionally, in $Chd7^{Ome/+}$ mice, goblet cells were found at higher density among other cells in the epithelium of the middle ear cavity (Figure 4B) and in the Eustachian tube duct (Figure 4D). By contrast, control mice exhibited few goblet cells in comparable sections of the mucosae of the middle ear cavity and Eustachian tube (Figure 4A and C). Hair cells and spiral ganglion cells were normal in both mutant and wild-type mice (Figure 3F, G). We also observed abnormal stapes in the mutant mice (Figure 3C). The head of the stapes in the mutant mouse was shifted toward the anterior crus and the obturator foramen was smaller because of inward growth of the footplate and anterior crus; the footplate was thinner and partially fused with surrounding bones. In studying the middle ear histology of P11 and P15 mice, we found that the onset of otitis media in the *Chd7* mutant mice can be as early as 11 days old (data not shown).

No bacteria known to cause otitis media detected in the mutant or wild-type mice

To assess whether the otitis media with effusion in $Chd7^{Ome/+}$ mice is caused by bacteria, we applied PCR identification [13] and bacterial culture techniques to detect pathogens in the $Chd7^{Ome/+}$ mice and wild-type mice. Three specific primer pairs for the three most common otitis media-associated pathogens were used in a diagnostic PCR reaction [13]. None of the three pathogens (*Streptococcus pneumoniae*, nontypeable *Haemophilus influenzae*, and *Moraxella catarrhalis*) were detected (n = 4 for each group) by diagnostic PCR. Nor were the three pathogens detected in cultures, but comparable levels of *Streptococci* were identified in both mutant and wild-type mice (four mice of each genotype were analyzed).

Decreased epithelial cilia density and increased goblet cell density in middle ears of mutant mice

In the middle ear cavity, the Eustachian tube, and other organs including the lung, cilia function in clearance of normal secretions

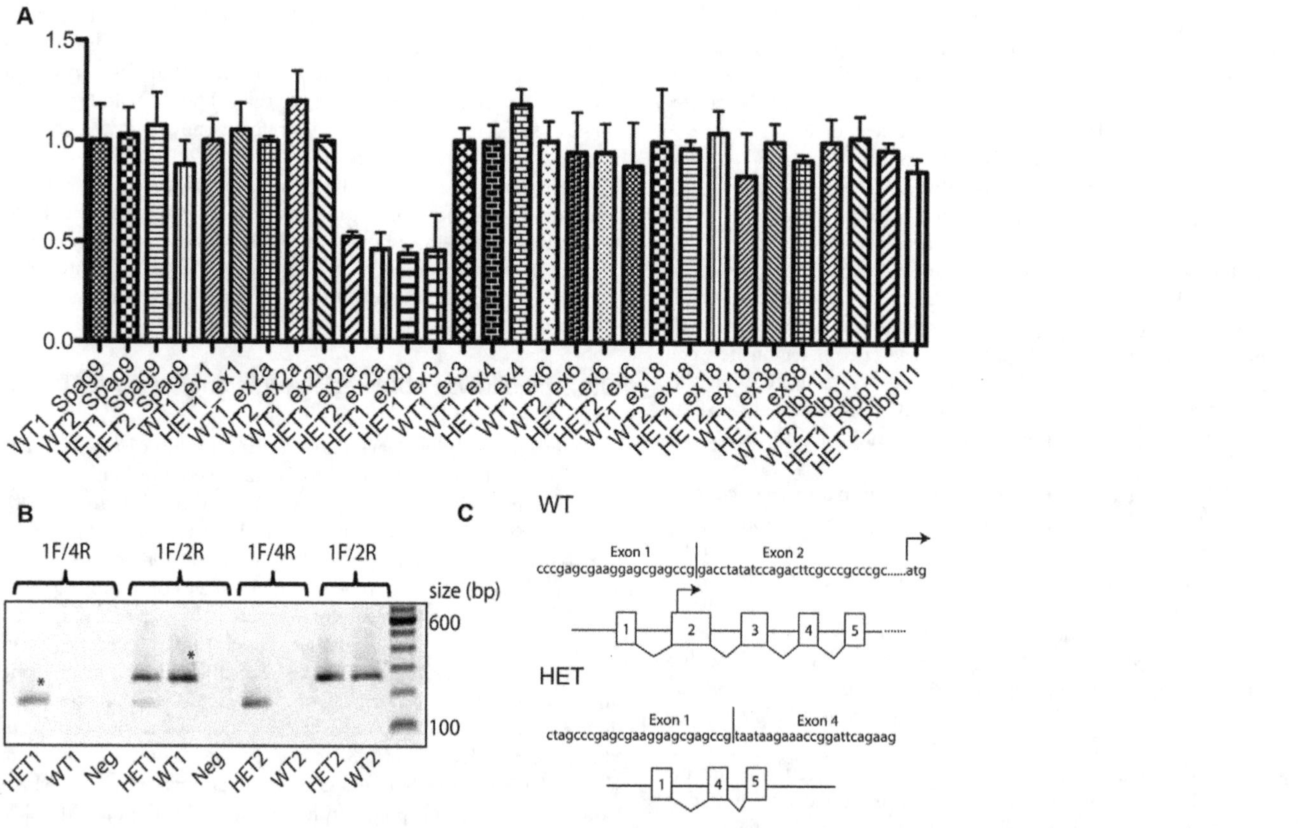

Figure 1. Identification of a heterozygous *Chd7* deletion mutation (*Chd7*$^{Ome/+}$) in circling mice. (**A**) Quantitative PCR analysis of *Chd7* exons 1, 2, 3, 4, 6, 18, and 38 on chromosome 4 using genomic DNA isolated from wild-type (WT1 and WT2) and heterozygous mutant mice (HET1 and HET2). Genomic regions corresponding to the *Spag9* (on Chr 11) gene and the *Rlbp1l1* gene (also known as *Clvs1*; located on Chr 4, downstream of *Chd7*) were also amplified and serve as additional controls. Data were normalized to *Spag9* and the band for this gene was assigned the value of 1.0 (*y* axis). (**B**) qPCR analysis of cDNA generated from wild-type and *Chd7* mutant mouse brain RNA. PCR primers anchored in exons 1 and 4 (1F/4R) yield a positive result only for cDNA from heterozygous mutant mice. This product fails to amplify from wild-type cDNA because of its large size (~2 kb). As expected for a heterozygous deletion mutation, PCR primers anchored in *Chd7* exons 1 and 2 (1F/2R) yield amplicons from both wild-type and mutant samples. "Neg" indicates a non-template control sample. A 100-bp standard was run in the lane near the right edge of the gel. Asterisks indicate bands that were isolated for sequencing in C. (**C**) Partial cDNA sequence of the bands isolated in panel B verifies that the mRNA transcribed from the mutant allele results from aberrant splicing of exons 1 and 4. The translation initiation codon is indicated in exon 2 of the wild-type allele, and has been deleted from the mutant allele.

and abnormal fluids [14]. Patients with impaired ciliary function have increased incidence of otitis media [15]. Using scanning electron microscopy, we assessed the integrity of the mucociliary epithelium in 1-month-old and 12-month-old wild-type and *Chd7*$^{Ome/+}$ mice (n = 3 each genotype). At 1 month, the cilia in mutant mice were indistinguishable in number and morphology from those in wild-type mice, indicating that *Chd7* mutation had no effect on development of the middle ear cilia. However, increased goblet cells and swollen epithelia were observed in the mutant mice despite normal ciliary morphology (Figure 4B, Figure 5B). In 12-month-old mutant mice, rarefied and shortened cilia and a high density of goblet cells were observed in the epithelia (Figure 5D). These results indicate that progressive loss of cilia is associated with otitis media.

Skull measurement reveals abnormalities in mutant mice

Craniofacial abnormalities are observed in CHARGE syndrome patients and are often related to increased OM incidence; thus, skull measurements were performed on age-matched mutant and control mice to detect whether mutant mice differ in skull

Table 1. Phenotype penetration in *Chd7*$^{Ome/+}$ mice.

Phenotype	Indicator	Mutant mice	Wild-type mice
Keratoconjunctivitis sicca	Gross examination	9/15 (60%)	2/16 (12.5%)
Mild growth retardation	Body mass at age P21 (mean)	10.3±2.7g*	12.4±2.0g
Hearing impairment	ABR threshold	10/10 (100%)	1/10 (10%)
Circling/ head bobbing	Gross examination	10/10 (100%)	0/10 (0%)

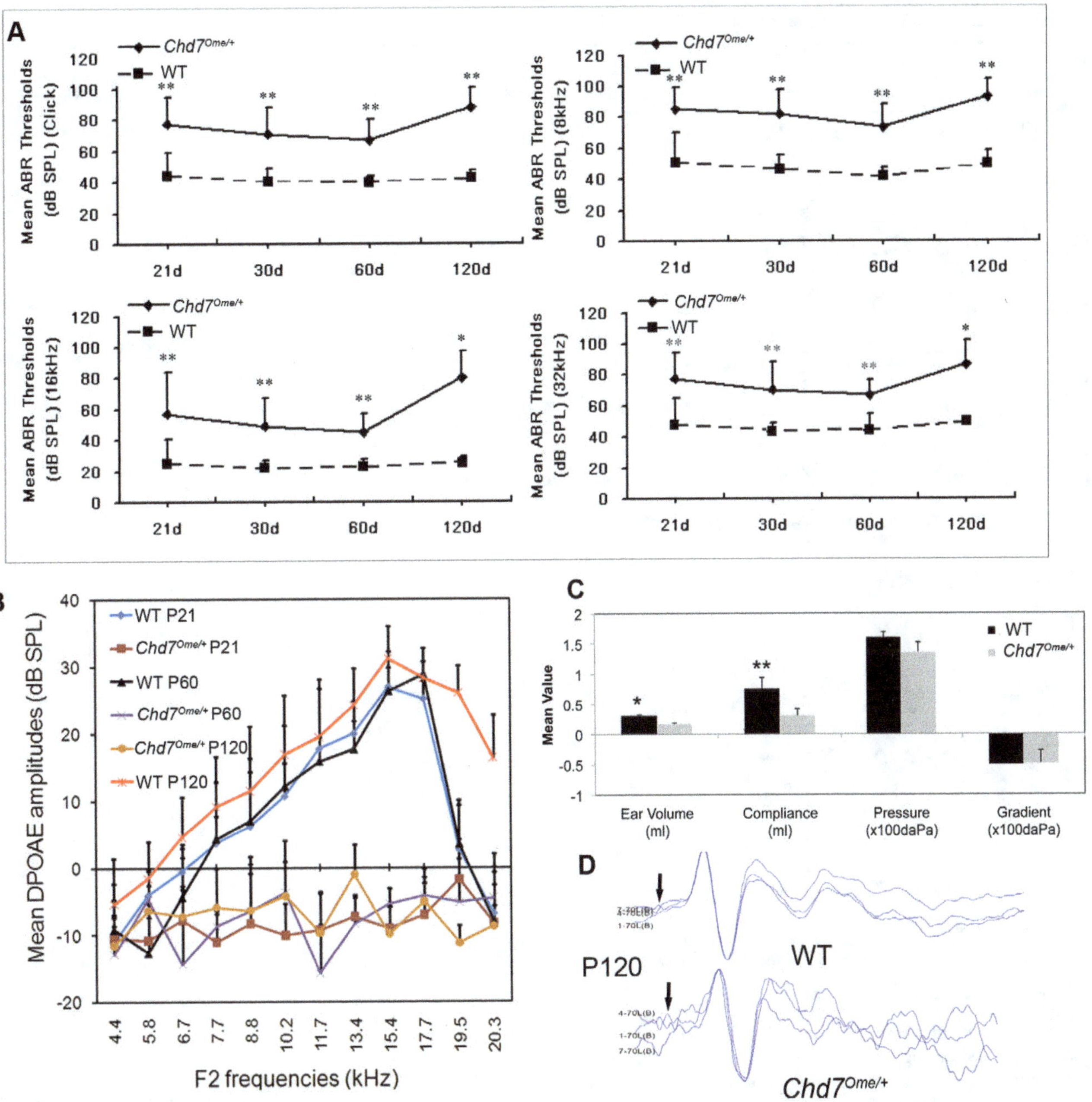

Figure 2. Evaluation of middle and inner ears in *Chd7* mutant and littermate control mice. (**A**) ABR thresholds in *Chd7*$^{Ome/+}$ and *Chd7*$^{+/+}$ littermate mice. *Chd7*$^{Ome/+}$ mice ranging in age from P21 to P120 (n = 13, 13, 7 and 3, respectively, in each age-group) and *Chd7*$^{+/+}$ littermate mice (n = 11, 17, 17 and 4, respectively, in each age-group) were assessed for ABR thresholds at click, 8 kHz, 16 kHz and 32 kHz. Mean ABR thresholds in *Chd7*$^{Ome/+}$ mice were about 20 dB SPL higher than mean thresholds of *Chd7*$^{+/+}$ littermate mice for all the frequencies tested, with significance indicated by asterisks (**P<0.01). (**B**) DPOAE amplitudes in a different set of mutant and wild-type mice at P21 (n = 4), P60 (n = 6) and P120 (n = 6). DPOAE amplitudes of mutant mice were undetectable at all three ages while control mice had normal DPOAE amplitudes. Error bars indicate standard deviation from the mean at each time point, for each mouse group. (**C**) Comparison of the values of tympanometry parameters in the right ears of *Chd7*$^{Ome/+}$ mice (n = 3) and littermate control mice (n = 4) at P90. Mean ear volume and compliance values in the mutant mice were significantly lower than those of littermate control mice (*, P<0.0001; **, P<0.05). (**D**) Both wild-type (WT) and *Chd7*$^{Ome/+}$ mice had normal CM recording, indicating normal inner ear function in the *Chd7* mutant mice even though DPOAE amplitudes were absent (data not shown). CM peaks from left ears of one mutant *Chd7*$^{Ome/+}$ mouse and one littermate control at 70 dB SPL are displayed.

dimension. Mutant mice showed a larger skull height/skull length, larger nose bone length/skull length ratio and a greater Eustachian tube angle when compared to littermate control mice (Figure 6), indicating craniofacial abnormalities in *Chd7* mutant mice.

Chd7 postnatal expression and cytokine expression in the middle ear

Studies have shown that *Chd7* is widely expressed during murine and human embryonic development [16,17]. Recently, *Chd7* was found to be expressed in the developing human and mouse

Table 2. Semi-quantitative evaluation of middle ear inflammation in $Chd7^{Ome/+}$ mice

Mouse	ID	Age	Effusion	Inflammatory cells	Tissue debris	Tissue proliferation
Wild type	1	22d	-	-	-	-
	2	27d	-	-	-	+
	3	29d	-	-	-	-
	4	31d	-	-	-	-
	5	31d	-	-	-	-
	6	35d	-	-	-	+
	7	35d	+	+	-	+
	8	35d	+	-	-	+
	9	35d	+	+	+	+
	10	35d	-	-	-	-
	11	37d	-	-	-	-
	12	77d	-	-	-	-
	13	77d	-	-	-	-
	14	77d	-	-	-	-
	15	77d	-	-	-	-
	16	77d	+	-	-	-
Mutant	1	21d	+++	++	++	++
	2	22d	+++	+	+	+++
	3	22d	++	+	+	+++
	4	22d	+	+	+	++
	5	22d	+++	++	++	+++
	6	27d	+++	++	++	+++
	7	33d	+	+	+	+++
	8	37d	+	+	+	+++
	9	37d	+	+	+	+++
	10	41d	+++	++	+	++
	11	61d	+++	++	+	+++
	12	77d	++	++	-	++

Mice from 21 to 77 days of age were used because of the early onset of otitis media in the mutant mice. Scoring system is described in the methods section. The total scored rate (85/144) of the four indicators in $Chd7^{Ome/+}$ mice was significantly higher than that (12/240) of the wild-type mice ($P<0.01$, chi-square test).

olfactory bulb and olfactory epithelium [18,19]. To detect whether *Chd7* is expressed during development of the middle ear cavity and whether this expression may be related to the incidence of otitis media, postnatal wild-type mouse tissues were stained with anti-*Chd7* antibody. Immunohistochemical staining revealed expression of the *Chd7* protein in the middle ear epithelia and in the inner ear organ of Corti, limbus, and spiral ganglion cells (Figure 7A–E). We also investigated the expression levels of *Muc5a*, *Muc5b*, *Tgf-β1* and *Tlr2* genes which have been reported to be involved in the development of otitis media and inflammation. Total RNA was generated from middle ear tissue of equal mass from mutant and wild-type littermate control mice (all were 2 months old). cDNA was synthesized by reverse transcription for semi-quantitative RT-PCR to profile the gene expression levels. Our study showed elevated expression levels of *Muc5a*, *Muc5b* and *Tgf-β1* in the mutant middle ears compared to that in wild-type samples (Figure 8). *Chd7* (detected with primers *Chd7F* and *Chd7R*) and *Tlr2* (detected with primers *Tlr2F* and *Tlr2R*) genes were expressed in mouse ears, but transcription levels varied both in mutants and in wild-type littermate controls and did not show significant differences between the two genotypes (N = 8, data not shown).

Discussion

Here we report the first spontaneous deletion mutation in the *Chd7* gene in mice. The phenotype and dominant inheritance of *Ome* mice are similar to those of mice with ENU mutagenesis-induced point mutations in the *Chd7* gene [19], including dizzy (*Dz*), eddy (*Edy*), and cyclone (*Cy*), and the unproven alleles wheels (*Whl*) and wheels-like (*Whll*). We report hearing loss in the $Chd7^{Ome}$ mutant mice and we provide evidence that otitis media is the major cause of hearing loss in this mouse model. The $Chd7^{Ome/+}$ mice also presented ocular abnormalities, balance defects, and growth retardation, all of which are consistent with the symptoms of human CHARGE syndrome patients and previously reported animal models for CHARGE syndrome [18,19,20,21,22,23].

Hearing loss was observed in the $Chd7^{Ome/+}$ mutant mice starting from the age of weaning, and this loss was relatively stable over time. At younger ages (1–2 months old), the inner ears of the *Chd7* mutant mice appeared normal compared to littermate controls. There was very little hair cell loss; the density of spiral ganglion cells was comparable to that in the control mice, and no stereocilia loss was evident at this stage. However, in the middle ear, both effusion and thickened epithelia were observed in most of

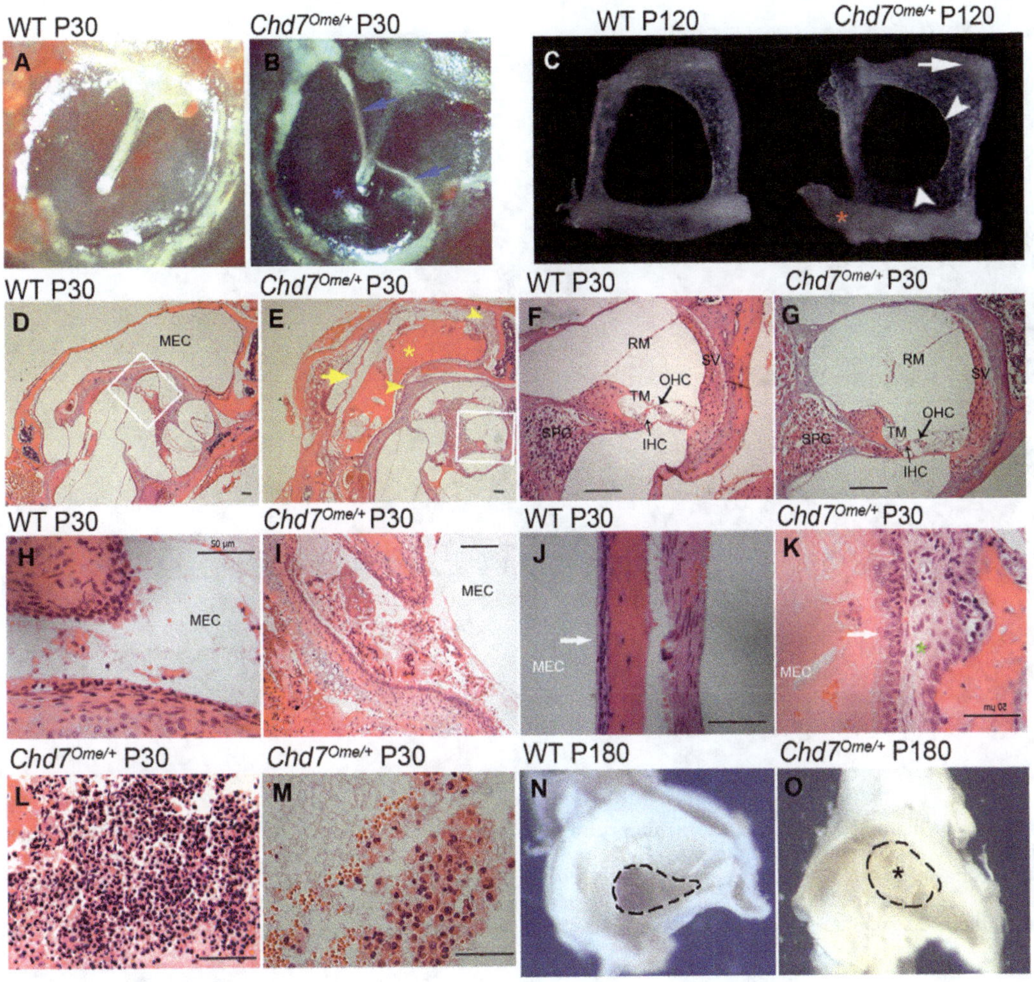

Figure 3. Middle ear and inner ear histology in *$Chd7^{Ome/+}$* mice. (**A–B**) Effusion (blue arrows) and tympanic membrane retraction (blue asterisk) can be seen in the mutant mice. (**C**) In the mutant mice, the head of the stapes is moved toward the anterior crus (white arrow); the obturator foramen is smaller because of inward growth of the footplate and anterior crus (white arrowheads); the footplate is thinner and partially fused with surrounding bones (red asterisk). (**D–E**) In mutant mice, effusion was evident with a small amount of inflammatory cells (yellow asterisk); the tympanic membrane (yellow arrow), middle ear epithelia (upper right yellow arrowhead) and round window ridge (central yellow arrowhead) were thickened. (**F–G**) Enlarged images from corresponding control and mutant mice (white rectangles in D and E) to show the inner ear morphology; SV, stria vascularis; RM, Reissner's membrane; TM, tectorial membrane; IHC, inner hair cell; OHC, outer hair cell; SPG, spiral ganglion neuron. (**H–I**) Eustachian tube openings in the control and mutant mice. MEC, middle ear cavity. (**J–K**) Dilated periostea (green asterisk) and thickened epithelia (white arrows) were observed in the mutant mice. (**L–M**) Inflammatory cells in the MEC of mutant mice. (**N–O**) Eustachian tube openings in six-month-old mutant mice and littermate control mice. Scale bars: D, E, F, G, I = 100 µm; H, J, K, L, M = 50 µm.

the mutant mice. Therefore, conductive hearing loss was dominant at this stage, which was also confirmed by the absence of DPOAE amplitudes in mutant mice. At an older age (7 months old), mutant mice observed by SEM exhibited hair-cell bundle loss from the cochlear basal turn, and this loss may have been caused by middle ear infection. At this stage, otitis media with effusion was predominant in the mutant mice; thus, mixed hearing loss caused by a combination of otitis media and stereocilia loss was dominant, in contrast to the earlier time point. Combining the results of histological and electrophysiological study, we conclude that hearing loss in the *Chd7* mutant mice is primarily caused by otitis media.

Otitis media is a multifactorial disease in which pathogenesis is affected by Eustachian tube structure and function, host immune status, innate mucosal defense, pathogen virulence, and strain and genetic susceptibility loci [3,24]. Any genetic deficiency that influences one or more of these factors can promote susceptibility to otitis media. *$Tlr2^{-/-}$* mice are more vulnerable to the challenge of gram-positive bacterium *S. pneumoniae* because of impaired bacterial clearance ability that leads to acute otitis media in this model [25]. *Eya4*-deficiency leads to Eustachian tube dysfunction and renders the mice susceptible to otitis media [2]. C3H/HeJ mice with a missense mutation in the *Tlr4* gene have a retarded response to endotoxin and an increased susceptibility to otitis media [26]. *Evi1*-null mice exhibited increased susceptibility to otitis media, caused by impaired transcriptional regulation of mucin genes in neutrophils through a TGF-β/SMAD signaling pathway [1]. Mutations in the *Fbxo11* gene discovered in *Jeff* mice lead to impaired regulation of TGF-β signaling and associated craniofacial abnormalities and thus cause impaired inflammatory responses in the middle ear [27,28,29]. In our study of *Chd7*-deficient mice, we found that abnormal Eustachian tube structure and function, dysregulated epithelial proliferation and decreased

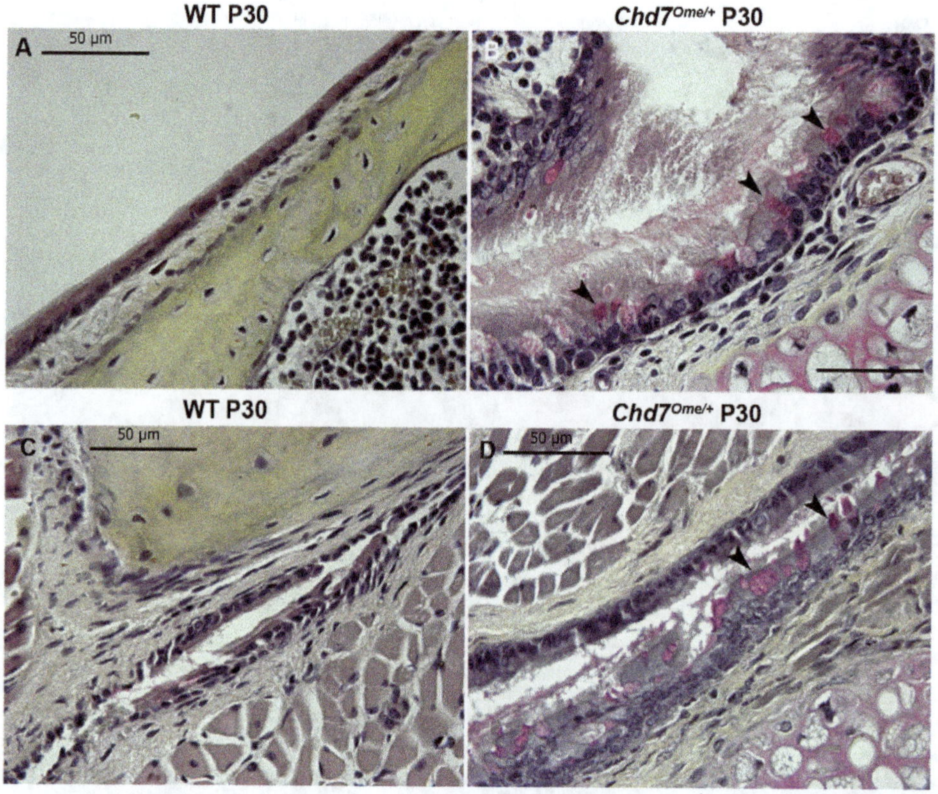

Figure 4. Representative sections of the middle ear and Eustachian tube mucosae of *Chd7*$^{+/+}$ and *Chd7*$^{Ome/+}$ littermates. Few goblet cells could be found in the middle ear (**A**) and Eustachian tube mucosae (**C**) of *Chd7*$^{+/+}$ littermate mice. By contrast, goblet cells were present at high density among other cells in the epithelium of the middle ear cavity (**B**) and the duct of the Eustachian tube (**D**) of *Chd7*$^{Ome/+}$ mice (typical goblet cells are indicated by arrows). Goblet cells have a distinctly polarized morphology in which the nucleus stains black in color at the cell base, and the mucus stains a deep rose color in the middle and apical portions of the cell. Scale bars = 50 μm.

middle ear cilia density rendered these mice susceptible to otitis media with effusion.

The Eustachian tube performs critical functions affecting the middle ear in regulation of pressure, protection from nasopharyngeal secretions and other foreign material, and clearance of middle ear secretions [30]. Craniofacial abnormalities are often related to structural and functional changes in the Eustachian tube, thus increasing susceptibility to otitis media [29]. Our study shows that when compared to wild-type control mice, *Chd7* mutant mice have abnormal skulls and Eustachian tubes of altered shape and larger tube angle, indicating possible Eustachian tube dysfunction. Further histological analysis of the middle ear cavity from mutant mice revealed a narrow Eustachian tube lumen caused by epithelial proliferation and a high density of goblet cells which together lead to increased mucus. These features are evidence of impaired structure and function of the Eustachian tube in mutant mice, and such changes would mechanically impede clearance of secretions in the middle ear cavity, therefore rendering the mice more susceptible to recurrent otitis media.

In addition to impaired Eustachian tube function, mucosal hyperplasia is a major feature of otitis media, contributing to symptoms and causing irreversible middle ear disease [31]. Middle ears of the mutant and wild-type mice examined by H&E staining indicated that 100% of the mutant mice had moderate to severe epithelial hyperplasia with or without effusion from as early as P11, while middle ear cavities (MECs) of wild-type mice were clear and showed no abnormalities of MEC epithelial layers. Immunohistochemical staining of middle ears from young postnatal mice indicated postnatal *Chd7* expression in the MEC epithelia during middle ear cavitation. Early onset of otitis media confirmed that middle ear epithelia dysmorphology corresponded to developmental expression of *Chd7*. In the mucociliary (respiratory) type of epithelium of the middle ear cavity, there are numerous mucin-secreting cells [32]. Mucins secreted by these cells play an important role in several processes that are crucial for the protection and function of the underlying epithelium. These processes include mechanical protection of the epithelium, mucociliary clearance of pathogens and particulate matter, antigen presentation, and prevention of pathogen adherence and host invasion [32]. These mucins interact with pathogens and protect the underlying epithelium from invasion and mechanical damage.

Effusion was seen in most *Chd7*$^{Ome/+}$ ears but the amount and composition of the effusions varied with age. At early ages, most effusion was aqueous with very few inflammatory cells. Excessive effusion, even without inflammatory cells, can impede mucociliary clearance leading to mucostasis and associated hearing loss. Especially when epithelial proliferation is severe, impaired epithelial function and consequent diminished ciliary density make this process irreversible, thus causing chronic otitis media with effusion.

Immunodeficiency has been reported in CHARGE syndrome patients and is characterized by hypogammaglobulinemia, IgG2 subclass deficiency, impaired specific antibody responses, and T-B cell and/or natural killer cell defects [33,34,35,36]. Bacterial culture indicated comparable bacteria levels in *Chd7* mutant mice and wild-type mice. Impaired immunity in the mutant mice could

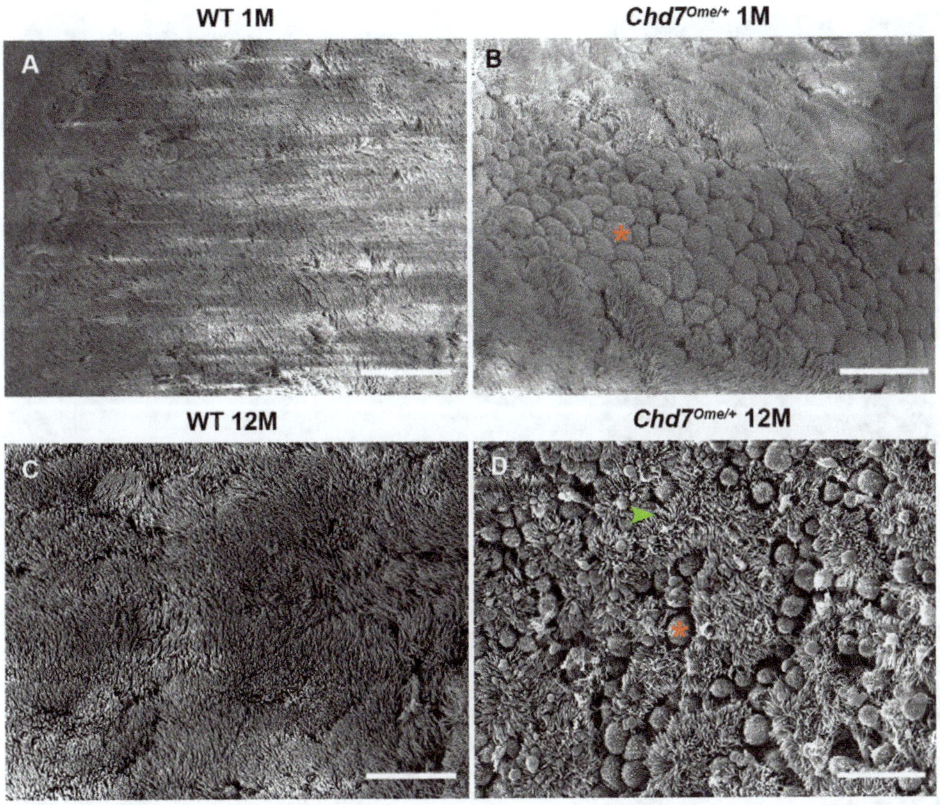

Figure 5. Scanning electron micrographs of middle ear cavities of *Chd7*$^{Ome/+}$ mice and littermate control mice. (**A, B**) Lateral views of Eustachian tube ostium epithelia in 1-month-old wild-type (**A**) and *Chd7*$^{Ome/+}$ (**B**) mice show increased goblet cells in *Chd7*$^{Ome/+}$ mice while ciliary morphology is indistinguishable from that in wild-type mice. Red asterisk identifies one of many goblet cells. (**C, D**) Rarefied cilia (green arrowhead) and scattered goblet cells (red asterisk) were observed in the mucociliary epithelia at the Eustachian tube ostia of 12-month-old *Chd7*$^{Ome/+}$ mice (**D**), while the cilia in age-matched wild-type mice (**C**) appeared normal. Scale bars = 15 μm.

explain the infections in middle ears of mutant mice in the presence of bacteria flora.

In previously reported mouse models for otitis media, expression of the mucin gene family [37,38] and the TGF signaling pathway [27] were affected. In this study, we profiled the expression levels of *Muc5ac* and *Muc5b* and *Tgf-β1* genes. Mucins are heavily glycosylated proteins that are considered primarily responsible for the gel-like characteristics of mucoid middle ear fluids. To date, 18 human mucin genes coding for mucin glycoproteins have been identified [39]. MUC5AC, MUC5B, and MUC2 are the key molecules that determine the properties of airway mucus gel [40]. These proteins participate in protecting the underlying middle ear epithelium from pathogen invasion and pathogen damage and assist with pathogen clearance. However, overproduction of these mucins can lead to increased viscosity of middle ear fluids, limited mucociliary clearance, and eventual mucin accumulation in the middle ear, ultimately leading to hearing loss. TGF-β1 is an important immunoregulatory mediator and participates in the middle ear inflammatory response and in other processes including apoptosis and tissue proliferation. Our discovery that mucin genes and TGF-β1 in the middle ear are upregulated is consistent with findings in human chronic otitis media patients [37,38,41]. These findings further support the *Chd7*$^{Ome/+}$ mutant mice as an ideal model to study the genetic pathways involved in human chronic otitis media. *Tlr2* gene expression was not significantly different between *Chd7*$^{Ome/+}$ mutant and control mice, suggesting that *Tlr2* is less involved in this chronic OM process. This result is consistent with the fact that no pathogenic bacteria were identified in this mutant though comparable levels of *Streptococci* were identified in both mutant and wild-type mice. In contrast, the TLR2-mediated immune response is significantly involved in *S. pneumoniae*-induced acute otitis media [25]. *Chd7* was expressed in mouse ears, which suggests that *Chd7* plays a direct role in ear development and ear disease processes including OM. *Chd7* transcript levels were not found to be significantly different between wildtype and *Chd7*$^{Ome/+}$ mutant mice, suggesting that the presence of the deletion mutation does not necessarily lead to non-sense mediated mRNA decay. However, due to a premature stop codon in the mutant transcript, the CHD7 protein level in heterozygous mice is predicted to be half that of the +/+ mice, and this haploinsufficiency of *Chd7* would lead to otitis media and other phenotypes.

Chd7$^{Ome/+}$ mice are a valuable model for human CHARGE syndrome because of a series of phenotypes that mimic human symptoms, including growth retardation, balance defects, otitis media, and hearing loss. Otitis media in *Chd7*$^{Ome/+}$ mice is characterized by Eustachian tube dysfunction, epithelial hyperplasia, middle ear effusion and associated hearing loss. All of these typical otitis media features make *Chd7*$^{Ome/+}$ mice a useful model for human otitis media. Further study of *Chd7*-associated genes that influence morphology and physiology of middle ear epithelia and the Eustachian tube may indicate new pathways with therapeutic potential for CHARGE syndrome and human otitis media.

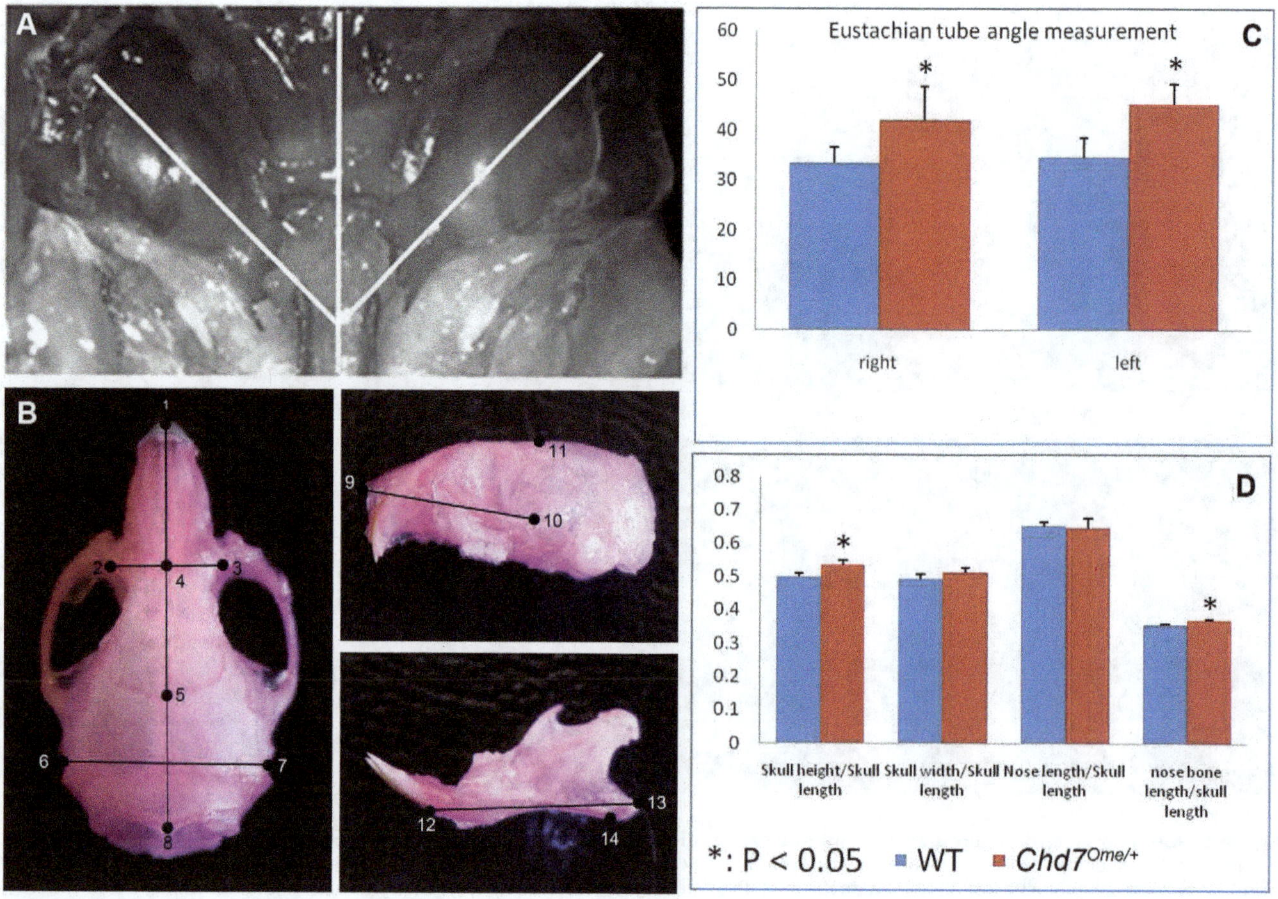

Figure 6. Skull and Eustachian tube measurement of *Chd7* mutant mice and littermate control mice. (**A, B**) Schematic diagrams superimposed on dissected skulls indicate the measured Eustachian tube angles (**A**) and skull dimensions (**B**). (**C, D**) Quantitative evaluation of the Eustachian tube angles and the skull dimensions in mutant and littermate control mice. Mutant mice have larger Eustachian tube angles of both ears than do the littermate control mice. Skull measurements indicated a greater skull height/skull length and nose bone length/skull length ratio in the mutant mice compared to littermate control mice.

Materials and Methods

Mice

Mice exhibiting head bobbling/circling behavior and with otitis media and eye defects (Ome mice) were first observed in at The Jackson Laboratory (JAX, Bar Harbor, Maine), then imported to Case Western Reserve University. Mating of an affected $Chd7^{Ome/+}$ male to a BALB/cByJ female revealed an autosomal dominant mode of inheritance. The mutant from a BALB/cByJ X CAST/Ei hybrid was backrossed 10 times to the BALB/cByJ background. Because circling females were not good breeders, mating pairs were usually arranged with a heterozygous male and a wild-type female. Mice were housed in ventilated racks at 21°C in a 12 h light–dark cycle with food and water given *ad libitum*. All animal protocols (R01DC009246, R01DC007392 and R21DC005846) were approved by the Institutional Animal Care and Use Committee of Case Western Reserve University.

Sequencing and Genotyping

We sequenced genomic DNA, amplifying each exon of all the 40 exons of the *Chd7* gene (or two exons when they were near each other) separately by standard PCR, then performed Sanger sequencing using BigDye Terminator v3.1 Cycle Sequencing chemistry (ABI) and gave the reactions to the sequencing core for electrophoresis on an ABI 3730 DNA Analyzer. Primer pairs (data not shown) flanking each exon are designed according mouse genomic sequence (NCBIM37) Chromosome 4: 8,617,553–8,794,806 forward strand (Chd7 ENSMUSG00000041235). No DNA sequence difference was detected between Ome/+ and +/+ mice. Then, we performed the real-time PCRs with genomic and cDNA (using SYBR green PCR mix (Applied Biosystems) in an Applied Biosystems 7300 Real-Time PCR system) to compare quantitive DNA differences between Ome/+ and +/+ mice. Then we sequenced cDNA only to show that exon 1 was spliced to exon 4.

Because the precise location of the mutation is unknown, RT-PCR was used to genotype the mice. Primers anchored in exons 1 and 4 yield a 150-bp band for cDNA made from the heterozygous mice. These primers do not amplify a detectable product from wild-type cDNA under standard PCR conditions because of the product's large size (~2 kb). Briefly, total RNA was prepared from the whole ear using the PureLink™ Micro-to-Midi™ Total RNA Purification System (Invitrogen). From each sample, 2 μg of total RNA template were used to synthesize cDNA using a SuperScript First-Strand Synthesis System. 1 μl of cDNA from each sample was subjected to PCR amplification in a Bio-Rad PTC-200 Peltier thermal cycler. Heterozygous mice were genotyped by detecting a truncated allele using a forward primer (1F, 5′-ctgactagcccgagcgaaggag-3′) and a reverse primer (4R, 5′-tggacacctgggtcttcgtc-3′) to

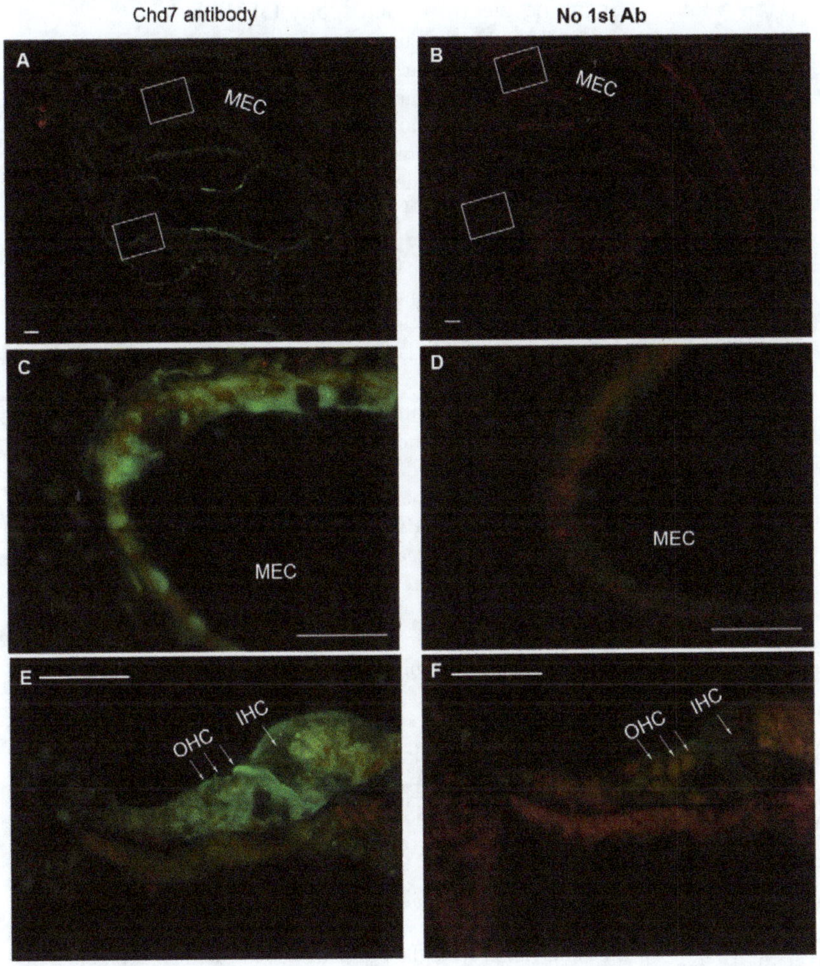

Figure 7. Immunohistochemical staining of *Chd7* protein in the developing middle ear. CHD7, revealed by green fluorescence, is expressed in the middle ear epithelium (**A, C**) and in the organ of Corti (**A, E**) in the inner ear of a wild-type mouse. MEC, middle ear cavity; IHC, inner hair cell; OHC, outer hair cell. Scale bars: A = 50 μm.

yield a ~150-bp band (Fig. 1). A second reverse primer (2R, 5′-cagactcccatcctcgccaaaaa-3′) anchored in exon 2 was used as positive control for the wild-type allele. Amplification conditions were 94 °C for 2 min; followed by 28 cycles of 94 °C for 30 s, 60 °C for 40 s and 72 °C for 50 s; followed by 5 min at 72 °C. Ten μl of the PCR products were subject to 2% agarose gel electrophoresis.

Comprehensive evaluation of hearing loss in *Chd7* mutant mice

Hearing was evaluated in anesthetized (Avertin, 0.5 mg/g mouse mass) wild-type and $Chd7^{Ome/+}$ mice by using auditory brainstem response (ABR, measures auditory nerve and brainstem pathways involved in hearing), distortion product otoacoustic emissions (DPOAE, measures outer hair-cell function and predicts conductive hearing loss [42]), and tympanometry (measures tympanic membrane and ossicle chain function). A computer-aided evoked potential system (Intelligent Hearing Systems) was used to measure mouse ABR thresholds and DPOAE amplitudes as previously described [42,43]. An Race Car tympanometer from Maico Diagnostics (Eden Prairie, MN, USA) was used to examine the tympaniogram following the procedures described previously [44].

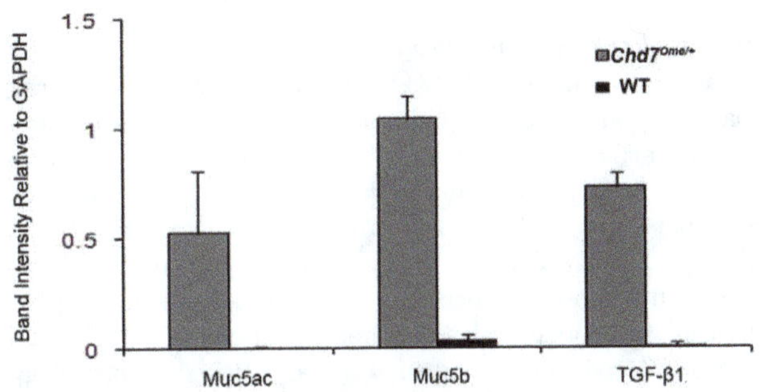

Figure 8. RT-PCR analysis of middle ears in $Chd7^{Ome/+}$ mice. Total RNA isolated from three $Chd7^{Ome/+}$ (mutant) and three wild-type littermate mice (control) were used to generate cDNA by reverse transcription. The cDNA was amplified using primers specific for *Gapdh*, *Muc5a*, *Muc5b* and *Tgf- β1*. The mutant mice showed significantly elevated expression levels for all three genes assayed, relative to *Gapdh* expression. Graph represents the digitized quantification of bands from an agarose gel. Error bars represent standard deviation from the mean, for each sample.

Table 3. Sequences of primers used for RNA analysis.

Primer	Oligonucleotide sequence (5′–3′)
GapdhF	AACTTTGGCATTGTGGAAGG
GapdhR	GGAGACAACCTGGTCCTCAG
Muc5aF	TGGAAGGATGCTATCCCAAG
Muc5aR	CACCAGCATTGTGGGTACAG
Muc5bF	GACACCATCTATGGGGTTGG
Muc5bR	CAGGACTGTTCACCCAGGTT
TGF-β1F	AGCCCGAAGCGGACTACTAT
TGF-β1R	TCCACATGTTGCTCCACACT
Tlr2F	GAGCGAGCTGGGTAAAGTAGAAA
Tlr2R	AGCCGAGGCAAGAACAAAGA
Chd7F	AGACGCTCCTAAAAACAAGGACT
Chd7R	AACCCTTTCTTCTCCTGTCAAAG

Histological analysis of middle and inner ears

Histological analyses of the middle and inner ears were performed following the methods described previously [45]. Briefly, middle and inner ears from *Chd7*$^{Ome/+}$ mice and wild-type mice were dissected after transcardial perfusion with 4% paraformaldehyde (PFA). Ear samples were immersed in 4% PFA for 48 h at 4°C, decalcified with 10% EDTA solution and embedded in paraffin. Sections (7 μm) were cut using an American Optical model 820 rotary microtome (American Optical, Buffalo, New York, USA), mounted onto Fisher Superfrost Plus slides (Fisher Scientific, Pittsburgh, PA) and counterstained in hematoxylin/eosin (H&E). Cryosections were prepared similarly but without dehydration, and instead, rinsed in a series of sucrose solutions and then embedded in Tissue-Tek OCT (Sakyra Finetek, Torrence, CA). Sections (10 μm) were cut with a Leica CM1900 cryostat microtome (Leica, Nussloch, Germany). Goblet cells, whose sole function is to secrete mucus, were identified by Mayer's Mucicarmine staining method following the protocol provided by Electron Microscopy Sciences (Catalog #26320).

Scoring system for pathology of middle ears

A scoring system of -/+/++/+++ was used to assess the severity of pathology in the middle and inner ears following a previously described method [25,45]. Histological analysis of the middle ears of control and mutant mice was performed using a light microscope (Leica DFC500, Germany). For the absence of pathology, a '–' symbol was assigned. When pathology was very scarce in the middle or inner ear, a '+' symbol was assigned. If pathology was more prevalent, but not to the point of spanning the entire middle or inner ear, then '++' was assigned. If pathology spanned the entire middle or inner ear, then '+++' was assigned. The pathologies being scored included middle ear effusion, inflammatory cell infiltration, tissue debris, and tissue proliferation. Both ears were examined in each mouse and only the one with more severe alteration was evaluated. Numerical scores were assigned to allow for semi-quantitative analysis of pathology (scoring 1 point for each +; for a total maximum possible score of 12 per mouse). A chi-square test was used to statistically evaluate the semi-quantitative data.

Scanning electron microscopy (SEM)

Middle and inner ears from *Chd7*$^{Ome/+}$ and wild-type mice were dissected after transcardial perfusion with 4% paraformaldehyde (PFA) and then immersed in 2.5% glutaraldehyde in 0.1 M phosphate buffered saline (PBS, pH = 7.2) for 4 hours at 4°C. Dissection was performed to expose the middle ear cavities and inner ear basilar membrane. After post-fixation in 1% OsO4 in 0.1 M PBS (pH = 7.2, 1 hour), samples were washed in 0.1 M PBS (pH = 7.2), dehydrated in increasing concentrations of ethanol, dried in a BAL-TEC CPD 030 critical point dryer (BAL-TEC GmbH, Witten, Germany) according to manufacturer's instructions and analyzed in a Hitachi S-4500 scanning electron microscope (Hitachi, Tokyo, Japan) at 5 kV.

Bacterial culture and identification

Bacterial culture and identification were performed following the protocol described previously [45]. Briefly, the bullae were removed and the middle ears were isolated under sterile conditions after ABR thresholds were determined. After microscopic examination, middle ears were washed with sterile PBS. 100 μl of the PBS lavage were inoculated onto a BBLTM Trypticase^{TM} Soy Agar plate with 5% sheep blood (TSA II, Fisher, Pittsburgh, PA, USA) and the plates were incubated at 37°C with 5% CO_2 for 18 h. Bacterial colonies were sorted by colony appearance, counted and subjected to further identification.

Immunohistochemistry

Cryosections were fixed in 1.5% PFA for 10 min. After being washed twice in 1x PBS and blocked in 5% bovine serum albumin for 1 h at room temperature, the samples were immersed in rabbit anti-*Chd7* polyclonal antibody (1:200 dilution, Abcam, Inc., ab31824, Cambridge, MA) and incubated at 4°C overnight. The samples were washed twice in 1x PBS for 5 min each, immersed in goat anti-rabbit secondary antibody conjugated to Alexa Fluor 488 (1:500 dilution; Invitrogen) and incubated at room temperature for 1 h. After counterstaining with PI for 15 min, the samples were mounted with Vectashield mounting medium (H-1000, Vector Laboratories). The samples were observed under an immunofluorescence microscope (Leica) and analyzed with Photoshop CS4 software.

Preparation of the skull and craniofacial measurement

To measure craniofacial dimensions in control and mutant mice, the skulls were dissected and removed from 5 mutant mice and 8 control mice at age 3 months. Skulls were macerated in 1% potassium hydroxide overnight to remove any soft tissue and then stained with alizarin red, as previously described [46]. After staining, the skulls were stored in undiluted glycerin until measurements were taken. To measure the dimensions of interest, a hand-held digital caliper (General Tools & Instruments, NY) with a resolution of 0.01 mm was used. These instruments provide a precise and accurate mode of measurement for small distances, necessary here because great precision and accuracy is needed to distinguish differences between control and mutant mice. Measurements were recorded in millimeters and results for control and mutant mice were graphed; this method has been previously validated for accuracy and precision [47,48]. Forty-four landmarks were adapted mostly from Dr. Joan Richtsmeier's paper on craniofacial dysmorphology in a Down syndrome mouse model [48], and from the standard measurement protocol in the Jackson Laboratory Craniofacial mutant source (Jackson Laboratory, Bar Harbor, ME http://craniofacial.jax.org/standard_protocols.html). Another measurement recorded was the angle between the midline of the skull base and the bony part of the Eustachian tube for both control and mutant mice. The skulls were then examined under an anatomical microscope and the skull base was photographed. The screen ruler software MB-Ruler 4.0 (Markus Bader, http://www.markus-bader.de/MB-Ruler/download.htm) was used to precisely locate the lines to be used for angle measurement and to measure the angles. The measurement data was statistically analyzed using the Student *t* test.

RNA analysis

The same cDNA template and PCR conditions from the previous genotyping step were used to profile mRNA accumulation of *Muc5ac*, *Muc5b* and *Tgf-β1* in the *Chd7* mice by methods previously described [49]. PCR products were subjected to electrophoresis and the gray intensity of each band on a 2% agarose gel was digitized using ImageJ software (NIH) and corrected by the coefficient of *Gapdh* (glyceraldehyde-3-phosphate dehydrogenase) gene expression level of the same sample. Primers used for RNA analysis are listed in Table 3.

Statistics

The Student *t* test was used for comparing mean ABR thresholds. Semi-quantitative data assessing ear pathology were analyzed by a chi-square test. A value of $P<0.05$ was considered significant.

Supporting Information

Video S1 A *Chd7*$^{Ome/+}$ mouse showing circling behavior in Video S1.

Video S2 A Chd7Ome/+ mouse showing poor swimming ability (Video S2).

Video S3 A Chd7+/+ mouse showing normal swimming ability with his nose above water (Video S3).

Acknowledgments

We thank Dr. Cynthia Benedict-Alderfer for preparing this manuscript and Linda Le English for proofreading the final version of this MS.

Author Contributions

Conceived and designed the experiments: QYZ. Performed the experiments: CT HY BY FH YZ CFB DS QYZ. Analyzed the data: QYZ PCS CT JEA. Contributed reagents/materials/analysis tools: PCS JEA QYZ. Wrote the paper: QYZ CT PCS.

References

1. Parkinson N, Hardisty-Hughes RE, Tateossian H, Tsai HT, Brooker D, et al. (2006) Mutation at the Evi1 locus in Junbo mice causes susceptibility to otitis media. PLoS Genet 2: e149.
2. Depreux FF, Darrow K, Conner DA, Eavey RD, Liberman MC, et al. (2008) Eya4-deficient mice are a model for heritable otitis media. J Clin Invest 118: 651–658.
3. Zheng QY, Hardisty-Hughes R, Brown SD (2006) Mouse models as a tool to unravel the genetic basis for human otitis media. Brain Res 1091: 9–15.
4. Vernacchio L, Lesko SM, Vezina RM, Corwin MJ, Hunt CE, et al. (2004) Racial/ethnic disparities in the diagnosis of otitis media in infancy. Int J Pediatr Otorhinolaryngol 68: 795–804.
5. Lalani SR, Safiullah AM, Fernbach SD, Harutyunyan KG, Thaller C, et al. (2006) Spectrum of CHD7 mutations in 110 individuals with CHARGE syndrome and genotype-phenotype correlation. Am J Hum Genet 78: 303–314.
6. Pagon RA, Graham JM Jr., Zonana J, Yong SL (1981) Coloboma, congenital heart disease, and choanal atresia with multiple anomalies: CHARGE association. J Pediatr 99: 223–227.
7. Zentner GE, Layman WS, Martin DM, Scacheri PC (2010) Molecular and phenotypic aspects of CHD7 mutation in CHARGE syndrome. Am J Med Genet A 152A: 674–686.
8. Schnetz MP, Handoko L, Akhtar-Zaidi B, Bartels CF, Pereira CF, et al. (2010) CHD7 targets active gene enhancer elements to modulate ES cell-specific gene expression. PLoS Genet 6: e1001023.
9. Zentner GE, Hurd EA, Schnetz MP, Handoko L, Wang C, et al. (2010) CHD7 functions in the nucleolus as a positive regulator of ribosomal RNA biogenesis. Hum Mol Genet 19: 3491–3501.
10. Schnetz MP, Bartels CF, Shastri K, Balasubramanian D, Zentner GE, et al. (2009) Genomic distribution of CHD7 on chromatin tracks H3K4 methylation patterns. Genome Res 19: 590–601.
11. Hurd EA, Adams ME, Layman WS, Swiderski DL, Beyer LA, et al. (2011) Mature middle and inner ears express Chd7 and exhibit distinctive pathologies in a mouse model of CHARGE syndrome. Hear Res 282: 184–195.
12. Buffone GJ, Darlington GJ (1985) Isolation of DNA from biological specimens without extraction with phenol. Clin Chem 31: 164–165.
13. Kaur R, Adlowitz DG, Casey JR, Zeng M, Pichichero ME (2010) Simultaneous assay for four bacterial species including Alloiococcus otitidis using multiplex-PCR in children with culture negative acute otitis media. Pediatr Infect Dis J 29: 741–745.
14. Borkowski G, Gurr A, Stark T, Philippou S, Sudhoff H (2000) [Functional and morphological defects of the mucociliary system in secretory otitis media]. Laryngorhinootologie 79: 135–138.
15. Roomans GM, Ivanovs A, Shebani EB, Johannesson M (2006) Transmission electron microscopy in the diagnosis of primary ciliary dyskinesia. Ups J Med Sci 111: 155–168.
16. Bajpai R, Chen DA, Rada-Iglesias A, Zhang J, Xiong Y, et al. (2010) CHD7 cooperates with PBAF to control multipotent neural crest formation. Nature 463: 958–962.
17. Aramaki M, Kimura T, Udaka T, Kosaki R, Mitsuhashi T, et al. (2007) Embryonic expression profile of chicken CHD7, the ortholog of the causative gene for CHARGE syndrome. Birth Defects Res A Clin Mol Teratol 79: 50–57.
18. Bergman JE, Bosman EA, van Ravenswaaij-Arts CM, Steel KP (2010) Study of smell and reproductive organs in a mouse model for CHARGE syndrome. Eur J Hum Genet 18: 171–177.
19. Layman WS, McEwen DP, Beyer LA, Lalani SR, Fernbach SD, et al. (2009) Defects in neural stem cell proliferation and olfaction in Chd7 deficient mice indicate a mechanism for hyposmia in human CHARGE syndrome. Hum Mol Genet 18: 1909–1923.
20. Vissers LE, van Ravenswaaij CM, Admiraal R, Hurst JA, de Vries BB, et al. (2004) Mutations in a new member of the chromodomain gene family cause CHARGE syndrome. Nat Genet 36: 955–957.
21. Bosman EA, Penn AC, Ambrose JC, Kettleborough R, Stemple DL, et al. (2005) Multiple mutations in mouse Chd7 provide models for CHARGE syndrome. Hum Mol Genet 14: 3463–3476.
22. Hurd EA, Capers PL, Blauwkamp MN, Adams ME, Raphael Y, et al. (2007) Loss of Chd7 function in gene-trapped reporter mice is embryonic lethal and associated with severe defects in multiple developing tissues. Mamm Genome 18: 94–104.
23. Randall V, McCue K, Roberts C, Kyriakopoulou V, Beddow S, et al. (2009) Great vessel development requires biallelic expression of Chd7 and Tbx1 in pharyngeal ectoderm in mice. J Clin Invest 119: 3301–3310.
24. Trune DR, Zheng QY (2009) Mouse models for human otitis media. Brain Res 1277: 90–103.
25. Han F, Yu H, Tian C, Li S, Jacobs MR, et al. (2009) Role for Toll-like receptor 2 in the immune response to Streptococcus pneumoniae infection in mouse otitis media. Infect Immun 77: 3100–3108.
26. MacArthur CJ, Hefeneider SH, Kempton JB, Trune DR (2006) C3H/HeJ mouse model for spontaneous chronic otitis media. Laryngoscope 116: 1071–1079.
27. Tateossian H, Hardisty-Hughes RE, Morse S, Romero MR, Hilton H, et al. (2009) Regulation of TGF-beta signalling by Fbxo11, the gene mutated in the Jeff otitis media mouse mutant. Pathogenetics 2: 5.
28. Hardisty-Hughes RE, Tateossian H, Morse SA, Romero MR, Middleton A, et al. (2006) A mutation in the F-box gene, Fbxo11, causes otitis media in the Jeff mouse. Hum Mol Genet 15: 3273–3279.
29. Hardisty RE, Erven A, Logan K, Morse S, Guionaud S, et al. (2003) The deaf mouse mutant Jeff (Jf) is a single gene model of otitis media. J Assoc Res Otolaryngol 4: 130–138.
30. Seibert JW, Danner CJ (2006) Eustachian tube function and the middle ear. Otolaryngol Clin North Am 39: 1221–1235.
31. Furukawa M, Ebmeyer J, Pak K, Austin DA, Melhus A, et al. (2007) Jun N-terminal protein kinase enhances middle ear mucosal proliferation during bacterial otitis media. Infect Immun 75: 2562–2571.
32. Kerschner JE, Li J, Tsushiya K, Khampang P (2010) Mucin gene expression and mouse middle ear epithelium. Int J Pediatr Otorhinolaryngol 74: 864–868.

33. Theodoropoulos DS, Theodoropoulos GA, Edwards BM, Kileny PR, Van Riper LA (2003) Immune Deficiency and Hearing Loss in CHARGE Association. Pediatrics 111: 711-a-712.
34. Chopra C, Baretto R, Duddridge M, Browning MJ (2009) T-cell immunodeficiency in CHARGE syndrome. Acta Paediatr 98: 408–410.
35. Hoover-Fong J, Savage WJ, Lisi E, Winkelstein J, Thomas GH, et al. (2009) Congenital T cell deficiency in a patient with CHARGE syndrome. J Pediatr 154: 140–142.
36. Gennery AR, Slatter MA, Rice J, Hoefsloot LH, Barge D, et al. (2008) Mutations in CHD7 in patients with CHARGE syndrome cause T-B + natural killer cell + severe combined immune deficiency and may cause Omenn-like syndrome. Clin Exp Immunol 153: 75–80.
37. Kerschner JE, Tripathi S, Khampang P, Papsin BC (2010) MUC5AC expression in human middle ear epithelium of patients with otitis media. Arch Otolaryngol Head Neck Surg 136: 819–824.
38. Preciado D, Goyal S, Rahimi M, Watson AM, Brown KJ, et al. (2010) MUC5B Is the predominant mucin glycoprotein in chronic otitis media fluid. Pediatr Res 68: 231–236.
39. Hoorens PR, Rinaldi M, Li RW, Goddeeris B, Claerebout E, et al. (2011) Genome wide analysis of the bovine mucin genes and their gastrointestinal transcription profile. BMC Genomics 12: 140.
40. Rousseau K, Kirkham S, McKane S, Newton R, Clegg P, et al. (2007) Muc5b and Muc5ac are the major oligomeric mucins in equine airway mucus. Am J Physiol Lung Cell Mol Physiol 292: L1396–1404.
41. Zhao SQ, Li J, Liu H, Zhang QG, Wang Y, et al. (2009) Role of interleukin-10 and transforming growth factor beta 1 in otitis media with effusion. Chin Med J (Engl) 122: 2149–2154.
42. Qin Z, Wood M, Rosowski JJ (2009) Measurement of conductive hearing loss in mice. Hear Res 263: 93–103.
43. Zheng QY, Johnson KR, Erway LC (1999) Assessment of hearing in 80 inbred strains of mice by ABR threshold analyses. Hear Res 130: 94–107.
44. Zheng QY, Tong YC, Alagramam KN, Yu H (2007) Tympanometry assessment of 61 inbred strains of mice. Hear Res 231: 23–31.
45. Han F, Yu H, Zhang J, Tian C, Schmidt C, et al. (2009) Otitis media in a mouse model for Down syndrome. Int J Exp Pathol 90: 480–488.
46. Selby PB (1987) A rapid method for preparing high quality alizarin stained skeletons of adult mice. Stain Technol 62: 143–146.
47. Mao M, Thedens DR, Chang B, Harris BS, Zheng QY, et al. (2009) The podosomal-adaptor protein SH3PXD2B is essential for normal postnatal development. Mamm Genome 20: 462–475.
48. Richtsmeier JT, Baxter LL, Reeves RH (2000) Parallels of craniofacial maldevelopment in Down syndrome and Ts65Dn mice. Dev Dyn 217: 137–145.
49. Han F, Yu H, Tian C, Chen HE, Benedict-Alderfer C, et al. (2010) A new mouse mutant of the Cdh23 gene with early-onset hearing loss facilitates evaluation of otoprotection drugs. Pharmacogenomics J.

11

Establishment of a Knock-In Mouse Model with the *SLC26A4* c.919-2A>G Mutation and Characterization of its Pathology

Ying-Chang Lu[1,2], Chen-Chi Wu[2,3,4], Wen-Sheng Shen[2], Ting-Hua Yang[2], Te-Huei Yeh[2], Pei-Jer Chen[3], I-Shing Yu[5], Shu-Wha Lin[5], Jau-Min Wong[1], Qing Chang[6], Xi Lin[6], Chuan-Jen Hsu[2,7]*

1 Institute of Biomedical Engineering, National Taiwan University, Taipei, Taiwan, **2** Department of Otolaryngology, National Taiwan University Hospital, Taipei, Taiwan, **3** Graduate Institute of Clinical Medicine, College of Medicine, National Taiwan University, Taipei, Taiwan, **4** Department of Medical Genetics, National Taiwan University Hospital, Taipei, Taiwan, **5** Transgenic Mouse Models Core (TMMC), Division of Genomic Medicine, Research Center for Medical Excellence, National Taiwan University, Taipei, Taiwan, **6** Department of Otolaryngology, Emory University School of Medicine, Atlanta, Georgia, United States of America, **7** Department of Otolaryngology, College of Medicine, National Taiwan University, Taipei, Taiwan

Abstract

Recessive mutations in the *SLC26A4* gene are a common cause of hereditary hearing impairment worldwide. Previous studies have demonstrated that different *SLC26A4* mutations may have different pathogenetic mechanisms. In the present study, we established a knock-in mouse model (i.e., *Slc26a4*$^{tm1Dontuh/tm1Dontuh}$ mice) homozygous for the c.919-2A>G mutation, which is a common mutation in East Asians. Mice were then subjected to audiologic assessment, a battery of vestibular evaluations, and inner ear morphological studies. All *Slc26a4*$^{tm1Dontuh/tm1Dontuh}$ mice revealed profound hearing loss, whereas 46% mice demonstrated pronounced head tilting and circling behaviors. There was a significant difference in the vestibular performance between wild-type and *Slc26a4*$^{tm1Dontuh/tm1Dontuh}$ mice, especially those exhibiting circling behavior. Inner ear morphological examination of *Slc26a4*$^{tm1Dontuh/tm1Dontuh}$ mice revealed an enlarged endolymphatic duct, vestibular aqueduct and sac, atrophy of stria vascularis, deformity of otoconia in the vestibular organs, consistent degeneration of cochlear hair cells, and variable degeneration of vestibular hair cells. Audiologic and inner ear morphological features of *Slc26a4*$^{tm1Dontuh/tm1Dontuh}$ mice were reminiscent of those observed in humans. These features were also similar to those previously reported in both knock-out *Slc26a4*$^{-/-}$ mice and *Slc26a4*$^{loop/loop}$ mice with the *Slc26a4* p.S408F mutation, albeit the severity of vestibular hair cell degeneration appeared different among the three mouse strains.

Editor: Mai Har Sham, The University of Hong Kong, China

Funding: This work was supported by research grants from the National Science Council of the Executive Yuan of the Republic of China (No. 96-2314-B-002-174-MY3). The funders had no role in study design, data collection and analysis decision to publish, or preparation of the manuscript.

Competing Interests: The authors have declared that no competing interests exist.

* E-mail: cjhsu@ntu.edu.tw

These authors contributed equally to this work.

Introduction

Mutations in the *SLC26A4* (*PDS*, GeneID 5172) gene are the second most frequent cause of human hereditary hearing impairment worldwide, following mutations in the *GJB2* (GeneID 2706) gene [1]. Recessive *SLC26A4* mutations are responsible for both non-syndromic hereditary hearing loss DFNB4 (MIM 600791) [2] and Pendred syndrome (PS, MIM 274600) [3], two disorders commonly encountered in patients with deafness. DFNB4 and PS are characterized by sensorineural hearing impairment accompanied by an enlarged vestibular aqueduct (EVA, MIM 603545) and/or incomplete partition of the cochlea (i.e., Mondini dysplasia), although the latter also includes development of goiter. *SLC26A4* encodes pendrin, an iodide/chloride/bicarbonate transporter expressed in the inner ear, thyroid, and kidney [4,5,6,7].

In recent years, the understanding of the pathogenesis of DFNB4 and PS has been facilitated by various studies performed in the knock-out mouse model *Slc26a4*$^{-/-}$ [8]. However, the phenotypes observed in *Slc26a4*$^{-/-}$ mice, such as unanimously profound hearing loss and the absence of thyroid pathology in all littermates, fail to completely reflect those observed in humans with various *SLC26A4* mutations. Clinically, patients with *SLC26A4* mutations have been shown to demonstrate a broad-spectrum of phenotypes, ranging from non-syndromic isolated EVA to full-blown PS with goiter and incomplete partition of the cochlea in addition to EVA. To date, more than 100 *SLC26A4* mutations have been identified (Pendred/BOR Homepage; www.healthcare.uiowa.edu/labs/pendredandbor). It was reported that patients with different *SLC26A4* genotypes were correlated to distinct clinical phenotypes, with PS patients more likely to have 2 *SLC26A4* mutant alleles than those with non-syndromic EVA [9,10]. Furthermore, cell line studies have demonstrated that certain *SLC26A4* mutations only impair the function of pendrin partially, instead of completely ablating the protein function [11,12]. These lines of evidence indicate that the pathogenetic mechanisms of *SLC26A4* mutations in humans to some extent differ from those mechanisms present in the *Slc26a4*$^{-/-}$ mouse model, in which exon 8 of the *Slc26a4* gene (GeneID 23985) is knocked out.

To elucidate the discrepancies in phenotypes observed between humans and *Slc26a4*$^{-/-}$ mice, it might be necessary to create knock-in mouse models that harbor the corresponding human *SLC26A4* mutations. Accordingly, the primary purpose of the present study was to establish a knock-in mouse model homozygous for the c.919A>G mutation, which is the most prevalent *SLC26A4* mutation in Chinese [13,14] individuals, and the second most prevalent mutation in Japanese [15] and Koreans [16]. We also characterized the associated audiological and vestibular phenotypes as well as the inner ear pathology in this model.

Results

Pathogenetic mechanisms of the c.919-2A>G mutation

In our previous study, the c.919-2A>G mutation was expected to lead to aberrant splicing, based on a computer-assisted analysis by the Neural Network at the Berkeley Drosophila Genome Project (BDGP; www.fruitfly.org/seq_tools/splice.html; splice score = 0 compared to 0.93 of the wild-type sequence [17]. In transformed lymphocytes, sequencing of the RT-PCR products revealed that *SLC26A4* transcripts from the allele with c.919-2A>G lose the entire exon 8, resulting in fusion of exons 7 and 9 [18]. In the present study, we confirmed that c.919-2A>G indeed led to a complete omission of exon 8 during the splicing process in inner ear and kidney (Fig. 1). The frameshift generated a new stop codon at position 348, resulting in prematurely truncated pendrin (347 amino acids). However, pendrin localization in the inner ear was not affected by the c.919-2A>G mutation, as shown by immunofluorescence studies (Fig. 2).

Audiological and vestibular phenotypes

A total of 45 mice (P35–P42), including 15 *Slc26a4*$^{+/+}$ mice, 15 *Slc26a4*$^{+/tm1Dontuh}$ mice and 15 *Slc26a4*$^{tm1Dontuh/tm1Dontuh}$ mice, were subjected to audiological evaluations. All *Slc26a4*$^{tm1Dontuh/tm1Dontuh}$ mice revealed profound hearing loss (>120 dB SPL) on ABR in all frequencies, whereas all *Slc26a4*$^{+/tm1Dontuh}$ and *Slc26a4*$^{+/+}$ mice revealed normal hearing (Fig. 3). These results indicate that the c.919-2A>G mutation of *Slc26a4* was inherited in an autosomal recessive manner in mice, as in humans. The audiological characteristics were observed until mice reached 12 months in age. We found no obvious change in hearing ability of these mice.

None of the *Slc26a4*$^{+/tm1Dontuh}$ or *Slc26a4*$^{+/+}$ mice revealed vestibular deficits, whereas 46% (23/50) of *Slc26a4*$^{tm1Dontuh/tm1Dontuh}$ mice demonstrated pronounced head-tilting and circling behaviors before reaching 3 weeks of age. The phenotype of circling behavior did not change until 12 months. A total of 60 mice, including 15 *Slc26a4*$^{+/+}$ mice, 15 *Slc26a4*$^{+/tm1Dontuh}$ mice, 15 *Slc26a4*$^{tm1Dontuh/tm1Dontuh}$ mice that did not exhibit circling and 15 *Slc26a4*$^{tm1Dontuh/tm1Dontuh}$ mice that did exhibit circling, were subjected to vestibular evaluations (Table 1). In general, *Slc26a4*$^{tm1Dontuh/tm1Dontuh}$ mice revealed impaired balancing ability compared to wild-type mice. The presence of circling behaviors was in complete accord with the presence of head-tilting in *Slc26a4*$^{tm1Dontuh/tm1Dontuh}$ mice. Furthermore, circling mice were associated with a significantly poorer performance on reaching, swimming, gripping, and rotorod tests. *Slc26a4*$^{tm1Dontuh/tm1Dontuh}$ mice without circling behaviors showed only a minor degree of vestibular dysfunction, yet their performance on the rotorod test was also poorer than wild-type mice. We also noted a significant difference in vestibular features, including reaching, swimming, gripping, and balancing on the rotorod, between *Slc26a4*$^{tm1Dontuh/tm1Dontuh}$ mice that exhibited circling and those that did not ($p<0.05$, in all cases).

Inner ear morphology: endolymphatic duct, vestibular aqueduct and sac

When observed with the naked eye, the orifice of vestibular aqueduct and fovea of endolymphatic sac were noticeably enlarged in *Slc26a4*$^{tm1Dontuh/tm1Dontuh}$ mice (Fig. 4B, as indicated by arrows and dot-dash line), as compared to those in *Slc26a4*$^{+/+}$ mice (Fig. 4A). This structural aberrance was also identified with histological studies by H&E staining (Fig. 4D vs. Fig. 4C).

Inner ear morphology: cochlea

Examination of the cochlear duct from 4-week-old mice revealed severe endolymphatic hydrops with dilatation of scala media in *Slc26a4*$^{tm1Dontuh/tm1Dontuh}$ mice (Fig. 5B), compared to *Slc26a4*$^{+/+}$ mice. A higher magnification view also showed degeneration of hair cells (Fig. 5B) and a significant atrophy of the stria vascularis (Fig. 5D) in all *Slc26a4*$^{tm1Dontuh/tm1Dontuh}$ mice by 6 weeks. Degeneration of inner and outer hair cells in the organ of Corti could also be confirmed by fluorescence confocal microscopy (Fig. 5H). Further investigation of the stria vascularis by TEM revealed that the most significant change was the diminished membrane invaginations of marginal cell with vacuolization changes or interstitial edema (Fig. 6).

Inner ear morphology: vestibular system

Morphological changes of the vestibular organs in *Slc26a4*$^{tm1Dontuh/tm1Dontuh}$ mice included deformity of otoconia and degeneration of the sensory epithelium. To be more specific, deformity included a decreased amount of otoconia present in the saccule and utricle (Fig. 7A), formation of "giant otoconia" in the saccule and utricle (Fig. 7D) and ectopic distribution of otoconia into the semicircular canal (Fig. 7F). Further investigation of the otoconia by SEM revealed that the giant otoconia in the saccule and utricle in *Slc26a4*$^{tm1Dontuh/tm1Dontuh}$ mice (Fig. 7H) as compared with wild-type mice (Fig. 7G). Furthermore, in contrast to the

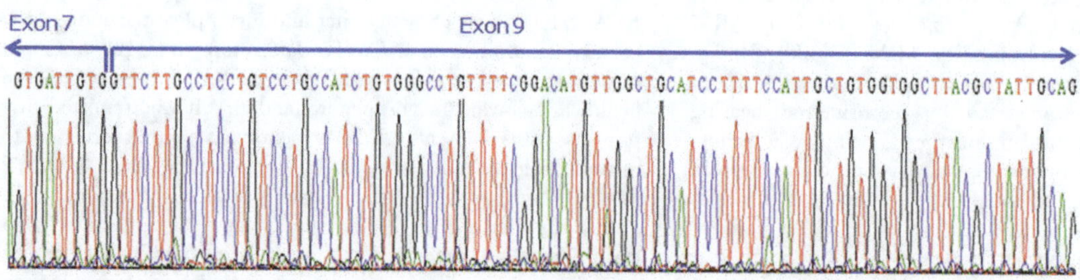

Figure 1. The *Slc26a4* transcripts from the allele with the c.919-2A>G mutation lead to a complete omission of exon 8 during the splicing process in *Slc26a4*$^{tm1Dontuh/tm1Dontuh}$ mice.

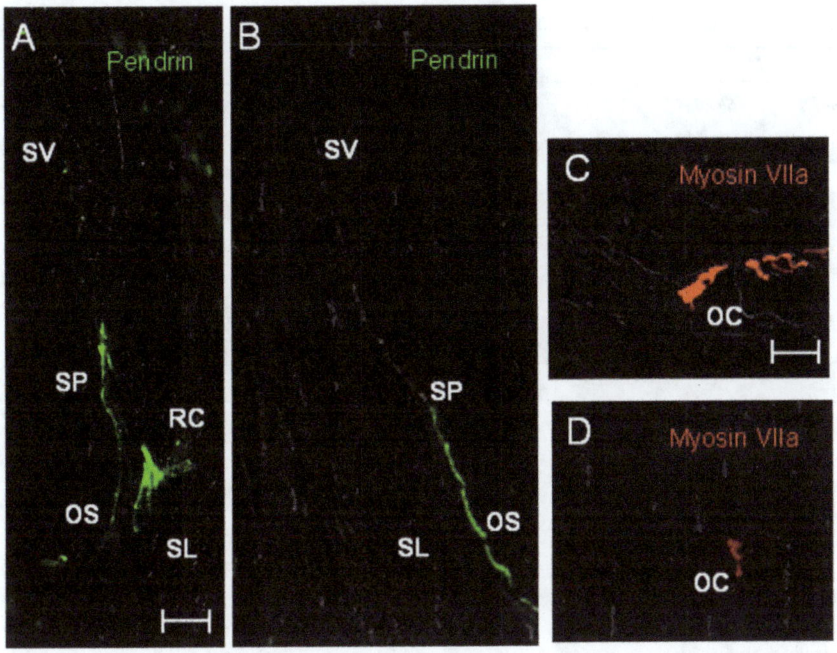

Figure 2. Immunolocalization of pendrin in *Slc26a4*$^{+/+}$ mice (A) and *Slc26a4*$^{tm1Dontuh/tm1Dontuh}$ mice (B). The expression of pendrin (stained in green) in spiral prominence and outer sulcus epithelial cells was not affected by the c.919-2A>G mutation. Degeneration of cochlear hair cells in *Slc26a4*$^{tm1Dontuh/tm1Dontuh}$ mice was revealed by fluorescence confocal microscopy (D). (OC, organ of Corti; OS, outer sulcus epithelial cells; RC, root cells; SP, spiral prominence; SL, spiral ligament; SV, stria vascularis). Bar = 50 μm.

consistent degeneration of cochlear hair cells seen in 6-weeks-old *Slc26a4*$^{tm1Dontuh/tm1Dontuh}$ mice, 8-week-old mice revealed a wide spectrum of hair cell loss and degeneration in the saccule (Fig. 7B), utricle (Fig. 7D & Fig. 7J) and semicircular canals (Fig. 7F). Of note, hair cells in the utricle appeared to be more affected than those in the saccule and semicircular canals. The morphological findings in the vestibular organs, including the abnormality of otoconia (defined by decreased amount of otoconia in the saccule and utricle, formation of giant otoconia in the utricle and ectopic distribution of otoconia in the semicircular canal), and the

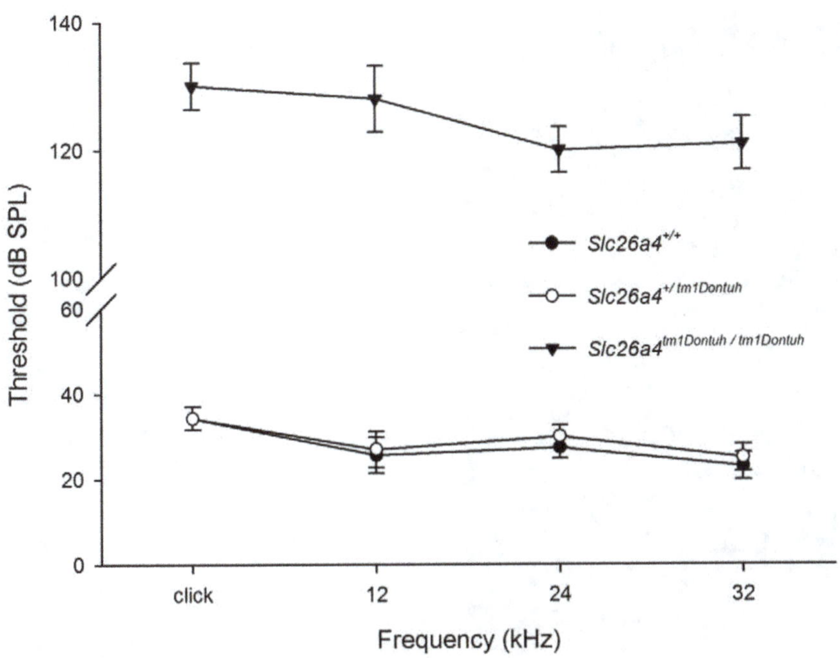

Figure 3. Audiological phenotypes of *Slc26a4*$^{tm1Dontuh/tm1Dontuh}$ mice. All *Slc26a4*$^{tm1Dontuh/tm1Dontuh}$ mice (n = 15) revealed profound hearing loss (>120 dB SPL) according to ABR at all frequencies, whereas all *Slc26a4*$^{+/tm1Dontuh}$ mice (n = 15) and all *Slc26a4*$^{+/+}$ mice (n = 15) revealed normal hearing.

Table 1. Comparison of vestibular features according to the genotypes and the circling behavior.

	$Slc26a4^{+/+}$ (n = 15)	$Slc26a4^{+/tm1Dontuh}$ (n = 15)	$Slc26a4^{tm1Dontuh/tm1Dontuh}$ (Non-circling) (n = 15)	$Slc26a4^{tm1Dontuh/tm1Dontuh}$ (Circling) (n = 15)
Head tilting* (n, abnormal/total)	0/15	0/15	0/15†,	15/15‡
Reaching§ (n, abnormal/total)	0/15	0/15	4/15†	11/15‡
Swimming§ (n, abnormal/total)	0/15	0/15	2/15†	11/15‡
Gripping§ (n, abnormal/total)	0/15	0/15	3/15†	13/15‡
Time on rod§ (sec)	164.7±13.9	159.3±18.1	66.3±8.9‡	4.0±1.6‡

*Observed at 3 weeks.
§Tested at 8 weeks.
†$p>0.05$ as compared to wild type.
‡$p<0.01$ as compared to wild type.

degeneration of hair cells (measured by calculating the number of areas of hair cell loss in 5 random sections per mouse), were then correlated to the vestibular phenotype of circling. As shown in Table 2, we detected no significant difference in the abnormality of otoconia between those mice that exhibited circling and those mice that did not, but the degeneration and loss of utricular hair cells were more significant in $Slc26a4^{tm1Dontuh/tm1Dontuh}$ mice that exhibited circling.

Thyroid and renal profiles

Goiter was not observed in $Slc26a4^{tm1Dontuh/tm1Dontuh}$ mice (n = 30) until 12 months in age. Total T_4 in 2-month-old (n = 10) and 6-month-old (n = 10) $Slc26a4^{tm1Dontuh/tm1Dontuh}$ mice were 3.34±0.14 μg/dl and 3.03±0.16 μg/dl, respectively; whereas total T_4 in 2-month-old (n = 10) and 6-month-old (n = 10) wild type mice were 3.46±0.20 μg/dl and 3.08±0.20 μg/dl, respectively, showing no difference between $Slc26a4^{tm1Dontuh/tm1Dontuh}$ and wild type mice. Similarly, $Slc26a4^{tm1Dontuh/tm1Dontuh}$ mice revealed normal renal functions up to 6 months. Blood urea nitrogen (BUN) in 2-month-old (n = 10) and 6-month-old (n = 10) $Slc26a4^{tm1Dontuh/tm1Dontuh}$ mice were 31.4±4.14 mg/dl and 33.3±5.18 mg/dl, respectively; whereas BUN in 2-month-old (n = 10) and 6-month-old (n = 10) wild type mice were 30.2±5.26 mg/dl and 32.4±4.20 mg/dl, respectively. Creatinine (CREA) in 2-month-old (n = 10) and 6-month-old (n = 10) $Slc26a4^{tm1Dontuh/tm1Dontuh}$ mice were 0.19±0.06 mg/dl and 0.21±0.04 mg/dl, respectively; whereas CREA in 2-month-old (n = 10) and 6-month-old (n = 10) wild type mice were 0.21±0.06 mg/dl and 0.22±0.02 mg/dl, respectively. There was no significant difference in BUN and CREA between $Slc26a4^{tm1Dontuh/tm1Dontuh}$ and wild type mice up to 6 months.

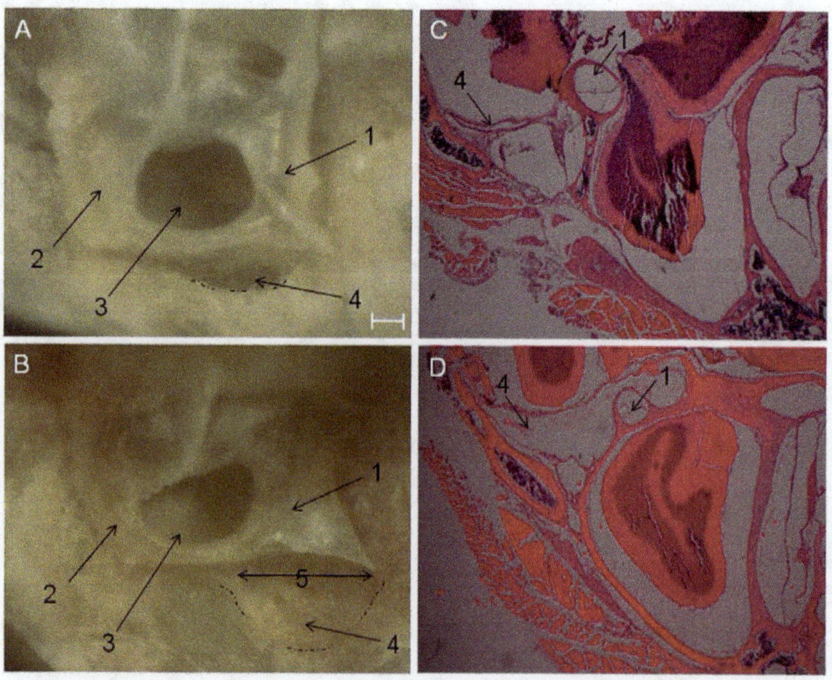

Figure 4. Structural aberrations of the vestibular aqueduct and endolymphatic sac in mice. The vestibular aqueduct and endolymphatic sac in the $Slc26a4^{tm1Dontuh/tm1Dontuh}$ mice were enlarged (B & D) compared to those in the $Slc26a4^{+/+}$ mice (A & C). (1, posterior semicircular canal; 2, superior semicircular canal; 3, subarcuate fossa; 4, fovea for endolymphatic sac (dot-dash line); 5, external orifice of vestibular aqueduct. Bar = 100 μm.

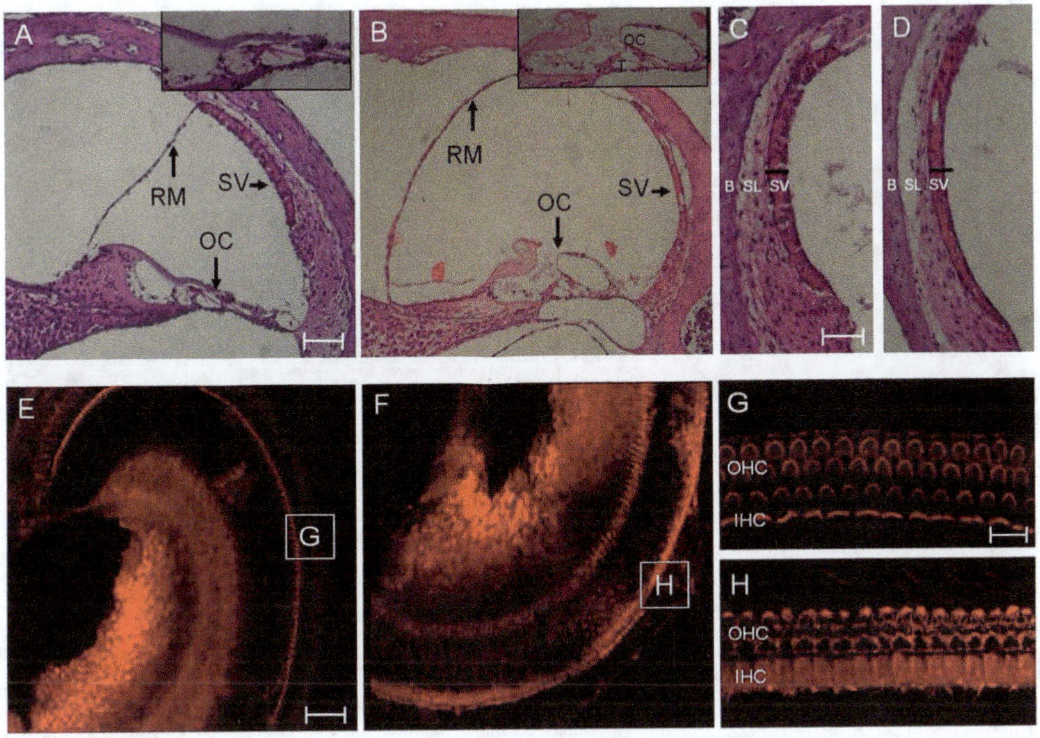

Figure 5. Comparison of cochlear morphology between *Slc26a4*$^{+/+}$ mice (A, C, E & G) and *Slc26a4*$^{tm1Dontuh/tm1Dontuh}$ mice (B, D, F & H). Microscopic examination of the cochlear duct revealed severe endolymphatic hydrops with dilatation of scala media, degeneration of hair cells (B) and a significant atrophy of the stria vascularis (D) in *Slc26a4*$^{tm1Dontuh/tm1Dontuh}$ mice. Degeneration of cochlear hair cells in *Slc26a4*$^{tm1Dontuh/tm1Dontuh}$ mice was also revealed by fluorescence confocal microscopy (H). G, H: magnification of boxes G and H from figures E and F, respectively. B, bone; IHC, inner hair cells; OC, organ of Corti; OHC, outer hair cells; RM, Reissner's membrane; SL, spiral ligament; SV, stria vascularis; T, tunnel of Corti. Bar = 150 μm (A & B), 50 μm (C, D, E & F), and 10 μm (G & H).

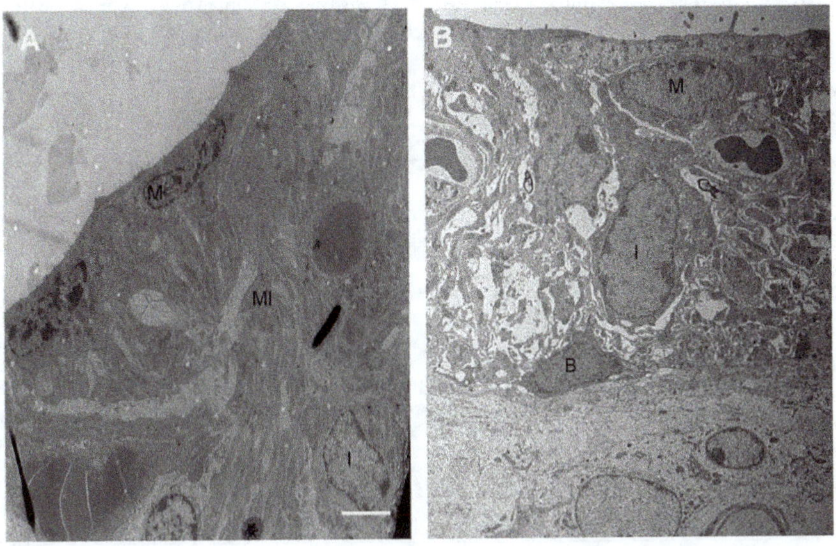

Figure 6. Transmission electron micrographs of the stria vascularis in *Slc26a4*$^{+/+}$ mice (A) and *Slc26a4*$^{tm1Dontuh/tm1Dontuh}$ mice (B). The most significant change in stria vascularis in *Slc26a4*$^{tm1Dontuh/tm1Dontuh}$ mice was diminished membrane invaginations of marginal cell with vacuolization changes. B, basal cell; I, intermediate cell; M, marginal cell; MI, membrane invaginations. Bar = 5 μm.

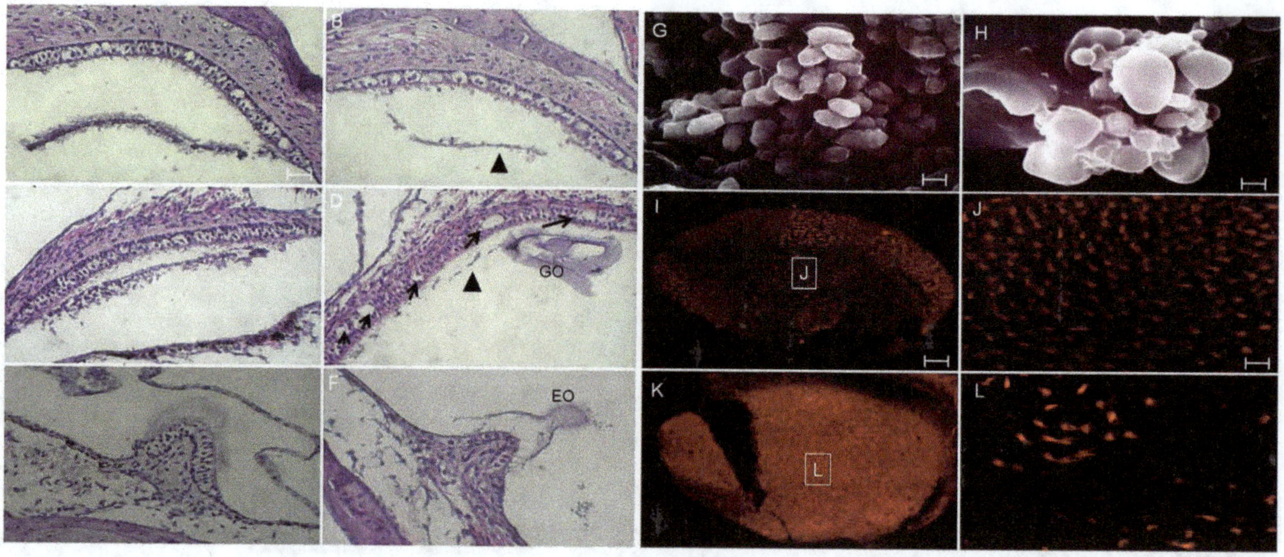

Figure 7. Comparison of vestibular morphology between *Slc26a4*$^{+/+}$ mice (A, saccule; C, utricle; E, semicircular canal; G, utricular macula) and *Slc26a4*$^{tm1Dontuh/tm1Dontuh}$ mice (B, saccule; D, utricle; F, semicircular canal; I, utricular macula). *Slc26a4*$^{tm1Dontuh/tm1Dontuh}$ mice revealed a decreased amount of otoconia in the saccule and utricle (B & D, arrowhead), formation of "giant otoconia" in the utricle (D & H), ectopic otoconia in the semicircular canal (F), as well as a wide spectrum of vestibular hair cell loss and degeneration (arrows) at 8 weeks of age. Scanning electron microscopy reveals the markedly enlarged otoconia at saccule and utricle in *Slc26a4*$^{tm1Dontuh/tm1Dontuh}$ mice (H) as compared with wild-type (G). Degeneration of vestibular hair cells in *Slc26a4*$^{tm1Dontuh/tm1Dontuh}$ mice was also revealed by fluorescence confocal microscopy (L). J, L: magnification of boxes J and L from figures I and K, respectively. EO, ectopic otoconia; GO, giant otoconia. Bar = 50 μm (A–F, I & K), and 10 μm (G, H, J & L).

Discussion

In this study, we generated a knock-in mouse model, denoted as *Slc26a4*$^{tm1Dontuh/tm1Dontuh}$ mice, which segregates a common deafness-associated mutation, c.919-2A>G, in humans. Phenotypic characterization of *Slc26a4*$^{tm1Dontuh/tm1Dontuh}$ mice revealed they had profound hearing impairment, impaired balancing ability, an enlarged vestibular aqueduct, degeneration of cochlear and vestibular hair cells and atrophy of stria vascularis. To our knowledge, there are only two other mouse mutants in the literature that harbor *Slc26a4* mutations: the knock-out *Slc26a4*$^{-/-}$ mouse model [8] and the *Slc26a4*$^{loop/loop}$ mouse, which segregates the *Slc26a4* p.S408F mutation generated by the ENU mutagenesis project [19]. From the pathogenetic perspective, *Slc26a4*$^{-/-}$ and *Slc26a4*$^{tm1Dontuh/tm1Dontuh}$ mice share a loss of exon 8 of the *Slc26a4* transcript, resulting in a truncated protein; whereas the p.S408F mutation of *Slc26a4*$^{loop/loop}$ mice leads to an aberrant protein. The audiological, vestibular, and inner ear morphological findings of *Slc26a4*$^{-/-}$, *Slc26a4*$^{loop/loop}$ and *Slc26a4*$^{tm1Dontuh/tm1Dontuh}$ mice are summarized in Table 3. Homozygous mice of all three strains revealed profound hearing loss, which indicates that the c.919-2A>G mutation of *Slc26a4* is inherited in an autosomal recessive manner. In contrast, the severity of vestibular phenotypes appeared variable: some mice showed marked vestibular deficits such as head-

Table 2. Comparison of vestibular morphological findings according to the vestibular phenotype of circling.

	Slc26a4$^{tm1Dontuh/tm1Dontuh}$ (Circling)	*Slc26a4*$^{tm1Dontuh/tm1Dontuh}$ (Non-circling)	*p*-value*
Saccule			
Areas of hair cell loss† (n of areas/animal)	0.6±0.9	0.4±0.9	$p>0.05$
Otoconia (n of animal, abnormal‡/total)	5/5	5/5	$p>0.05$
Utricle			
Areas of hair cell loss (n of areas/animal)	9.6±5.9	1.6±3.0	$p<0.05$
Otoconia (n of animal, abnormal‡/total)	5/5	5/5	$p>0.05$
Semicircular canal			
Areas of hair cell loss (n of areas/animal)	2.4±2.2	1.6±2.2	$p>0.05$
Ectopic otoconia (n of animal, abnormal‡/total)	4/5	5/5	$p>0.05$

*Fisher's exact test for categorical variables and Student's *t*-test for continuous variables.

†Measured by calculating the number of areas of hair cell loss in 5 random sections pre mouse.

‡Defined by decreased amount of otoconia in the saccule and utricle, formation of giant otoconia in the utricle and ectopic distribution of otoconia in the semicircular canal.

Table 3. Comparison of phenotypes among mouse strains segregating different slc26a4 mutations.

	Slc26a4$^{-/-}$	*Slc26a4*$^{loop/loop}$	*Slc26a4*$^{tm1Dontuh/tm1Dontuh}$
Audiological phenotypes	Profound hearing loss (>100 dB SPL)	Profound hearing loss (>100 dB SPL)	Profound hearing loss (>120 dB SPL)
Vestibular phenotypes	Vestibular deficits, including head-tilting, head-bobbing unsteadiness, circling and abnormal reaching response in ~50% mice.	Variable vestibular deficits, including unsteady gait, circling, absence of reaching response and tilted body. Proportion of mice with vestibular deficits not reported.	46% of mice with head-tilting and circling. Poorer vestibular function in *Slc26a4*$^{tm1Dontuh/tm1Dontuh}$ mice, esp. in those with circling.
Inner Ear Morphology			
Vestibular aqueduct	Enlarged	ND	Enlarged
Scala media	Enlarged	ND	Enlarged
Stria vascularis	Atrophic	ND	Atrophic
Cochlear hair cells	Severe degeneration of inner and outer hair cells by P30.	ND	Severe degeneration of inner and outer hair cells at 6 wks.
Vestibular hair cells	Severe degeneration of vestibular hair cells by P30.	Normal morphology of vestibular hair cells at 2 m.	Loss and degeneration of utricular hair cells correlated to the vestibular phenotypes
Otoconia	Almost complete absence of otoconia with occasional presence of giant otoconia.	Giant otoconia in the utricle from P0 to 10 m; gradual change in otoconia composition to calcium oxalate in the saccule from P0 to 10 m; ectopic otoconia in the semicircular canal.	Decreased amount of otoconia in the saccule and utricle, formation of giant otoconia in the saccule and utricle, and ectopic distribution of otoconia into the semicircular canal

ND, not described.
**Slc26a4*$^{loop/loop}$: mice homozygous for the p.S408F mutation.

tilting and circling behaviors, whereas the others remained relatively normal.

It has been reported that mice with different *Slc26a4* mutations revealed different degrees of vestibular degeneration. In particular, the morphology of utricular hair cells in 2-month-old *Slc26a4*$^{loop/loop}$ mice was found to be normal [19], whereas *Slc26a4*$^{-/-}$ mice show severe utricular hair cell degeneration by the age of 1 month [8]. As demonstrated in the present study, *Slc26a4*$^{tm1Dontuh/tm1Dontuh}$ mice seem to have an intermediate grade of morphological changes, with the severity of vestibular hair cell degeneration related to the presence of vestibular deficits. These findings suggest that a genotype-phenotype correlation can be deduced among mice with different *Slc26a4* mutations. In humans, it has been reported that PS patients are more likely to have 2 *SLC26A4* mutant alleles than those with non-syndromic EVA [9,10]. Moreover, the number of *SLC26A4* mutant alleles is also significantly correlated to the severity of hearing loss in individuals with EVA [20]. However, because of its diverse mutation spectrum, it is difficult to delineate the phenotypes associated with a specific *SLC26A4* mutation in humans. Consequently, determination of the pathogenetic role of each specific *SLC26A4* mutation largely relies on functional studies performed in cell lines [11,12,21]. The observation that mice with distinct *Slc26a4* mutations reveal different phenotypes indicates that transgenic mice may serve as an appropriate, direct model to investigate corresponding *SLC26A4* mutations in humans.

Recent studies have provided excellent insights into how *SLC26A4* mutations lead to hearing impairment. It has been proposed that *Slc26a4*$^{-/-}$ mice develop deafness via several mechanisms. First, loss of cochlear HCO_3^- secretion results in the acidification of endolymph, which consequently increases Ca^{2+} concentration in the endolymph by inhibiting Ca^{2+} reabsorption [22,23] leads to free radical stress-mediated loss of *Kcnj10* protein expression in stria vascularis, ultimately abolishing the production of endocochlear potential [24]. Second, local hypothyroidism in the cochlea may contribute to delays in cochlear development, which can lead to the inability to develop hearing [25]. In addition to the degeneration of cochlear hair cells, *Slc26a4*$^{-/-}$ and *Slc26a4*$^{tm1Dontuh/tm1Dontuh}$ mice show atrophy of stria vascularis, which is uncommon in other mouse models for hereditary hearing impairment. According to a previous study, atrophy of stria vascularis may cause degeneration of hair cells by alteration in endolymph composition [26]. Since *Slc26a4* mutant mice revealed normal cochlear hair cells at a younger age (P7) (Fig. S1), it is conceivable that the pathology in the stria vascularis plays a pivotal role in the later degeneration of cochlear hair cells associated with *SLC26A4* mutations. In the present study, we investigated the morphology of stria vascularis using TEM, and identified that the most significant change in *Slc26a4*$^{tm1Dontuh/tm1Dontuh}$ mice was the disappearance of marginal cell invaginations with vacuolization changes. Interestingly, ablation of primary and secondary processes of marginal cells with normal appearing intermediate cells and basal cells has been documented as an end-stage strial change in presbycusic gerbils [27]. It is suggested that the basal part of marginal cells endure a greater exposure to free radicals by virtue of harboring abundant mitochondria, thus being more vulnerable to aging-related injury [27]. The similar morphological strial changes seen in *Slc26a4*$^{tm1Dontuh/tm1Dontuh}$ mice support the previous hypothesis that free radicals are crucial for the development of stria vascularis atrophy and the ensuing degeneration of cochlear hair cells.

In comparison to hearing loss, less is known concerning the vestibular dysfunction associated with *SLC26A4* mutations, despite the fact that as many as 70% of patients with *SLC26A4* mutations suffer from episodes of vertigo [28,29]. In their pioneer study, Everett *et al.* observed giant otoconia at utricle and saccule in *Slc26a4*$^{-/-}$ mice [30]. Dror *et al.* investigated the mineral composition and morphology of otoconia in *Slc26a4*$^{loop/loop}$ mice, and identified abnormal giant carbonate minerals in the utricle of mice at all ages, a gradual change in mineral composition leading to the formation of calcium oxalate in the saccule in adult mice, as well as ectopic giant otoconia in semicircular canals. The authors postulated that the variability of the defective vestibular behavior in *Slc26a4*$^{loop/loop}$ mice, ranging from very mild to severe, can be partially explained by the variable position of dislocated mineralized bodies [19]. In the present study, we did not detect a correlation between abnormal otoconia and the presence of circling behavior in *Slc26a4*$^{tm1Dontuh/tm1Dontuh}$ mice, but we noted an association between circling behavior and the degeneration of utricular hair cells (Table 2). The underlying factors leading to the degeneration, nevertheless, remain to be clarified.

Although *Slc26a4*$^{-/-}$, *Slc26a4*$^{loop/loop}$, and *Slc26a4*$^{tm1Dontuh/tm1Dontuh}$ mice revealed phenotypes reminiscent of those observed in humans, there are some discrepancies that limit direct extrapolation of these results from animal studies into clinical medicine. First, the hearing impairment was profound in these mice, although patients with *SLC26A4* mutations demonstrate a wide variety in audiological features. Some patients exhibit a milder hearing impairment that deteriorates with time, either progressively or after attacks of fluctuating hearing loss [31,32]. Second, a significant proportion of mutant mice revealed severely impaired vestibular function, but patients with *SLC26A4* mutations usually do not complain of vestibular symptoms, except during attacks of vertigo. Accordingly, further modifications of these mutant mice are necessary to better simulate phenotypes in humans. We submit two possible methods that may alleviate the phenotypes of mice. The first approach includes establishment of a knock-in mouse model with a missense *Slc26a4* mutation other than p.S408F, instead of a mutation that leads to a truncated protein, might result in more minor phenotypes. It has been reported previously that truncating mutations may be associated with a more severe phenotype in certain types of genetic hearing impairments [33]. Alternatively, conditional knock-in mice models that modulate the expression of the *Slc26a4* gene after birth might be helpful in generating animals that are not congenitally deaf.

Materials and Methods

Construction of *Slc26a4*$^{tm1Dontuh/tm1Dontuh}$ knock-in mice

The mutation gene-targeting vector was constructed using a recombineering approach previously developed by Dr. Copeland's group [34,35]. From the bMQ323G13 BAC clone (Sanger institute, UK), which carried the entire mouse *Slc26a4* locus, we subcloned a 12.47-kb fragment spanning introns 3 to 10 of *Slc26a4* into the PL253 plasmid (Fig. S2). The subcloned genomic 12.47-kb region was modified in a subsequent targeting round by inserting the neomycin (*neo*) cassette from the PL451 plasmid and creating the c.919-2A>G mutation in intron 7. The conditional targeting vector was then linearized by *Not*I digestion and electroporated into R1 embryonic stem (ES) cells. G418 (240 μg/ml) and Ganciclovir (2 μM) double-resistant clones were analyzed by Southern blot hybridization. The retained *neo* cassette flanked by *FRT* sites was excised *in vivo* by transfecting the targeted clone with plasmid transiently expressing the FLPe recombinase. Established ES clones were then identified by polymerase chain reaction (PCR) screening and subsequently injected into C57BL/6 blastocysts to produce chimeras. Chimeric males were bred with C57BL/6 females to produce *Slc26a4*$^{+/tm1Dontuh}$ mice. *Slc26a4*$^{+/tm1Dontuh}$ mice (F1) were mated with each other to produce *Slc26a4*$^{+/+}$, *Slc26a4*$^{+/tm1Dontuh}$ and *Slc26a4*$^{tm1Dontuh/tm1Dontuh}$ mice littermates (F2), and then *Slc26a4*$^{tm1Dontuh/tm1Dontuh}$ mice were maintained in C57BL/6 background. All animal experiments were carried out in accordance with animal welfare guidelines and approved by the Institutional Animal Care and Use Committee (IACUC) of National Taiwan University College of Medicine (approval no. 20070077)

Determination of the pathogenesis of the c.919-2A>G mutation

The pathogenetic mechanisms of the c.919-2A>G mutation were determined by investigating both the mRNA product of mice with this mutation and the consequences of the mutation on pendrin expression. To examine the mRNA product, we purified kidney and inner ear mRNA from both *Slc26a4*$^{+/+}$ and *Slc26a4*$^{tm1Dontuh/tm1Dontuh}$ mice using Trizol reagent (Invitrogen Carlsbad, CA, USA) according to the manufacturer's instructions. Subsequently, 2 μg of total RNA was reverse-transcribed with a Transcription High Fidelity cDNA Synthesis Kit(RocheDiagnostics Gmbh, Mannheim, Germany), and reverse transcription-PCR (RT-PCR) was carried out using the forward primer 5′-ATCGTGCTCAATGTTTCAACC-3′ and the reverse primer 5′-ATCCAGAGAAGACGTTGCTTATCC-3′. The PCR product length of the wild-type mRNA was determined to be 478 bp encompassing exon 6 (partially) to exon 10 (partially).

For pendrin expression experiments, we prepared tissue sections (5 μm) from the inner ears of *Slc26a4*$^{+/+}$ and *Slc26a4*$^{tm1Dontuh/tm1Dontuh}$ mice. Tissue sections mounted on silane-coated glass slides were then deparaffinized in xylene and rehydrated via graded ratios of ethanol to water. After antigen heat retrieval (500 W microwave oven, in 10 mM citric buffer, pH 6.0, for 20 min), slides were incubated overnight at 4°C with primary antibodies in PBST (phosphate buffer saline & Tween) [rabbit anti-pendrin, 1:100 (H195); mouse anti-Myosin VIIa, 1:100 (C-5) (Santa Cruz Biotechnology, Santa Cruz, CA)]. Slides were then washed and incubated for 1 h at 25°C with appropriate secondary antibodies at a 1:1000 dilution in PBST (donkey anti-rabbit Alexa 488). After incubation, slides were washed with PBST, mounted with ProLong Antifade kit (Molecular Probes, Eugene, OR, USA) for 20 min at room temperature. Images of tissues were obtained using a laser scanning confocal microscope (Zeiss LSM 510, Germany).

Audiological evaluations

Mice were anesthetized with sodium pentobarbital (35 mg/kg) delivered intraperitoneally and maintained in a head-holder within an acoustically and electrically insulated and grounded test room. We used an evoked potential detection system (Smart EP 3.90, Intelligent Hearing Systems, Miami, FL, USA) to measure the thresholds of the auditory brainstem response (ABR) in mice. Click sounds as well as 8, 16, and 32 kHz tone bursts at varying intensity (from 10 to 130 dB SPL), were given to evoke ABRs of mice. The response signals were recorded with a subcutaneous needle electrode inserted ventrolaterally into the ears of the mice.

Vestibular evaluations

Mice were subjected to a battery of vestibular evaluations, including observation of their circling behavior and head-tilting (performed at 3 weeks of age), a reaching test, a swimming test, a gripping test, and a rotorod test (all performed at 8 weeks of age). The reaching responses of mice were recorded after suspending animals by their tails and observing the reaction of their limbs and head-bobbing behaviors. Mice that extended their forelimbs and tried to reach a surface were considered normal (i.e., in terms of reaching response), whereas animals that either clasped their forelimbs or exhibited head-bobbing behavior were classified as abnormal. For the swimming test, mice were observed for 15–20 s, and those that maintained themselves well at the water surface were classified as normal, whereas those that failed to stay near the surface were considered abnormal. For the gripping test, mice were placed on the lower end of a 45-cm-long metal stick, and those that required more than 15 s to reach the top of the stick were classified as abnormal (i.e., <15 s were normal). For the rotorod test, mice were assessed for their ability to balance on a revolving rod (i.e., rotorod) of 3.5 cm diameter. For each test, the mouse was placed on the rod rotating at 50 rpm, and the time required for the mouse to fall was recorded. Each mouse was tested 5 times, and the results were averaged.

Inner ear morphology studies

Tissues from inner ears of *Slc26a4*$^{+/+}$, *Slc26a4*$^{+/tm1Dontuh}$ and *Slc26a4*$^{tm1Dontuh/tm1Dontuh}$ mice were subjected to hematoxylin and eosin (H&E) staining, and the morphology of each sample was examined with a Leica optical microscope. For light microscopy, transmission electron microscopy (TEM) and scanning electron microscopy (SEM) studies, inner ears from adult mice were fixed by perilymphatic perfusion with 4% paraformaldehyde (PFA) in phosphate-buffered saline (PBS) through round and oval windows and a small fenestra in the apex of the cochlear bony capsule. Specimens were subsequently rinsed in PBS buffer and decalcified in 4% PFA with 0.35 M EDTA at 4°C for 1 week. For light microscopy studies, samples were dehydrated and embedded in paraffin. Subsequently, serial sections (7 μm) were stained with H&E. For TEM studies, samples were post-fixed for 2 h in 2% OsO_4 in 0.1 M PBS, dehydrated through graded ethanol solutions, and embedded in Epon. Ultrathin sections (70 nm thickness) were collected on copper grids, doubly stained with uranyl acetate and lead citrate, and examined with a Hitachi 7100 electron microscope (Hitachi, Tokyo, Japan). For SEM studies, samples were dehydrated in ethanol, critical point dried, gold sputter coated, and then examined in a field emission scanning electron microscope (S-4500; Hitachi, Tokyo, Japan).

Whole-mount studies of mouse inner ear specimens were performed as previously described [36], with some minor modification. Briefly, after perfusion with 4% PFA, the cochleae were postfixed in the same solution for 2 h at room temperature and washed in PBS. Segments of stria vascularis and organ of Corti together with Reissner's membrane were dissected out of the inner ear specimens using a fine needle. Samples were permeabilized in 1% Triton X-100 for 30 min and washed with PBS, followed by overnight incubation at 4°C in blocking solution. The tissues were then stained with rhodamine-phalloidin (1:100 dilution; Molecular Probes, Eugene, OR, USA). After washing in PBS, the tissues were mounted using the ProLong Antifade kit (Molecular Probes, Eugene, OR, USA) for 20 min at room temperature. Images of tissues were obtained using a laser scanning confocal microscope (Zeiss LSM 510, Germany).

Thyroid and renal serum biochemistry

Terminal blood samples were obtained from mice at 2 months and 6 months. Total T_4 was measured in undiluted serum (25 μl) by RIA (Diagnostic Products Corp., Los Angeles, CA). Blood urea nitrogen (BUN) and serum creatinine (CREA) were measured by research services of National Taiwan University Hospital.

Data analyses

Data are presented as mean ± SD, unless indicated otherwise. Statistical analyses included the $\chi 2$ or Fisher's exact test for categorical variables and Student's *t*-tests or ANOVA for continuous variables. A p value of <0.05 was considered statistically significant. All analyses were performed using SPSS/Windows software 15.0 (SPSS Science, Chicago, IL, USA).

Supporting Information

Figure S1 ***Slc26a4***$^{tm1Dontuh/tm1Dontuh}$ **mice revealed normal cochlear hair cells at P7.** IHC, inner hair cells; OHC, outer hair cells Bar = 50 μm.

Figure S2 Plasmid construct of the c.919-2A>G mutation. A BAC clone (clone no. bMQ23G13 Geneservice^{TM}) from the 129S7/AB2.2 BAC library containing mouse *Slc26a4* genomic region was used to construct the targeting vector. The BAC was transferred into the modified *Escherichia coli* strain EL350 by electroporation. Two homology arms flanking the genomic area of *Slc26a4* to be subcloned by gap repair were PCR amplified using BAC DNA from clone bMQ23G13 as the template, digested with *Not*I and *Hind*III (5′ arm) or *HindIII* and *Spe*I (3′ arm) and three-way ligated into *Not*I- and *Spe*I-digested PL253. The primers used for amplification of the 5′ and 3′ homology arms were as follows: 5′ arm F, 5′-ATAGCGGCCGCTTAAATGCTGTTTTCTC-CATA-3′; 5′ arm R, 5′-AGCAAGCTTAGTCTTAAGTTGG-CAGGGATGGTGAGTG-3′; 3′ arm F, 5′-TATAAGCTTAA-GAGCAGCCAGTGCTCTTAACC-3′; and 3′ arm R, 5′-ATTACTAGTGTTTGGGCCTGAAGTGTAACAGC-3′. This retrieval vector was linearized by *Afl*II and *Hind*III digestion, gel purified and transformed into heat-shocked and electrocompetent EL350 cells containing the bMQ23G13 BAC clone. The genomic 12.47-kb region was modified in the next targeting round by inserting the neomycin (*neo*) cassette from PL451 and creating the c.919-2A>G mutation (blue asterisk) in intron 7. A *neo*/kanamycin cassette (from PL451) containing homology to a region between intron 6 and exon 8 of *Slc26a4* was inserted. The primers used to amplify the 5′ homology arm were as follows: targeting 5′ arm F, 5′-ATGGTCGACTTTCCTTGAGCTTGTTAATCTGC-3′ and targeting 5′ arm R, 5′-ATAGCGGCCGCTAGGTGCCATT-TTGTGGGGTTTTG-3′. The primers used to amplify the 3′ c.919-2A>G mutation homology arm were as follows: targeting 3′ arm F, 5′-AGCGAATTCATCTTACCAGGACAATTTTTAG-GATTTTTCTTTTTGATAAGACTCACATGTGCTGTTTG-ATGTGATATGACTTTTCCTGTGGGAGAATTG-3′; targeting 3′ arm R, 5′-ATAGCGGCCGCAAAATATATATGAGAA-GATGGCTT-3′; and mutation R, 5′-ATAGGTACCACC-CACTTGGGATGGACTTAACAATGCCAGCATTGTAGTT-CTTTTCCAAGTTGG-3′. Homology arms were digested with *Sal*I and *Bam*HI (5′ arm) and *Eco*RI and *Not*I (3′ arm), and four-way ligated with the *Eco*RI- and *Bam*HI-digested *neo* cassette from PL451 and *Sal*I- and *Not*I-digested PL451 backbone. The targeting cassette was released by *Sal*I and *Not*I digestion and inserted into the retrieved *Slc26a4* fragment by recombineering.

Author Contributions

Conceived and designed the experiments: YCL CCW PJC. Performed the experiments: YCL WSS ISY TH. Yang. Analyzed the data: CCW SWL JMW TH. Yeh. Contributed reagents/materials/analysis tools: TH. Yang TH. Yeh QC XL. Wrote the paper: YCL CCW CJH.

References

1. Hilgert N, Smith RJ, Van Camp G (2009) Forty-six genes causing nonsyndromic hearing impairment: Which ones should be analyzed in DNA diagnostics? Mutat Res 681: 189–196.
2. Li XC, Everett LA, Lalwani AK, Desmukh D, Friedman TB, et al. (1998) A mutation in PDS causes non-syndromic recessive deafness. Nat Genet 18: 215–217.

3. Everett LA, Glaser B, Beck JC, Idol JR, Buchs A, et al. (1997) Pendred syndrome is caused by mutations in a putative sulphate transporter gene (PDS). Nat Genet 17: 411–422.
4. Everett LA, Morsli H, Wu DK, Green ED (1999) Expression pattern of the mouse ortholog of the Pendred's syndrome gene (Pds) suggests a key role for pendrin in the inner ear. Proc Natl Acad Sci U S A 96: 9727–9732.
5. Bidart JM, Mian C, Lazar V, Russo D, Filetti S, et al. (2000) Expression of pendrin and the Pendred syndrome (PDS) gene in human thyroid tissues. J Clin Endocrinol Metab 85: 2028–2033.
6. Royaux IE, Wall SM, Karniski LP, Everett LA, Suzuki K, et al. (2001) Pendrin, encoded by the Pendred syndrome gene, resides in the apical region of renal intercalated cells and mediates bicarbonate secretion. Proc Natl Acad Sci U S A 98: 4221–4226.
7. Royaux IE, Belyantseva IA, Wu T, Kachar B, Everett LA, et al. (2003) Localization and functional studies of pendrin in the mouse inner ear provide insight about the etiology of deafness in pendred syndrome. J Assoc Res Otolaryngol 4: 394–404.
8. Everett LA, Belyantseva IA, Noben-Trauth K, Cantos R, Chen A, et al. (2001) Targeted disruption of mouse Pds provides insight about the inner-ear defects encountered in Pendred syndrome. Hum Mol Genet 10: 153–161.
9. Pryor SP, Madeo AC, Reynolds JC, Sarlis NJ, Arnos KS, et al. (2005) SLC26A4/PDS genotype-phenotype correlation in hearing loss with enlargement of the vestibular aqueduct (EVA): evidence that Pendred syndrome and non-syndromic EVA are distinct clinical and genetic entities. J Med Genet 42: 159–165.
10. Azaiez H, Yang T, Prasad S, Sorensen JL, Nishimura CJ, et al. (2007) Genotype-phenotype correlations for SLC26A4-related deafness. Hum Genet 122: 451–457.
11. Scott DA, Wang R, Kreman TM, Andrews M, McDonald JM, et al. (2000) Functional differences of the PDS gene product are associated with phenotypic variation in patients with Pendred syndrome and non-syndromic hearing loss (DFNB4). Hum Mol Genet 9: 1709–1715.
12. Choi BY, Stewart AK, Madeo AC, Pryor SP, Lenhard S, et al. (2009) Hypo-functional SLC26A4 variants associated with nonsyndromic hearing loss and enlargement of the vestibular aqueduct: genotype-phenotype correlation or coincidental polymorphisms? Hum Mutat 30: 599–608.
13. Wu CC, Yeh TH, Chen PJ, Hsu CJ (2005) Prevalent SLC26A4 mutations in patients with enlarged vestibular aqueduct and/or Mondini dysplasia: A unique spectrum of mutations in Taiwan, including a frequent founder mutation. Laryngoscope 115: 1060–1064.
14. Wang QJ, Zhao YL, Rao SQ, Guo YF, Yuan H, et al. (2007) A distinct spectrum of SLC26A4 mutations in patients with enlarged vestibular aqueduct in China. Clin Genet 72: 245–254.
15. Tsukamoto K, Suzuki H, Harada D, Namba A, Abe S, et al. (2003) Distribution and frequencies of PDS (SLC26A4) mutations in Pendred syndrome and nonsyndromic hearing loss associated with enlarged vestibular aqueduct: a unique spectrum of mutations in Japanese. Eur J Hum Genet 11: 916–922.
16. Park HJ, Lee SJ, Jin HS, Lee JO, Go SH, et al. (2005) Genetic basis of hearing loss associated with enlarged vestibular aqueducts in Koreans. Clin Genet 67: 160–165.
17. Wu CC, Chen PJ, Hsu CJ (2005) Specificity of SLC26A4 mutations in the pathogenesis of inner ear malformations. Audiol Neurootol 10: 234–242.
18. Yang JJ, Tsai CC, Hsu HM, Shiao JY, Su CC, et al. (2005) Hearing loss associated with enlarged vestibular aqueduct and Mondini dysplasia is caused by splice-site mutation in the PDS gene. Hear Res 199: 22–30.
19. Dror AA, Politi Y, Shahin H, Lenz DR, Dossena S, et al. (2010) Calcium oxalate stone formation in the inner ear as a result of an Slc26a4 mutation. J Biol Chem 285: 21724–21735.
20. King KA, Choi BY, Zalewski C, Madeo AC, Manichaikul A, et al. (2010) SLC26A4 Genotype, But Not Cochlear Radiologic Structure, Is Correlated With Hearing Loss in Ears With an Enlarged Vestibular Aqueduct. Laryngoscope 120: 384–389.
21. Rebeh IB, Yoshimi N, Hadj-Kacem H, Yanohco S, Hammami B, et al. (2010) Two missense mutations in SLC26A4 gene: a molecular and functional study. Clin Genet 78: 74–80.
22. Wangemann P, Nakaya K, Wu T, Maganti RJ, Itza EM, et al. (2007) Loss of cochlear HCO3− secretion causes deafness via endolymphatic acidification and inhibition of Ca2+ reabsorption in a Pendred syndrome mouse model. Am J Physiol Renal Physiol 292: F1345–1353.
23. Nakaya K, Harbidge DG, Wangemann P, Schultz BD, Green ED, et al. (2007) Lack of pendrin HCO3− transport elevates vestibular endolymphatic [Ca2+] by inhibition of acid-sensitive TRPV5 and TRPV6 channels. Am J Physiol Renal Physiol 292: F1314–1321.
24. Singh R, Wangemann P (2008) Free radical stress-mediated loss of Kcnj10 protein expression in stria vascularis contributes to deafness in Pendred syndrome mouse model. Am J Physiol Renal Physiol 294: F139–148.
25. Wangemann P, Kim HM, Billings S, Nakaya K, Li X, et al. (2009) Developmental delays consistent with cochlear hypothyroidism contribute to failure to develop hearing in mice lacking Slc26a4/pendrin expression. Am J Physiol-Renal 297: F1435–F1447.
26. Johnsson LG, Hawkins JE, Jr. (1972) Strial atrophy in clinical and experimental deafness. Laryngoscope 82: 1105–1125.
27. Spicer SS, Schulte BA (2005) Pathologic changes of presbycusis begin in secondary processes and spread to primary processes of strial marginal cells. Hear Res 205: 225–240.
28. Suzuki H, Oshima A, Tsukamoto K, Abe S, Kumakawa K, et al. (2007) Clinical characteristics and genotype-phenotype correlation of hearing loss patients with SLC26A4 mutations. Acta Otolaryngol 127: 1292–1297.
29. Sugiura M, Sato E, Nakashima T, Sugiura J, Furuhashi A, et al. (2005) Long-term follow-up in patients with Pendred syndrome: vestibular, auditory and other phenotypes. Eur Arch Otorhinolaryngol 262: 737–743.
30. Everett LA, Belyantseva IA, Noben-Trauth K, Cantos R, Chen A, et al. (2001) Targeted disruption of mouse Pds provides insight about the inner-ear defects encountered in Pendred syndrome. Hum Mol Genet 10: 153–161.
31. Zhou G, Gopen Q, Kenna MA (2008) Delineating the hearing loss in children with enlarged vestibular aqueduct. Laryngoscope 118: 2062–2066.
32. Wu CC, Chen YS, Chen PJ, Hsu CJ (2005) Common clinical features of children with enlarged vestibular aqueduct and mondini dysplasia. Laryngoscope 115: 132–137.
33. Snoeckx RL, Huygen PL, Feldmann D, Marlin S, Denoyelle F, et al. (2005) GJB2 mutations and degree of hearing loss: a multicenter study. Am J Hum Genet 77: 945–957.
34. Lee EC, Yu D, Martinez de Velasco J, Tessarollo L, Swing DA, et al. (2001) A highly efficient Escherichia coli-based chromosome engineering system adapted for recombinogenic targeting and subcloning of BAC DNA. Genomics 73: 56–65.
35. Su KY, Chien WL, Fu WM, Yu IS, Huang HP, et al. (2007) Mice deficient in collapsin response mediator protein-1 exhibit impaired long-term potentiation and impaired spatial learning and memory. J Neurosci 27: 2513–2524.
36. Belyantseva IA, Adler HJ, Curi R, Frolenkov GI, Kachar B (2000) Expression and localization of prestin and the sugar transporter GLUT-5 during development of electromotility in cochlear outer hair cells. J Neurosci 20: RC116.

12

Internet Video Telephony Allows Speech Reading by Deaf Individuals and Improves Speech Perception by Cochlear Implant Users

Georgios Mantokoudis*, Claudia Dähler, Patrick Dubach, Martin Kompis, Marco D. Caversaccio, Pascal Senn

University Department of Otorhinolaryngology, Head & Neck Surgery, Inselspital, Bern, Switzerland

Abstract

Objective: To analyze speech reading through Internet video calls by profoundly hearing-impaired individuals and cochlear implant (CI) users.

Methods: Speech reading skills of 14 deaf adults and 21 CI users were assessed using the Hochmair Schulz Moser (HSM) sentence test. We presented video simulations using different video resolutions (1280×720, 640×480, 320×240, 160×120 px), frame rates (30, 20, 10, 7, 5 frames per second (fps)), speech velocities (three different speakers), webcameras (Logitech Pro9000, C600 and C500) and image/sound delays (0–500 ms). All video simulations were presented with and without sound and in two screen sizes. Additionally, scores for live Skype^{TM} video connection and live face-to-face communication were assessed.

Results: Higher frame rate (>7 fps), higher camera resolution (>640×480 px) and shorter picture/sound delay (<100 ms) were associated with increased speech perception scores. Scores were strongly dependent on the speaker but were not influenced by physical properties of the camera optics or the full screen mode. There is a significant median gain of +8.5%pts (p = 0.009) in speech perception for all 21 CI-users if visual cues are additionally shown. CI users with poor open set speech perception scores (n = 11) showed the greatest benefit under combined audio-visual presentation (median speech perception +11.8%pts, p = 0.032).

Conclusion: Webcameras have the potential to improve telecommunication of hearing-impaired individuals.

Editor: Stefan Kiebel, Max Planck Institute for Human Cognitive and Brain Sciences, Germany

Funding: This study was supported by a grant of the foundation "Stiftung für die Erforschung von Hör- und Sprachstörungen", Bern. Logitech Europe S.A. provided the webcameras. The funders had no role in study design, data collection and analysis, decision to publish, or preparation of the manuscript.

Competing Interests: The company Logitech Europe S.A. provided commercially available products for this study.

* E-mail: mantokoudis@gmx.ch

Introduction

For many years the use of videophones for transmission of sign language or lip motion over telephone networks was either expensive or of low image quality, thereby limiting its use [1]. Short message service (SMS), instant messaging services or teletypewriters have therefore become the main long-distance communication modes among hearing-impaired and deaf individuals in the last two decades [2]. Written communication, however, is usually slower and less ideal to transport emotional content compared to audio-visual (AV) communication. The relative lack of long-distance communication options among hearing-impaired and deaf individuals contributes to a reduction of social connectivity and is associated with increased morbidity and mortality [3,4]. Recently, Internet infrastructure and communication software tools have been rapidly developing and now allow both audio and audio-visual Internet communication with ever-improving quality. In comparison to conventional telephony, Internet telephony also offers broader sound frequency ranges and improved conservation of audio quality. These technical advantages of Internet over conventional telephony have translated into improved speech perception by hearing-impaired and normal hearing adults in recent, laboratory-based studies by our group [5,6]. Earlier studies were limited to transmission of audio signals through Internet telephony, and to our knowledge, no reports on speech perception with Internet transmission of audio and visual content have been published. The current study aims to address the value of added visual content. There is evidence that cochlear implant (CI) users improve speech perception performance if visual cues are presented together with an auditory input [7–9]. In addition, CI users maintain their speech reading capacities after implantation [7–11].

Video telephony as provided by Skype^{TM} and other Internet communication companies offer a broadband transmission of voice and image over an Internet protocol (IP) network. The Internet software sends small packets of encoded data over the

Table 1. Demographic and technical data of cochlear implanted individuals.

ID	Age at implantation	Age at test	Gender	Etiology of deafness	CI-Device	Speech Processor	Communication mode
npCI1	4	26	F	Meningitis	Nucleus 22 Series	ESPrit 3G	Total communication*
npCI2	50	56	F	Sudden deafness	PULSARci100	OPUS2	Auditory-oral**
npCI3	45	58	F	Progressive	C40	OPUS2	Total communication
npCI4	11	25	F	Rubella embryopathy	CI24M Nucleus 24	Freedom SR	Total communication
npCI5	20	25	F	Meningitis	PULSARci100	OPUS2	Total communication
npCI6	17	30	M	Meningitis	C40	CIS PRO+	Auditory-oral
npCI7	17	22	F	Congenital	PULSARci100	OPUS2	Total communication
npCI8	61	69	M	Streptomycin	PULSARci100	OPUS2	Auditory-oral
npCI9	15	26	F	Progressive	SONATAti100	OPUS2	Auditory-oral
npCI10	52	61	F	Progressive	PULSARci100	OPUS2	Auditory-oral
npCI11	48	55	M	Progressive	HiRES90K	Auria Harmony	Auditory-oral
pCI12	21	24	F	Progressive	Freedom Implant (straight)	Freedom SP	Auditory-oral
pCI13	34	40	F	Progressive	PULSARci100	OPUS2	Auditory-oral
pCI14	41	49	F	Progressive	PULSARci100	OPUS2	Auditory-oral
pCI15	63	70	F	Progressive	C40+	OPUS2	Auditory-oral
pCI16	61	64	F	Sudden deafness	SONATAti100	OPUS2	Auditory-oral
pCI17	12	24	M	Congenital	C40+	OPUS2	Total communication
pCI18	3	24	F	Meningitis	CI22M	ESPrit 3G/N22	Total communication
pCI19	57	62	F	Meningitis	PULSARci100	OPUS2	Auditory-oral
pCI20	11	24	F	Congenital	C40+	OPUS2	Total communication
pCI21	14	18	M	Meningitis	PULSARci100	OPUS2	Auditory-oral

*Total communication includes hearing, speech reading and sign language.
**Auditory-oral communication includes hearing and speech reading.

Internet guided via the IP. Each data packet takes a unique pathway through the network before arriving at a receiver computer that uses the same software as the sender. The receiver's software then collects, reconstructs and decodes all data packets before finally converting them back into an analog signal that is presented to the end-user.

Despite its potential benefits, the quality of internet video telephony transmission may be hampered by congested internet lines [12], inadequate infrastructure or insufficient bandwidth, which lead to data packet loss or delay, frame rate reduction, audio-visual asynchrony [13], or decreased signal-to-noise ratio of the video signal [14]. The web camera properties (lenses, resolution, camera software) may also influence video quality. To what extent these parameters influence speech perception, particularly by hearing-impaired individuals, has not been sufficiently addressed. Additionally, the potential of rapidly-improving Internet communication technology for helping hearing-impaired individuals remains largely unknown. The first aim of this study was therefore to test the hypothesis that current Internet technology allows sufficient transmission of lip and face motion images for adequate speech reading. The second aim was to assess the range of parameters within which visual contributions are suitable for improving communication over the Internet.

Materials and Methods

Ethics Statement

The study protocol was approved by the local institutional review board (Kantonale Ethikkomission Bern, Switzerland); all patients gave written informed consent.

Test Subjects

All tests were conducted between March 2010 and July 2011 at the Department of Otorhinolaryngology-Head and Neck Surgery, Inselspital, University of Bern, Switzerland. In total, 14 deaf adults and 21 CI users participated in the study. We chose deaf individuals as a reference for the assessment of speech reading and CI users for the assessment of both speech reading and audiovisual gain. Deaf individuals were recruited from deaf community organizations ("IGGH Interessegemeinschaft Gehörlose und Hörbehinderte der Kantone Bern und Freiburg" and "proaudito, Schwerhörigenverein Bern"). Eight individuals had congenital deafness (rubella embryopathy, mumps and unknown), four had prelingual deafness (2 with meningitis, 1 with mumps and 1 unknown) and two individuals lost their hearing at the age of 22 and 44 y (progressive hearing loss). The mean age of this group was 41.6 years (range 23–63 years). All 14 deaf adults used sign language and speech reading in daily communication. They had normal vision or normal corrected vision.

CI users were recruited through a database of the audiological department of our tertiary referral center. The mean age of CI users at time of cochlear implantation was 31.3 years (range 3–63 years) and 40.6 years at the time of testing (range 18–70 years). All CI users were therefore experienced, with a mean CI-listening experience of 9.3 years (range 4–22 years). All 21 CI users had bilateral profound hearing loss, normal vision or normal corrected vision, and used an auditory-oral or total communication mode in daily life. Table 1 summarizes the clinical data of CI users included in this study. Eligible CI users had an aided minimum monosyllabic word discrimination score of 20% at 60 dB sound pressure level (SPL). Prior to testing, CI users were divided into two subgroups based on speech perception scores obtained by the HSM sentence test [15]. The subgroup of non-proficient CI users (npCI; n = 11) scored <70% correct, whereas the subgroup of proficient CI users (pCI; n = 10) scored 70% or higher in the sentence test at a SPL of 60 dB.

Speech Reading Test Procedure

We performed three series of experiments to assess speech reading cues transmitted over the Internet. A first set of experiments assessed speech reading in deaf adults under controlled conditions. Factors hypothesized to influence Internet speech communication such as different speech velocities (different speakers), camera properties (resolution, different lenses), screen properties (resolution) and Internet transmission rates (resulting in a specific frame per second [fps]) were tested by a video simulation. We presented video simulations using three different speakers (CD, 97 words/min; SF, 178 words/min; JB, 161 words/min), four screen resolutions (1280×720 px, 640×480 px, 320×240 px, 160×120 px), two screen sizes (original resolution size versus full screen mode), five frame rates (5, 7, 10, 20 and 30 fps), and three web cameras (Logitech Pro9000, Carl Zeiss lens, 2 Megapixel; Logitech C600, 2 Megapixel; Logitech C500, 1.4 Megapixel). Details about the digital generation of audio-visual video files for the simulation are shown in Text S1.

A second set of experiments tested speech reading skills in deaf individuals and CI users under real but controlled conditions (efficacy trial) by using a Skype™ Internet connection (250 kBps download and 3 kBps upload speed) between two rooms. A telephonometric communication (two persons communicate in the same room at 1 m distance) served as a reference standard. [16] This test condition is also referred as a face-to-face communication mode. Settings about a live Skype™ video transmission and its monitoring are described in Text S2.

A third set of experiments on CI users aimed to assess audiovisual cues transmitted by Internet video telephony. Auditory and combined AV stimuli with different AV-delays (0–500 ms) were used under simulated and real network conditions. Patients were asked about their overall experience with AV delay and whether they felt they required both auditory and visual stimuli or relied on either auditory or visual stimuli alone.

The German "HSM" sentence test [15] was used to assess speech perception for all test experiments across all conditions. This open set speech recognition test provides 30 lists with 20 sentences and 106 words per list. One unique list for each test condition was used to avoid learning effects. Testing was performed in a sound treated room in the free sound field using standardized equipment. Audio and video signals were delivered to the loudspeaker/laptop screen at ear level (speech signal calibrated at 60 dB SPL), at a distance of 1 m in front of the participant's head. To balance difficulty level across subject groups and test procedures, npCI-users were tested in quiet and pCI-users were tested with simultaneous competing noise (CCITT) at a constant SPL of 50 dB for AV testing (signal-to-noise ratio (SNR) of 10 dB SPL) or 55 dB for AV-delay testing (SNR of 5 dB SPL). Subjects were asked to repeat aloud the presented words or sentences as quickly as possible or to write down. No feedback was given to the participants. Subjects were given a five-minute training session prior to testing. The percentage of correctly repeated words was used for comparison of performance across conditions. Normal hearing adults usually have a speech perception score between 90–100% in noise (SNR of 10 dB SPL) [17] [15], whereas CI users have an expected average score of 70% [18] Subjects were assigned randomly to different test sequences. To avoid order effects, different test sequences were constructed by permutation. Subjects and investigator were blinded to the different video qualities used.

All CI users were tested monaurally using the same ear throughout the entire test battery. Bilateral CI users were asked to remove the device on the poorer hearing side in order to obtain more homogenous data across subjects. The opposite ear canal was occluded with an ear plug (E.A.R. classic, Aearo Ltd., Stockport, UK) if residual low-frequency hearing was present. The specified average attenuation of these earplugs is 24.6 to 41.6 dB in the range of 250 to 4000 Hz. For the live speech reading test (Skype™ versus face-to-face) without acoustical input (visual only), CI users were required to power off their devices and to use ear plugs bilaterally.

Testing was performed in a single session with a total testing time per subject of approximately 2 hours including breaks.

Statistics

Robust nonparametric analyses were performed to assess the potentially non-normally distributed speech perception scores from this small study population. We used the Spearman correlation test to assess the relationship between speech perception and camera properties (frame rate and resolution [megapixel]). To evaluate speech reading performance, we first used the Friedman test to identify possible differences at a 0.05 significance level in each of the following parameters: camera types, communication modes, speakers and AV-modes. Then, we used the two-tailed Wilcoxon matched pairs signed-rank test to compare groups within the parameters that were identified as different from the Friedman test. Bonferroni correction was performed for multiple testing (P_{Bonf}).

Results

Speech Reading Performance by Deaf Adults

All 14 deaf adults had measurable speech reading abilities (face-to-face without sign language) with speech perception scores ranging from 41.5%–97.2% (median 74.5%). When video files were presented, scores were lower and ranged from 1.9% to 75.5% (median 51.9%), depending on the speaker. The slower speaking individual 'CD' (97 words/s) was better understood and this resulted in substantially higher scores (median 52.4%) compared to presentations of files by the other two speakers (median 17%, JB and 11.4%, SF, respectively). The score differences from speaker 'CD' to 'JB' and 'SF' were statistically significant (Figure 1A).

Similarly, the communication mode influenced speech perception by deaf individuals as shown in Figure 1B. The scores obtained with video presentation from the same speaker on a high-definition screen were statistically lower than a face-to-face communication mode (Figure 1B, p = 0.002). There was a significant loss of speech reading scores (up to 50%pts) obtained in the live Skype™ video transmission mode compared to a face-to-face communication mode (Figure 1B, p = 0.0005) or to video presentation mode (Figure 1B, p = 0.001). The median speech

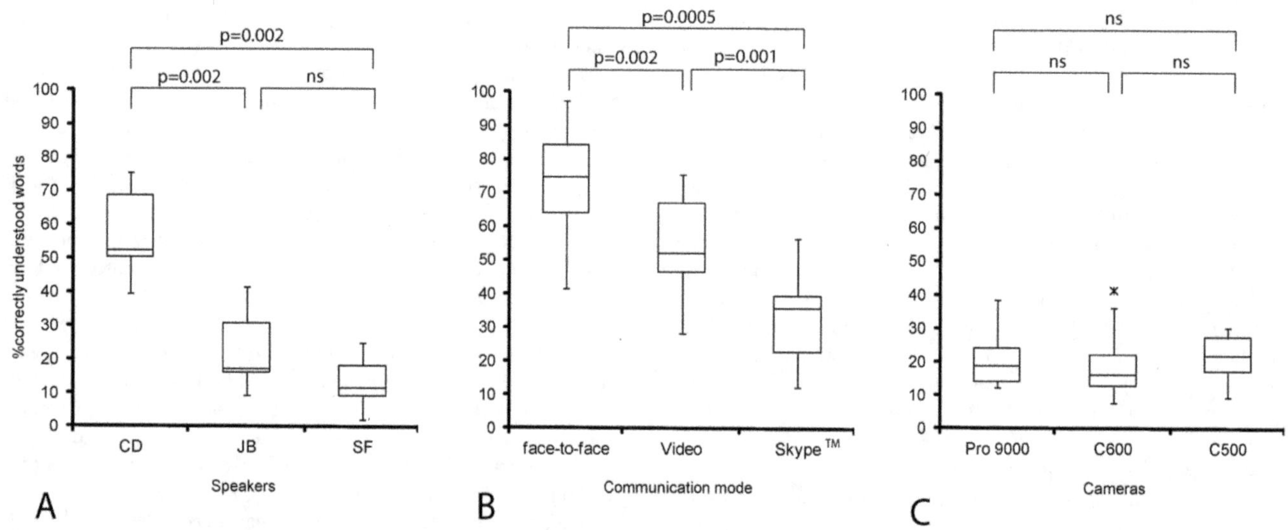

Figure 1. Boxplots demonstrating lower quartile, median, and upper quartile, and whiskers representing 1.5 times the interquartile range (X = outliers): Speech reading performance (correctly-repeated words in percent) from 14 deaf individuals by using (A) the same high definition web camera (Logitech Pro9000) and different speakers (CD, medical student, 97 words/s; JB, actress, 161 words/s; SF, speech therapist, 178 words/s), (B) the same speaker (CD) but different communication modes and (C) the same speaker (SF) with 3 different webcams: Logitech Pro9000, Logitech C600, and Logitech C500.

perception scores of deaf adults using a Skype™ transmission for speech reading alone (without using sign language) was 35.9% (range 12.3%–56.6%), which was not sufficient for satisfactory communication.

Camera hardware, resolution, frame rate and screen size. The type of camera hardware did not greatly influence speech reading scores by deaf individuals; none of the comparisons across camera types reached statistical significance (Figure 1C, $p = 0.79$). In contrast, higher camera resolutions (Figure 2A, $p = 0.0025$, Spearman $r = 0.56$) and higher transmitted frame rates (Figure 2B, $p < 0.0001$, Spearman $r = 0.66$) were associated with statistically significant higher speech reading scores. The screen size for video presentation did not greatly influence the speech reading scores. No statistical significant difference was found when comparing full screen mode vs. the video's original size ($p = 0.79$, data not shown).

Speech Reading Performance by CI-users

All CI users could understand speech based on speech reading (visual only mode, Figure 3), particularly in the face-to-face communication mode. Speech perception scores were significantly lower for the Skype™ visual only transmission mode as compared to face-to-face communication without the implant activated (pCI $p = 0.0029$; npCI $p = 0.0015$). Non-proficient (npCI) CI users were generally better speech readers compared to proficient (pCI) CI users, regardless of the communication mode (median scores of 61.3% vs. 56.7% in the face-to-face communication mode and 50.9% vs. 45.8% in the Skype™ transmission mode, figure 3).

Overall, CI users are not as good as deaf subjects at speech reading (median 61.3% vs. 74.5%), however, deaf individuals showed greater degradation of speech reading performance during a Skype™ video call (median 50.9% for npCI versus 35.9% for deaf subjects).

Audio-visual gain. Figure 4 shows speech perception scores for audio only vs. audio-visual (AV) presentation for the Skype™ transmission mode. For all CI users (pCI and npCI combined), there is a significant overall median gain in speech perception scores of +8.5%pts (range −18% to 51%, $p = 0.009$) if live webcam images are added to the audio signal. NpCI users showed the greatest benefit of combined AV presentation (Figure 4). For this group, the median speech discrimination gain was +11.8%pts (−18% to 45.3%, $p = 0.032$) compared to the audio only presentation. A smaller, and statistically insignificant gain of +3.8%pts (−8.5 to 51%, $p = 0.13$) was found for the pCI-group.

Audio-visual asynchrony. Audio-visual asynchrony was associated with lower speech perception scores by CI users. The association between duration of the AV-delay and the speech perception scores are directly correlated for short delays (0–300 ms for pCI-users; 0–200 ms for npCI-users; Figure 5). Interestingly, the two groups behaved differently for longer delays, when the two signals could no longer be fused and only one stimulus could be considered for speech perception. Whereas pCI-users reported to exclusively rely on auditory signals, the npCI-users fully relied on visual stimuli. Therefore, after 300 ms and 200 ms, respectively, the speech perception scores were again higher, once the participants no longer tried to fuse the two stimuli.

Discussion

This study demonstrates that current Internet communication technology already provides sufficient quality of video transmission for speech reading by deaf individuals. When using Internet communication, cochlear implant users show improved speech perception scores when using combined audio and visual input as compared to audio input alone. In addition, several technical parameters were identified that are associated with improved speech perception: frame rates above 15 fps, camera resolution above 640×480 px, slower speaker and shorter audio-visual delay (<100 ms). To our knowledge, this is the first study investigating speech perception using Internet video telephony technology available on the market.

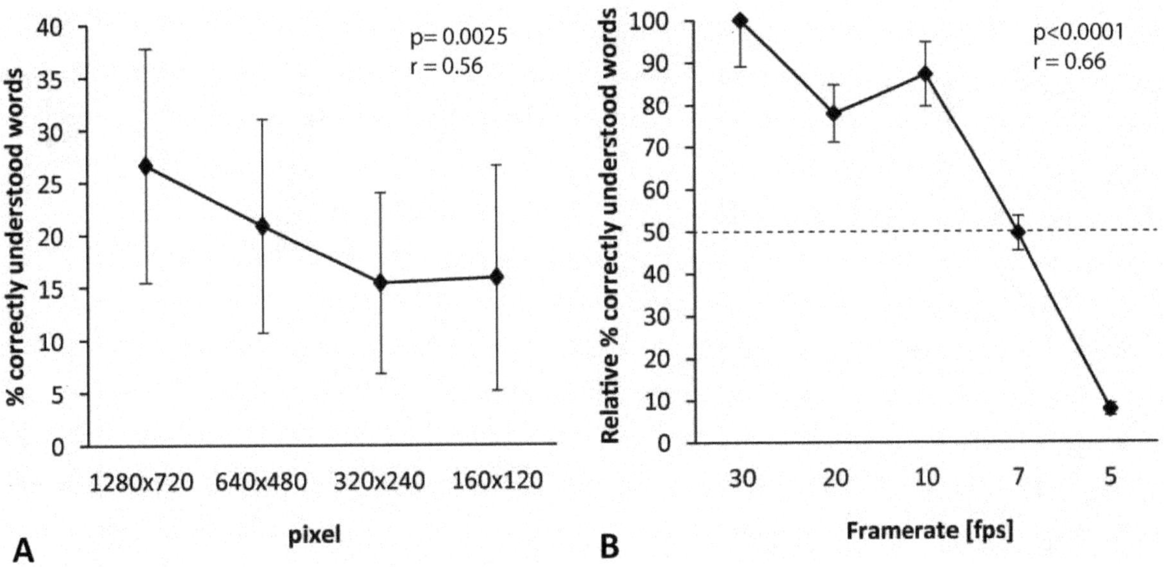

Figure 2. Speech reading performance (mean +/−1 SD) by n = 14 deaf individuals for 4 different spatial resolutions (A) and 5 different frame rates (B). In B, the maximum achieved speech perception at 30 fps is set to 100% (relative data). Mean speech perception scores remained above 80% until the frame rate of 10 images per second. Frame rates <10 fps were associated with a substantial reduction of the speech reading performance and frame rates at 7 fps led to a 50% reduction of the initial performance at optimal video quality. Speech reading at 5 fps was almost impossible.

Background and Comparison with Other Studies

Communication mode, speaker and audiovisual gain. Speech reading is often used in conjunction with sign language or with an auditory input (AV-mode) if applicable. A multimodal communication mode increases speech perception performance by deaf and CI-using individuals. Audio-visual speech perception depends on several factors such as speech reading abilities, auditory performance and capacity of AV-fusion. CI users rely on bimodal speech comprehension, especially for face-to-face communication under noisy conditions where the

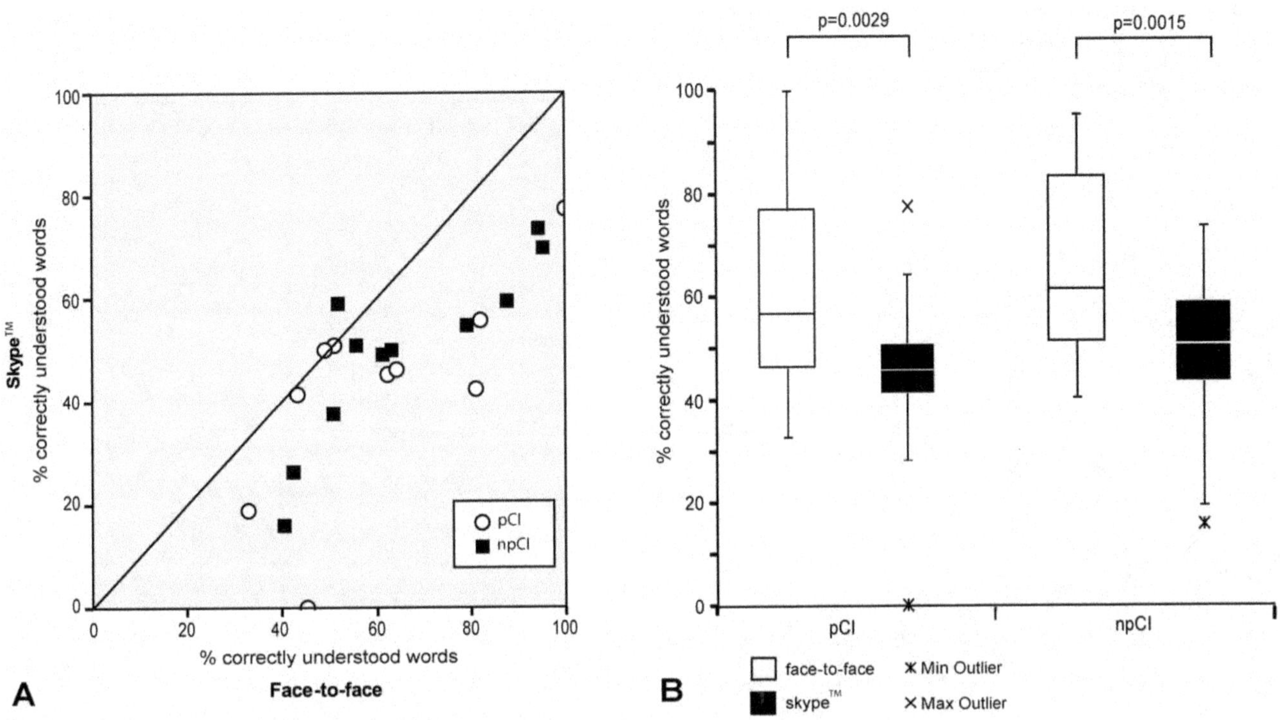

Figure 3. Speech reading capability of cochlear implant users. A. Comparison of speech perception scores in the absence of auditory input for n = 10 proficient (pCI) and n = 11 non-proficient (npCI) CI users for two visual communication modes (face-to-face without their implant activated vs. Skype™ video only). B. Boxplots showing speech reading scores for each condition and group.

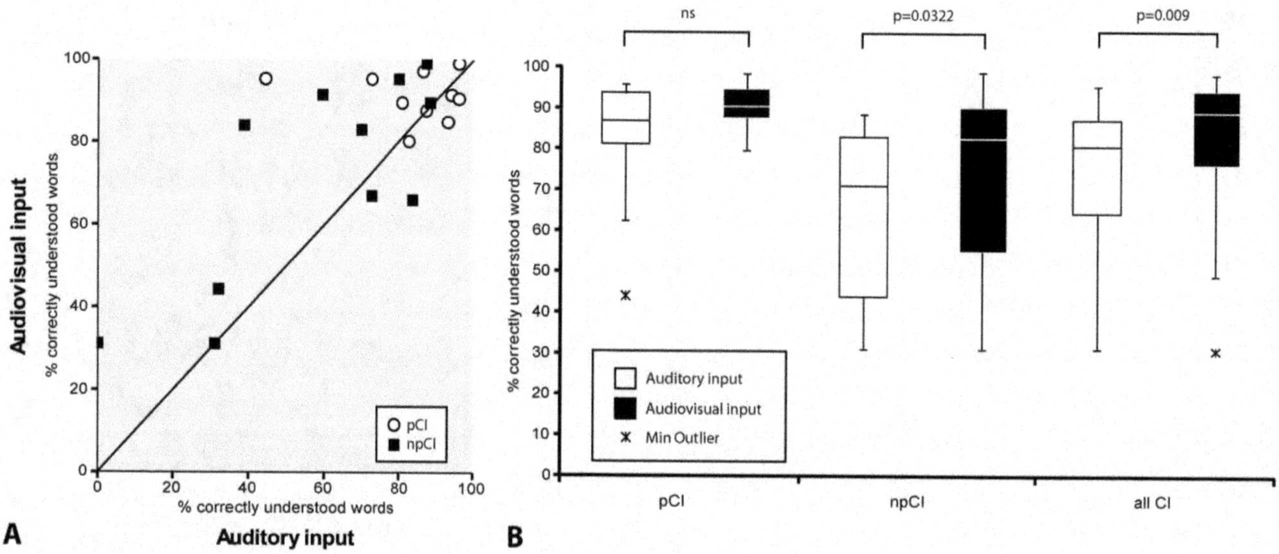

Figure 4. CI-users and audio-visual gain for Skype™ transmission. A. Speech perception scores of n = 10 proficient (pCI) and n = 11 non-proficient (npCI) CI users for exclusive auditory input vs. audio-visual input. B. Non-proficient CI users and the two groups combined (all CI) showed a statistically significant audio-visual gain (Boxplots). Proficient CI users showed a non-significant trend for AV-gain.

auditory speech signal is degraded. Speech reading is still possible after cochlear implantation and does not change within the first postoperative year with recruiting of visual and audio-visual brain areas during communication [10].

Together with directional microphones, AV cues improve speech perception performance under adverse listening conditions [19,20], a phenomenon which is also a known for hearing aid users [21,22]. Enhancement of speech perception in noisy conditions by visual cues is also described for normal-hearing individuals [23] and even for deaf individuals under an exposure of multimodal congruent information [24]. Speech perception based on speech reading alone usually remains poorer in comparison to a bimodal speech information transmission, because live spoken speech transmits lip shape information at a frame rate of 25 Hz, which is 4 times lower than a pure acoustical stimulation rate [25]. Our results are consistent with the literature, in that most of the listeners experienced an audio-visual gain if congruent visual cues were transmitted, however, the two tested subgroups of CI users behaved differently. Whereas non-proficient CI users benefitted from the combined AV-mode, proficient CI users only showed a trend toward better speech perception scores. Non-proficient users showed a mean reduction of error of 26% in comparison to 3% error reduction in proficient users. One reason for this difference could be that proficient CI users experience a ceiling effect by achieving higher scores by hearing alone, leaving little room for improvement. Another reason could be a loss of speech reading skills following successful implantation; however, a longitudinal study showed that speech reading abilities remain un-

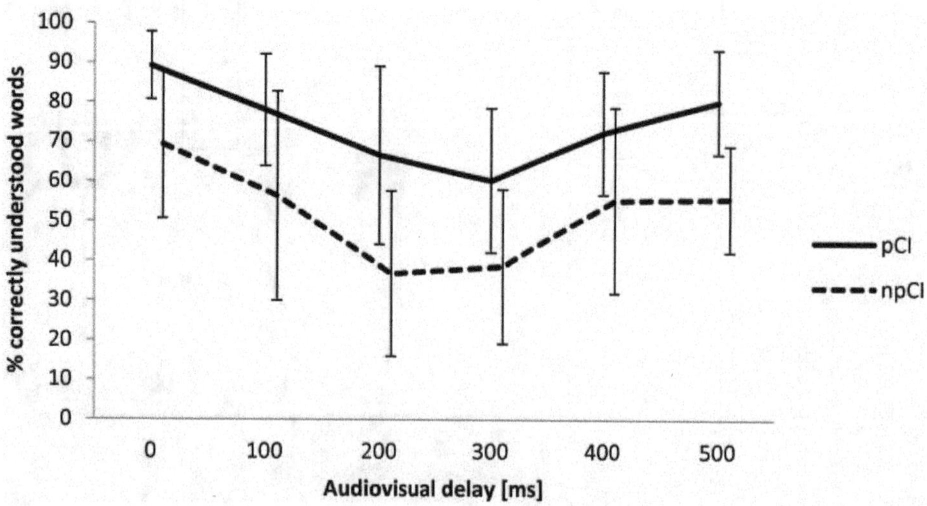

Figure 5. Audiovisual delay. Bimodal mean speech perception (+/−1 SD) is plotted against audio-visual delay (auditory signal proceeds image) for n = 10 proficient (pCI) and n = 11 non-proficient (npCI) CI users. Fusion of incongruent auditory and visual stimuli is not possible after 200 ms for npCI and 300 ms for pCI users. Intelligibility improved again after long AV delays because CI users did not try to fuse both incongruent signals and relied on either one of the stimuli.

changed after implantation even after several years [8]. All CI users in this study had a long listening experience ranging from 4–22 years and half of them (pCI group, n = 10) were mainly orally communicating in their daily lives. It is conceivable that pCI-users keep their compensatory speech reading skills in case they are exposed to difficult listening conditions.

Furthermore, the transmission of speech reading cues over a video screen or via Skype™ transmission led to lower speech perception scores in comparison to a face-to-face communication mode (Figures 1B and 3). There was always a loss of information observed probably because of the lack of depth of field, missed 3D perception and degradation of the signal during Internet transmission. While speech reading abilities during a live face-to-face conversation remain excellent, deaf individuals experience more speech perception difficulties during a Skype™ video call compared to CI users. It seems conceivable that deaf individuals evaluate more facial details during speech reading than CI users, who rely more on auditory signals and pay less attention to other facial cues than lip motion. In fact, it could be shown that deaf individuals have a better visual cognition compared to hearing controls [26]. Speech reading performance of our test subjects was strongly dependent on the individual speaker (Figure 1A). The factors contributing to this variability include speech velocity, lip shapes, skin, facial hair or different visual articulation, as reported earlier [25].

Frame rate. Foulds et al. [27] suggested a minimal frame rate of at least12 images per second for sufficient sign language transmission. For video transmission of speech reading cues, the United Nations Specialized Agency "ITU" recommended 10 years ago a frame rate of 20 fps or more [28] but with some constraints, a frame rate of 12 fps and higher could be used. A frame rate of more than 15 fps still increases speech perception performance, but to a lesser extent [22]. Theoretically, 10 phonemes per second have to be transmitted which requires a frame rate of at least 20 fps [28]. Trained and experienced lip readers, however, will achieve sufficient speech understanding by speech reading alone even under adverse network conditions with reduced frame rate (<15 fps) because of sentence reconstruction of guessed words and redundancy. Frame rates lower than 8 fps are not considered sufficient for speech reading [28]. With current Internet technology, the recommendation by the ITU-T seems to be met, since our live Skype™ video calls transmitted a mean frame rate of 15 fps (range 12–30 fps). All participants showed a benefit on speech understanding by using speech reading cues even under adverse network conditions with decreased frame rates. Speech perception was, as mentioned previously, dependant on the speaker and her speed of speaking (Figure 1A). Faster speech requires higher frame rates compared to slower speech to allow adequate transmission. The findings in this study add evidence to the strong relationship between frame rate and speech reading performance.

Spatial resolution and camera properties. It has been reported that communication by speech reading and sign language at a resolution of 176×144 pixels is possible despite losing many facial details [28]. The display size seems not to be the main limiting factor for speech reading [22]. Our results suggest the use of higher spatial resolutions in order to improve speech performance (Figure 2B). Video conversations at small spatial resolutions (lower than 640×480 px) should be performed in full screen mode because the lip shape information is still preserved. However, current Skype™ versions support the transmission of high definition images (720 p). Better camera properties like expensive camera lenses were not associated with better speech comprehension. Hence, even cameras affordable for a smaller budget are sufficient for audio-visual modes of speech reading.

Bandwidth. According to Luca De Cicco et al [29] a minimum bit rate of 40 kbps is mandatory to engage in a video Skype™ call. One decade ago, Internet communication technology did not provide sufficient bandwidth for real-time video transmission over communication networks [1]. Many attempts were made to transmit real-time video at lower bandwidths by using modern algorithms with data compression, image size reduction or intelligent recognition of hand and face movements [30–32]. These solutions, however, have lost importance recently with improving broadband Internet infrastructure ensuring stable and fast data connections. The latest version of Skype™ (>4.2 Beta) supports broadband transmission of high-definition video (1280×720 px), which further enhances the communication experience.

Signal delay. End-to-end video delay should be kept below 0.4 s [28] similar to the requirements for audio conversations in order to ensure an agreeable communication. Roundtrip time (RTT) measures the time needed for a data packet to be transmitted from the sender to the receiver plus the time back for the acknowledgment of the received packet. Current 100 MBit connections by Ethernet have normally a RTT less than 1 ms, while the RTT for wireless Internet connections (WLAN 802.11 g/n) is prolonged (<5 ms). Mean RTT for the Skype™ connection measured in this study was <1 ms (range 0–15 ms), which is an acceptable RTT length. RTT depends also on internet infrastructure and the geographical location of both sender and receiver [33].

Audiovisual asynchrony. AV signals are often synchronized by a form of interlaced video and audio data or by explicit AV synchronization by time-stamping [34]. Different audio and video paths can lead to a variable AV-sync delay (AV asynchrony). An incongruent AV signal is often associated with a degradation of speech perception performance. CI users have the ability to fuse incongruent auditory and visual information [11] regardless of hearing impairment or age [13,35] which could be shown for both CI-study groups, pCI and npCI. The fusion process, however, depends on the duration of the AV-delay (Figure 5). Recent data suggests that CI users have an increased ability for cross-modal central interaction between visual and auditory processing compared to normal hearing listeners [10]. Speech perception performance of non-proficient CI users depends more on visual cues in cases of incongruent visual and auditory cues (AV conflict) [11]. Figure 5 represents this phenomenon for npCI users experiencing AV conflict (minimal speech reading performance at 200 ms intermodal delay), whereas pCI users were more resistant up to 300 ms. NpCI users reported to rely only on visual cues if unable to fuse incongruent AV information (>200 ms, Figure 5). An over-reliance on visual cues may affect speech perception performance under asynchronous AV conditions because visual stimuli could impair auditory processing based on cross-modal plasticity in cochlear implant users [36]. Therefore, a time delay between audio and image transmission over the IP-network should be kept to a minimum. Baskent and Bazo [13] demonstrated, that an intermodal delay of −108 to +203 msecs was not detectable for more than half of normal hearing test subjects. Estimates of the minimal detectable asynchrony (sound leads the image) vary widely in the literature (20 ms –150 ms) [37], however, a time window for possible AV integration of asynchronous signals ranges between 40 to 600 ms [38]. In our study, subject speech perception performance with an AV-delay of at least 100 ms fell below the performance levels of speech reading or hearing alone. The recommended acceptable time delays of up to 100 ms [28] are in line with our findings.

AV asynchrony may be related to calculation delay in the cochlear implant system, however we did not test this. Based on manufacturer data, the processing time in the implant or speech processor is negligible compared to the AV-delays occurring in video telephony.

One limitation of the presented study is the fact that only speech reading based speech perception by deaf individuals was assessed. The effects of sign language or bimodal communication (lip movements and sign language combined) on speech perception through video-transmission have not been considered. The main reason for focusing on speech reading was that all participants (deaf individuals and CI users) had some experience reading lip reading cues. Not all tested CI users were able to understand sign language. In addition, this study aimed to understand the potential of current technology for transmitting lip motion cues over the network, which is more delicate compared to hand and finger motion cues [28]. Another limitation is that our data cannot be generalized for all Internet video telephony services on the market. We have analyzed only one popular service (Skype™); nevertheless, the present study may be used as a reference for other services or similar studies, because the codecs used in Skype ™ are produced by Google's subsidiary company On2 Technologies, the world market leader providing most modern video codecs for other Internet communication services.

Potential Implications

Internet video telephony (in particular Skype™) offers direct communication benefit for deaf and cochlear-implanted individuals at minimal cost. We believe the four main advantages of this new technology for CI users are: 1. Bilateral hearing is possible either in free field with PC active loudspeakers or with headphones, 2. the auditory signal can be amplified up to a comfort level, while the conventional telephone is adjustable only to a limited extent, 3. broadband voice quality is near CD-quality in comparison to a low-pass filtered signal in conventional telephony [5] and 4. visual cues are available to the end-user through the web camera. The advantage of Skype™ video transmission in comparison to pre-existing videophones (based on ISDN or other networks) is the worldwide and widespread use of this free available software with more than 2.4 billion software downloads, more than 700 million registered users and more than 30 million online users. Cochlear-implanted individuals may therefore communicate with numerous normal hearing users without previous investments in communication devices. Additionally, Skype™ conference calls may be helpful for deaf individuals by using sign language interpreters. Therefore, professionals dealing with hard of hearing and deaf individuals, should recommend the use of Internet video calls for an enhanced communication experience.

Conclusions

The present study identified several factors associated with improved speech reading performance over Internet video telephony, such as frame rates above 15 fps, camera resolution above 640×480 px, slower speaker and shorter audio-visual delay (<100 ms). Overall, Internet video telephony transmits sufficient lip shape information for speech reading by deaf and cochlear-implanted individuals. There are significant audio-visual benefits observed for CI users; however, bimodal cues with the addition of sign language for deaf individuals or auditory input for cochlear-implanted patients are still recommended for engaging in meaningful video-conversation over the web.

Acknowledgments

The authors would like to thank all test subjects for their participation in the study and the non-profit organisations "IGGH Interessegemeinschaft Gehörlose und Hörbehinderte der Kantone Bern und Freiburg" and "proaudito, Schwerhörigenverein Bern". Further, we would like to thank the company Logitech Europe S. A., Morges, Switzerland, for providing the web cameras, Christoph Schmid, Benjamin von Gunten, engineers and Christian Güder, computer scientist, for technical support and Bryan Kevin Ward, MD, for proofreading the text.

Author Contributions

Conceived and designed the experiments: GM CD PD MK MDC PS. Performed the experiments: GM CD. Analyzed the data: GM CD PS. Contributed reagents/materials/analysis tools: GM MK MDC PS. Wrote the paper: GM CD PD MK MDC PS.

References

1. Hellstrom Delevert, Revelius (1997) Quality requirements on Videotelephony for Sign Language; Stockholm, Sweden.
2. Bowe FG (2002) Deaf and hard of hearing Americans' instant messaging and e-mail use: a national survey. Am Ann Deaf 147: 6–10.
3. Dalton DS, Cruickshanks KJ, Klein BE, Klein R, Wiley TL, et al. (2003) The impact of hearing loss on quality of life in older adults. Gerontologist 43: 661–668.
4. Barnett S, Franks P (1999) Deafness and mortality: analyses of linked data from the National Health Interview Survey and National Death Index. Public Health Rep 114: 330–336.
5. Mantokoudis G, Kompis M, Dubach P, Caversaccio M, Senn P (2010) How internet telephony could improve communication for hearing-impaired individuals. Otol Neurotol 31: 1014–1021.
6. Mantokoudis G, Dubach P, Pfiffner F, Kompis M, Caversaccio M, et al. (2012) Speech perception benefits of internet versus conventional telephony for hearing-impaired individuals. J Med Internet Res 14: e102.
7. Bergeson TR, Pisoni DB, Davis RA (2005) Development of audiovisual comprehension skills in prelingually deaf children with cochlear implants. Ear Hear 26: 149–164.
8. Strelnikov K, Rouger J, Barone P, Deguine O (2009) Role of speechreading in audiovisual interactions during the recovery of speech comprehension in deaf adults with cochlear implants. Scand J Psychol 50: 437–444.
9. Rouger J, Lagleyre S, Fraysse B, Deneve S, Deguine O, et al. (2007) Evidence that cochlear-implanted deaf patients are better multisensory integrators. Proc Natl Acad Sci U S A 104: 7295–7300.
10. Rouger J, Fraysse B, Deguine O, Barone P (2008) McGurk effects in cochlear-implanted deaf subjects. Brain Res 1188: 87–99.
11. Tremblay C, Champoux F, Lepore F, Theoret H (2010) Audiovisual fusion and cochlear implant proficiency. Restor Neurol Neurosci 28: 283–291.
12. Farrera MP, Fleury M, Guild K, Ghanbari M (2010) Measurement and analysis Study of Congestion Detection for Internet Video Streaming. Journal of Communications 5: 169–177.
13. Baskent D, Bazo D (2011) Audiovisual Asynchrony Detection and Speech Intelligibility in Noise With Moderate to Severe Sensorineural Hearing Impairment. Ear Hear 32: 582–592.
14. Pavel M, Sperling G, Riedl T, Vanderbeek A (1987) Limits of visual communication: the effect of signal-to-noise ratio on the intelligibility of American Sign Language. J Opt Soc Am A 4: 2355–2365.
15. Hochmair-Desoyer I, Schulz E, Moser L, Schmidt M (1997) The HSM sentence test as a tool for evaluating the speech understanding in noise of cochlear implant users. Am J Otol 18: S83.
16. ITU-T Handbook on Telephonometry (1992). Geneva: International Telecom-

munication Union.

17. Lenarz M, Sonmez H, Joseph G, Buchner A, Lenarz T (2012) Effect of gender on the hearing performance of adult cochlear implant patients. Laryngoscope 122: 1126–1129.
18. Lenarz M, Sonmez H, Joseph G, Buchner A, Lenarz T (2012) Long-term performance of cochlear implants in postlingually deafened adults. Otolaryngol Head Neck Surg 147: 112–118.
19. Wu YH, Bentler RA (2010) Impact of visual cues on directional benefit and preference: Part I–laboratory tests. Ear Hear 31: 22–34.
20. Wu YH, Bentler RA (2010) Impact of visual cues on directional benefit and preference: Part II–field tests. Ear Hear 31: 35–46.
21. Erber NP (1969) Interaction of audition and vision in the recognition of oral speech stimuli. J Speech Hear Res 12: 423–425.
22. Frowein HW, Smorrenburg GF, Pyters L, Schinkel D (1991) Improved speech recognition through videotelephony: experiments with the hard of hearing. IEEE Journal on Selected Areas in Communications 9: 611–616.
23. Ross LA, Saint-Amour D, Leavitt VM, Javitt DC, Foxe JJ (2007) Do you see what I am saying? Exploring visual enhancement of speech comprehension in noisy environments. Cereb Cortex 17: 1147–1153.
24. Alegria J, Lechat J (2005) Phonological processing in deaf children: when lipreading and cues are incongruent. J Deaf Stud Deaf Educ 10: 122–133.
25. Luettin J. Towards Speaker Independent Continuous Speechreading; 1997 22–25 September; Rhodes, Greece. EUROSPEECH. 1991–1994.
26. Bavelier D, Dye MW, Hauser PC (2006) Do deaf individuals see better? Trends Cogn Sci 10: 512–518.
27. Foulds RA (2004) Biomechanical and perceptual constraints on the bandwidth requirements of sign language. IEEE Trans Neural Syst Rehabil Eng 12: 65–72.
28. ITU-T Recommendations (1999) H-Series: Application profile - Sign language and lip-reading real-time conversation using low bit rate video communication. International Telecommunication Union.
29. De Cicco L, Mascolo S, Palmisano V. Skype Video Responsiveness to Bandwidth Variations; 2008 28/05/2008; Braunschweig, Germany.
30. Cavender A, Vanam R, Barney DK, Ladner RE, Riskin EA (2008) MobileASL: intelligibility of sign language video over mobile phones. Disabil Rehabil Assist Technol 3: 93–105.
31. Ciaramello F, Hemami S (2011) A computational intelligibility model for assessment and compression of American Sign Language video. IEEE Trans Image Process 20: 3014–3027.
32. Saxe DM, Foulds RA (2002) Robust region of interest coding for improved sign language telecommunication. IEEE Trans Inf Technol Biomed 6: 310–316.
33. Skoglund J, Kozica E, Linden J, Hagen R, Kleijn WB (2008) Voice over IP: Speech Transmission over Packet Networks. Handbook of Speech processing. Heidelberg: Springer. 307–330.
34. ITU-T Recommendations (2009) H-Series: Packet-based multimedia communications systems. International Telecommunication Union.
35. Tye-Murray N, Sommers MS, Spehar B (2007) Audiovisual integration and lipreading abilities of older adults with normal and impaired hearing. Ear Hear 28: 656–668.
36. Champoux F, Lepore F, Gagne JP, Theoret H (2009) Visual stimuli can impair auditory processing in cochlear implant users. Neuropsychologia 47: 17–22.
37. Summerfield Q (1992) Lipreading and audio-visual speech perception. Philos Trans R Soc Lond B Biol Sci 335: 71–78.
38. Colonius H, Diederich A (2011) Computing an optimal time window of audiovisual integration in focused attention tasks: illustrated by studies on effect of age and prior knowledge. Exp Brain Res.

13

Burden of Disease Caused by Otitis Media

Lorenzo Monasta[1]*, Luca Ronfani[1], Federico Marchetti[2], Marcella Montico[1], Liza Vecchi Brumatti[3], Alessandro Bavcar[4], Domenico Grasso[5], Chiara Barbiero[1], Giorgio Tamburlini[3]

1 Epidemiology and Biostatistics Unit, Institute for Maternal and Child Health - IRCCS "Burlo Garofolo", Trieste, Italy, **2** Department of Paediatrics, Institute for Maternal and Child Health - IRCCS "Burlo Garofolo", Trieste, Italy, **3** Research Direction, Institute for Maternal and Child Health - IRCCS "Burlo Garofolo", Trieste, Italy, **4** Unit for Health Services Research and International Health, Institute for Maternal and Child Health - IRCCS "Burlo Garofolo", Trieste, Italy, **5** Ear, Nose and Throat Unit, Department of Paediatric Surgery, Institute for Maternal and Child Health - IRCCS "Burlo Garofolo", Trieste, Italy

Abstract

Background: Otitis media (OM) is a leading cause of health care visits and drugs prescription. Its complications and sequelae are important causes of preventable hearing loss, particularly in developing countries. Within the Global Burden of Diseases, Injuries, and Risk Factors Study, for the year 2005 we estimated the incidence of acute OM, chronic suppurative OM, and related hearing loss and mortality for all ages and the 21 WHO regional areas.

Methods: We identified risk factors, complications and sequelae of OM. We carried out an extensive literature review (Medline, Embase, Lilacs and Wholis) which lead to the selection of 114 papers comprising relevant data. Data were available from 15 of the 21 WHO regions. To estimate incidence and prevalence for all countries we adopted a two stage approach based on risk factors formulas and regression modelling.

Results: Acute OM incidence rate is 10.85% i.e. 709million cases each year with 51% of these occurring in under-fives. Chronic suppurative OM incidence rate is 4.76‰ i.e. 31million cases, with 22.6% of cases occurring annually in under-fives. OM-related hearing impairment has a prevalence of 30.82 per ten-thousand. Each year 21thousand people die due to complications of OM.

Conclusions: Our study is the first attempt to systematically review the available information and provide global estimates for OM and related conditions. The overall burden deriving from AOM, CSOM and their sequelae is considerable, particularly in the first five years of life and in the poorest countries. The findings call for incorporating OM-focused action within preventive and case management strategies, with emphasis on the more affected.

Editor: Ann M. Moormann, University of Massachusetts Medical School, United States of America

Funding: For this work, financial support was received by the University of Edinburgh and by the Institute for Maternal and Child Health - Istituto Di Ricovero e Cura a Carattere Scientifico "Burlo Garofolo" (n.31/09). The funders had no role in study design, data collection and analysis, decision to publish, or preparation of the manuscript.

Competing Interests: The authors have declared that no competing interests exist.

* E-mail: monasta@burlo.trieste.it

Introduction

Acute otitis media (AOM) is a very common condition and a leading cause of health care visits and antibiotic prescription [1]. Studies carried out in developed countries show that by their third birthday 80% of children will have experienced at least one episode of AOM [2,3] and 40% will have six or more recurrences by the age of seven years [4]. As with most infectious diseases, the burden of AOM varies substantially across countries, the main differences residing in the frequency of suppurative complications such as mastoiditis and meningitis and of sequelae such as hearing loss due to chronic suppurative otitis media (CSOM) [1,3]. CSOM is an important cause of preventable hearing loss, particularly in the developing world [5], and a reason of serious concern, particularly in children, because it may have long-term effects on early communication, language development, auditory processing, psychosocial and cognitive development, and educational progress and achievement [6].

Based on prevalence surveys, which vary widely in disease definition, sampling methods, and methodological quality, WHO estimated that 28 thousand deaths every year are attributable to complications of OM [6]. OM and CSOM can lead to death mainly through meningitis and brain abscess. In addition WHO estimated that between 65 and 330 million individuals suffer from CSOM (show signs of CSOM), 50% of whom suffer from hearing impairment [6].

In industrialised countries, hearing loss (both conductive and sensorineural) is known to be the third most prevalent chronic condition in older adults after hypertension and arthropathy with considerable implications on physical and mental health [7,8]. Information on the adult population of less industrialised countries is scanty [5]. A better knowledge of the incidence and prevalence of AOM and its complications across ages and geographical regions is necessary to adequately assess the need for interventions aimed at reducing its health, social and economic burden.

As members of the Expert Group on pneumonia, meningitis, sepsis, otitis media, pertussis and influenza of the Global Burden of Diseases, Injuries, and Risk Factors Study, we estimated the global burden of otitis media for all ages for all of the 21 WHO regional areas [9], for the year 2005, through a systematic, transparent and comprehensive literature review.

Methods

All aspects of the methods are described in more detail in Text S1.

Identification of risk factors, complications and sequelae of OM was the starting point (Figure 1, Table 1). Given the complexity of the causal pathways, the frequent overlapping of conditions, the lack of clear and consistent definitions and the fact that conditions included may have a mild and temporary nature or be rare, we focused in our review on AOM, CSOM, and on permanent Hearing Impairment (HI, both conductive and sensorineural) caused by OM (Figure S1). This simplification is consistent with that adopted in previous estimates of the OM GBD [10].

We searched for all articles presenting original data on incidence or prevalence of AOM or CSOM, and linking HI data with CSOM (proportion of HI caused by CSOM, or proportion of CSOM cases causing HI), published from 1980 to 2008. We did not formally define nor register a review protocol. The systematic review covering AOM, CSOM, HI and related risk factors was carried out on Medline (PubMed, last search 11/08/2008), Embase (last search 23/07/2008), Lilacs (last search 11/08/2008), Wholis (last search 11/08/2008), without any language restriction (details in Table S1). We retrieved 9356 records that became 7168 after duplication removal (Figure 2 for the complete flow diagram). We carried out a two-step evaluation to identify relevant papers:

1) by titles, abstract and keywords, aimed at identifying papers on epidemiology and risk factors of OM and reviews on OM (Figure S2). Papers on risk factors were used to review and complete the risk factors diagram (Figure S3).
2) by full text, when available, aimed at identifying papers on epidemiology of AOM, CSOM and HI. All articles with original data on AOM, CSOM or HI incidence or prevalence were included.

Information on mortality was collected through WHO vital registration databases, when available and reliable, or estimated for countries and areas where data were unavailable or unreliable.

Both the selection of relevant papers and data extraction were carried out independently by two of the authors (respectively by

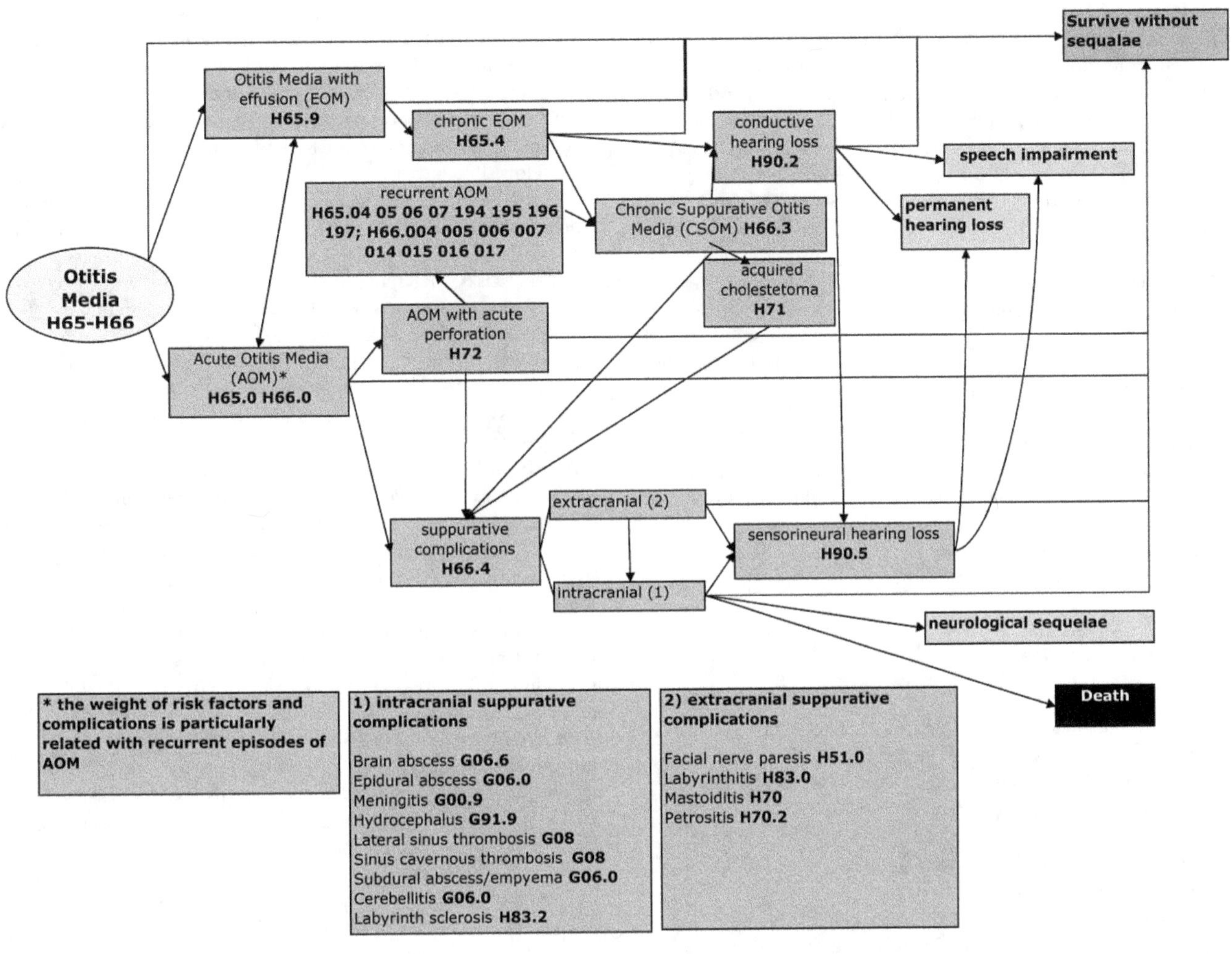

Figure 1. Sequelae of OM (complete scheme) with ICD-10-CM diagnosis codes.

Table 1. Definitions of main conditions involved in the sequelae of otitis media.

Otitis media is the generic term for all types of inflammation of the middle ear [60,61].
Acute otitis media (AOM) is usually a short-term inflammation of the middle ear, characterised by the rapid onset of one or more signs or symptoms of acute inflammation in the middle ear such as earache, tugging at the ear, fever, or irritability in the presence of a middle-ear effusion. It is often preceded by upper respiratory symptoms, including a cough and rhinorrhoea [39,60,61].
Chronic suppurative otitis media (CSOM) is defined as a persistent inflammatory process associated with a perforated tympanic membrane draining exudate for more than 6 weeks [62]. It is often associated with a cholesteatoma.
Hearing impairment (HI): is the total or partial inability to hear sound in one or both ears [63]. WHO defines disabling hearing impairment as having permanent unaided hearing threshold in the better ear of more than 30 dB in children aged up to 15 years, or more than 40 dB in adults at frequencies of 0.5, 1, 2, and 4 kHz [64].
- **Conductive hearing loss (CHL)** is the total or partial inability to hear sound in one or both ears because of some mechanical problem in the external or middle ear. The three tiny bones of the ear (ossicles) may fail to conduct sound to the cochlea, or the eardrum may fail to vibrate in response to sound. Fluid in the middle ear can cause CHL [63].
- **Sensorineural hearing loss (SNHL)** is the total or partial inability to hear sound in one or both ears resulting from a dysfunction of the inner ear. It most often occurs when the tiny hair cells (called cilia) that transmit sound through the ear are injured. This type of hearing loss is sometimes called "nerve damage," although this is not accurate [63].

LM and AB or CB, and by LM and MM, LVB or CB). Any disagreement were resolved through discussion involving a third author (LR).

Estimation process: incidence of AOM and CSOM

When only prevalence data were available, prevalence was transformed into incidence based on the average duration of AOM and CSOM. Although studies show that clinically symptomatic AOM usually has a shorter duration [11,12] we assumed a duration of 21 days because when both prevalence and incidence data were available the actual duration, including the effusion was shown to be around 21 days [13]. This was the only real evidence on duration of AOM we could rely on. The average duration of CSOM in adults is 10 years [14–19].

The estimation process was divided into two phases. In the first and second phase all estimations were done by country within a specific area, the only exception being Oceania, for which we extrapolated country specific data to the whole region. As described below, while phase one estimations were carried out using a formula based on risk factors, the second phase was based on exponential regression models. Phase one, in fact, generated estimates for countries in regions in which we had original data. Phase two allowed us to expand the estimates to regions with no data and in general to fine tune all previously elaborated estimates.

Estimates were done by all age groups [9]. We did not calculate estimates by gender, since evidence on gender differences is scanty and conflicting.

AOM and CSOM estimates: first phase. The first phase was carried out by the following formula based on risk factors:

- $N_{e/cy} = (Pop_{new}) \times (Inc_{Ref}) \times \{1 + \sum_{(i=1 \to n)} [(Prev_{RF.new.i} - Prev_{RF.Ref.i}) \times [RR_{RF.i} - 1]]\}$

Were $N_{e/cy}$ is the number of cases, Pop_{new} is the population, Inc_{Ref} is the incidence in the reference population, $Prev_{RF.new.i}$ is the prevalence of a specific risk factor i in the new population, $Prev_{RF.Ref.i}$ is the prevalence of the i risk factor in the reference population, $RR_{RF.i}$ is the risk ratio for risk factor i.

Incidence in the reference population refers to the incidence for those countries for which data were available from the literature.

Risk estimates were extracted from the literature review [20–22] and in particular from day care center attendance (RR 2.45), exclusive bottle-feeding vs. exclusive breastfeeding up to six months (RR 2.00), parental smoking (RR 1.66), and malnutrition (RR 3.48).

The choice of limiting the list of risk factors to the ones above was determined, among the more relevant, by two fundamental reasons. The first being that we needed good quality data on risk ratios and, thus, we focused on data from meta-analyses. Malnutrition was an exception but we considered it to be a key factor in developing countries. The second reason is that we needed risk factors for which we could have reliable information for each country. Malnutrition was included only for developing countries (no data on malnutrition is available for developed countries and malnutrition is certainly more important in developing countries), while day-care centre attendance was only included for developed countries (no data on day-care centre is available for developing countries and is certainly more important in developed countries).

We used two different sets of risk factors. For Western Europe, North America High Income, Asia Pacific High Income and Australasia we used the following risk factors and associated Relative Risks (RRs): adults smoking (RR 1.66), exclusive breastfeeding at six months (RR 2.00), day-care attendance (RR 2.45). Data for these risk factors, for the year 2005, were taken from WHO, UNICEF and OSCE reports and databases [23–27] (www.oecd.org/els/social/family/database). For all other areas, day-care was substituted with under five children underweight (RR 3.48).

AOM and CSOM estimates: second phase. Areas for which we did not have any data were: Europe Central, Europe Eastern, Oceania, Asia East, Asia Central, Latin America Southern and Latin America Andean. To be able to cover these areas and to fine tune the estimates elaborated in phase one, we adopted a more robust strategy.

Phase two was based on exponential regression models. A model for AOM and a model for CSOM incidence rates were built for less industrialised areas. These models were based on the following factors: [23–25] prevalence of Acute Respiratory Infections (ARI) in children under five (ARI-U5), underweight prevalence in under five children (U-U5), under five mortality rate (MR-U5), proportion of children under six months exclusively breastfed (EBF), prevalence of adults smoking (AS). These models were based on data and phase one estimates from 45 countries and helped estimate AOM and CSOM incidence for the age group 1–4 years and validate the estimates of all countries. These models had an R^2 of 0.83 for AOM and 0.85 for CSOM:

- $AOM = 35.1859 * (1.0235^{ARI\text{-}U5}) * (1.0060^{U\text{-}U5}) * (0.9979^{AS}) * (1.0079^{MR\text{-}U5}) * (0.9846^{EBF})$

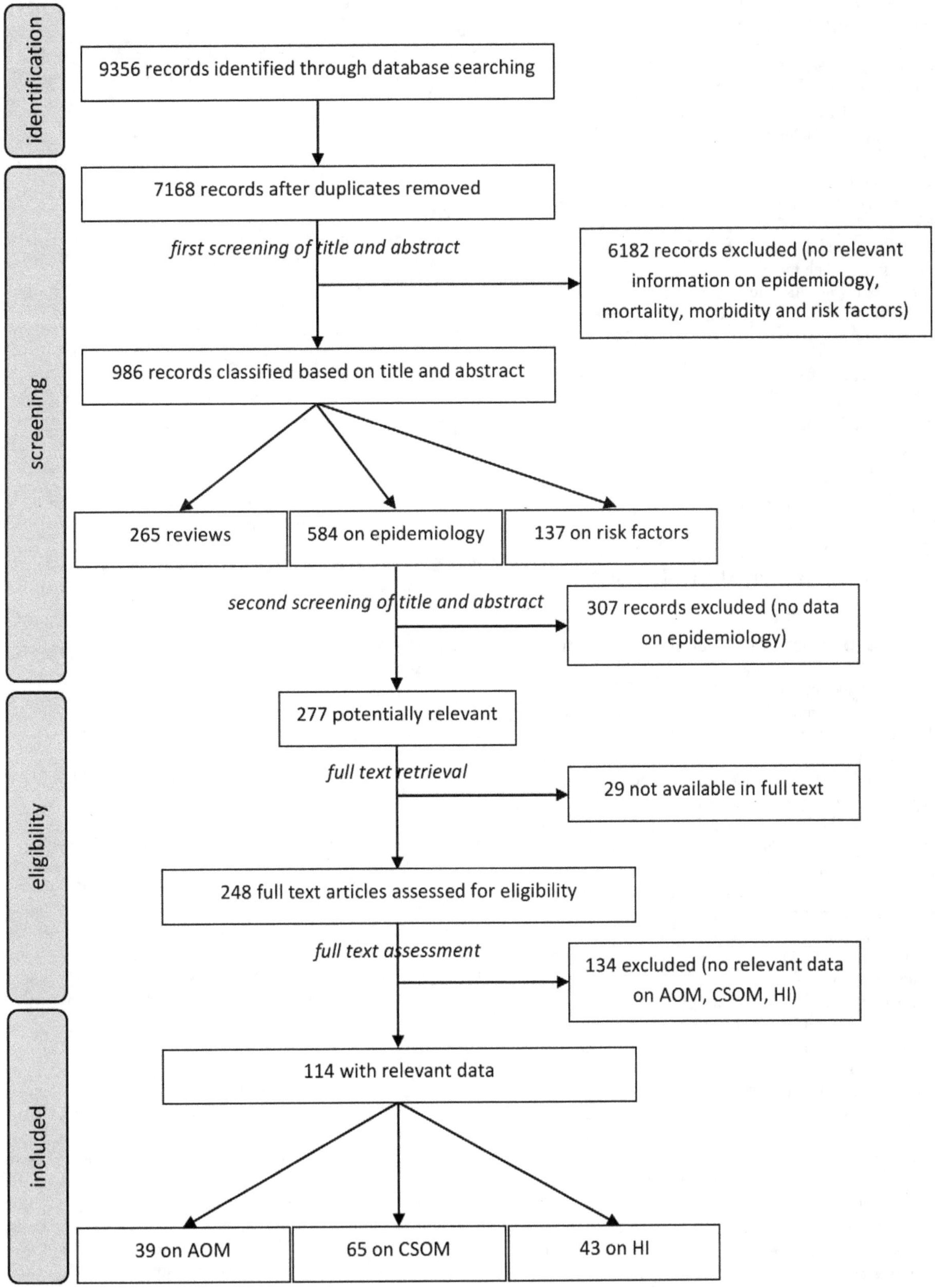

Figure 2. Screening process of articles on epidemiology of AOM, CSOM and HI, according to the PRISMA 2009 Flow Diagram. AOM: Acute Otitis Media; CSOM: Chronic Suppurative Otitis Media; HI: Hearing Impairment.

- $CSOM = 4.8451 * (1.0152^{ARI\text{-}U5}) * (1.0298^{U\text{-}U5}) * (1.0055^{AS}) * (1.0021^{MR\text{-}U5}) * (0.9872^{EBF})$

We should not be surprised to see that single risk factors have coefficients that vary from >1 to <1 in different models (i.e. AS in the models above and EBF in the ones below), if we take into account the possibility of different interrelations between risk factors considered simultaneously.

For more industrialised areas (Europe Western, North America High Income and Australasia) we built exponential models to estimate AOM and CSOM for 1–4 years old children based on breastfeeding, adults smoking, day-care attendance (DCA) and under five mortality rate. The models were based on 22 countries Europe Western countries and helped re-estimate the other countries and validate the estimates of all countries. The R^2 for these models were 0.61 for AOM and 0.79 for CSOM:

- $AOM_{1\text{-}4} = 20.9264 * (0.9882^{EBF}) * (1.0124^{DCA}) * (1.0008^{AS}) * (0.9998^{MR\text{-}U5\hat{}3})$
- $CSOM_{1\text{-}4} = 0.8572 * (1.0010^{EBF}) * (1.0110^{DCA}) * (1.0123^{AS}) * (1.0022^{MR\text{-}U5\hat{}3})$

The estimates of AOM and CSOM for Australia, Greenland and New Zealand were calculated as a weighted average of the estimates for aboriginals and non-aboriginals, with weight based on proportion of aboriginals to non-aboriginals by age group. For Asia Pacific High Income we kept the estimates based on the first phase model.

Estimation process: prevalence of Hearing Impairment

According to the WHO definitions [28,29] (Table S2), we estimated the prevalence of HI for all four degrees (slight, moderate, severe and profound). We used the following assumption to extend the estimates to the four degrees of HI or to estimate the WHO thresholds from other thresholds used (pg.6): "Where non-WHO thresholds used, the prevalence of hearing impairment at the WHO thresholds was interpolated assuming the log of the cumulative prevalence is linear with threshold. This relationship holds reasonably well in most studies [29]."

Again, a two phases estimation process was adopted in order to elaborate robust estimates. Details on the assumptions made and on both estimation phases are described in the Text S1.

HI estimates: first phase. We estimated cases of HI due to otitis media on the basis of the Oman age distribution of HI [30]. The Oman study was the only one reporting a complete age distribution of HI due to OM. The Oman distribution included HI caused by presbyacusis and accidents, thus we corrected this distribution to only include HI due to CSOM, and on the basis of the 0.19% of the population affected by HI due to CSOM calculated from Oman but adjusted to Europe, using Finland (0.001232%).

- Prevalence of HI>35 dB in best ear was extrapolated to countries on the basis of cases of CSOM per age group.
- Prevalence was cumulated to calculate cumulated cases and then cases by age group.
- Total for Western Europe were then calculated adding all cases per country and age group.

This was done for all regions for which we had countries with data: Brazil [19], China [31], India [32,33], Malaysia [34], Nigeria [35], Oman [30] and South Africa [36].

HI estimates: second phase. Two regression models were used in the second phase: one model was used to estimate the prevalence of slight HI (25 dB to 40 dB), and another to estimate moderate HI (40 dB to 60 dB), using estimates from respectively 11 and 10 countries (China, India, Japan, Malaysia, Australia, Oman, Finland, Brazil, United States of America, South Africa, Nigeria) for which we had more reliable data and/or estimates. In the 40 dB model we used estimates from the same countries but excluding Malaysia, which did not have a good fit in the model compared with the other countries. The models, with regressors and coefficients, are reported in Text S1.

Mortality estimates

We selected a number of countries for which we had reliable WHO 2005 Vital Registration data. Using these data and regressors such as incidence of AOM, CSOM, AOM in 1–4, CSOM in 1–4 and under five mortality rate, we developed and evaluated three different regression models. Models and reasons for choosing different models for different areas are described in detail in Text S1.

The 1st model was based on overall otitis mortality rate ×10million from 12 countries and four regressors (U5 mortality, overall CSOMx1000, CSOM 1–4, AOM 1–4) had a R^2 of 0.954 and a Standard Error (SE) of 8.09:

- $MORT_1 = -107.3699 + 0.0804 * U5\text{-}MR + 34.0711 * CSOM - 0.3516 * CSOM1\text{-}4 - 0.4326 * AOM1\text{-}4$

The 2nd was based on nine countries and two regressors (U5 Mortality rate and adult mortality): had a R^2 of 0.996 and an SE of 2.60:

- $MORT_2 = 8.4023 + 0.5101 * U5\text{-}MR - 0.1222 * Adult\text{-}MR + 0.0168 * (U5\text{-}MR)^2$

The 3rd model was based on seven countries and the same four regressors as model one: had a R^2 of 0.997 and an SE of 0.32:

- $MORT_3 = -7.8715 + 0.5709 * U5\text{-}MR + 2.3664 * CSOM + 0.0776 * CSOM1\text{-}4 - 0.0382 * AOM1\text{-}4$

For all areas but five we selected the average of two models (1st and 3rd). For Asia Pacific High Income we selected an average between the 2nd and the 3rd models. For Latin America Andean we used the 3rd model. Australasia used the 2nd model. The choice of the models to adopt for each area were made on the basis of models fitting vital registration data when available – even if less reliable than the ones used for the generation of the models – or on the basis of unreliable or negative estimates generated by the other models.

Uncertainty bounds

For AOM and CSOM incidence and HI prevalence, uncertainty bounds were calculated using the standard error (SE) of the second phase regression models. Further sources of uncertainty for AOM and CSOM estimates derive from the data selected from original studies, from the adoption of estimates generated by the model used in phase one, from the decision on how to estimate the age distributions, and from the approach taken to convert prevalence to incidence. For HI estimates, uncertainty also derives from the use of previously estimated AOM and CSOM incidence, the adoption of WHO formulas to estimate different degrees of HI, the decisions on how to transpose original data on worst to best year, the use of data selected from original studies (including the heterogeneity in methods used to establish HI in different studies and the uncertainty of survey data) and finally the adoption of the Oman distribution in the estimation of HI by age. For mortality estimates, uncertainty bounds were calculated using the

SE of the regression models. Further uncertainty derives from the methodology used to estimate the age distribution, and from the use of estimates of AOM and CSOM as regressors, which for their nature are subject to imprecision. To account for all sources of uncertainty, we increased the confidence level to 99%. It is, however, important to emphasise that the increase from 95% to 99% should be considered as a way to include other sources of uncertainty and that by no means these bounds should be considered to express 99% confidence.

Results

Out of 584 papers on OM epidemiology, 307 were excluded because they were clearly not providing information relevant to our study. Out of the remaining 277, 29 were not available in full text. We then evaluated the 248 papers available in full text and excluded further 134 because not relevant for our study. Out of the remaining 114 papers, 39 contained data on AOM, 65 on CSOM and 43 on HI (Figure 2).

Data on AOM were available from six regions, the majority of the studies (32 of 44) being carried out in Europe Western and North America High Income (Table S3). Data on HI/CSOM were available for a greater number of regions. We were able to find data on CSOM from 15 regions, data on proportion of CSOM causing HI from 10 regions and data on proportion of HI caused by OM from 11 regions. Data covering all four classes of indicators were available only for three regions, whilst for six regions no data were found. Overall, our review was able to collect some data on AOM, CSOM or HI from 15 out of 21 regions, while only three areas had data on all three conditions: Europe Western, North Africa/Middle East and North America High Income.

In Tables 2 and 3 (Table S4) and Figures 3, 4, 5, 6 we report global estimates for AOM, CSOM, HI and attributable mortality.

AOM

Global AOM incidence rate (new episodes per hundred people per year) is, according to our estimates, 10.85% i.e. 709 million cases each year with 51% of these occurring in children under five years of age (U5) (Tables 2 and 3). Global incidence rate ranges from 3.64 for Europe Central (40% of cases occurring in children 0–5) to 43.36 and 43.37 for Sub-Saharan Africa West (56% in U5) and Central (58% in U5) respectively. Other areas with incidence lower than 5 are Asia Pacific High Income (3.75), Asia East (3.93), Europe Eastern (3.96) and Latin America Southern (4.25).

Global incidence rate is highest in the age group 1–4 (60.99%) and in the first year of life (45.28%). Incidence lowers to a minimum of 1.49 in the age group 35–44 and raises again to 2.3% after 75 years of age.

Areas with an incidence rate higher than 100% in the 1–4 age group are Oceania (114.98%), Sub-Saharan Africa Central (143.87%) and West (154.12%). An incidence rate of over 100% means we expect children in this age group to have an average of more than one episode of AOM in a one year time. In such age group four areas have an incidence below 30%: Latin America Andean (29.39%) and Southern (25.56%), Asia East (27.38%) and Asia Pacific High Income (24.21%).

CSOM

Global estimated CSOM incidence rate is 4.76 per thousand people for a total of 31 million cases, with 22.6% of these cases occurring annually in U5 children. Latin America Andean is the area with the lowest incidence (1.70 per thousand), followed by Asia Pacific High Income (3.02) and North America High Income (3.06). Oceania has the highest incidence with 9.37, while two other areas have an incidence higher than 7: Sub-Saharan Africa Central (7.56) and West (7.22).

Globally, CSOM incidence rate is highest is the first year of life (15.40 per thousand) and reaches its lowest value after 65 years of age (2.51).

In the first year of life, Asia Pacific High Income has the lowest incidence rate (1.59 per thousand), while Oceania has the highest (35.96). The proportion of cases occurring in U5 vary from 1.8% in the Asia Pacific High Income, to 38.9% in Oceania and 41.0% in Sub-Saharan Africa Central.

Hearing Impairment

HI caused by OM, defined as permanent hearing loss for best ear >25 dB, has a prevalence of 30.82 per ten thousand, with Europe Western, Australasia, North America High Income and Asia Pacific High Income all having a prevalence below 2 per ten thousand. Asia South has by far the highest prevalence (97.04), followed by Oceania (51.23) and then by Sub Sahara Africa West, East and Central all in the range of 30 to 35.

Prevalence increases with age, with 9.34 per ten thousand in the first year of life and a highest prevalence of 45.05 in the age group 65–74.

In Asia South, by the age of five, six out of one thousand children (6.02 per thousand) have a HI of at least 25 dB in the best ear caused by sequelae of OM. Oceania follows with 3.02 per thousand, then Sub-Saharan Africa West, East and Central with 2.21, 1.95 and 1.92 respectively. On the opposite extreme, less than one child per ten thousand suffers from HI by the age of five in Europe Western (0.55 per ten thousand), Australasia (0.62) North America High Income (0.64) and Asia Pacific High Income (0.80).

Mortality

According to our estimates, globally, each year approximately 21 thousand people, i.e. 33 per 10 million people, die due to the complications of OM. Mortality is higher in the first year of life (85.4 per 10 million) and in the age group 1–4 years of age (90.5). it lowers to 13.6 in the 25–34 years age group and raises again to the highest values after 75 years of age (160.5).

North America High Income shows the lowest mortality (1.6 per 10 million), followed by Asia Pacific High Income (1.7), Europe Western (2.8) and Australasia (3.7). Oceania has the highest mortality with 101.1 deaths each year per 10 million, followed by Sub-Saharan Africa Central (96.2) and West (91.8). Other areas with a mortality higher than 50 per 10 million are Sub-Saharan Africa East (73.49) and Asia South (68.88).

Discussion

Our study is the first attempt to systematically review the available information and provide global estimates for the incidence of AOM and CSOM, the prevalence of OM-related HI, and for OM-related mortality.

In our review we had to face a number of difficulties, the main ones being the scarcity or absence of data from some geographical areas and age groups and the heterogeneity of the available information, due to heterogeneity in study design, measurements and definitions. We provide estimates for 21 geographical sub-regions and 13 age groups. Since we were able to collect data on either AOM, CSOM or HI from 15 out of 21 regions, some of our estimates are based on modelling. In other cases we extrapolated to sub-regional level data that were collected in only a few

Table 2. AOM and CSOM incidence rate, HI prevalence and mortality estimates for the year 2005, by WHO areas.

Areas	AOM% incidence			CSOM‰ incidence			HI>25 dB best ear °/°°° prevalence			Deaths °/°°°°°°		
	AOM	MIN	MAX	CSOM	MIN	MAX	HI	MIN	MAX	Deaths	MIN	MAX
Asia Central	7.90	7.21	8.59	4.05	3.53	4.56	8.60	7.96	9.24	18.88	12.24	30.98
Asia East	3.93	3.24	4.61	3.67	3.16	4.18	9.69	9.05	10.32	9.32	9.04	9.62
Asia Pacific High Income	3.75	3.31	4.19	3.02	2.17	3.88	1.91	1.28	2.54	1.72	1.00	2.49
Asia South	14.52	13.84	15.21	6.56	6.05	7.08	97.04	96.37	97.71	68.88	68.21	69.02
Asia South East	8.15	7.47	8.84	4.69	4.17	5.20	14.67	14.03	15.31	27.16	25.18	29.81
Australasia	7.25	6.81	7.69	3.41	2.56	4.26	1.36	0.75	1.99	3.69	0.00	9.83
Caribbean	9.08	8.40	9.77	4.18	3.67	4.70	7.32	6.68	7.96	18.60	12.57	78.84
Europe Central	3.64	2.95	4.32	3.69	3.17	4.20	5.02	4.39	5.65	4.97	2.61	16.08
Europe Eastern	3.96	3.28	4.65	3.75	3.24	4.26	5.30	4.67	5.93	5.72	4.73	9.31
Europe Western	5.91	5.88	5.99	3.39	3.24	3.57	1.34	0.72	1.96	2.82	2.53	3.11
Latin America Andean	5.39	5.02	6.07	1.70	1.19	2.21	5.30	4.64	5.96	12.72	12.32	12.72
Latin America Central	6.78	6.10	7.47	3.92	3.40	4.43	5.28	4.65	5.91	12.36	9.16	16.96
Latin America Southern	4.25	3.56	4.93	3.60	3.09	4.12	5.15	4.52	5.79	6.00	3.94	13.53
Latin America Tropical	5.90	5.21	6.59	3.74	3.23	4.25	4.95	4.32	5.58	9.60	8.82	10.58
North Africa Middle East	8.67	7.98	9.35	4.41	3.90	4.92	8.63	7.99	9.27	21.96	18.48	27.17
North America High Income	5.46	5.40	5.53	3.06	2.82	3.30	1.41	0.79	2.04	1.63	1.23	1.90
Oceania	28.56	27.87	29.24	9.37	8.86	9.88	51.23	50.57	51.88	101.07	86.63	112.17
Sub-Saharan Africa Central	43.37	42.69	44.06	7.56	7.04	8.07	30.20	29.57	30.84	96.20	90.27	102.71
Sub-Saharan Africa East	22.81	22.13	23.50	6.06	5.55	6.57	31.91	31.26	32.56	73.49	68.30	78.20
Sub-Saharan Africa Southern	14.71	14.02	15.40	4.79	4.27	5.30	9.37	8.73	10.00	33.96	29.11	43.66
Sub-Saharan Africa West	43.36	42.68	44.05	7.22	6.71	7.74	34.37	33.74	35.00	91.82	85.26	98.34
Total	10.85	10.25	11.46	4.76	4.27	5.24	30.82	30.18	31.47	32.78	31.07	35.30

Table 3. Global AOM and CSOM incidence rate, HI prevalence and mortality estimates for the year 2005, by WHO age groups.

Age Groups	AOM% incidence			CSOM‰ incidence			HI>25 dB best ear °/°°° prevalence			Deaths °/°°°°°°		
	AOM	MIN	MAX	CSOM	MIN	MAX	HI	MIN	MAX	Deaths	MIN	MAX
0–11 m.	45.28	44.63	45.93	15.40	14.82	15.97	9.34	8.72	9.99	85.42	73.06	85.10
1–4	60.99	60.32	61.65	10.13	9.59	10.67	22.84	22.20	23.49	90.54	86.46	97.28
5–9	22.15	21.51	22.80	8.31	7.77	8.84	26.28	25.63	26.93	38.86	37.21	41.85
10–14	18.50	17.86	19.15	3.89	3.35	4.43	26.95	26.30	27.59	32.50	31.00	34.75
15–19	3.53	2.90	4.16	3.36	2.88	3.85	26.87	26.22	27.51	19.47	19.01	21.17
20–24	3.14	2.52	3.77	4.80	4.25	5.38	29.68	29.04	30.32	13.72	12.86	14.84
25–34	1.56	0.95	2.17	3.31	2.80	3.82	30.61	29.96	31.25	13.56	12.88	14.72
35–44	1.49	0.90	2.08	3.17	2.71	3.64	32.85	32.21	33.49	19.12	18.02	20.91
45–54	1.77	1.20	2.35	4.10	3.62	4.60	35.32	34.68	35.96	14.82	14.00	16.04
55–64	1.92	1.37	2.47	3.74	3.34	4.14	39.58	38.94	40.22	23.36	22.14	25.28
65–74	2.10	1.57	2.65	2.47	2.12	2.77	45.05	44.42	45.69	49.26	46.88	53.72
75–84	2.34	1.86	2.83	2.55	2.28	2.77	43.24	42.60	43.88	156.19	149.09	168.15
85+	2.27	1.86	2.68	2.73	2.56	2.83	37.73	37.10	38.37	179.01	167.26	200.77
Total	10.85	10.25	11.46	4.76	4.27	5.24	30.82	30.18	31.47	32.78	31.07	35.30

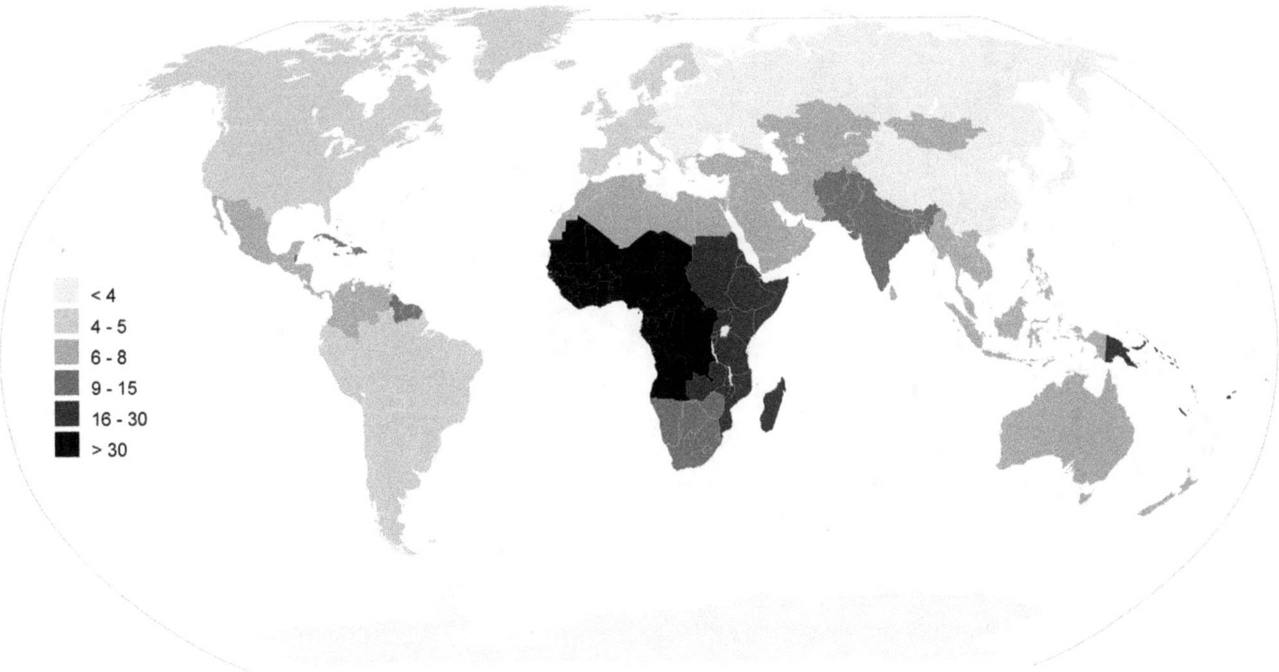

Figure 3. AOM incidence rate estimates for the year 2005 per hundred people, by the 21 WHO regions.

countries. Data were particularly scarce on incidence/prevalence of AOM and CSOM in adult and elderly age groups.

While there are no other global estimates of AOM, our findings related to CSOM, HI and OM-related mortality can be compared with the estimates released by the WHO in 2004 [6]. It is noteworthy that our point estimate for CSOM prevalence (200.8 million cases) (Table S4) falls in between the range of estimates provided by WHO (65.5 to 328.2 million cases). Since we had no access to methods used by WHO to calculate previous estimates and we avoided any comparison or adjustment with WHO data while elaborating our methods and estimates, this may be considered as a reciprocal validation of both estimates. Our HI

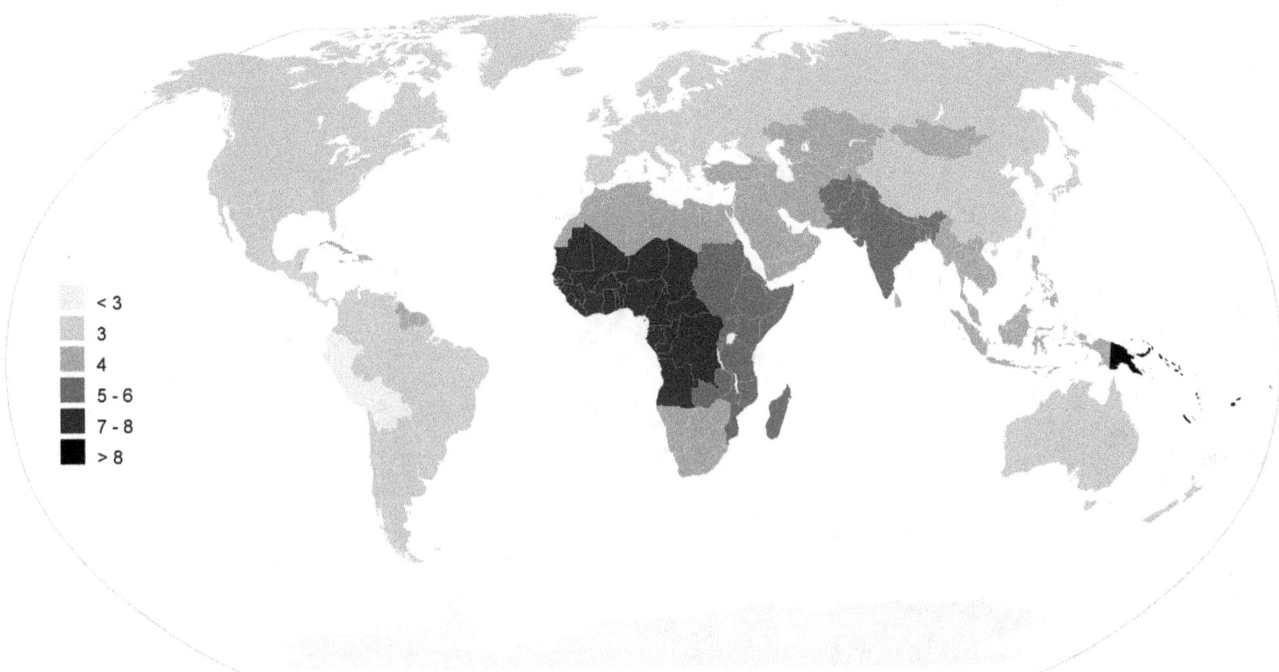

Figure 4. CSOM incidence rate estimates for the year 2005 per thousand people, by the 21 WHO regions.

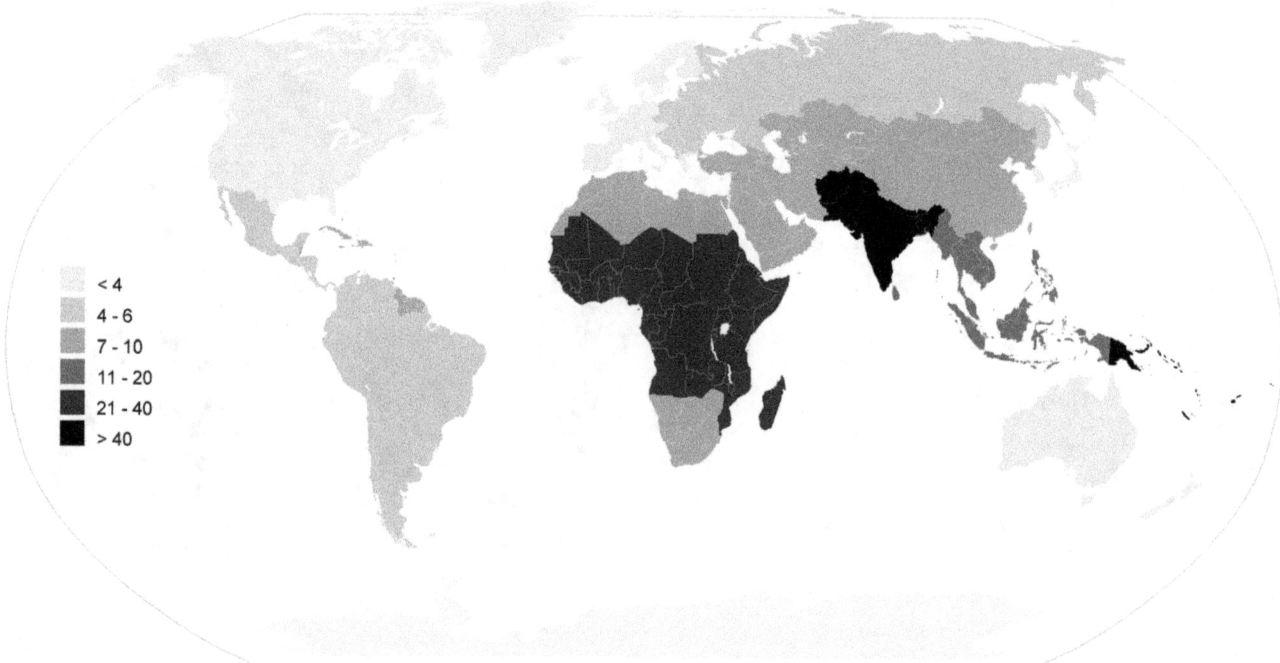

Figure 5. OM-associated HI (>25 dB for best ear) prevalence rate estimates for the year 2005 per ten thousand people, by the 21 WHO regions.

prevalence estimates, on the contrary, are much lower than those reported by WHO. Adding up the HI prevalent cases for all HI degrees (25 dB, 40 dB, 60 dB and 80 dB for best ear) we calculated a global estimate of 20.1 million cases. The WHO report provides an estimate, of 164.1 million people with CSOM-associated, but this was obtained by simply calculating 50% of CSOM prevalence. Our estimates of HI are based on a more complex and, in our opinion, more reliable model. In addition, our definition of HI includes only permanent HI while the WHO report does not explicitly exclude temporary HI. Finally, our mortality estimate (21.4 thousand deaths due to AOM, CSOM and related complications) is close to that reported by WHO (28 thousand) [6] which includes only mortality due to CSOM, but

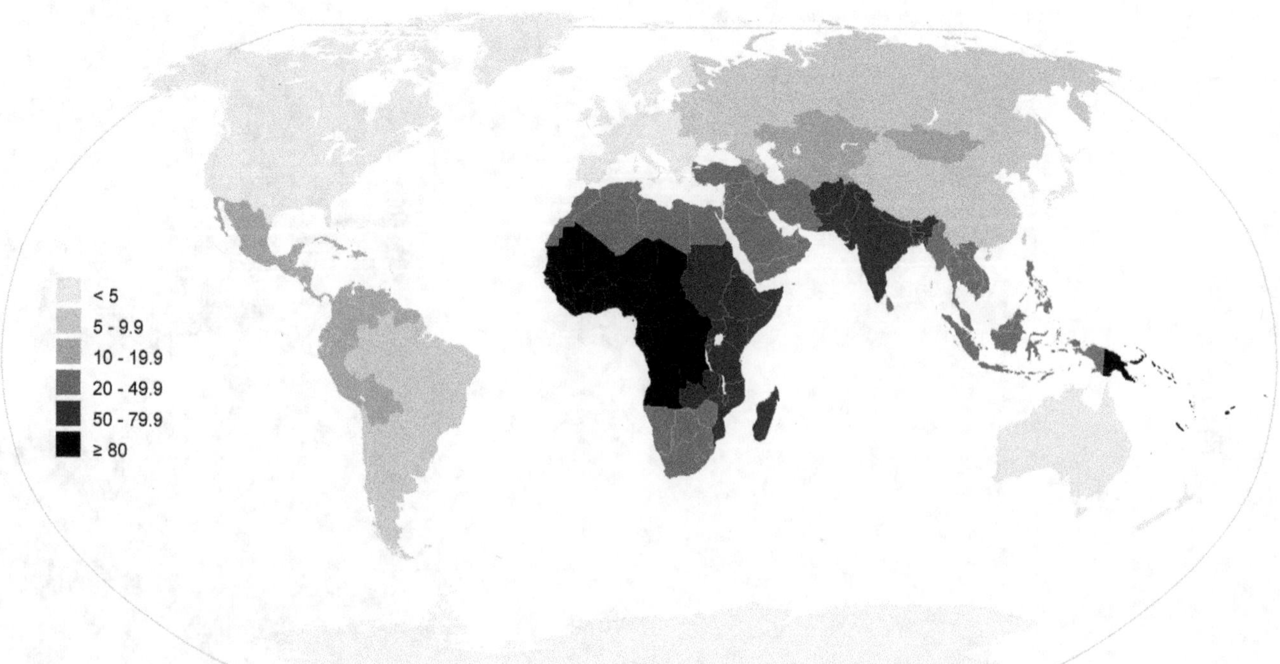

Figure 6. OM-associated mortality estimates for the year 2005 per ten million people, by the 21 WHO regions.

much higher than the one reported in the GBD 2001 and 2004 update (4 and 5 thousand respectively) [10,37].

Not surprisingly, the incidence of AOM and, to a lesser extent, of CSOM is particularly high in the first five years – when its incidence is more than double that of pneumonia [38] – and in Sub-Saharan Africa and South Asia. The prevalence of HI follows a similar geographical distribution, but although it becomes significant quite early, it increases gradually to reach its maximum in the elderly population. Mortality attributable to OM is relatively low as compared to other causes. However, the overall burden deriving from the combination of AOM, CSOM and their sequelae is considerable, particularly in the first five years of life and in the poorest countries. AOM, CSOM and HI significantly contribute to temporary disability, suffering, use of health services and drug prescription and self-medication, particularly of non-steroidal anti-inflammatory drugs and antibiotics [39]. The direct and indirect costs of AOM, CSOM and related HI for health systems and households, the consequences on learning and working performances [40,41] and the cost and adverse effects of drugs at both individual and population level represent an important burden for societies.

The findings of our review represent a serious challenge for health authorities. Early diagnosis and treatment of AOM, including the rational use of antibiotics should be improved, by incorporating clinical algorithms in current outpatient guidelines and by supporting the use of otoscopy in primary care practice. By doing this, prevention of complications and long term sequelae of AOM will be greatly strengthened. This is especially important for children under five, who bear 51% of all cases of AOM, and are particularly affected by the consequences on language development and school performance of early onset HI [42–44]. It is also particularly relevant for the poorest countries. We found that AOM incidence in Sub-Saharan Africa, South Asia and Oceania is two to eight times higher than in the remaining regions (Table 2, Figure 3). Here, co-morbidity with malnutrition, HIV and exposure to contaminated water greatly increases the risk of developing CSOM and its complications [45].

Health policies and programmes should incorporate preventive interventions as well as improved care seeking and access to effective treatment for common conditions such as AOM and CSOM.

Breastfeeding, smoking avoidance during and after pregnancy, and reduction of exposure to indoor air pollution are the pillars of prevention of AOM and its complications and sequelae [46–48] as well as of many other infant and child conditions. Vaccines against Streptococcus pneumoniae and HiB have been introduced to reduce the burden of child mortality consequent to meningitis and pneumonia. Although Hib vaccines (anti-capsular) do not target NTHi (non-capsular) which cause OM, a recent anti-Streptococcus pneumoniae capsular vaccine conjugated to a NTHi protein may be expected to reduce the incidence of AOM [49], and this should be taken into account when estimating and comparing the cost-effectiveness of vaccines [50] as well as of other preventive strategies.

Early diagnosis and treatment based on prompt care-seeking remain crucial particularly in the first years of life, also as a way to prevent HI. In developing countries, there have been attempts to standardize diagnosis and treatment of sick children through the IMCI strategy [51,52]. Although IMCI does not focus explicitly on AOM, it ensures, when effectively implemented, effective treatment on a pragmatic basis to children with nonspecific signs and symptoms that may be caused by AOM, but it does not call for attention to the ear when examining the child to search for ear discharge. The family and community component of IMCI is supposed to improve care-seeking [52] for children with nonspecific signs and symptoms. Improved care-seeking needs to be combined with affordable access and effective care, which are still an utopia in most of the poorest countries and for the most disadvantaged groups [53]. There is the need to implement in clinical practice what we know about indications to antibiotic treatment of AOM in children, by adapting evidence from research studies [54–56] to local health system and risk factors. However, appropriately designed studies are necessary in order to assess to which extent strategies proven effective in developed countries (i.e. the wait and see strategy) [57,58] are applicable in totally different contexts. Uncertainties still existing about treatment of CSOM in children should also be addressed [59].

In conclusion, our review calls for incorporating OM-focused action within preventive and case management strategies, with emphasis on high burden countries and for more research on epidemiology of OM and related conditions, focusing on high burden countries.

Supporting Information

Text S1 Expanded Methods Section.

Figure S1 Sequelae of OM, simplified scheme.

Figure S2 1st screening by titles, abstract and keywords.

Figure S3 Risk factor diagram.

Table S1 Search strategies and results.

Table S2 WHO grades of hearing impairment.

Table S3 Data coverage.

Table S4 AOM and CSOM incidence and prevalence, HI cases and prevalence estimates, and Mortality estimates, by age groups and WHO region.

Acknowledgments

We thank Harry Campbell (University of Edinburgh Medical School, UK) and Igor Rudan (Croatian Centre for Global Health, Split, Croatia), leaders of the Global Burden of Disease Expert Group on pneumonia, meningitis, sepsis, otitis media, pertussis and influenza, for their support, guidance and advice. We carried out study as members of this Expert Group and in the context of the new *Global Burden of Diseases, Injuries, and Risk Factors Study* (GBD Study), led by a consortium including Harvard University, the Institute for Health Metrics and Evaluation at the University of Washington, Johns Hopkins University, the University of Queensland, and the World Health Organization.

Author Contributions

Conceived and designed the experiments: LM LR MM GT FM DG. Performed the experiments: LM LR AB MM LVB CB. Analyzed the data: LM LR MM AB LVB CB. Contributed reagents/materials/analysis tools: LM LR AB. Wrote the paper: LM LR FM GT FM.

References

1. Klein JO (2000) The burden of otitis media. Vaccine 19 Suppl 1: S2–S8.
2. Teele DW, Klein JO, Rosner B (1989) Epidemiology of otitis media during the first seven years of life in children in greater Boston: a prospective, cohort study. J Infect Dis 160: 83–94.
3. Vergison A, Dagan R, Arguedas A, Bonhoeffer J, Cohen R, et al. (2010) Otitis media and its consequences: beyond the earache. Lancet Infect Dis 10: 195–203.
4. Casselbrant ML, Mandel EM (2003) Epidemiology. In: Rosenfeld RM, Bluestone CD, eds. Evidence-based otitis media. Hamilton, (ON): BC Decker. pp 147–162.
5. Berman S (1995) Otitis media in developing countries. Pediatrics 96: 126–131.
6. Acuin J (2004) Chronic suppurative otitis media - Burden of Illness and Management Options. Geneva: World Health Organization.
7. Cruickshanks KJ, Wiley TL, Tweed TS, Klein BE, Klein R, et al. (1998) Prevalence of hearing loss in older adults in Beaver Dam, Wisconsin. The Epidemiology of Hearing Loss Study. Am J Epidemiol 148: 879–886.
8. Yueh B, Shapiro N, MacLean CH, Shekelle PG (2003) Screening and management of adult hearing loss in primary care: scientific review. JAMA 289: 1976–1985.
9. Harvard University, Institute for Health Metrics and Evaluation at the University of Washington, Johns Hopkins University, University of Queensland, World Health Organization (2009) GBD Study Operations Manual – Final Draft Jan. 2009.
10. Mathers CD, Lopez AD, Murray CJL (2006) The burden of disease and mortality by condition: data, methods and results for 2001. In: Lopez AD, Mathers CD, Ezzati M, Jamison DT, Murray CJL, eds. Global Burden of Disease and Risk Factors. Washington, (DC): World Bank. pp 45–240.
11. Little P, Gould C, Williamson I, Moore M, Warner G, Dunleavey J (2001) Pragmatic randomised controlled trial of two prescribing strategies for childhood acute otitis media. BMJ 322: 336–342.
12. NICE Short Clinical Guidelines Technical Team (2008) Respiratory tract infections – antibiotic prescribing. Prescribing of antibiotics for self-limiting respiratory tract infections in adults and children in primary care. London: National Institute for Health and Clinical Excellence.
13. Mandel EM, Doyle WJ, Winther B, Alper CM (2008) The incidence, prevalence and burden of OM in unselected children aged 1–8 years followed by weekly otoscopy through the "common cold" season. Int J Pediatr Otorhinolaryngol 72: 491–499.
14. Osma U, Cureoglu S, Hosoglu S (2000) The complications of chronic otitis media: report of 93 cases. J Laryngol Otol 114: 97–100.
15. Cusimano F, Cocita VC, D'Amico A (1989) Sensorineural hearing loss in chronic otitis media. J Laryngol Otol 103: 158–163.
16. Sade J, Halevy A (1976) The natural history of chronic otitis media. J Laryngol Otol 90: 743–751.
17. Papp Z, Rezes S, Jokay I, Sziklai I (2003) Sensorineural hearing loss in chronic otitis media. Otol Neurotol 24: 141–144.
18. Tüz M, Dogru H, Uygur K, Aynali G (2006) Sensorineural Hearing Loss Associated with Chronic Otitis Media. S D Ü Týp Fak Derg 13: 1–2.
19. Fernandes de Azevedo A, Pinto DC, de Souza NJ, Greco DB, Goncalves DU (2007) Sensorineural hearing loss in chronic suppurative otitis media with and without cholesteatoma. Braz J Otorhinolaryngol 73: 671–674.
20. Uhari M, Mantysaari K, Niemela M (1996) A meta-analytic review of the risk factors for acute otitis media. Clin Infect Dis 22: 1079–1083.
21. Ip S, Chung M, Raman G, Chew P, Magula N, et al. (2007) Breastfeeding and maternal and infant health outcomes in developed countries. Evid Rep Technol Assess (Full Rep). pp 1–186.
22. Lasisi AO, Olaniyan FA, Muibi SA, Azeez IA, Abdulwasiu KG, et al. (2007) Clinical and demographic risk factors associated with chronic suppurative otitis media. Int J Pediatr Otorhinolaryngol 71: 1549–1554.
23. World Health Organization (2008) World Health Statistics 2008.
24. World Health Organization (2009) World Health Statistics 2009.
25. UNICEF (2006) The State of the World's Children 2007: The Double Dividend of Gender Equality.
26. OECD (2008) OECD in Figures 2008. Available: http://www.oecd.org/dataoecd/44/17/41733586.pdf. Accessed 2012 Mar 19.
27. OECD (2008) OECD Health Data 2008. Available: http://stats.oecd.org/index.aspx?DataSetCode = HEALTH_STAT. Accessed 2012 Mar 19.
28. WHO-PDH (1991) Report of the Informal Working Group on Prevention of Deafness and Hearing Impairment, Programme Planning. Geneva, 18–21 June 1991. WHO/PDH/91.1.
29. Mathers CD, Smith A, Concha M Global Burden of hearing loss in the year 2000 - GBD 2000 Working Paper.
30. Al Khabori M, Khandekar R (2004) The prevalence and causes of hearing impairment in Oman: a community-based cross-sectional study. Int J Audiol 43: 486–492.
31. Liu C, Bu XK, Xing GQ, Zhou L, Xu X, et al. (2006) [Epidemiologic study on hearing impairment and ear diseases in old people]. Zhonghua Er Bi Yan Hou Tou Jing Wai Ke Za Zhi 41: 661–664.
32. Bansal R, Raj A (1998) Hearing loss in rural population: The etiology. Indian Journal of Otolaryngology and Head and Neck Surgery 50(2)()(pp 147–155), 1998 Date of Publication: 1998 147–155.
33. Jacob A, Rupa V, Job A, Joseph A (1997) Hearing impairment and otitis media in a rural primary school in south India. Int J Pediatr Otorhinolaryngol 39: 133–138.
34. Elango S, Purohit GN, Hashim M, Hilmi R (1991) Hearing loss and ear disorders in Malaysian school children. Int J Pediatr Otorhinolaryngol 22: 75–80.
35. Lasisi AO, Sulaiman OA, Afolabi OA (2007) Socio-economic status and hearing loss in chronic suppurative otitis media in Nigeria. Ann Trop Paediatr 27: 291–296.
36. Prescott CA, Kibel MA (1991) Ear and hearing disorders in rural grade 2 (Sub B) schoolchildren in the Western Cape. S Afr Med J %19;79: 90–93.
37. World Health Organization (2008) The global burden of disease. 2004 update p.
38. Rudan I, Tomaskovic L, Boschi-Pinto C, Campbell H (2004) Global estimate of the incidence of clinical pneumonia among children under five years of age. Bull World Health Organ 82: 895–903.
39. Rovers MM, Schilder AG, Zielhuis GA, Rosenfeld RM (2004) Otitis media. Lancet 363: 465–473.
40. Teele DW, Klein JO, Chase C, Menyuk P, Rosner BA (1990) Otitis media in infancy and intellectual ability, school achievement, speech, and language at age 7 years. Greater Boston Otitis Media Study Group. J Infect Dis 162: 685–694.
41. Arlinger S, Lunner T, Lyxell B, Pichora-Fuller MK (2009) The emergence of cognitive hearing science. Scand J Psychol 50: 371–384.
42. Williams CJ, Jacobs AM (2009) The impact of otitis media on cognitive and educational outcomes. Med J Aust 191: S69–S72.
43. Roberts J, Hunter L, Gravel J, Rosenfeld R, Berman S, et al. (2004) Otitis media, hearing loss, and language learning: controversies and current research. J Dev Behav Pediatr 25: 110–122.
44. Bennett KE, Haggard MP, Silva PA, Stewart IA (2001) Behaviour and developmental effects of otitis media with effusion into the teens. Arch Dis Child 85: 91–95.
45. Taipale A, Pelkonen T, Taipale M, Bernardino L, Peltola H, Pitkaranta A (2011) Chronic suppurative otitis media in children of Luanda, Angola. Acta Paediatr.
46. Paradise JL, Rockette HE, Colborn DK, Bernard BS, Smith CG, et al. (1997) Otitis media in 2253 Pittsburgh-area infants: prevalence and risk factors during the first two years of life. Pediatrics 99: 318–333.
47. Cook DG, Strachan DP (1999) Health effects of passive smoking-10: Summary of effects of parental smoking on the respiratory health of children and implications for research. Thorax 54: 357–366.
48. Bruce N, Perez-Padilla R, Albalak R (2000) Indoor air pollution in developing countries: a major environmental and public health challenge. Bull World Health Organ 78: 1078–1092.
49. Prymula R, Peeters P, Chrobok V, Kriz P, Novakova E, et al. (2006) Pneumococcal capsular polysaccharides conjugated to protein D for prevention of acute otitis media caused by both Streptococcus pneumoniae and non-typable Haemophilus influenzae: a randomised double-blind efficacy study. Lancet 367: 740–748. S0140-6736(06)68304-9 [pii];10.1016/S0140-6736(06)68304-9 [doi].
50. Boonacker CW, Broos PH, Sanders EA, Schilder AG, Rovers MM (2011) Cost effectiveness of pneumococcal conjugate vaccination against acute otitis media in children: a review. Pharmacoeconomics 29: 199–211.
51. Victora CG, Hanson K, Bryce J, Vaughan JP (2004) Achieving universal coverage with health interventions. Lancet 364: 1541–1548.
52. Hill Z, Kendall C, Arthur P, Kirkwood B, Adjei E (2003) Recognizing childhood illnesses and their traditional explanations: exploring options for care-seeking interventions in the context of the IMCI strategy in rural Ghana. Trop Med Int Health 8: 668–676.
53. Gunasekera H, Morris PS, Daniels J, Couzos S, Craig JC (2009) Otitis media in Aboriginal children: the discordance between burden of illness and access to services in rural/remote and urban Australia. J Paediatr Child Health 45: 425–430.
54. Damoiseaux RA, Rovers MM (2011) AOM in children. Clin Evid (Online) 2011. Available: http://bestpractice.bmj.com/best-practice/evidence/0301.html. Accessed 2012 Mar 19.
55. Hoberman A, Paradise JL, Rockette HE, Shaikh N, Wald ER, et al. (2011) Treatment of acute otitis media in children under 2 years of age. N Engl J Med 364: 105–115. 10.1056/NEJMoa0912254 [doi].
56. Tahtinen PA, Laine MK, Huovinen P, Jalava J, Ruuskanen O, Ruohola A (2011) A placebo-controlled trial of antimicrobial treatment for acute otitis media. N Engl J Med 364: 116–126. 10.1056/NEJMoa1007174 [doi].
57. Rovers MM, Glasziou P, Appelman CL, Burke P, McCormick DP, et al. (2006) Antibiotics for acute otitis media: a meta-analysis with individual patient data. Lancet 368: 1429–1435.
58. Marchetti F, Ronfani L, Nibali SC, Tamburlini G (2005) Delayed prescription may reduce the use of antibiotics for acute otitis media: a prospective observational study in primary care. Arch Pediatr Adolesc Med 159: 679–684.
59. Acuin J (2007) Chronic suppurative otitis media. Clin Evid (Online) 2007. Available: http://www.ncbi.nlm.nih.gov/pmc/articles/PMC2943814/pdf/2007-0507.pdf. Accessed 2012 Mar 19.
60. SIGN (2003) Diagnosis and management of childhood otitis media in primary care - A national clinical guideline.

61. Gates GA, Klein JO, Lim DJ, Mogi G, Ogra PL, et al. (2002) Recent advances in otitis media. 1. Definitions, terminology, and classification of otitis media. Ann Otol Rhinol Laryngol Suppl 188: 8–18.
62. Alberta Clinical Practice Guidelines Working Group (2000) Diagnosis and Treatment of Acute Otitis Media in Children - 2008 Update.
63. Medline plus enciclopedia (2011) Hearing loss. National Library of Medicine - National Institutes of Health. Available: http://www.nlm.nih.gov/medlineplus/ency/article/003044.htm. Accessed 2012 March 19.
64. World Health Organization (2001) International classification of functioning, disability and health: ICF.

14

Wolfram Syndrome: New Mutations, Different Phenotype

Concetta Aloi[1,§], Alessandro Salina[1,§], Lorenzo Pasquali[1,2], Francesca Lugani[1,3,4], Katia Perri[1], Chiara Russo[1], Ramona Tallone[1], Gian Marco Ghiggeri[4], Renata Lorini[1], Giuseppe d'Annunzio[1]*

1 Pediatric Clinic, University of Genoa, IRCCS G. Gaslini Institute, Genoa, Italy, **2** Centro de Investigacion Biomedica en Red (CIBER) de Diabetes y Enfermedades Metabolicas Asociadas (CIBERDEM), Barcelona, Spain, **3** Division of Nephrology, Department of Medicine, Columbia University, New York, New York, United States of America, **4** Laboratory on Pathophysiology of Uremia and Department of Nephrology, IRCCS G. Gaslini Institute, Genoa, Italy

Abstract

Background: Wolfram Syndrome (WS) is an autosomal recessive neurodegenerative disorder characterized by Diabetes Insipidus, Diabetes Mellitus, Optic Atrophy, and Deafness identified by the acronym "DIDMOAD". The WS gene, *WFS1*, encodes a transmembrane protein called Wolframin, which recent evidence suggests may serve as a novel endoplasmic reticulum calcium channel in pancreatic β-cells and neurons. WS is a rare disease, with an estimated prevalence of 1/550.000 children, with a carrier frequency of 1/354. The aim of our study was to determine the genotype of WS patients in order to establish a genotype/phenotype correlation.

Methodology/Principal Findings: We clinically evaluated 9 young patients from 9 unrelated families (6 males, 3 females). Basic criteria for WS clinical diagnosis were coexistence of insulin-treated diabetes mellitus and optic atrophy occurring before 15 years of age. Genetic analysis for *WFS1* was performed by direct sequencing. Molecular sequencing revealed 5 heterozygous compound and 3 homozygous mutations. All of them were located in exon 8, except one in exon 4. In one proband only an heterozygous mutation (A684V) was found. Two new variants c.2663 C>A and c.1381 A>C were detected.

Conclusions/Significance: Our study increases the spectrum of *WFS1* mutations with two novel variants. The male patient carrying the compound mutation [c.1060_1062delTTC]+[c.2663 C>A] showed the most severe phenotype: diabetes mellitus, optic atrophy (visual acuity 5/10), deafness with deep auditory bilaterally 8000 Hz, diabetes insipidus associated to reduced volume of posterior pituitary and pons. He died in bed at the age of 13 years. The other patient carrying the compound mutation [c.409_424dup16]+[c.1381 A>C] showed a less severe phenotype (DM, OA).

Editor: Tadafumi Kato, RIKEN Brain Science Institution, Japan

Funding: The authors have no support or funding to report.

Competing Interests: The authors have declared that no competing interests exist.

* E-mail: giuseppedannunzio@ospedale-gaslini.ge.it

§ These authors contributed equally to this work.

Introduction

Wolfram Syndrome (WS), also known as DIDMOAD (Diabetes Insipidus, Diabetes Mellitus, Optic Atrophy and Deafness), is an autosomal recessive neurodegenerative disease usually diagnosed in childhood when non autoimmune diabetes occurs with optic atrophy [1,2]. The condition is very rare with an estimated prevalence of one in 550.000 of children, [3] and with a carrier frequency of one in 354. Mortality is $\sim$65% before age 35 years, due to central respiratory failure with brainstem atrophy and renal failure secondary to infections [4]. Recently WS was described in a 44 year old patient with diabetes mellitus, central respiratory failure, cognitive impairment, ataxia and parkinsonism [5].

The nuclear gene for WS, *WFS1*, mapped on chromosome 4p16.1 [6], is composed of eight exons: the first is noncoding, the 2nd to the 7th are coding exons, and the 8th is 2.6 kb long spanning 33.4 kb of genomic DNA. The 3.6-kb mRNA encodes an 890-aminoacid hydrophobic and tetrameric protein named Wolframin [7], composed by nine transmembrane segments and large hydrophilic regions at both termini [8]. WFS1 mRNA is expressed in pancreas, brain, heart, skeletal muscle, placenta, lung, liver and kidney. Biochemical studies in cultured cells indicate *WFS1* to be an integral, endoglycosidase H-sensitive membrane glycoprotein that primarily localizes in the endoplasmic reticulum. Evidence suggests that *WFS1* is either a novel endoplasmic reticulum calcium channel or a regulator of channel activity [9,10].

In 2000 a second locus, *WFS2*, has been mapped on chromosome 4q22-q24 following the linkage analysis of four consanguineous Jordanian families [11]. These patients were not affected by diabetes insipidus, but showed upper gastrointestinal ulceration and bleeding. The ZCD2-encoded protein, ERIS (Endoplasmic Reticulum Intermembrane Small protein), is also shown to localize to the endoplasmic reticulum but does not interact directly with Wolframin.

The aim of our study was to evaluate clinical and molecular observations in nine patients with WS from nine different families and their follow-up in order to establish a genotype/phenotype correlation.

Materials and Methods

Etical Statement

The research was conducted according to Declaration of Helsinki and approved by IRCCS Giannina Gaslini Institute Ethical Committee.

Subjects

We clinically evaluated nine unrelated patients (six males and three females) from nine unrelated families, referred to our Pediatric Clinic. Basic criteria for the Wolfram Syndrome diagnosis were the coexistence of insulin-treated, juvenile-onset Diabetes Mellitus (DM) and Optic Atrophy (OA) occurring before 15 years of age. All analyses were performed after informed written consent obtained from patients or their parents.

Biochemical and clinical analyses

Autoantibodies against pancreatic β-cells (anti-glutamic acid decarboxylase: GADA, anti-thyrosin phosphatase-like protein: IA-2A, anti-insulin: IAA) were detected by RIA [12], and the analysis of HLA-DQA1 and -DQB1 polymorphisms at genomic levels was performed by polymerase chain reaction/sequence specific primers technique [13]. OA was confirmed by the presence of white papilla with regular and well-demarcated borders at the ophthalmoscope. As regards microangiopathic complications, peripheral neuropathy was assessed by electrophysiological examination, retinopathy was detected by fundoscopy and nephropathy screening was performed by overnight albumin excretion rate. Brain nuclear magnetic resonance (NMR) imaging was performed to assess posterior pituitary and brain structures. Structural renal tract abnormalities were assessed by ultrasonography and intravenous urography. Diagnosis of Diabetes Insipidus (DI) was based on the clinical findings of polyuria, polydipsia, an osmolality of less than 300 mOsm per kilogram of water, or a specific gravity of less than 1010 in a 24 hour urine sample without glycosuria and ketonuria [14]. Hearing impairment was assessed by audiograms across a range of frequencies (125–8000 Hz), and by brainstem auditory evoked potentials to explore the central conduction time of the auditory pathways.

Molecular analyses

DNA from probands, parents and controls were extracted from whole blood using High Pure PCR Template Preparation Kit (Roche, Mannheim, Germany). Exons and flanking regions of *WFS1* were amplified by PCR using previously described primers [15]. Amplicons were purified with exonuclease I and shrimp alkaline phosphatase (ExoSap-IT, USB Corporation, Staufen, Germany) and then sequenced for both sense and antisense strands using an automated fluorescent sequencing method (Big Dye Terminator Kit v1.1, Applied Biosystems). The products were separated on a ABI PRISM sequencing apparatus 3730 (Applied Biosystems). All variation were validated by sequencing both DNA strand of three independent PCR products.

Results

Main clinical data of each our patients are reported in Table 1.

Mutational screening, conducted in our Laboratory, revealed a total of 14 distinct variants (7 missense, 2 nonsense, 5 frameshift) all located in exon 8 except the c. 409_424dup16 in exon 4. Twelve were already described (c.1628T>G, c.2104 G>A, c.1060_1062delTTC, c.1620delGTG, c.2020 G>A, c.1885C>T, c.1230_1233delCTCT, c.1582 T>G, c.2106_2113del8n, c.2051C>T, c.1456 C>T, c.409_424dup16) [15,16,17,15,18,19,20,21,21–22,23,15,24] and two: the c.2663 C>A, p. S888X; and the c.1381 A>C, p. T461P were novel (Table 2). In order to establish the correct allelic segregation, DNA of parents were sequenced in all cases except in parents of proband 7, whose DNA sample was not available when molecular investigation was performed. None *WFS1* mutations was found in the 100 normal unrelated controls screened by sequencing. None of these mutations has been described in our previous work [25].

Case 1

A male patient, with surgically repaired Tetralogy of Fallot at age of 3 years, received a diagnosis of OA and DM without ketoacidosis at the age of 10 and 11 years respectively. B-cells autoantibodies were absent. Molecular analysis of HLA-DR and HLA-DQ regions revealed 0 heterodimers for type 1 DM susceptibility. He had a sudden anxiety with psychotic hints. The patient carried compound heterozygous mutation: the c.1628T>G, leading to substitution of Leucine with Arginine at codon 543 (L543R), this amino acid change was located in the sixth transmembrane domain of Wolframin. The G702S caused by G>A transition at nucleotide 2104, resulting in the substitution of Glycine with Serine at codon 702.

Table 1. Clinical features and age at diagnosis in nine patients with Wolfram Syndrome.

Patient n°	Sex (M/F)	Current Age (years)	DM (age)	OA (age)	DI (age)	D (age)	Renal tract abnormalities	Neurologic abnormalities
1	M	23	11	10	-	-	-	Anxiety with psychotic hints
2	M	13	4	9 ½	9 ½	9 ½	-	Reduced volume of posterior pituitary
3	M	15	11	14	-	-	-	-
4	F	12	9	9	-	-	-	-
5	M	17	10	7	16	16	-	-
6	F	12	7	11	-	-	double left district	-
7	F	15	14	14	-	10 months	-	Mild cognitive impairment
8	M	12	4	6	7	7	-	Posterior pituitary absence
9	M	17	9	16	-	-	-	-

(Patient n° 2 suddenly died at the age of 13 years).
DM: diabetes mellitus; OA: optic atrophy; DI: diabetes insipidus; D: deafness.
Current age: 2011.

Table 2. Mutations in the *WFS1* gene (new identified *WFS1* mutations are presented in bold).

Family	Exon	Nucleotide change	Amino acide change	Type of mutation	Reference
1	8	c.1628T>G;	L543R;	Missense;	Colosimo et al.[2003]
		c.2104 G>A	G702S	missense	Gasparin et al. [2009]
2	8	c.1060_1062delTTC;	F354del;	Frameshift;	Hardy et al. [1999]
		c.2663 C>A	**S888X**	**nonsense**	**This study**
3	8	c.1620delGTG;	V540del;	Frameshift;	Colosimo et al.[2003]
		c.2020G>A	G674R	missense	Khanim et al. [2001]
4	8	c.1885C>T;	R629W;	Missense;	Kadayifci et al.[2001]
		c.1230_1233delCTCT	V412fsX440	frameshift;	Giuliano et al. [2005]
5	8	c.1582 T>G	Y528D	Missense	Zalloua et al. [2008]
6	8	c.2106_2113del8nt	F646fs708X	Frameshift	Zalloua et al. [2008]
					Rigoli et al. [2011]
7	8	c.2051 C>T	A684V	Missense	Tessa et al. [2001]
8	8	c.1456 C>T	Q486X	Nonsense	Colosimo et al.[2003]
9	4	c. 409_424dup16	V142fsX251	Frameshift;	Gomez-Zaera et al. [2001]
	8	**c.1381 A>C**	**T461P**	**missense**	**This study**

(Patient 7 carried only one heterozygous mutation).

Case 2

A male patient with the most severe phenotype, died in bed at the age of 13 years. He showed DM with glycosuria, chetonuria, in absence of ketoacidosis at age of 4 years. B-cells autoantibodies were absent. Molecular analysis of HLA-DR and HLA-DQ regions revealed 0 heterodimers of susceptibility for type 1 DM. Celiac disease was diagnosed at age of 8 years and gluten free diet was prescribed. At age of 9 years he started to suffer from nocturnal apnea. OA (visual acuity 5/10) was diagnosed by fundoscopy at age of 9.5 years. Brain NMR revealed reducing the volume of posterior pituitary and optic nerve atrophy. Also DI and deafness (D) with hearing impairment at the 8000 Hz bilaterally were diagnosed at the age of 9.5 years. He harbored in-frame 3-bp deletion, nucleotides 1060_1062, in exon 8, that results in the loss of Phenylalanine 354 residue. According to the predicted structure of the Wolframin protein [17] residues 350 and 354 are likely to be located in the first transmembrane domain. However, the ultimate effect of these deletions cannot be anticipated yet. He also carried a novel nonsense mutation in exon 8 c.2663 C>A leading to S888X, causing a premature stop codon at residue 888 which removes 2 high conserved aminoacids from the carboxy tail.

Case 3

A male patient developed insulin treated DM without ketoacidosis at 11 years of age. B-cells autoantibodies were absent. Molecular analysis of HLA-DR and HLA-DQ regions revealed 0 heterodimers for type 1 DM susceptibility. OA was diagnosed at the age of 14 years. DI and D were absent up to now. He harbored an in-frame deletion, 1620delGTG, causing the loss of one Valine residue (V540del) and a missense mutation G674R resulting in the substitution of Glycine with Arginine at codon 674.

Case 4

A female patient developed insulin-treated DM and OA at the age of 9 years. B-cells autoantibodies were absent. Molecular analysis of HLA-DR and HLA-DQ regions revealed 0 heterodimers of susceptibility for type 1 DM. DI and D were not present up to now. She was found to be compound heterozygous: the R629W that converted Arginine in Tryptophan at codon 629 and the in-frame deletion of four nucleotides at position 1230 resulting in a premature stop codon, predicting a truncated protein of 450 aminoacids (V412fsX440).

Case 5

A male patient presented at the age of 7 years impaired vision, mild papillary pallor, presence some microaneurysms at fundoscopy, diffuse reduction of sensitivity: genetic testing for Leber's optic atrophy was positive. He suffered from insulin-treated DM with glycosuria, chetonuria, ketoacidosis since the age of 10 years. B-cells autoantibodies were absent. Molecular analysis of HLA-DR and HLA-DQ regions revealed 1 heterodimer for type 1 DM susceptibility. At the age of 16 years D with loss of sensorineural hearing for high tones, confirmed by audiometric test, and DI were diagnosed. He carried a homozygous missense mutation, inherited from both his parents, c.1582 T>G resulting in the substitution of Tyrosine with Aspartic Acid at codon 528 (Y528D).

Case 6

A female patient developed insulin treated DM at 7 years of age. B-cells autoantibodies were absent. Molecular analysis of HLA-DR and HLA-DQ regions revealed 2 heterodimers for type 1 DM susceptibility. At the age of 11, OA was diagnosed by fundoscopy; brain NMR signs of optic nerve impairment. DI, D were absent up to now. Urinary tract ultrasonography showed a double left district. She was found to have a homozygous 8-bp deletion from both alleles, nucleotides 2106_2113 in exon 8, resulting in a frameshift at codon 646 (Phenylalanine) and an early STOP codon, predicting a truncated protein of 708 amino acids missing part of the transmembrane domains and its hydrophilic carboxy tail.

Case 7

A female patient had profound deafness from the age of 10 months confirmed by audiometric test; at age of 5 years a cochlear implant was inserted. She showed insulin-treated DM, with glycosuria, chetonuria, ketoacidosis, and OA at 14 years of age. B-cells autoantibodies were absent. Molecular analysis of HLA-DR and HLA-DQ regions revealed 0 heterodimers of susceptibility for type 1 DM. DI is absent up to now. She showed mild cognitive impairment. Only one heterozygous mutation was found: the A684V caused by C>T transition at nucleotide 2051 resulting in the substitution of Alanine with Valine at codon 684. She also carried 10 polymorphisms (rs1801213 CG Het, rs1801212 AG Het, rs1801206 CT Het [V395V associated with DM1[26]], rs1801208 GA Het [R456H, associated with risk of Type 2 Diabetes [27], suicide [28] non autoimmune Diabetes [29]] rs1801214 CT Het, rs1046314 AG Het and rs1046316 AG Het [K811K and S855S, associated with DM1 [26]], rs1046317 CT Het, rs1046319 CT Het, rs1802453 GA Het). The A684V could not be confirmed in her parents since no DNA sample from their was available at the time of the screening of *WFS1* gene.

Case 8

A male patient showed all the clinical features of the syndrome: he suffered from insulin-treated DM since the age of 4. B-cells autoantibodies were absent. Molecular analysis of HLA-DR and HLA-DQ regions revealed 0 heterodimers for type 1 DM susceptibility. At the age of 6 years, OA was found and at age of 7 years, bilateral sensoneurial deafness and DI were diagnosed. Brain NMR revealed reducing the thickness of the nerve and chiasm and optic tracts, a nodule of heterotopic gray matter in the left anterior frontal periventricular. The posterior pituitary was not present. He resulted to be homozygous for the nonsense mutation 1456 C>T leading to a premature stop codon at residue 468 (Q486X), inherited from both his parents. This variant is predicted to give rise to an abnormal protein, missing part of the transmembrane domains and its hydrophilic carboxy tail.

Case 9

A male patient suffered from insulin-treated DM since the age of 9 years. Autoantibodies against β-cells were absent. Molecular analysis of HLA-DR and HLA-DQ regions revealed 0 heterodimers for type 1 DM susceptibility. At the age of 16 years OA was diagnosed. DI and D were absent up to now. He carried a compound heterozygous mutation: the 409_424dup16 in exon 4 is predicted to produce an aberrant protein; assuming that no splicing alterations occur, translation will follow until residue 251, where a stop codon is created [24]. The other identified change was a novel missense mutation c.1381 A>C resulting in the substitution of Treonine with Proline at codon 461.

Discussion

We report clinical and molecular observations about nine unrelated patients with WS and their follow-up. Up to now a wide spectrum of *WFS1* mutations were described [22]. In our study 14 different molecular defects were found. Thirteen were identified in both alleles: five probands carried compound heterozygous for *WFS1* mutations; three had *WFS1* defects in homozygous state. In one proband (patient 7) only an heterozygous mutation (A684V) was detected. Two novel mutations the S888X, and the T461P were found in patients 2 and 9 respectively (Table 2). All cases exhibited the main clinical features of WS.

The median age of the patients at the time of DNA analysis was 15,1 years (range 12–23).

Diabetes Mellitus is usually the first symptom occurring before age of 10 years, with optic atrophy at a median age of 11 years [30]. In our series, the average age at onset of diabetes was 8,7 years (range 4–14). WS-associated DM shows clear differences respect to autoimmune type 1 diabetes. WS-associated DM is due to loss of pancreatic β-cell function and number, as confirmed by autoptic studies, without markers for an autoimmune process [31].

Optic Atrophy occurs by definition in all patients with WS and is progressive. All our patients had OA and its identification was concomitant or after diabetes diagnosis except in case n° 1 and 5: where OA occurred before DM diagnosis. OA was diagnosed and confirmed by brain NMR in the first decade of life in 5 cases and between 11 and 16 years of age in the other 4. Although our patients are genetically heterogeneous, ophthalmological findings and age at detection are similar to other series [4,32,33]. The pathogenesis of OA could result from the effects of WS mutation on the survival of retinal ganglion cells, and in that case the mutation would lead to anterograde atrophy of retinal axons and shrinkage of the optic nerve. Retinal ganglion cells and optic nerve glial cells were found to be strongly labelled, suggesting that dual dysfunction of Wolframin in these cells might explain the progressive optic nerve atrophy reported in WS [34].

The development of polyuria and/or enuresis can indicate diabetes insipidus, which usually appears during the second decade. In our series only three patients showed DI at younger age (n° 2, 5, 8 at age of $9_{1/2}$, 16, 7 years respectively). (Table 1).

Sensorineural Deafness, confirmed by audiograms, was diagnosed in three patients at a mean age of 10.8 years (range $7–9_{1/2}$). Proband 7 had profound deafness from infancy requiring a cochlear implant. Such early onset of severe deafness has not been usually reported in Wolfram Syndrome. Hearing impairment reported in 66% of WS patients, ranging from congenital deafness to mild, progressive hearing impairment. Other case series reported deafness at a median age of 16 years in 60% of cases [35]. Audiometric features include a severe auditory threshold shift, more evident for the medium/high frequencies. Auditory impairment could be a consequence not only of a dysfunction of cochlear neurons and VII nerve fibers, but also of the central nervous pathways in brainstem and inferior colliculus [36].

Involvement of urinary tract represents another serious complication in WS patients and is estimated to occur in up to 90% of patients, being diagnosed during adolescence [37] or adulthood [38]. In our cases has been found only one patient (n° 6) with renal tract abnormalities: the ultrasonography of the urinary tract showed a double left district.

Neuropsychiatric manifestations are reported in the third decade. However Chaussenot A et al, who showed that the onset of neurologic symptoms, with a median age of 15 years, is much earlier than previously reported (mean age 30 years) [39]. In the majority of our patients behavioral problems or depression were evident at much younger ages. This could be due to the fact that previous studies focused on cerebellar ataxia and brainstem involvement as main neurological involvement in WS.

In many cases, it can be difficult to tease out the effect of multiple disabilities and reactive depression from a true depressive illness. It is important to involve a pediatric psychiatrist as part of the multidisciplinary team, particularly if there is a seminal event such as a first seizure. Such events can have devastating psychological consequences for an adolescent.

Wolframin *in vivo* is organized as a tetramer which originates a membrane Ca^{2+} channel of the Endoplasmic Reticulum (ER) and lack of function of *WFS1* determines apoptotic input signaling [40]. The ER has many roles, which include post-translational modification, folding and assembly of newly synthesized proteins such as insulin. Perturbations in ER function cause an imbalance

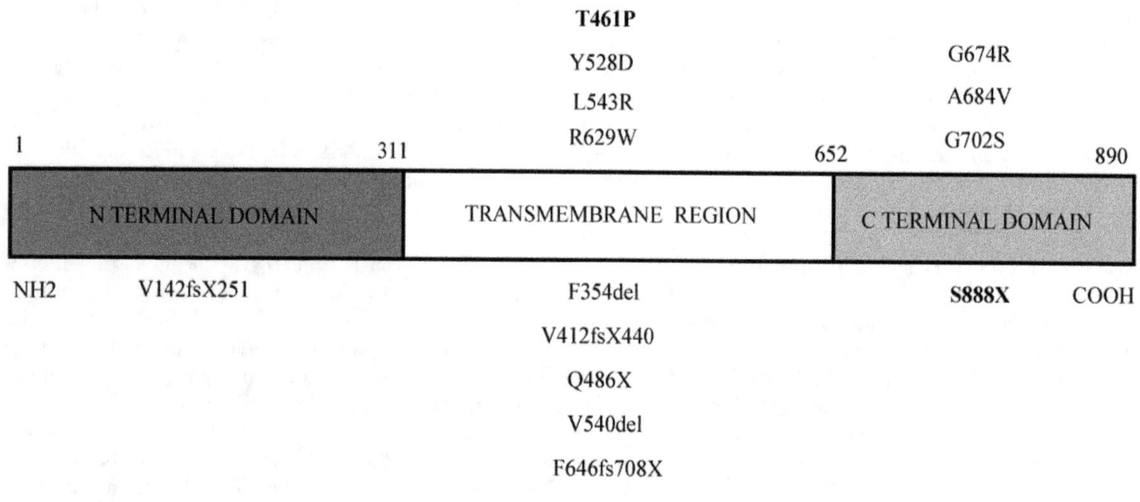

Figure 1. Schematic representation of Wolframin showing all our identified mutations. The novel are in boldface.

between these processes, leading to accumulation of misfolded and unfolded proteins in +the organelle, a state called ER stress [41].

Except the V142fsX251 found in exon 4, all the detected mutations are located in exon 8, corresponding to the transmembrane region and carboxytail of Wolframin protein. The majority of mutations described in our study were localized to the predicted transmembrane domains (64,3%, n = 9/14). Mutations in the amino-terminal domain were identified on 1 (7,1%) and in the carboxy-tail on 4 (28,6%) respectively (Fig. 1). This is in agreement with other studies in Italian and world-wide populations [15]. All causative mutations were identified on both alleles except in one case in which only one heterozygous mutation was found.

The predicting information that genetic analysis can give regards the difference between inactivating and non-inactivating mutations. The age at onset of DM was chosen as an indicator of disease severity. Missense mutations and 3 bp deletions, resulting in a deletion of one amino acid, were considered non-inactivating mutations. Nonsense, frameshift mutations, deletions and insertions of more than 3 bp were considered inactivating mutations [42]. Among the five patients with *WFS1* compound heterozygous mutation, two carried 2 non-inactivating mutations, three carried 1 inactivating and 1 non-inactivating. Their ages at diabetes clinical onset were 11 years and 7,3 years, respectively.

Among the three patients with *WFS1* homozygous mutation two carried inactivating and one non-activating; their mean ages at onset of diabetes were 5,5 and 10 years respectively.

Patient 7 carried only one non-inactivating mutation and the age at onset of diabetes was 14 years.

However, the only patient harbouring one mutations outside exon 8 showed a mild phenotype: the onset of diabetes mellitus and optic atrophy was 9 and 16 years respectively. A hearing deficit, diabetes insipidus, renal tract and neurologic abnormalities were absent. We could observe in our study that inactivating mutation give a more severe phenotype that non inactivating mutation, although clinical symptoms are different, according to a previous observation [9].

In our study, seven cases among 9 cases were identified mutations already published elsewhere. To clarify the actual genotype/phenotype correlation, we compared clinical manifestaions of the subjects sharing the same mutations. The clinical features caused by the missense mutation Y528D and the delection F646fs708X, both found in homozygous state in proband P5 and in P6, respectively; were similar to what reported by Zalluoa 2008 and Zalluoa 2008-Rigoli 2011. Unfortunately, the combination of compound heterozygous defects found in our series has never been reported in literature. So, it is difficult to compare the phenotype these our patients with what reported in other studies. However, validation of any genotype–phenotype correlation must await detailed functional analysis of mutations on a cellular and molecular level.

If the mutation causing the syndrome in a family is known, it is possible to offer genetic counselling and prenatal diagnosis. Prenatal diagnosis is possible analyzing DNA extracted from fetal cells by amniocentesis at approximately 15–18 weeks gestation or chorionic villus sampling at approximately 10–12 weeks gestation. [43,44].

WS is a progressive neurodegenerative disorder, that usually appears in adolescence and requires careful endocrinological evaluation aimed to start an early and adequate hormonal substitutive therapy. Even if WS is characterized by a wide differential diagnosis including other causes of neurodegeneration, it should be suspected in a young with diabetes mellitus and optic atrophy, hearing loss, polyuria and polydipsia but adequate glucose control [44]. Genetic test represents the best opportunity to confirm the clinical diagnosis and to propose prenatal diagnosis.

In conclusion, we have analyzed the *WFS1* in nine WS patients. Our study increases the spectrum of *WFS1* mutations with two novel variants.

Acknowledgments

The authors wish to thank the following collaborators of this study: Franco Cerutti M.D., Ivana Rabbone M.D. (Turin), Sonia Toni M.D. (Florence), Riccardo Lera M.D. (Alessandria), Anna Paola Frongia M.D., Margherita Chessa M.D. (Cagliari), Nicoletta Milani M.D. (Milan), Franco Meschi M.D., Elena Grechi M.D. (Milan) and Andrea Mascagni Mr (Genoa).

Author Contributions

Conceived and designed the experiments: CA AS LP RL GDA. Performed the experiments: CA AS LP. Analyzed the data: CA AS FL. Contributed reagents/materials/analysis tools: CA AS KP CR RT GMG. Wrote the paper: CA AS RL GDA.

References

1. Wolfram DJ (1938) Diabetes mellitus and simple optic atrophy among siblings. A report of four cases. Proc Mayo Clin 13: 715–718.
2. Strom TM, Hortnagel K, Hofmann S, Gekeler F, Scharfe C, et al. (1998) Diabetes insipidus, diabetes mellitus, optic atrophy and deafness (DIDMOAD) caused by mutations in a novel gene (Wolframin) coding for a predicted transmembrane protein. Hum Mol Genet 7: 2021–2028.
3. Kumar S (2010) Wolfram syndrome: important implications for pediatricians and pediatric endocrinologists. Pediatr Diabetes 11: 28–37.
4. Barrett TG, Bundey SE, Macleod AF (1995) Neurodegeneration and diabetes: UK nationwide study of Wolfram (DIDMOAD) syndrome. Lancet 346: 1458–1463.
5. Waschbisch A, Volbers B, Struffert T, Hoyer J, Schwab S, et al. (2011) Primary diagnosis of Wolfram syndrome in an adult patient-case report and description of a novel pathogenic mutation. J Neurol Sci 300: 191–193.
6. Inoue H, Tanizawa Y, Wasson J, Behn P, Kalidas K, et al. (1998) A gene encoding a transmembrane protein is mutated in patients with diabetes mellitus and optic atrophy (Wolfram syndrome). Nat Genet 20: 143–148.
7. Takeda K, Inoue H, Tanizawa Y, Matsuzaki Y, Oba J, et al. (2001) WFS1 (Wolfram syndrome 1) gene product: predominant subcellular localization to endoplasmic reticulum in cultured cells and neuronal expression in rat brain. Hum Mol Genet 10: 477–484.
8. Hofmann S, Philbrook C, Gerbitz KD, Bauer MF (2003) Wolfram syndrome: structural and functional analyses of mutant and wild-type Wolframin, the *WFS1* gene product. Hum Mol Genet 12: 2003–2012.
9. Osman AA, Saito M, Makepeace C, Permutt MA, Schlesinger P, et al. (2003) Wolframin expression induces novel ion channel activity in endoplasmic reticulum membranes and increases intracellular calcium. J Biol Chem 278: 52755–52762.
10. Riggs AC, Bernal-Mizrachi E, Ohsugi M, Wasson J, Fatrai S, et al. (2005) Mice conditionally lacking the Wolfram gene in pancreatic islet beta cells exhibit diabetes as a result of enhanced endoplasmic reticulum stress and apoptosis. Diabetologia 48: 2313–2321.
11. El-Shanti H, Lidral AC, Jarrah N, Druhan L, Ajlouni K (2000) Homozygosity mapping identifies an additional locus for Wolfram syndrome on chromosome 4q. Am J Hum Genet 66: 1229–1236.
12. Naserke HE, Dozio N, Ziegler AG, Bonifacio E (1998) Comparison of a novel micro-assay for insulin autoantibodies with the conventional radiobinding assay. Diabetologia 41: 681–683.
13. Lorini R, Orecchia G, Martinetti M, Dugoujon JM, Cuccia M (1992) Autoimmunity in vitiligo: relationship with HLA, Gm and Km polymorphisms. Autoimmunity 11: 255–260.
14. Maghnie M, Cosi G, Genovese E, Manca-Bitti ML, Cohen A, et al. (2003) Central diabetes insipidus in children and young adults. N Engl J Med 343: 998–1007.
15. Colosimo A, Guida V, Rigoli L, Di Bella C, De Luca A, et al. (2003) Molecular detection of novel WFS1 mutations in patients with Wolfram syndrome by a DHPLC-based assay. Hum Mutat 21: 622–629.
16. Gasparin MR, Crispim F, Paula SL, Freire MB, Dalbosco IS, et al. (2009) Identification of novel mutations of the WFS1 gene in Brazilian patients with Wolfram syndrome. Eur J Endocrinol 160: 309–316.
17. Hardy C, Khanim F, Torres R, Scott-Brown M, Seller A, et al. (1999) Clinical and molecular genetic analysis of 19 Wolfram syndrome kindreds demonstrating a wide spectrum of mutations in WFS1. Am J Hum Genet 65: 1279–1290.
18. Khanim F, Kirk J, Latif F, Barrett TG (2001) WFS1/wolframin mutations, Wolfram syndrome, and associated diseases. Hum Mutat 17: 357–367.
19. Kadayifci A, Kepekci Y, Coskun Y, Huang Y (2001) Wolfram syndrome in a family with variable expression. Acta Medica 44: 115–118.
20. Giuliano F, Bannwarth S, Monnot S, Cano A, Chabrol B, et al. (2005) Wolfram syndrome in French population: characterization of novel mutations and polymorphisms in the WFS1 gene. Hum Mutat 25: 99–100.
21. Zalloua PA, Azar ST, Delépine M, Makhoul NJ, Blanc H, et al. (2008) WFS1 mutations are frequent monogenic causes of juvenile-onset diabetes mellitus in Lebanon. Hum Mol Genet 17: 4012–4021.
22. Rigoli L, Lombardo F, Di Bella C (2011) Wolfram syndrome and WFS1 gene. Clin Genet 79: 103–117.
23. Tessa A, Carbone I, Matteoli MC, Bruno C, Patrono C, et al. (2001) Identification of novel WFS1 mutations in Italian children with Wolfram syndrome. Hum Mutat 17: 348–349.
24. Gómez-Zaera M, Strom TM, Rodríguez B, Estivill X, Meitinger T, et al. (2001) Presence of a major WFS1 mutation in Spanish Wolfram syndrome pedigrees. Mol Genet Metab 72: 72–81.
25. d'Annunzio G, Minuto N, D'Amato E, De Toni T, Lombardo F, et al. (2008) Wolfram Syndrome (Diabetes Insipidus, Diabetes, Optic Atrophy, and Deafness). Diabetes Care 31: 1743–1745.
26. Domènech E, Gómez-Zaera M, Nunes V (2002) WFS1 mutations in Spanish patients with diabetes mellitus and deafness. Eur J Hum Genet 10: 421–426.
27. Fawcett KA, Wheeler E, Morris AP, Ricketts SL, Hallmans G, et al. (2010) Detailed Investigation of the Role of Common and Low-Frequency *WFS1* Variants in Type 2 Diabetes Risk. Diabetes 59: 741–746.
28. Sequeira A, Kim C, Seguin M, Lesage A, Chawky N, et al. (2003) Wolfram Syndrome and Suicide: Evidence for a Role of WFS1 in Suicidal and Impulsive Behavior. Am J Med Genet B Neuropsychiatr Genet 119: 108–113.
29. Awata T, Inoue K, Kurihara S, Ohkubo T, Inoue I, et al. (2000) Missense Variations of the Gene Responsible for Wolfram Syndrome (*WFS1/wolframin*) in Japanese: Possible Contribution of the Arg456His Mutation to Type 1 Diabetes as a Nonautoimmune Genetic Basis. Biochem Biophys Res Commun 268: 612–616.
30. Casey JA. Smith (2004) Phenotype-Genotype Correlations in a Series of Wolfram Syndrome Families. Diabetes Care 27: 2003–2009.
31. Kinsley BT, Dumont RH, Swift M, Swift RG (1995) Morbidity and mortality in the Wolfram syndrome. Diabetes Care 187: 1566–1570.
32. Simsek E, Simsek T, Tekgul S, Hosal S, Seyrantepe V, et al. (2003) Wolfram (DIDMOAD) symdrome: a multidisciplinary clinical study in nine Turkish patients and review of literature. Acta Paediatr 92: 55–61.
33. Medlej R, Wasson J, Baz P, Azar S, Salti I, et al. (2004) Diabetes mellitus and optic atrophy: a study of Wolfram syndrome in the Lebanese population. J Clin Endocrinol Metab 89: 1656–1661.
34. Yamamoto H, Hofmann S, Hamasaki DI, Yamamoto H, Kreczmanski P, et al. (2006) Wolfram Syndrome 1 (WFS1) protein expression in retinal ganglion cells and optic nerve glia of the cynomolgus monkey. Exp Eye Res 83: 1303–1306.
35. Megighian D, Savastano M (2004) Wolfram syndrome. Int J Ped Otorhinolaryngol 68: 243–247.
36. Genis D, Davalos A, Molins A, Ferrer I (1997) Wolfram syndrome: a neuropathological study. Acta Neuropathol 93: 426–429.
37. Tekgul S, Oge O, Simsek E, Yordam N, Kendi S (1999) Urological manifestations of the Wolfram Syndrome: observations in 14 patients. J Urol 161: 616–617.
38. Piccoli GB, Mezza E, Jeantet A, Segoloni JP (2003) An uncommon genetic syndrome with acute renal failure in a 30-year-old diabetic patient. Nephrol Dial Transplant 18: 206–208.
39. Chaussenot A, Bannwarth S, Rouzier C, Vialettes B, Mkadem SA, et al. (2011) Neurologic features and genotype-phenotype correlation in wolfram syndrome. Ann Neurol 69: 501–508.
40. Philbrook C, Fritz E, Weiher H (2005) Expressional and functional studies of Wolframin, the gene function deficient in Wolfram Syndrome, in mice and patient cells. Exper Gerontol 40: 671–678.
41. Fonseca SG, Ishigaki S, Oslowski CM, Lu S, Lipson KL, et al. (2010) Wolfram syndrome 1 gene negatively regulates ER stress signaling in rodent and human cells. J Clin Invest 120: 744–755.
42. Cryns K, Sivakumaran TA, Van den Ouweland JM, Pennings RJ, Cremers CW, et al. (2003) Mutational spectrum of the WFS1 gene in Wolfram syndrome, nonsyndromic hearing impairment, diabetes mellitus, and psychiatric disease. Hum Mut 22: 275–287.
43. Tranebjaerg L, Barrett T, Rendtorff ND (2009) WFS1-Related Disorders. Gene Reviews 24.
44. Domenech E, Kruyer H, Gomez C, Calvo MT, Nunes V (2004) First prenatal diagnosis for wolfram syndrome by molecular analysis of the WS1 gene. Prenat Diagn 24: 787–789.

15

Regeneration of Stereocilia of Hair Cells by Forced Atoh1 Expression in the Adult Mammalian Cochlea

Shi-Ming Yang[1]*, Wei Chen[2], Wei-Wei Guo[1], Shuping Jia[3], Jian-He Sun[1], Hui-Zhan Liu[3], Wie-Yen Young[1], David Z. Z. He[3]*

1 Department of Otolaryngology—Head and Neck Surgery, Institute of Otolaryngology, Chinese PLA General Hospital, Beijing, China, **2** Department of Otolaryngology—Head and Neck Surgery, PLA Air Force General Hospital, Beijing, China, **3** Department of Biomedical Sciences, Creighton University School of Medicine, Omaha, Nebraska, United States of America

Abstract

The hallmark of mechanosensory hair cells is the stereocilia, where mechanical stimuli are converted into electrical signals. These delicate stereocilia are susceptible to acoustic trauma and ototoxic drugs. While hair cells in lower vertebrates and the mammalian vestibular system can spontaneously regenerate lost stereocilia, mammalian cochlear hair cells no longer retain this capability. We explored the possibility of regenerating stereocilia in the noise-deafened guinea pig cochlea by cochlear inoculation of a viral vector carrying Atoh1, a gene critical for hair cell differentiation. Exposure to simulated gunfire resulted in a 60–70 dB hearing loss and extensive damage and loss of stereocilia bundles of both inner and outer hair cells along the entire cochlear length. However, most injured hair cells remained in the organ of Corti for up to 10 days after the trauma. A viral vector carrying an EGFP-labeled *Atoh1* gene was inoculated into the cochlea through the round window on the seventh day after noise exposure. Auditory brainstem response measured one month after inoculation showed that hearing thresholds were substantially improved. Scanning electron microscopy revealed that the damaged/lost stereocilia bundles were repaired or regenerated after Atoh1 treatment, suggesting that Atoh1 was able to induce repair/regeneration of the damaged or lost stereocilia. Therefore, our studies revealed a new role of Atoh1 as a gene critical for promoting repair/regeneration of stereocilia and maintaining injured hair cells in the adult mammal cochlea. Atoh1-based gene therapy, therefore, has the potential to treat noise-induced hearing loss if the treatment is carried out before hair cells die.

Editor: Li I. Zhang, University of Southern California, United States of America

Funding: This work was supported by grants from the Major State Basic Research Development Program of China (973 Program #2011CBA01000), the National Basic Research Program of China (973 Program #2012CB967900), National Hi-Tech Research and Development Program of China (863 Program #2007AA02Z150), the National Natural Science Foundation of China (#30871398, 30730040) to SMY, and by National Institutes of Health (NIH) grants R21 DC 009908 and R01 DC 004696 to DH from the National Institute on Deafness and Other Communication Disorders (NIDCD). The funders had no role in study design, data collection and analysis, decision to publish, or preparation of the manuscript.

Competing Interests: The authors have declared that no competing interests exist.

* E-mail: yangsm301@263.net (SMY); hed@creighton.edu (DZZH)

Introduction

Noise-induced hearing loss (NIHL) is a major health problem. Acoustic trauma causes NIHL when permanent cochlear damage results from exposure to high-intensity sounds, such as explosions, gunfire, and firecrackers. NIHL is usually due to destruction of cochlear hair cells and/or damage to their hair bundles [1]. Cochlear hair cells transduce mechanical stimuli into electrical activity [2]. The hair bundle, a staircase array of stereocilia of different heights, is the site of mechanoelectrical transduction [3]. The delicate hair bundle is susceptile to both acoustic trauma and ototoxic drugs. While hair cells in lower vertebrates and mammalian vestibular systems can spontaneously regenerate lost stereocilia [4–6], mammalian cochlear hair cells no longer retain this capability [7]. The inability of stereocilia to self-repair can subsequently lead to hair cell death and permanent hearing loss. Injured neonatal gerbil hair cells can live for 10 to 12 days *in vitro* after their stereocilia are destroyed [7]. If adult cochlear hair cells can likewise survive for a number of days after loss of stereocilia due to exposure to impulsive noise or ototoxic drugs, this window of opportunity could be crucial for potentially rescuing and repairing hair cells using therapeutic genetic or chemical interventions.

The transcription factor *atonal* belongs to the family of basic helix-loop-helix (bHLH)-containing proteins and plays an essential role in the development of the *Drosophila* nervous system [8]. In mammals, Atoh1 (also known as math1) has been shown to be essential for neurogenesis in the central and peripheral nervous system [9–12], and for the formation of several non-neural cell types [13,14]. In the auditory system, Atoh1 plays a critical role for hair cell differentiation during development [15–17]. Embryonic Atoh1-null mice fail to generate cochlear and vestibular hair cells, as indicated by the absence of stereocilia and other hair cell-specific markers [15]. Furthermore, overexpression (or misexpression) of Atoh1 in *in vitro*, *in vivo*, and *in utero* cochleae results in the production of ectopic hair cells derived from non-sensory supporting cells [18–21]. These studies suggest that Atoh1 is important for hair cell genesis or apical specialization (i.e., stereocilia development and formation). We questioned whether forced expression of Atoh1 in the noise-deafened cochlea can promote repair/regeneration of the stereocilia destroyed by impulsive noise.

Materials and Methods

1. Animals

Care and use of the animals in this study was approved by the Institutional Animal Care and Use Committee of the Chinese PLA General Hospital. Healthy (250–300 g) adult albino guinea pigs of either sex were used for the experiments. Hearing in both ears was measured using auditory brainstem responses (ABR) before and seven days after noise exposure. Only those animals whose hearing thresholds were normal before exposure and significantly elevated (≥60 dB SPL at all frequencies tested) after noise exposure, with no obvious sign of middle ear infection and damage, were selected for further experiments.

2. Impulsive Noise Exposure

Animals were put in a specially designed cage with their heads constrained. The cage was housed inside a sound isolation room. Each animal was continuously exposed to 200 rounds of simulated gunfire inside the soundproof room. The sound source was placed 20 cm away from each ear. The peak sound pressure level measured near the ear canal was approximately 164 dB SPL (C-frequency weighting). The impulse had B-duration of 10 ms. The interval between each pulse was 10 seconds.

3. Viral Construct and Inoculation

Replication-deficient recombinant adenoviruses (Ad5) with deleted E1 and E3 regions were used to construct Ad.*Atoh1-GFP* and Ad.*GFP* using the Adeno-X expression system (K1650-1, Clontech). Dr. W. Q. Gao from Genentech, San Francisco, CA, kindly provided us with the *Atoh1* plasmids. The sequence and other information about the constructs have been published elsewhere [18,20,21]. Animals were anesthetized with xylazine and ketamine, and kept warm using a 37°C warm pad. Viral vectors were inoculated into the cochlea through the round window either seven days or one month after noise exposure. 5 μl of viral suspension with concentration of 1×10^{10} total particles of purified virus per milliliter was inoculated.

4. Immunocytochemistry and Scanning Electron Microscopy

Cochleae were perfused with 4% formaldehyde in phosphate buffered saline (PBS) and treated with 0.2% Triton X-100/PBS. Goat serum (10%) was used to block nonspecific binding. The tissue was then incubated with an anti-C-mPres antibody [22] and washed with PBS, followed by incubation with secondary antibodies. To visualize the stereocilia, F-actin was labeled with rhodamine-phalloidin, as described previously [7]. An anti-myosin 7a antibody was also used to label the hair cells as described elsewhere [21]. A sample was mounted on glass slides with antifade solution (Prolong Antifade Kit, Invitrogen, Carlsbad, CA) before imaging on an Olympus FluoView FV1000 Confocal Microscope (Olympus (China)., Ltd., Beijing).

For scanning electron microscopy (SEM), the cochleae were fixed with 2.5% glutaraldehyde in 0.1 M sodium cacodylate buffer (pH 7.4) containing 2 mM $CaCl_2$, washed in PBS, then post-fixed for 15 minutes with 1% OsO_4 in the same buffer and washed. The tissues were dehydrated in an ethanol series, critical point dried from CO_2, and sputter-coated with gold. The tissue was then examined using a Hitachi S-3700N scanning electron microscope.

5. ABR and Cochlear Microphonic Measurements

Details of ABR and cochlear microphonic (CM) measurements are described as previously performed [22]. During ABR and CM measurements, guinea pigs were anaesthetized with xylazine and ketamine. For ABR, needle electrodes were inserted at the vertex and pinna. ABRs were evoked with clicks and/or 5-ms tone pips (0.5 ms rise–fall, at 30/sec) with frequencies of 4, 8, 16, and 20 kHz. The response was amplified, filtered, and averaged using the Intelligent Hearing System (Intelligent Hearing System Corp., Miami, FL). Sound level was raised in 20- and/or 5-dB steps. At each level, 1,024 responses were averaged. Hearing threshold was determined by visual inspection. For CM measurement, a silver wire electrode was placed near the round window membrane. Responses to a 4-kHz tone burst were amplified, filtered, and averaged using the Intelligent Hearing System.

Results

Adult guinea pigs were exposed to 200 rounds of simulated gunfire. We measured the CM to monitor the damage to the hair cells in some animals. The CM, an electrical potential generated in the cochlear hair cells in response to acoustic stimulation, primarily reflects mechanotransduction in the stereocilia of outer hair cells [23]. The CM response before and after 1, 10, and 200 rounds of gunfire was recorded. As examples, Figure 1A shows the CM response waveforms at three high sound intensity levels before, during, and after noise exposure. As shown, the magnitude of CM responses at saturation levels was reduced by as much as 26% after exposure to just one round of gunfire. After exposures to 10 and 200 rounds of gunfire, the magnitude decreased by 66% and 97%, respectively. The magnitude-intensity (input-output) function of the CM (Fig. 1B) shows that there was at least a 60 dB elevation in sound pressure level for the same magnitude of the CM after noise exposure. The reduction represents a significant disruption of outer hair cell (OHC) mechanotransduction after noise exposure. We measured hearing thresholds (Fig. 1C) before and seven days after noise exposure, using sound-evoked ABRs [22]. ABRs, frequently used to monitor hearing loss, are electrical signals evoked from the brainstem during presentation of an acoustic signal. ABR thresholds were obtained from both ears of 19 animals at 4, 8, 16, and 20 Hz using tone pips. The means and standard deviations of the thresholds before and seven days after noise exposure are presented in Figure 1C. Consistent with CM measurements, hearing thresholds for both ears were elevated by more than 60 dB for all frequencies tested. Since the ABR thresholds were measured at seven days after noise exposure to minimize the effect of temporary threshold shift, this threshold elevation should represent the permanent hearing loss. Only those animals whose hearing thresholds were elevated by more than 60 dB were used for further experiments.

We examined the morphological integrity of the stereocilia along the entire cochlear length at seven days after noise exposure using SEM. Figure 2 (A–F) shows examples obtained from three cochlear locations. Extensive stereocilia damage and loss of both inner and outer hair cells in the first, second, and third turns were observed. Sporadic hair cell death, as indicated by scar formation (marked by arrows in Fig. 2B), was also seen. Notably, injured hair cells remained in the organ of Corti despite severe bundle damage/loss. This is indicated by the presence of rootlets of the truncated stereocilia in the reticular lamina (Fig. 2G, H) and/or by the presence of OHC somas sandwiched between reticular lamina and the Deiters' cells (Fig. 2I).

To examine the fate of hair cells after stereocilia damage/loss, prestin immunoreactivity combined with confocal microscopy was used. Prestin is the motor protein of OHCs [24] and is only expressed in the plasma membrane [25]. Therefore, prestin immunoreactivity can be used as an assay to probe the status of

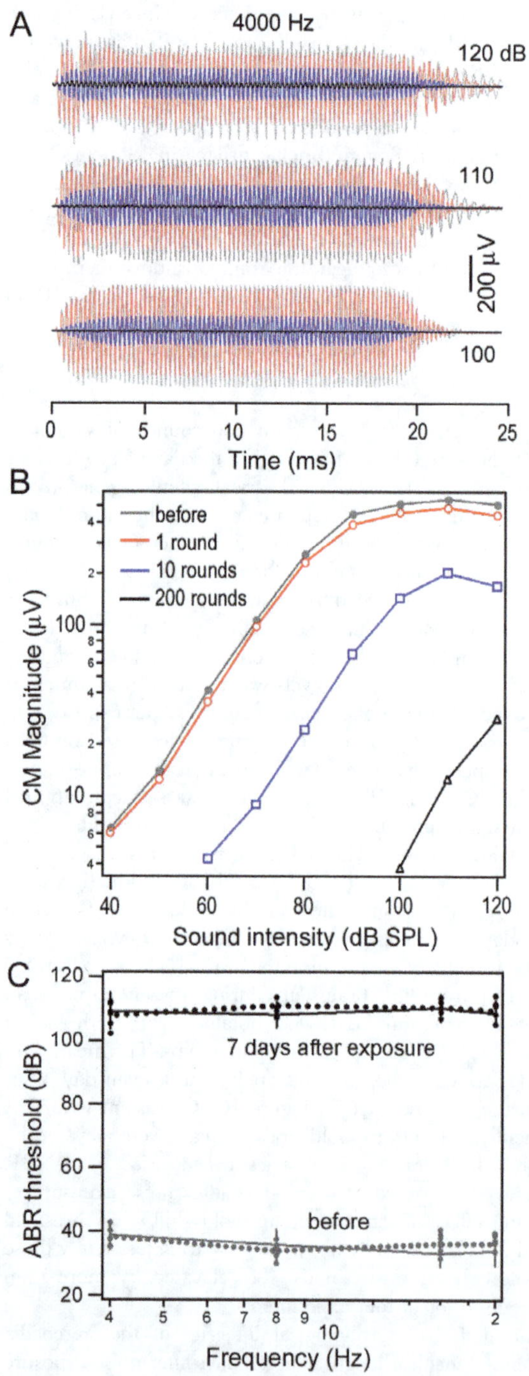

Figure 1. Hearing loss after exposure to simulated gunfire. *A:* Three examples of CM responses obtained before, during, and immediately after noise exposure. *B:* CM magnitude as a function of sound level before, during, and after noise exposure. Note the magnitude is plotted on log scale. *C:* Tone pip-evoked ABR thresholds (mean ± SD, n = 19) for both ears before and seven days after noise exposure. No statistical difference (student's t-test) in thresholds at each frequency was found between left (dot lines) and right (solid lines) ears either before or after noise exposure ($p>0.05$).

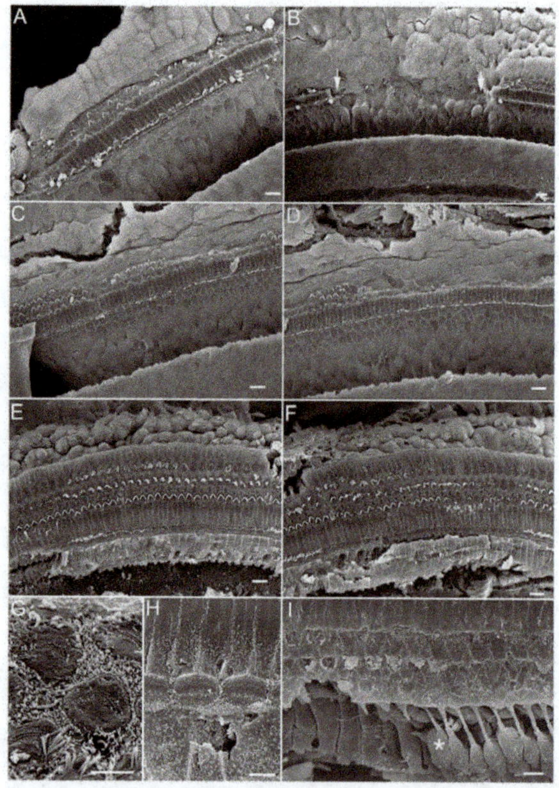

Figure 2. SEM images of the hair bundles seven days after exposure to impulsive noise. *A–F:* Images of hair bundle damage/loss obtained from representative locations in the basal (*A,B*), second (*C,D*), and third (*E,F*) turns. An area with hair cell death and scar formation is marked by arrows. *G,H:* High-magnification pictures of OHCs and IHCs with complete loss of stereocilia bundles. *I:* Image of complete loss of OHC stereocilia bundles in a second turn region. Note that the OHCs still remained in the organ of Corti despite loss of stereocilia bundles. A Deiters' cell is marked with an asterisk. Scale bars: 20 μm (*A–F*), 5 μm (*G,H*), and 10 μm (*I*).

OHCs. Absence of staining or presence of membrane debris would suggest cell death. To simultaneously visualize the hair bundle, rhodamine-phalloidin was used to label F-actin-containing stereocilia [7]. Figure 3A shows a composite confocal image obtained from a cochlea 10 days after noise exposure. As shown, the "V"-shaped OHC bundles (in red) were missing in the outmost (third) row and in some second row OHCs. However, the bundleless hair cells remained in the organ of Corti, although some sporadic hair cell loss was also observed (evidenced by empty space between prestin-labeled OHCs). Figure 3B shows a 3-D prestin-immunolabeled image (stacked along the z-axis) from a different cochlear location. This, again, shows that most OHCs survived the acoustic trauma despite sporadic OHC death (e.g., membrane debris and missing OHCs in Fig. 3B). Consistent with a previous study using the cultured organ of Corti [7], we concluded that noise-damaged OHCs with bundle damage/loss could survive up to at least 10 days after exposure.

Since the bundleless hair cells could remain in the organ of Corti for at least 10 days, this window could be crucial for intervention to repair hair bundles and to prevent the eventual death of hair cells. We explored the possibility of rescuing and repairing the injuried hair cells by overexpressing Atoh1. A viral vector carrying an EGFP-labeled *Atoh1* gene was inoculated into the cochlea through the round window on the seventh day after noise exposure. We chose the left ear for viral inoculation and the right (contralateral) ear as the control in eight animals. In another six animals, viral vectors carrying only the EGFP gene were inoculated into the left cochlea (seven days after noise exposure) as

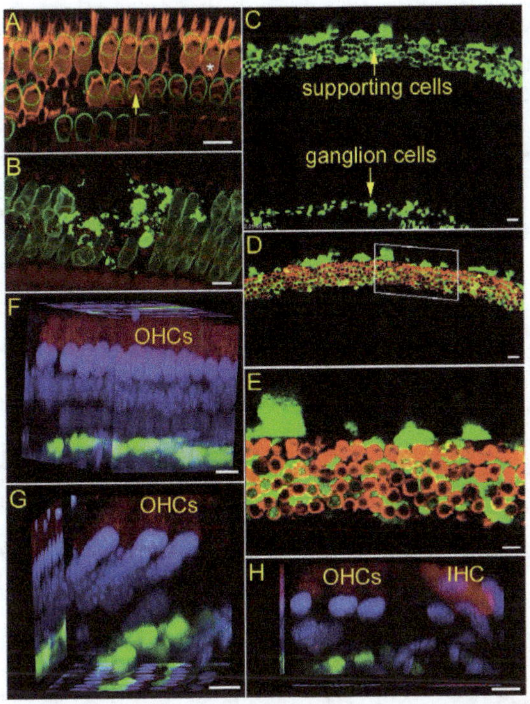

Figure 3. Confocal images of the stereocilia and prestin immunoactivity, and the pattern of Atoh1-EGFP expression in the organ of Corti. *A:* Stereocilia bundles in one cochlear location. The hair bundle was labeled with rhodamine-phalloidin (in red). The "V"-shaped OHC bundles were missing in the outmost (third) rows of OHCs. One bundleless OHC is indicated by an asterisk. One "V"-shaped hair bundle is marked by a yellow arrow. Prestin immunoactivity was labeled in green. Scale bar: 10 µm. *B:* Z-axis stack image of prestin immunoactivity at another cochlear location. Scale bar: 10 µm. All the images in *A* and *B* were obtained from cochleae 10 days after noise exposure. *C:* Confocal image of Atoh1-expression in a cochlea. *D:* Composite images of hair cells (labeled with myo7a antibody, in red) and EGFP-positive cells (from the same location as shown in panel *C*). The images were acquired seven days after Ad.*Atoh1-EGFP* inoculation in the noise-damaged cochlea (second turn). A magnified image of the area marked by white lines is presented in panel *E*. Scale bar: 20 µm for *C* and *D*. *E:* High magnification image of Atoh1 and myo7a expression in the organ of Corti. Scale bar: 10 µm. *F:* Confocal image obtained from optical sectioning from a basal turn location at 3 days after Atoh1 treatment. Hair cells were labeled with myo7a (in red) and the nuclei were labeled with DAPI. Most preparations examined at 3 days after transfection showed weak or no expression of EGFP in the organ of Corti. For those that expressed EGFP, the expression was in the area of Deiters' cells. *G, H:* Confocal image using optical sectioning from a basal turn location at 7 and 14 days after Atoh1 treatment. Scale bars (*F,G, H*): 10 µm.

an additional control. Expression of Atoh1 by the EGFP expression was examined by confocal microscopy seven days after inoculation. Figure 3C exhibits a survey confocal image obtained from the basal turn in a whole-mount preparation. As shown, intense EGFP-positive labeling was observed in the areas of the organ of Corti and spiral ganglion neurons. To determine where the forced expression of Atoh1 occured in the organ of Corti, we used a myo7a antibody to label hair cells. Figure 3D shows that EGFP and myo7a were expressed in the different cell types in the organ of Corti. High magnification images show that EGFP expression was not in the hair cells (Fig. 3E). To further confirm that forced Atoh1 expression was not in hair cells, we took a series of optical sections to reconstruct 3-D images of the organ of Corti at 7 days after transfection. Reconstruction from the obtained images confirmed that forced Atoh1 expression was not seen in the hair cells, but rather in the supporting cells (Fig. 3G). To determine whether forced Atoh1 expression ever occurred in the hair cells at different time points after transfection, we also examined EGFP expression at 3 (Fig. 3F) and 14 (Fig. 3H) days after Atoh1 inoculation. As shown, forced Atoh1 expression was confined to the supporting cells and was not detected in the hair cells.

The morphology of stereocilia at three cochlear locations was examined in the control (right) and Atoh1-treated (left) ears using SEM at one month after viral inoculation. In the control ears without Atoh1 inoculation after noise exposure, the reticular lamina was mostly flat with a few remaining stereocilia bundles (Fig. 4A–C). The remaining bundles had obvious signs of damage such as truncation, fusion, and folding. In contrast, most hair bundles in the Atoh1-treated ears appeared to have a normal appearence. Although hair cells with damaged or lost bundles were also sporadically observed along the entire length of the cochlea in the Atoh1-treated ears, most areas contained four rows of stereocilia (i.e., one row of IHCs and three rows of OHCs) on the reticular lamina (Fig. 4D–F). The Deiters' cells were coupled to the synaptic poles of OHCs (Fig. 4E). The presence of both OHCs and Deiters' cells suggests that the architectural relationship between OHCs and Deiters' cells was maintained in the "recovered" organ of Corti.

To quantify bundle repair/regeneration after Atoh1 treatment, we counted the total number of bundles from three cochlear locations (each 1 mm in length) from three normal (i.e., without noise exposure) cochleae as reference. Cochleae from Atoh1-treated left ears, as well as from control (right) ears, at one month after inoculation were also examined. The three sites were approximately 14.5–15.5, 10.5–11.5, and 4.0–5.0 mm from the basal end of the basilar membrane. Although the characteristic

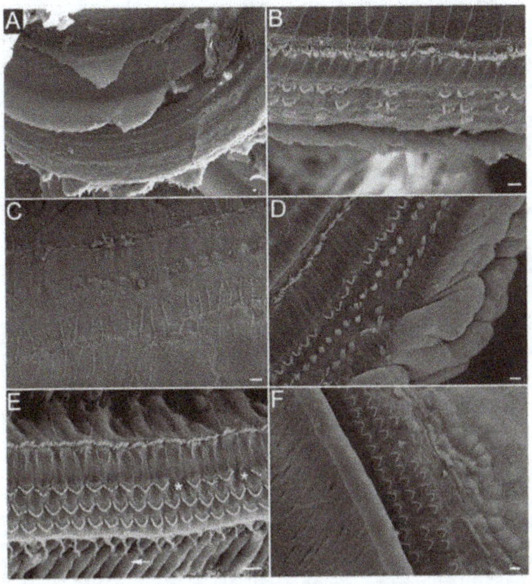

Figure 4. Representative SEM pictures obtained from different cochlear locations from Atoh1-treated and untreated (control) ears one month after viral inoculation. *A–C:* SEM images showing different extent and severity of damage from the control cochleae. *D–F:* SEM pictures of hair bundles from the Atoh1-treated ears. Missing hair bundles in panel *E* are marked by asterisks. The arrow indicates a Deiters' cell. Scale bars: 20 µm (*A*) and 10 µm (*B* to *F*).

frequencies of these locations were unknown due to the lack of a place-frequency map of the guinea pig cochlea [26], we estimated the characteristic frequency of these three locations based on recordings of inner hair cell (IHC) receptor potentials near these locations. Cheatham and colleague [27,28] have determined that locations 17 (in the fourth turn), 15 (in the third turn), and 10 (in the second turn) mm from the basal end of the cochlea correspond to the characteristic frequencies of 270, 1000, and 4000 Hz, respectively. Based on this information, we estimated that the three locations we chose encompassed the areas that had the characteristic frequencies of roughly 1000, 4000, and 15,000 Hz, respectively. Three cochleae for each group of normal, Atoh1-treated, and untreated ears were used for bundle count. Status of the bundles was determined by visual inspection of the bundles under the scanning electron microscope. Hair bundles that had obvious signs of damage such as truncation (Fig. 5A), fusion (Fig. 5B), or folding were excluded in the bundle count. Although tip-links are known to be vulnerable to noise damage [29,30], tip-link integrity was not considered in the bundle count.

Figure 5 (D and E) exhibits the means and standard deviations of the total numbers of bundles of IHCs and OHCs at three cochlear locations. As shown, noise exposure caused a significant reduction in the number of the hair bundles of both inner and outer hair cells in the untreated (right) ears ($p<0.01$ for both IHCs and OHCs at all three locations, student's t-test). After Atoh1 treatment, the numbers of bundles of both IHCs and OHCs were significantly greater than those of the untreated cochleae ($p<0.01$ for all cases). However, these numbers were still significantly less than in the normal cochlea, suggesting that a large number of damaged/lost bundles were not repaired. Transfection efficacy and hair cell death likely occurred before Atoh1 treatment were responsible for the disparity seen between the normal and Atoh1-treated ears.

We measured hearing thresholds from both (Atoh1-treated and contralateral) ears from eight animals using click-evoked ABRs at two weeks, three weeks, and one and two months after viral inoculation. As an additional control, hearing thresholds were also measured from noise-deafened animals with inoculation of the EGFP vector alone in the right ear. The results are presented in Figure 6A. Atoh1-treated ears showed an approximately 35–40 dB (SPL) threshold improvement (comparing to the contralateral ears) 30 days after Atoh1 treatment. We measured tone pip-evoked ABR thresholds at 4, 8, 16, and 20 kHz at one month after viral inoculation. Significant threshold improvement was seen at all freqeuncies tested (Fig. 6B). In contrast, thresholds in the contralateral ears without Atoh1 treatment were only improved by about 10–15 dB. Although thresholds of the contralateral ears also recoverd somewhat (Fig. 6A,B), this improvement was likely due to neural input from the cross (nerve) fibers originating from the Atoh1-treated ears [20] since the improvement disappeared when the middle ear strcutures in Atoh1-treated ears were intentionally damaged (in two ears, data not shown). ABR thresholds measured from noise-deafened ears with inoculation of the EGFP vector alone did not show any improvement one month after inoculation (Fig. 6B). To determine whether Atoh1 treatment was still effective after hair cell death, we introduced the *Atoh1* gene into the cochleae one month after noise exposure. None of the four animals showed any improvement in ABR thresholds examined at one month after the "delayed" treatment (Fig. 7). SEM showed that the hair cells were completely lost and the reticular lamina was flat with no signs of any normal-looking stereocilia bundles (Fig. 7). The absence of sensory epithelia and lack of improvement in hearing threshold after the delayed

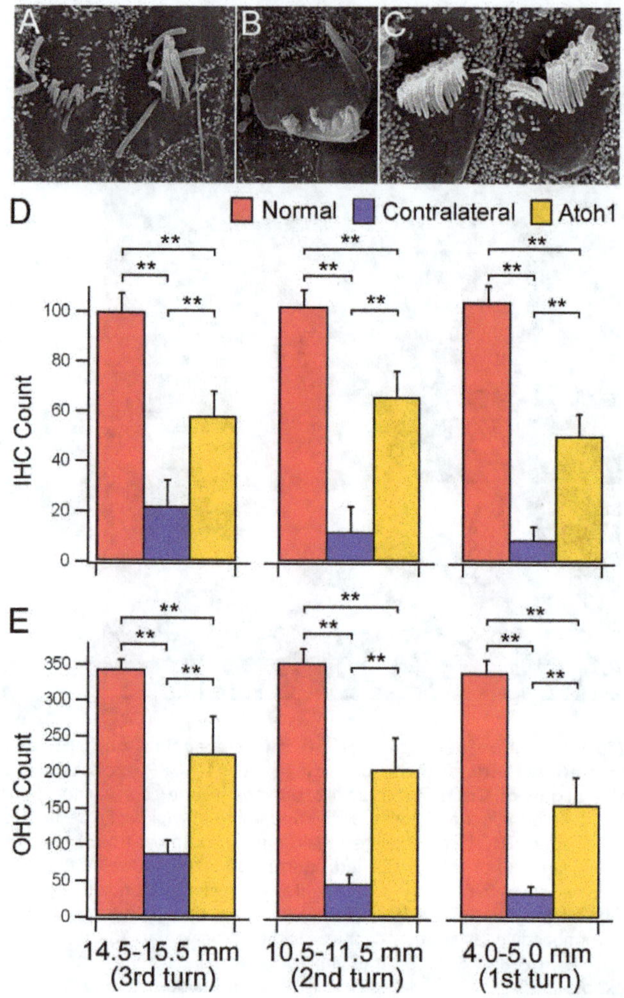

Figure 5. Stereocilia bundle counts in the normal (without noise exposure), Atoh1-treated and untreated cochleae. *A–B*: Examples of damaged bundles. *C*: Examples of normal-looking bundles. Scale bar represent 5 μm for all images in panels from *A* to *C*. *D, E*: Counts of IHC and OHC bundles in three different cochlear locations, each 1 mm in length. Three cochleae were used for each group (normal, Atoh1-treated, and untreated). Status of the bundles was determined by visual inspection of the bundles under scanning electron microscope. Hair bundles with no clear signs of trunction, fusion, or folding were included in the bundle count. Student's t-test was used for statistical analysis. Two asterisks represent statistical significance with a p-value less than 0.01.

treatment suggest that the Atoh1-based gene therapy was effective only when injured hair cells were still present in the organ of Corti.

Discussion

In this study, we show for the first time that introduction of the Atoh1 gene into a noise-damaged adult cochlea one week after noise exposure was able to substantially improve the hearing thresholds. Morphological examinations revealed that the numbers of stereocilia bundles of both IHCs and OHCs in the Atoh1-treated animals were significantly greater than those of the untreated cochleae. The re-emergence of stereocilia bundles after Atoh1 treatment suggests that Atoh1 is able to induce repair/regeneration of the damaged and/or lost stereocilia in the noise-deafened cochlea. We speculate that the new bundles originated

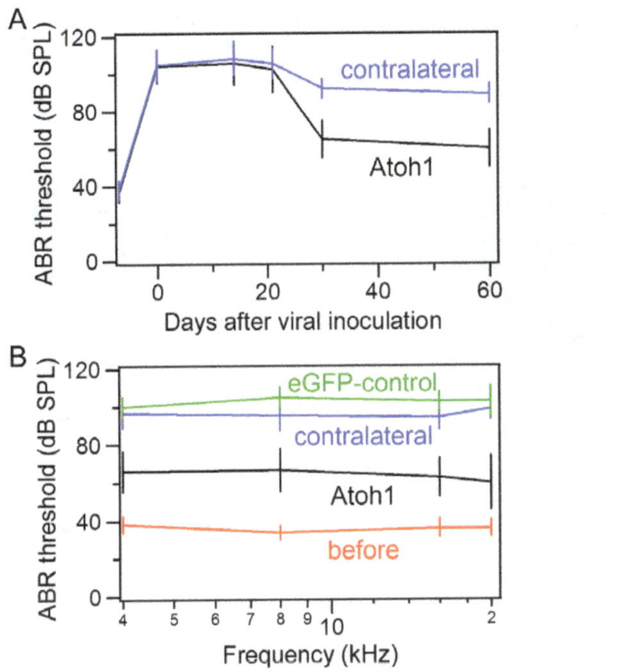

Figure 6. ABR thresholds measured from Atoh1-treated and control ears. *A:* ABR thresholds (means ± SD, n = 8) were measured at different days after the viral vector carrying the *Atoh1* gene was introduced. Contralateral ears were used as control. Click was used to evoke ABRs. *B:* ABR thresholds (means ± SD) of the Atoh1-treated ears (n = 8), contralateral ears (n = 8), and EGFP vector-treated ears (n = 6) at one month after cochlear inoculation. Tone pips with frequencies of 4, 8, 16, and 20 kHz were used to evoke ABRs.

from elongation of the truncated stereocilia, since the roots of truncated stereocilia were still present (Fig. 2G,H). It is also possible that regeneration originated from the microvilli. Gorelik et al. [31] show that microvilli may act as an elementary "building block" for the assembly of the specialized structures on the apical surface of cells. The mechanism(s) by which Atoh1 alone can promote repair/regeneration of the hair bundles with a functional mechanotransduction apparatus in both types of hair cells is unknown. It appears Atoh1 does not exert direct influence on hair cells, because forced Atoh1 expression was not detected in the hair cells (Fig. 3). However, supporting cells with forced Atoh1 expression may release diffusible factor(s) that may then influence adjacent hair cell repair.

It has been shown that the structure of the hair bundle is dynamically maintained by regulating the turnover of the actin filaments in a process described as treadmilling [32]. Recent evidence suggests that myosin-3a can facilitate hair bundle elongation by transporting espin-1 to the plus ends of actin filaments [33] and that the interaction of myosin-15a and whirlin is important for hair bundle morphogenesis and elongation [34–35]. Thus, it is possible that forced Atoh1 expression in the supporting cells may ultimately influence genes involved in hair bundle morphogenesis and elongation in the adjacent injured hair cells. Alternatively, the factor(s) released by supporting cells may stabilize the injured hair cells, allowing them to live long enough to repair themselves by upregulating genes involved in hair bundle elongation [33–35]. This notion that Atoh1 is important for maintaining hair cell viability in the adult cochlea is supported by a recent study [36]. We should point out that the molecular mechanism of how and why Atoh1 is critical for hair cell

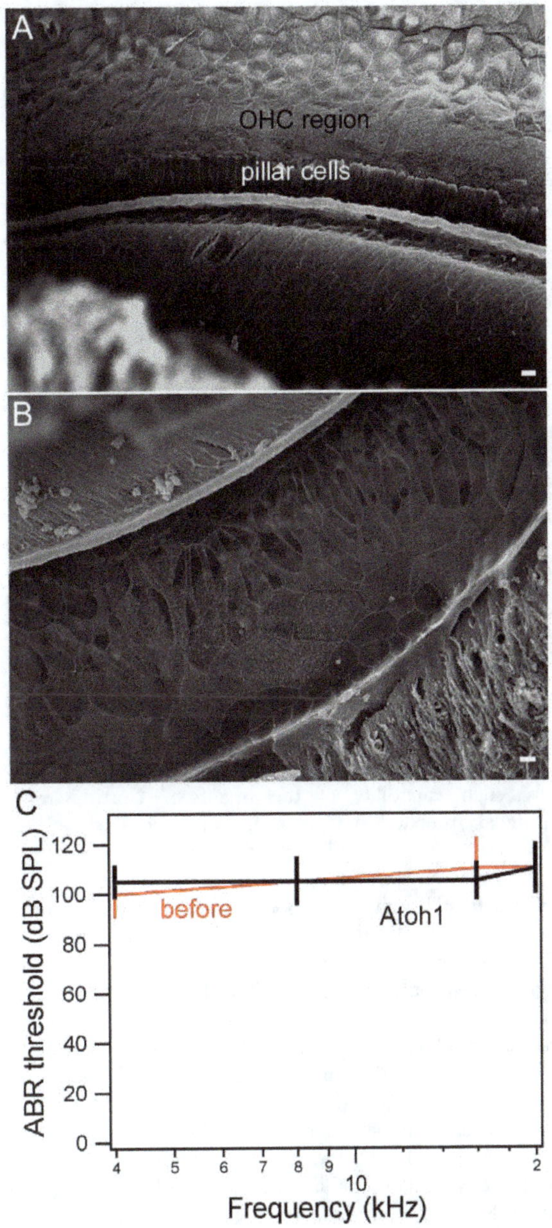

Figure 7. Representative SEM pictures and ABR thresholds obtained from cochleae treated with the Atoh1 gene one month after noise deafening. *A, B:* SEM images obtained from basal and middle turns. The reticular lamina was flat with no sign of stereocilia. Bars represent 10 µm. *C:* ABR thresholds (means ± SD, n = 4) measured from control and Atoh1-treated ears one month after the treatment.

differentiation is not clear, despite the fact that its critical role in hair cell morphogenesis was discovered some 13 years ago [15]. Regardless of whatever the mechanisms may be, our study reveals a role of Atoh1 that has not been revealed before. This new role in maintaining injured hair cells and subsequently promoting repair of damaged stereocilia in the adult mammalian cochlea has the potential to treat hearing loss after exposure to impulsive noise if gene therapy can be applied shortly after acoustic trauma.

It is important to distinguish between hair bundle repair/regeneration and transdifferentiation of supporting cells into hair cells after forced Atoh1 expression. Izumikawa et al. have shown that Atoh1 is able to induce hair cell regeneration in cochleae deafened by ototoxic drugs [20]. According to their study, the newly generated hair cells are likely formed by phenotypic conversion of supporting cells that remained in the deafened cochlea. However, there are no follow-up studies to determine how long the hair cells converted from supporting cells can live without supporting cells. Hair cells and supporting cells in the organ of Corti depend on each other; malfunction or apoptosis of one population can trigger degeneration of the other. Follow-up studies to determine whether a critical period during which the Atoh1-based treatment is effective are also lacking.

Our proposed mechanism for repair/regeneration is different from that of Izumikawa et al. [20]. In our model, we demonstrated that it was the regeneration/repair of the stereocilia rather than transdifferention of supporting cells. The strongest evidence to support this notion is based on the fact that both hair cells and supporting cells were present and that the architectural relationship between OHCs and Deiters' cells was maintained in the "recovered" cochleae after the treatment (Fig. 4E). If Deiters' cells had been converted to hair cells without mitosis, we would not have seen both supporting cells and hair cells in the Atoh1-treated cochlea. Furthermore, it has long been known that hair cells and supporting cells depend on each other for survival in the organ of Corti. Hair cell death can rapidly trigger signaling pathways that lead to supporting cell death [37,38]. Thus, it is inconceivable that either supporting cells or transdiffferentiated hair cells could survive alone in the adult mammalian cochlea. Besides, although supporting cells have the capability for phenotypic conversion to hair cells, such capability of the organ of Corti is only demonstrated in prenatal and neonatal preparations where hair cells and supporting cells are still under development [18,21,22]. It is not clear whether supporting cells in the adult mammalian organ of Corti still retain the potential to transdifferentiate, although interdental cells may be able to convert to ectopic hair cells after *Atoh1* gene transfer [19]. Finally, regeneration of stereocilia occurred only when Atoh1 inoculation was performed before hair cell death. Atoh1 treatment at one month after noise exposure could no longer rescue hair cells and restore hearing.

We should point out that there are substantial differences in how the *Atoh1* gene was introduced into the cochlea and how the animals were deafened between our experiments and those of Izumikawa et al. [20]. In our study, Atoh1 was inoculated through the round window and entered into the perilymph, which bathed both hair cells and Deiters' cells. In contrast, Izumikawa et al. inoculated the gene into the endolymph via the scala media. In our study the animals were deafened by impulsive noise, while Izumikawa et al. used ototoxic drugs to destroy hair cells. These differences may explain different underlying mechanisms for the two studies. However, it is known that individual susceptibility to ototoxic drugs varies significantly among animals (i.e., lethal dosage for one animal may be only sublethal to another) and that sublethal dosage of ototoxic drugs often only destroys stereocilia [5,6]. Thus, we entertain the possibility that the hearing recovery observed by Izumikawa et al. could also be the result of hair bundle repair/regeneration after Atoh1 treatment.

We are fully aware that there are other mechanical and metabolic injuries (besides stereocilia damage) to hair cells, supporting cells, ganglion neurons, the stria vascularis, and Reissner's membrane after noise trauma [39–48]. The severity and extent of damage depends on the type (continuous vs. impulsive), level, duration, and interval of the noise [40–48]. In this study, possible damage to structures other than the stereocilia was not examined since our focus was the damage and repair in the hair bundles. However, we were aware that damage to other structures may cause subsequent hair cell death and hearing loss. We also note that the total number of bundles of inner and outer hair cells in the Atoh1-treated ears was significantly less than that of the intact cochlea (Fig. 5D and E). The reduction in the number of functional stereocilia bundles, together with possible damage to the Reissner's membrane and stria vascularis, may explain why the hearing threshold was not fully recovered with Atoh1 treatment. We measured ABR thresholds at 4, 8, 16, and 20 kHz, representing the locations that are most vulnerable to impulsive noise in the animal models [41,46–48]. Impulsive noise has a relatively wide spectrum and does more damage in the higher frequency region than in the lower frequency region [41,46–48]. The frequencies we have measured represent a large area in the basilar membrane, sufficient to demonstrate the damage and the subsequent recovery, and to rule out any site-specific variability.

Some evidence suggests hair cell apoptosis resulting from continuous and/or low-level noise is likely caused by metabolic dysfunction [49], while damage to the basilar membrane (and the organ of Corti) and Reissner's membrane by impulsive noise usually originates directly from mechanical trauma [41,46–48]. Thus, Atoh1-based gene therapy may not be suitable for the treatment of all types of noise-induced hearing loss. However, if Atoh1 treatment can stabilize injured hair cells and directly or indirectly promote repair, such treatment may be effective for treating both noise- and drug-induced hearing loss. In the context of acoustic trauma, this could be especially important for the prevention/treatment of hearing impairment in the allied troops serving in Afghanistan, where the duration of their combat missions could be arranged based on a seven- to 10-day treatment window after exposure to impulsive weapon noise.

Author Contributions

Conceived and designed the experiments: DH SMY. Performed the experiments: SMY WC WWG SPJ JHS HZL WYY DH. Analyzed the data: WC WWG SPJ JHS HZL WYY DH. Wrote the paper: DH.

References

1. Liberman MC, Dodds LW (1984) Single-neuron labeling and chronic cochlear pathology. III. Stereocilia damage and alterations of threshold tuning curves. Hear Res 16: 55–74.
2. Hudspeth AJ, Corey DP (1977) Sensitivity, polarity, and conductance change in the response of vertebrate hair cells to controlled mechanical stimuli. Proc Natl Acad Sci USA 74: 2407–2411.
3. Fettiplace R, Hackney CM (2006) The sensory and motor roles of auditory hair cells. Nat Rev Neurosci 7: 19–29.
4. Baird RA, Burton MD, Fashena DS, Naeger RA (2000) Hair cell recovery in mitotically blocked cultures of the bullfrog saccule. Proc Natl Acad Sci USA 97: 11722–11729.
5. Gale JE, Meyers JR, Periasamy A, Corwin JT (2002) Survival of bundleless hair cells and subsequent bundle replacement in the bullfrog's saccule. J Neurobiol 50: 81–92.
6. Zheng JL, Keller G, Gao WQ (1999) Immunocytochemical and morphological evidence for intracellular self-repair as an important contributor to mammalian hair cell recovery. J Neurosci 19: 2161–2170.
7. Jia SP, Yang S, Guo W, He DZ (2009) Fate of mammalian cochlear hair cells and stereocilia after loss of the stereocilia. J Neurosci 29: 15277–15285.
8. Jarman AP, Grau Y, Jan LY, Jan YN (1993) Atonal is a proneural gene that directs chordotonal organ formation in the Drosophila peripheral nervous system. Cell 73: 1307–1321.
9. Akazawa C, Ishibashi M, Shimizu C, Nakanishi S, Kageyama R (1995) A mammalian helix-loop-helix factor structurally related to the product of Drosophila proneural gene atonal is a positive transcriptional regulator expressed in the developing nervous system. J Biol Chem 270: 8730–8738.
10. Ben-Arie N, Bellen HJ, Armstrong DL, McCall AE, Gordadze PR, et al. (1997) Math1 is essential for genesis of cerebellar granule neurons. Nature 390: 169–172.

11. Helms AW, Johnson JE (1998) Progenitors of dorsal commissural interneurons are defined by math1 expression. Development 125: 919–928.
12. Bermingham NA, Hassan BA, Wang VY, Fernandez M, Banfi S, et al. (2001) Proprioceptor pathway development is dependent on Math1. Neuron 30: 411–422.
13. Yang Q, Bermingham NA, Finegold MJ, Zoghbi HY (2001) Requirement of Math1 for secretory cell lineage commitment in the mouse intestine. Science 294: 2155–2158.
14. Van Keymeulen A, Mascre G, Youseff KK, Harel I, Michaux C, et al. (2009) Epidermal progenitors give rise to Merkel cells during embryonic development and adult homeostasis. J Cell Biol 187: 91–100.
15. Bermingham NA, Hassan BA, Price SD, Vollrath MA, Ben-Arie N, et al. (1999) Math1: an essential gene for the generation of inner ear hair cells. Science 284: 1837–1841.
16. Chen P, Johnson JE, Zoghbi HY, Segil N (2002) The role of Math1 in inner ear development: Uncoupling the establishment of the sensory primordium from hair cell fate determination. Development 129: 2495–2505.
17. Woods C, Montcouquiol M, Kelley MW (2004) Math1 regulates development of the sensory epithelium in the mammalian cochlea. Nat Neurosci 7: 1310–1318.
18. Zheng JL, Gao WQ (2000) Overexpression of Math1 induces robust production of extra hair cells in postnatal rat inner ears. Nat Neurosci 3: 580–586.
19. Kawamoto K, Ishimoto S, Minoda R, Brough DE, Raphael Y (2003) Math1 gene transfer generates new cochlear hair cells in mature guinea pigs *in vivo*. J Neurosci 23: 4395–4400.
20. Izumikawa M, Minoda R, Kawamoto K, Abrashkin KA, Swiderski DL, et al. (2005) Auditory hair cell replacement and hearing improvement by Atoh1 gene therapy in deaf mammals. Nat Med 11: 271–276.
21. Gubbels SP, Woessner DW, Mitchell JC, Ricci AJ, Brigande JV (2008) Functional auditory hair cells produced in the mammalian cochlea by *in utero* gene transfer. Nature 455: 537–541.
22. Kelly MC, Chang Q, Pan A, Lin X, Chen P (2012) Atoh1 directs the formation of sensory mosaics and induces cell proliferation in the postnatal mammalian cochlea *in vivo*. J Neurosci 32:6699–6710.
23. Liberman MC, Gao J, He DZ, Wu X, Jia S, et al. (2002) Prestin is required for electromotility of the outer hair cell and for the cochlear amplifier. Nature 419: 300–304.
24. Dallos P (1992) The active cochlea. J Neurosci 12: 4575–4585.
25. Zheng J, Shen W, He DZ, Long KB, Madison LD, et al. (2000) Prestin is the motor protein of cochlear outer hair cells. Nature 405: 149–155.
26. Belyantseva IA, Adler HJ, Curi R, Frolenkov GI, Kachar B (2000) Expression and localization of prestin and the sugar transporter GLUT-5 during development of electromotility in cochlear outer hair cells. J Neurosci 20: RC116 (1–5).
27. Greenwood DD (1990) A cochlear frequency-position function for several species–29 years later. J Acoust Soc Am 87: 2592–2605.
28. Cheatham MA, Dallos P (1993) Longitudinal comparisons of IHC ac and dc receptor potentials recorded from the guinea pig cochlea. Hearing Res 68: 107–114.
29. Cheatham MA (1993) Cochlear function reflected in mammalian hair cell responses. Prog Br Res 97: 13–19.
30. Pickles JO, Osborne MP, Comis SD (1987) Vulnerability of tip links between stereocilia to acoustic trauma in the guinea pig. Hear Res 25: 173–183.
31. Gorelik J, Shevchuk AI, Frolenkov GI, Diakonov IA, Lab MJ, et al. (2003) Dynamic assembly of surface structures in living cells. Proc Natl Acad Sci USA 100: 5819–5822.
32. Schneider ME, Belyantseva IA, Azevedo RB, Kachar B (2002) Rapid renewal of auditory hair bundles. Nature 418: 837–838.
33. Salles FT, Merritt RC Jr, Manor U, Dougherty GW, Sousa AD, et al. (2009) Myosin IIIa boosts elongation of stereocilia by transporting espin 1 to the plus ends of actin filaments. Nat Cell Biol 11: 443–50.
34. Delprat B, Michel V, Goodyear R, Yamasaki Y, Michalski N, et al. (2005) Myosin XVa and whirlin, two deafness gene products required for hair bundle growth, are located at the stereocilia tips and interact directly. Hum Mol Genet 14: 401–410.
35. Belyantseva IA, Boger ET, Naz S, Frolenkov GI, Sellers JR, et al. (2005) Myosin-XVa is required for tip localization of whirlin and differential elongation of hair-cell stereocilia. Nat Cell Biol 7: 148–156.
36. Pan N, Jahan I, Kersigo J, Duncan JS, Kopecky B, et al. (2012) A novel Atoh1 "self-terminating" mouse model reveals the necessity of proper Atoh1 level and duration for hair cell differentiation and viability. PLoS One. 7(1): e30358.
37. Matsui JI, Gale JE, Warchol ME (2004) Critical signaling events during the aminoglycoside- induced death of sensory hair cells in vitro. J Neurobiol 61: 250–266.
38. Manuela M, Gale JE (2008) Damage-induced activation of ERK1/2 in cochlear supporting cells is a hair cell death-promoting signal that depends on extracellular ATP and calcium. J Neurosci 28: 4918–4928.
39. Wang Y, Hirose K, Liberman MC (2002) Dynamics of noise-induced cellular injury and repair in the mouse cochlea. J Assoc Res Otolaryngol 3: 248–268.
40. Hamernik RP, Patterson JH, Salvi RJ (1987) The effect of impulse intensity and the number of impulses on hearing and cochlear pathology in the chinchilla. J Acoust Soc Am 81: 1118–1129.
41. Liang ZA (1992) Parametric relation between impulse noise and auditory damage. In: Dancer A, Salvi RJ, Henderson D, editors. Noise-Induced Hearing Loss. St Louis: Mosby Year Book. pp 325–335.
42. Harding GW, Bohne BA (2004) Noise-induced hair-cell loss and total exposure energy: analysis of a large data set. J Acoust Soc Am 115: 2207–2220.
43. Hu BH, Henderson D, Nicotera TM (2006) Extremely rapid induction of outer hair cell apoptosis in the chinchilla cochlea following exposure to impulse noise. Hear Res 211: 16–25.
44. Price GR (2007) Predicting mechanical damage to the organ of Corti. Hear Res 226: 5–13.
45. Kujawa SG, Liberman MC (2009) Adding insult to injury: cochlear nerve degeneration after "temporary" noise-induced hearing loss. J Neurosci 29: 14077–14085.
46. Hamernik RP, Turrentine G, Roberto M, Salvi R, Henderson D (1984) Anatomical correlates of impulse noise-induced mechanical damage in the cochlea. Hear Res 13: 229–247.
47. Hamernik RP, Ahroon WA, Patterson JH (1988) Threshold recovery functions following impulse noise trauma. J Acoust Soc Am 84: 941–950.
48. Henderson D, Hamernik RP (1986) Impulse noise: a critical review. J Acoust Soc Am 80: 569–584.
49. Hu BH, Henderson D, Yang WP (2008) The impact of mitochondrial energetic dysfunction on apoptosis in outer hair cells of the cochlea following exposure to intense noise. Hear Res 236: 11–21.

Sickness Absence due to Otoaudiological Diagnoses and Risk of Disability Pension

Emilie Friberg[1]*, Catarina Jansson[1], Ellenor Mittendorfer-Rutz[1], Ulf Rosenhall[2,3], Kristina Alexanderson[1]

1 Division of Insurance Medicine, Department of Clinical Neuroscience, Karolinska Institutet, Stockholm, Sweden, 2 Department of Clinical Neuroscience, Center for Hearing and Communication Research, Karolinska Institutet, Stockholm, Sweden, 3 Department of Audiology, Karolinska University Hospital, Stockholm, Sweden

Abstract

Background: Hearing difficulties are a large public health problem. Knowledge is scarce regarding risk of disability pension among people who have been sickness absent due to these difficulties.

Methods: A cohort including all 4,687,756 individuals living in Sweden in 2005, aged 20–64, and not on disability or old-age pension, was followed through 2009. Incidence rate ratios (RR) of disability pension with 95% confidence intervals (CI) were estimated using Cox proportional hazard models.

Results: In multivariable models, individuals who had a sick-leave spell due to otoaudiological diagnoses in 2005 had a 1.52-fold (95% CI: 1.43–1.62) increased risk of being granted a disability pension compared to individuals on sick leave due to other diagnoses. Hearing and tinnitus sick-leave diagnoses were associated with risk of disability pension: RR 3.38, 95% CI: 3.04–3.75, and 3.30, 95% CI: 2.95–3.68, respectively. No association was observed between sick leave due to vertigo diagnoses and disability pension whereas otological diagnoses and no sick leave were inversely associated with risk of disability pension compared to non-otoaudiological sick-leave diagnoses. Sick leave due to otoaudiological diagnoses was positively associated with risk of disability pension due to otoaudiological diagnoses and sick leave due to a tinnitus diagnosis was also associated with risk of disability pension due to mental diagnoses. The risk of disability pension among individuals with hearing or tinnitus sick-leave diagnoses was highest in the age group 35–44. Moreover, men had a slightly higher risk.

Conclusion: This large cohort study suggests an increased risk of disability pension among those with sickness absence due to otoaudiological diagnoses, particularly hearing and tinnitus diagnoses, compared to those with sickness absence due to non-otoaudiological diagnoses.

Editor: Roberta W. Scherer, Johns Hopkins Bloomberg School of Public Health, United States of America

Funding: This study was financed by the Swedish Council for Working Life and Social Research Center on Hearing Disabilities in Working Life and Society, by the Swedish Council for Working Life and Social Research, and by the Swedish Research Council. The funders had no role in study design, data collection and analysis, decision to publish, or preparation of the manuscript.

Competing Interests: The authors have declared that no competing interests exist.

* E-mail: Emilie.Friberg@ki.se

Introduction

Hearing difficulties are a public health concern [1] with increasing prevalence according to several studies [1,2,3,4,5]. Other otoaudiological diagnoses, such as vertigo and balance problems, are also important health problems that might cause long-term disability and exclusion from the labor market. In Sweden, approximately half of the persons with hearing difficulties are of working ages [6]. Gender differences have been suggested, i.e. hearing difficulties are more common among men but the prevalence of hearing difficulties is increasing to a larger extent among women [6]. It has been suggested that people with hearing difficulties are overrepresented among those on long-term sick leave [7].

Evidence regarding consequences of being on sick-leave due to different otoaudiological diagnoses is scarce [8]. To our knowledge, there are only two previous studies regarding sickness absence due to hearing difficulties in relation to disability pension [9,10]. One study examined only vertigo [9] and in the other we found that those who in 1985 had at least one new sick-leave spell due to an otoaudiological diagnosis (mainly vertigo diagnoses) had a higher risk of disability pension compared to individuals on sick leave due to all other diagnoses [10]. In the present, more recent and much larger, nationwide, prospective cohort study we further examine this finding, for the first time adjusting for a large variety of sociodemographic and health variables. The larger number of individuals admits a more specific diagnosis categorization, and, in addition, further possibilities for stratifications. Furthermore, this is the first study examining the association between sick leave due to otoaudiological diagnoses and risk of diagnosis-specific disability pension.

Thus, the objective was to assess if being on sick-leave due to different otoaudiological diagnoses is associated with risk of all-cause disability pension as well as diagnosis-specific disability pension, compared to sickness absence with non-otoaudiological diagnoses, in a Swedish, nationwide, prospective cohort study. Further, the aim was to assess if the potential associations differ with age or sex.

Methods

All 4 687 756 individuals living in Sweden during 2005 and aged 20–64, and not on disability pension (560 912 individuals) or early old-age pension (29 011 individuals) were included in the cohort. For each individual we had the following annual data: From Statistics Sweden; information on sex, age, educational level, family situation, type of living area, country of birth, migration, and old-age pension. From the Swedish Social Insurance Agency: data on all sick-leave spells compensated in 2005, and disability pension granted in 2006–2009, information includes diagnosis, and old-age pension. Information from the National Patient Register on number of days hospitalized during 2000–2005 and from the national Causes of Death Register on date of death. The unique Personal Identity Number, assigned to all residents in Sweden, was used to link data from the different registers. In Sweden, a sickness certificate issued by a physician is required to obtain sickness benefits after the 7th day of a sick-leave spell. All individuals in Sweden receiving an income from work or from unemployment benefits are covered by the same public sickness insurance. For most employed people, the sickness benefits are compensated by the employer for the first 14 sick-leave days and from the Social Insurance Agency from the 15th day. Disability pension may be granted to those with a medical work incapacity that is predicted to be long term. The old-age retirement age is generally 65 years but may be taken in younger ages. Sickness benefits cover about 80% of lost income and disability and old-age pension at least 65%.

The sick-leave diagnoses were classified according to the International Statistical Classification of Diseases and Related Health Problems, version 10 (ICD-10) [11] (table S1). The exposure was categorized as either: 1) having at least one prevalent (i.e. on-going or new) sick-leave spell during 2005 due to otoaudiological diagnoses (ICD-10 chapter VIII, H60–H95); 2) having at least one prevalent sick-leave spell during 2005 due to non-otoaudiological diagnoses (or no registered diagnosis), reference category), or 3) having no sick-leave day compensated by the Social Insurance Agency during 2005. All individuals with an otoaudiological sick-leave spell were included in the first category, even if they also had non-otoaudiological sick-leave spells during 2005.

Moreover, for detailed analyses, the otoaudiological diagnoses were further categorized as (replacing the category otoaudiological diagnoses in the model): mainly "otological" (H60–H75, H80, H92, H94, H95), "hearing" (H83, H90, H91), "vertigo" (H81, H82), or "tinnitus" (H93). Twenty-seven individuals had more than one sick-leave spell due to two different otoaudiological diagnoses and were thus included in both categories.

The outcome, i.e. disability pension, was defined as incident disability pension, i.e. a disability pension granted during 2006–2009. We studied all-cause disability pension and disability pension due to the following diagnoses: otoaudiological (ICD-10; H60–H95), circulatory (ICD-10;I00-I99), cancer (ICD-10; C00-D48), and mental (ICD-10; F00-F95) diagnoses.

Statistical analysis

We calculated person-time of follow-up for each individual from January 1, 2006 to the date of disability pension, death, migration, 65 years of age, or December 31, 2009, whichever came first. Incidence rate ratios (RRs) for all cause and diagnosis-specific disability pension and 95% confidence intervals (CIs) were estimated by Cox proportional hazards models, using person-time of follow-up as the underlying time scale. The data conformed to the proportional hazards assumption.

We performed crude, age-adjusted, and multivariable analyses. In the main analysis, we adjusted for age, sex, family situation, type of living area, country of birth, educational level, and number of days hospitalized (inpatient) in 2000–2005. Furthermore, the risk of diagnosis-specific disability pension associated with sick leave due to different otoaudiological diagnoses was assessed. Moreover, analyses stratified by age and sex was performed for all-cause disability pension since both age and sex have been reported to influence the risk of both sick-leave and disability pension [12]. All individuals with missing information on any of the variables included in the models were excluded from the analyses.

All statistical analyses were performed using SAS software (version 9.2; SAS Institute, Cary, NC).

The study was approved by the Regional Ethical Committee in Stockholm, Sweden.

Results

The 4 687 756 individuals together contributed 17 918 476 person-years during the mean follow-up of 3.8 years (2006–2009). In total, 123 473 individuals were granted disability pension of which 1709 individuals were granted disability pension due to otoaudiological diagnoses. The mean age when granted disability pension (due to all diagnoses) was 50 (±11) and due to an otoaudiological diagnosis 55 (±8). In table 1, baseline characteristics of the cohort, in total and by the different categories of sick-leave diagnoses, are presented. Individuals with at least one sick-leave spell during 2005 due to an otoaudiological diagnosis were on average older, more often married/cohabiting, born in another country than Sweden, less often living in a large city or hospitalized compared to individuals with a sick-leave spell with non-otoaudiological diagnoses in 2005. Individuals with a hearing or tinnitus sick-leave diagnosis had on average a higher educational level compared to both other sickness absentees and to those with no sickness absence benefits in 2005. Among those with sickness absence in 2005, the proportion absent due to otoaudiological diagnoses increased with age (figure 1).

Overall, we observed that individuals with sick-leave due to any otoaudiological diagnosis had an increased risk of being granted a disability pension (RR 1.52, 95% CI 1.43–1.62) compared to individuals with sick-leave due to non-otoaudiological diagnoses (table 2). Especially sickness absence due to hearing and tinnitus diagnoses were associated with high risk increases of disability pension; RR 3.38 (95% CI 3.04–3.75) and 3.30 (95% CI 2.95–3.68), respectively. Sick leave due to vertigo diagnoses was associated with modest risk increases in the crude models, but not in the multivariable adjusted models and sickness absence due to otological diagnoses was inversely associated with risk of disability pension compared to sickness absence due to non-otoaudiological diagnoses. Inverse associations were observed between no sick-leave days and risk of disability pension compared to those with non-otoaudiological sick leave.

In the analyses of diagnosis-specific disability pension (table 3), we observed strongly increased risks of incident disability pension due to otoaudiological diagnoses among those sickness absent due to these diagnoses. Although the inverse association between no sick leave benefits and risk of disability pension due to otoaudiological diagnoses compared to sickness absence due to

Table 1. Baseline characteristics for all individuals (n = 4 687 756) included in the cohort in 2005.

Characteristic	All	No sick leave in 2005[a]	Sick-leave due to non-otoaudiological diagnoses[a]	Sick-leave due to otoaudiological diagnoses[ab]				
				All	Otological[c]	Hearing[d]	Vertigo[e]	Tinnitus[f]
N	4 687 756	4 078 640	604 951	4 165	1 283	770	1 372	767
(%)	(100)	(87.01)	(12.90)	(0.009)	(0.0002)	(0.0002)	(0.0003)	(0.0002)
Women (%)	48	46	61	58	59	63	61	47
Mean age (years)	41	41	44	48	45	52	48	50
Education >12years (%)	36	37	27	32	26	42	31	41
Living in larger cities (%)	38	38	35	35	38	29	36	31
Not born in Sweden (%)	14	14	15	14	18	12	13	10
Married or cohabiting (%)	56	56	58	57	61	56	64	58
Days hospitalized in 2000–2005	1.85	1.30	5.61	3.41	3.94	3.41	3.66	1.95

[a]Values other than for age and sex have been directly standardized according to the age distribution of the cohort.
[b]Twenty-seven individuals had more than one spell of sick leave and two different otoaudiological diagnoses and thus are included in two categories.
[c]ICD10: H60–H75, H80, H92, H94, H95.
[d]ICD10: H83, H90, H91.
[e]ICD10: H81, H82.
[f]ICD10: H93.

non-otoaudiological diagnoses were strong, it was weaker than in the analyses of disability pension due to other outcomes. A sick-leave diagnosis of tinnitus was associated with an increased risk of disability pension due to mental diagnoses (RR 1.69, 95% CI 1.27–2.25), while the other otoaudiological diagnoses categories were not. Very few individuals with a sick-leave spell due to otoaudiological diagnoses were granted a disability pension due to circulatory (20 individuals) or cancer (10 individuals) diagnoses. A sick-leave spell due to otoaudiological diagnoses was associated with decreased risks of disability pension due to circulatory (RR 0.42, 95% CI 0.27–0.65) and cancer (RR 0.43, 95% CI 0.23–0.79) diagnoses.

Finally, in the analyses of all disability pension stratified by age and sex, respectively, we observed relatively small differences (table 4). The risk of being granted a disability pension among individuals with a hearing or tinnitus diagnosis was highest in the age-group 35–44. Men who were sickness absent due to otoaudiological diagnoses had a slightly higher risk of disability pension than women sickness absent with these diagnoses.

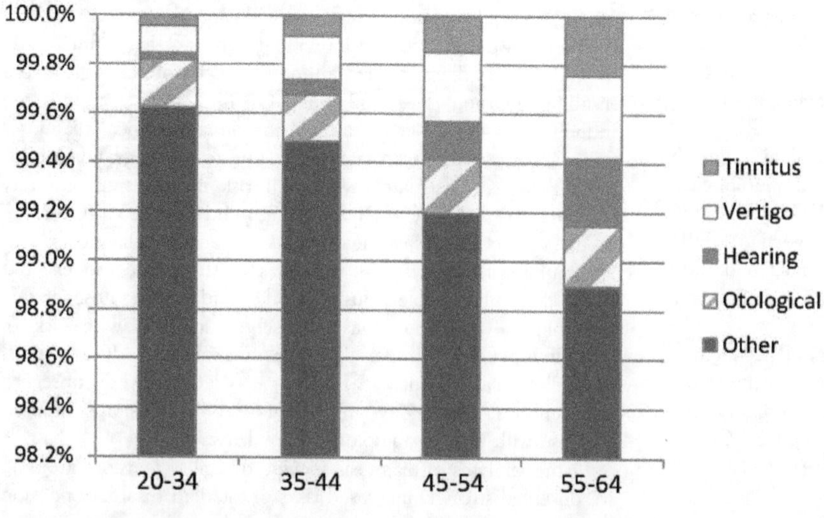

Figure 1. Distribution (%) of individuals sickness absent due to different sick-leave diagnoses in four different age groups. Otological: (ICD10) H60–H75, H80, H92, H94, H95. Hearing: (ICD10) H83, H90, H91. Vertigo: (ICD10) H81, H82. Tinnitus: (ICD10) H93. Other: all non-otoaudiological sick-leave diagnoses.

Table 2. Sickness absence due to otoaudiological diagnoses and incidence rate ratios (RRs) and 95% confidence intervals (CIs) for disability pension.

	Number of people granted disability pension	Person-years	Crude RR (95% CI)	Age-adjusted RR (95% CI)[a]	Multivariable RR (95% CI)[b]	Multivariable RR (95% CI)[c]
Non-otoaudiological sick-leave diagnoses	89 044	2 121 525	1.00 (ref)	1.00 (ref)	1.00 (ref)	1.00 (ref)
No sick leave	33 435	15 783 423	0.05 (0.05–0.05)	0.06 (0.06–0.06)	0.06 (0.06–0.06)	0.07 (0.07–0.07)
All otoaudiological sick-leave diagnoses	994	13 528	1.73 (1.62–1.84)	1.45 (1.36–1.54)	1.52 (1.43–1.62)	1.52 (1.43–1.62)
Otological[d]	90	4 799	0.44 (0.36–0.55)	0.41 (0.34–0.51)	0.42 (0.34–0.52)	0.40 (0.33–0.49)
Hearing[e]	352	1 979	3.93 (3.54–4.36)	2.90 (2.61–3.22)	3.20 (2.88–3.56)	3.38 (3.04–3.75)
Vertigo[f]	249	4 694	1.24 (1.09–1.40)	1.04 (0.92–1.18)	1.06 (0.93–1.20)	1.03 (0.91–1.16)
Tinnitus[g]	318	2 126	3.34 (2.99–3.73)	2.61 (2.34–2.91)	2.97 (2.65–3.31)	3.30 (2.95–3.68)

[a]Adjusted for age (20–34, 35–44, 45–54, 55–64).
[b]Further adjusted for sex (female, male); family situation (married/cohabiting, married/cohabiting with children, single, single with child, child living with parent); type of living area (larger cities, medium sized cities, smaller places); birth region (Sweden, Nordic countries, Europe, Other world), years of education (0–9, 10–12, 12<), excluding 292 403 observations due to missing data on education and/or family situation.
[c]Further adjusted hospitalization days (summarized days 2000–2005; 0, 1–4, >4), excluding 292 403 observations due to missing data on education and/or family.
[d]ICD10: H60–H75, H80, H92, H94, H95.
[e]ICD10: H83, H90, H91.
[f]ICD10: H81, H82.
[g]ICD10: H93.

Table 3. Sickness absence due to otoaudiological diagnosis and incidence rate ratios (RR) with 95% confidence intervals (CI) for diagnosis specific disability pension in 2006–2009 among individuals living in Sweden.

	Number of people granted diagnosis-specific disability pensions	Crude RR (95% CI)	Multivariable RR (95% CI)[a]
Disability pension due to otoaudiological diagnoses	(1709)		
All non-otoaudiological sick-leave diagnoses	509	1.00 (ref)	1.00 (ref)
No sick leave	523	0.14 (0.12–0.16)	0.15 (0.13–0.17)
All otoaudiological sick-leave diagnoses	677	205.72 (183.37–230.79)	147.76 (131.45–166.10)
Otological[b]	35	12.01 (8.57–16.82)	11.08 (7.90–15.54)
Hearing[c]	288	168.29 (146.01–193.98)	107.56 (93.16–124.18)
Vertigo[d]	138	51.06 (42.66–61.10)	43.24 (36.14–51.73)
Tinnitus[e]	229	118.41 (101.47–138.19)	74.24 (63.57–86.69)
Disability pension due to mental diagnoses	(45 234)		
All non-otoaudiological sick-leave diagnoses	31 182	1.00 (ref)	1.00 (ref)
No sick leave	13 933	0.06 (0.06–0.06)	0.07 (0.07–0.07)
All otoaudiological sick-leave diagnoses	119	0.59 (0.49–0.71)	0.58 (0.48–0.69)
Otological[b]	14	0.20 (0.12–0.34)	0.19 (0.11–0.32)
Hearing[c]	24	0.78 (0.52–1.16)	0.78 (0.52–1.16)
Vertigo[d]	33	0.48 (0.34–0.67)	0.45 (0.32–0.64)
Tinnitus[e]	48	1.48 (1.12–1.97)	1.69 (1.27–2.25)

[a]Adjusted for age (20–34, 35–44, 45–54, 55–64); sex (female, male); family (married/cohabiting, married/cohabiting with children, alone, alone with child, child living with parent); type of living area (larger cities, medium sized cities, smaller places); birth region (Sweden, Nordic countries, Europe, Other world); years of education (0–9, 10–12, >12); hospitalization days (summarized days 2000–2005; 0, 1–4, >4), excluding 292 403 observations due to missing data on education and/or family.
[b]ICD10: H60–H75, H80, H92, H94, H95.
[c]ICD10: H83, H90, H91.
[d]ICD10: H81, H82.
[e]ICD10: H93.

Table 4. Multivariable incidence rate ratios[a] with 95% confidence intervals for disability pension in 2006–2009 among individuals with sickness absence due to otoaudiological diagnosis in 2005, stratified by age and sex.

	N	Non-otoaudiological sick-leave diagnoses	No sick leave	Otoaudiological sick-leave diagnoses				
				All	Otological[b]	Hearing[c]	Vertigo[d]	Tinnitus[e]
Age								
20–34	1 368 888	1.00 (ref)	0.07	1.52	0.31	1.17	0.71	2.21
			(0.07–0.08)	(1.43–1.62)	(0.14–0.69)	(0.38–3.62)	(0.34–1.49)	(0.99–4.93)
35–44	1 153 491	1.00 (ref)	0.05	1.17	0.37	3.70	0.75	3.48
			(0.05–0.06)	(0.97–1.42)	(0.22–0.62)	(2.66–5.15)	(0.51–1.11)	(2.50–4.85)
45–54	995 615	1.00 (ref)	0.06	1.46	0.41	3.19	1.15	3.19
			(0.06–0.06)	(1.30–1.64)	(0.28–0.60)	(2.61–3.89)	(0.93–1.41)	(2.58–3.95)
55–64	877 059	1.00 (ref)	0.07	1.70	0.42	3.34	1.04	3.17
			(0.07–0.07)	(1.57–1.85)	(0.31–0.56)	(2.92–3.83)	(0.87–1.24)	(2.75–3.66)
Sex								
Women	2 146 123	1.00 (ref)	0.06	1.48	0.45	3.23	1.01	3.17
			(0.06–0.07)	(1.36–1.60)	(0.35–0.58)	(3.84–4.67)	(0.86–1.18)	(2.70–3.71)
Men	2 248 930	1.00 (ref)	0.07	1.60	0.32	3.80	1.06	3.50
			(0.07–0.07)	(1.45–1.77)	(0.22–0.46)	(3.16–4.56)	(0.86–1.29)	(3.00–4.09)

[a]Adjusted for age (20–34, 35–44, 45–54, 55–64) or sex (female, male) when applicable, and family (married/cohabiting, married/cohabiting with children, alone, alone with child, child living with parent); type of living area (larger cities, medium sized cities, smaller places); birth region (Sweden, Nordic countries, Europe, Other world); years of education (0–9, 10–12, >12); hospitalization days (summarized days 2000–2005; 0, 1–4, >4).
[b]ICD10: H60–H75, H80, H92, H94, H95.
[c]ICD10: H83, H90, H91.
[d]ICD10: H81, H82.
[e]ICD10: H93.

Discussion

In this population-based cohort including all individuals living in Sweden, aged 20–64 years, and not on old-age or disability pension in 2005, we found that the risk of being granted a new disability pension was 52% higher among individuals having at least one sick-leave spell due to an otoaudiological diagnosis compared to individuals with sickness absence due to non-otoaudiological diagnoses. The risk increase was most pronounced among individuals with a hearing or tinnitus diagnosis, where more than threefold increased risks of being granted a disability pension compared to those with non-otoaudiological sick-leave diagnoses were observed. As expected, the risk of diagnosis-specific disability pension due to otoaudiological diagnoses was very strongly associated with sick-leave due to otoaudiological diagnoses. The associations did not differ substantially across different age groups or between men and women.

Only a few prior cohort studies have presented data on sick leave or disability pension in relation to hearing difficulties or diagnoses [9,10,13,14,15,16,17]. The majority of previous studies include small groups [9,13,14,16] or only focus on specific occupational groups [15,17]. Most previous studies [9,10,15,16] have indicated an increased risk of disability pension among individuals with a hearing difficulty. The results of this study confirms and extends previous results from a Swedish cohort study including 40 786 individuals living in a county in southern Sweden, where we found that individuals with sick leave due to an otoaudiological diagnosis had a 42% higher risk of disability pension compared to individuals with sick leave spells due to non-otoaudiological diagnoses [10].

One explanation for our findings is that hearing difficulties lead to increased levels of stress. Even a minor hearing difficulty might decrease an individual's possibilities to be involved in ordinary conversation, especially if there is several persons talking at the same time or if there is a lot of background noise, the need to constantly strain to hear might be stressful [6].

As in all studies on sick leave due to specific diagnoses the number of persons on sick leave with a specific diagnosis cannot directly be translated to all who have that disease. Most people with different diseases, including hearing difficulties, are not sickness absent due to them [18,19]. Most likely, a majority of people with hearing difficulties have different aids or adapted work conditions which means that they may be able to work regardless of their hearing difficulties or their hearing difficulties does not impair their work capacity. Moreover, for some individuals with multi-morbidity, hearing difficulties might not have been the main reason for their sick leave, but contributed to their work incapacity. This means that our results might be an underestimation of the associations observed between being on sick-leave due to otoaudiological diagnoses and risk of disability pension.

Major strengths of this study include its population-based nationwide design, comprising the whole Swedish population of working ages, not a sample, the prospective study design, and the complete follow-up (i.e. no drop out). Other strengths are the high quality of the population-based registers, that data were not self-reported [20,21], and our adjustments for a wide range of potential confounders such as age, sex, family situation, type of living area, birth region, years of education and, hospitalization days. The prospective design and the register-based information including the whole Swedish population limit the risk of selection bias. Another strength is that detailed information regarding sick-leave diagnoses was available. Such information is often not available in large population-based studies. The validity of sick-leave diagnoses is often discussed, however, seldom studied. A study of the validity of sick-leave diagnoses comparing them to medical charts report good validity [22].

A limitation is that for employed individuals, information about most sick-leave spells shorter than 15 days are not included. However, the majority of shorter sick-leave spells are due to different types of infections, migraine etc. [12]. If such sick-leave spells had been included, the associations would probably have been even stronger. Another limitation is that we excluded persons who already had received or were granted disability pension during 2005. This might have underestimated the risk of being granted a disability pension. The relatively short follow-up of four years has advantages and disadvantages, but a 52% risk increase of all cause disability pension among those on sick leave due to otoaudiological diagnoses warrants attention. The register-based data does not include lifestyle factors that might influence the risk of being granted a disability pension, thus the possibility of uncontrolled or residual confounding cannot be entirely eliminated. However, we have adjusted for multiple potential confounders, and we observed only very small differences in the risk estimates between the crude models and the adjusted models.

In absolute numbers, the number of individuals with sick-leave spells due to audiological diagnoses (i.e. hearing loss or tinnitus) might not be considered very large, but the risk of exclusion from the labor market and the adverse consequences must be recognized. In our study, many individuals aged 35–40 years with such sick-leave diagnoses were granted disability pension. This observation is consistent with the notion that many of the subjects could have early onset hearing loss that may progress into profound hearing loss, or profound hearing loss with adult onset [23]. The severe consequences of a disrupted ability to communicate due to late deafness are well known [24]. Awareness of the importance to introduce work adjustments or comprehensive rehabilitation measures is warranted.

In conclusion, this large nationwide population-based cohort study suggests an increased risk of disability pension among those sickness absent due to otoaudiological diagnoses compared to those sickness absent due to non-otoaudiological diagnoses. The risk increase was most pronounced among individuals with a hearing or a tinnitus sick-leave diagnosis. This finding emphasizes the importance of initiating preventive measures among people with sick leave due to otoaudiological diagnoses in order to prevent disability pension.

Supporting Information

Table S1 Categorization of otoaudiological diagnoses (Chapter VIII. Diseases of the ear and mastoid process) in accordance with the International Statistical Classification of Diseases and Related Health Problems 10th Revision (ICD-10).

Author Contributions

Conceived and designed the experiments: EF KA. Performed the experiments: EF. Analyzed the data: EF. Contributed reagents/materials/analysis tools: KA. Wrote the paper: EF. Critically revised the manuscript for important intellectual content: CJ EMR UR KA. Participated in the interpretation of the data: EF CJ EMR UR KA. Approved the final version of the paper: EF CJ EMR UR KA.

References

1. Mathers CD, Loncar D (2006) Projections of global mortality and burden of disease from 2002 to 2030. PLoS Med 3: 2011–2030.
2. Kochkin S (2005) MarkeTrak VII: Hearing loss population tops 31 million people. Hearing-impaired population continues to increase - along with satisfaction ratings for hearing instruments. Hearing Review 12: 16–29.
3. Wallhagen MI, Strawbridge W, Cohen RD, Kaplan GA (1997) An increasing prevalence of hearing impairment and associated risk factors over three decades of the Alameda County Study. Am J Public Health 87: 440–442.
4. Agrawal Y, Platz EA, Niparko J (2008) Prevalence of hearing loss and differences by demographic characteristics among US adults: data from the National Health and Nutrition Examination Survey, 1999–2004. Arch Intern Med 168: 1522–1530.
5. Sorri M, Roine R (2001) Age-adjusted prevalence of hearing impairment has significantly increased during the last two decades. Scand Audiol Suppl: 5–7.
6. Hörselskadades Riksförbund. Årsrapport. (The Swedish Association of Hard of Hearing People, yearly report). (In Swedish) Stockholm: Sweden.
7. Danermark B (2005) A review of the psychosocial effects of hearing impairment in the working-age population. In: Stephens D, Jones L, eds. The impact of genetic hearing impairment. London: Whurr. pp 106–136.
8. Alexanderson K, Norlund A (2004) Swedish Council on Technology Assessment in Health Care (SBU). Chapter 12. Future need for research. Scand J Public Health Suppl 63: 256–258.
9. Skoien AK, Wilhemsen K, Gjesdal S (2008) Occupational disability caused by dizziness and vertigo: a register-based prospective study. Br J Gen Pract 58: 619–623.
10. Gustafsson K, Backenroth-Ohsako G, Rosenhall U, Ternevall-Kjerulf E, Ulfendahl M, et al. (2011) Future risk for disability pension among people with sickness absence due to otoaudiological diagnoses; a population-based cohort study with a 12-year follow-up. Scand J Public Health Online March 7.
11. (1992) International Statistical Classification of Diseases and Related Health Problems, Tenth Revision (ICD-10). World Health Organization (WHO).
12. Alexanderson K, Norlund A (2004) Sickness absence - causes, consequences, and physicians sickness cerification practice. A systematic literature review by the Swedish Council on Technology Assessment in Health Care. Scand J Public Health 32(Suppl 63): 1–263.
13. Bjorne A, Agerberg G, Bjorne A, Agerberg G (2003) Reduction in sick leave and costs to society of patients with Meniere's disease after treatment of temporomandibular and cervical spine disorders: a controlled six-year cost-benefit study. Cranio 21: 136–143.
14. Andersson G (2000) Longitudinal follow-up of occupational status in tinnitus patients. Int Tinnitus J 6: 127–129.
15. Ide C (2007) Hearing loss, accidents, near misses and job losses in firefighters. Occup Med (Lond) 57: 203–209.
16. Rudin R, Svardsudd K (1987) Otitis media and well-being in a male population in Gothenburg. The study of men born in 1913. Acta Otolaryngol 104: 454–462.
17. Sewell RK, Song C, Bauman NM, Smith RJ, Blanck P (2004) Hearing loss in Union Army veterans from 1862 to 1920. Laryngoscope 114: 2147–2153.
18. Marmot M, Feeney A, Shipley M, North F, Syme SL (1995) Sickness absence as a measure of health status and functioning: from the UK Whitehall II study. J Epidemiol Community Health 49: 124–130.
19. Alexanderson K (1998) Women's health at work. In: Kilbom Å, Messing K, Thorbjörnsson B, eds. Measuring health, indicators for working women. Solna: National Institute for Working Life. pp 121–161.
20. Hensing G (2004) Swedish Council on Technology Assessment in Health Care (SBU). Chapter 4. Methodological aspects in sickness-absence research. Scand J Public Health Suppl 63: 44–48.
21. Svedberg P, Ropponen A, Lichtenstein P, Alexanderson K (2010) Are self-report of disability pension and long-term sickness absence accurate? Comparisons of self-reported interview data with national register data in a Swedish twin cohort. BMC Public Health 10: 763.
22. Ljungdahl LO, Bjurulf P (1991) The accordance of diagnoses in a computerized sick-leave register with doctor's certificates and medical records. Scand J Soc Med 19: 148–153.
23. Hallam R, Ashton P, Sherbourne K, Gailey L (2006) Acquired profound hearing loss: mental health and other characteristics of a large sample. Int J Audiol 45: 715–723.
24. Barlow JH, Turner AP, Hammond CL, Gailey L (2007) Living with late deafness: insight from between worlds. Int J Audiol 46: 442–448.

17

Dual Sensory Impairment in Older Adults Increases the Risk of Mortality

Bamini Gopinath[1], Julie Schneider[2], Catherine M. McMahon[3,4], George Burlutsky[1], Stephen R. Leeder[2], Paul Mitchell[1]*

1 Centre for Vision Research, Department of Ophthalmology and Westmead Millennium Institute, University of Sydney, New South Wales, Australia, **2** Menzies Centre for Health Policy, University of Sydney, Sydney, New South Wales, Australia, **3** HEARing Co-operative Research Centre, University of Melbourne, Melbourne, Victoria, Australia, **4** Centre for Language Sciences, Linguistics Department, Macquarie University, Sydney, New South Wales, Australia

Abstract

Although concurrent vision and hearing loss are common in older adults, population-based data on their relationship with mortality is limited. This cohort study investigated the association between objectively measured dual sensory impairment (DSI) with mortality risk over 10 years. 2812 Blue Mountains Eye Study participants aged 55 years and older at baseline were included for analyses. Visual impairment was defined as visual acuity less than 20/40 (better eye), and hearing impairment as average pure-tone air conduction threshold greater than 25 dB HL (500–4000 Hz, better ear). Ten-year all-cause mortality was confirmed using the Australian National Death Index. After ten years, 64% and 11% of participants with DSI and no sensory loss, respectively, had died. After multivariable adjustment, participants with DSI (presenting visual impairment and hearing impairment) compared to those with no sensory impairment at baseline, had 62% increased risk of all-cause mortality, hazard ratio, HR, 1.62 (95% confidence intervals, CI, 1.16–2.26). This association was more marked in those with both moderate-severe hearing loss (>40 dB HL) and presenting visual impairment, HR 1.84 (95% CI 1.19–2.86). Participants with either presenting visual impairment only or hearing impairment only, did not have an increased risk of mortality, HR 1.05 (95% CI 0.61–1.80) and HR 1.24 (95% CI 0.99–1.54), respectively. Concurrent best-corrected visual impairment and moderate-severe hearing loss was more strongly associated with mortality 10 years later, HR 2.19 (95% CI 1.20–4.03). Objectively measured DSI was an independent predictor of total mortality in older adults. DSI was associated with a risk of death greater than that of either vision loss only or hearing loss alone.

Editor: Linda Chao, University of California, San Francisco, United States of America

Funding: The Blue Mountains Eye and Hearing Study were supported by the Australian National Health and Medical Research Council (Grant Nos. 974159, 991407, 211069, 262120). The authors also acknowledge the financial support of the National Health and Medical Research Council (NHMRC) Partnerships for Better Health (grant no. 571449) and the HEARing CRC, established and supported under the Australian Government's Cooperative Research Centres Program. Bamini Gopinath is supported by an NHMRC Centre for Clinical Research Excellence (grant no 529923). The funders had no role in study design, data collection and analysis, decision to publish, or preparation of the manuscript.

Competing Interests: The authors have declared that no competing interests exist.

* E-mail: paul_mitchell@wmi.usyd.edu.au

Introduction

Impaired vision and hearing are common among older adults [1,2] and can occur separately or in combination [3]. Visual loss impacts negatively on functional independence, mental health and cognition, and reduces quality of life, as well as increasing the need for support services [4–7]. Age-related hearing loss is more frequent and is associated with an increased risk of depression, and impairs quality of life and the ability to conduct activities of daily living, as well as leading to an increased reliance on community and informal supports [2,8–13].

There are also prospective data to suggest that vision loss was associated with a greater mortality risk in older adults [14–16]. In a US study of 2520 adults aged between 65–84 years old, worse baseline acuity was associated with a 5% higher mortality rate. Recently, Karpa et al. [14] showed in the Blue Mountains Eye Study (BMES) of adults aged 49 years and over that the presence of presenting visual impairment increased the risk of all-cause mortality by 29%, after adjusting for potential confounders. Age-related hearing loss has also been shown to be associated with a greater risk of all-cause mortality in older adults [17]. In the Blue Mountains Hearing Study of adults aged 55 years and over, indirect path analyses showed that any level of hearing loss (>25 dB HL) was associated with increased all-cause mortality via three mediating variables: disability in walking, cognitive impairment and self-rated health [17].

There is a lack of population-based studies that have examined the association between the presence of objectively measured hearing and vision impairment, i.e. dual sensory impairment (DSI) and mortality risk. In the US National Health and Nutrition Examination Survey of 5444 adults aged 55–74 years, clinically confirmed DSI, however, was not found to be associated with an increased risk of mortality [18]. In an Italian study of 1140 adults aged 70–75 years, a significant association between DSI and 6-year total mortality was observed in men but not in women [19]. In this study, hearing loss was not measured objectively using pure-tone audiometry (i.e. 'gold-standard'), but using the free-field whispered voice test. Finally, results from the US National Health Interview Survey of adults aged 18 years and older, showed that self-reported DSI was associated with a higher risk of all-cause mortality among men and women as compared to those reporting either visual impairment alone or hearing impairment alone [20,21]. Many previous studies that have assessed the association between DSI and mortality had a relatively small number of participants with DSI at baseline and/or did not adequately adjust for mortality risk markers (e.g., cardiovascular diseases, diabetes, cognitive impairment and self-rated health) [18,19,22].

In the present study, we aimed to address previous gaps in knowledge, by examining the association between clinically confirmed DSI with 10-year mortality risk in a large cohort of adults aged 55 years and older, after adjusting for potential confounders such as self-rated health, walking disability and cognitive impairment, in addition to traditional mortality risk markers.

Methods

Study Population

The BMES is a population-based cohort study of common eye diseases and other health outcomes in a suburban Australian population located west of Sydney. Study methods and procedures have been described elsewhere [23]. Following a door-to-door census of the region, baseline examinations of 3654 residents aged >49 years were conducted during 1992-4 (BMES-1, 82.4% participation rate). Of the baseline participants, 2335 (75.1% of survivors) returned for 5-year follow-up examinations during 1997-9 (BMES-2), and 1952 participants (53.4% of the original cohort, or 76.6% of survivors) returned for 10-year follow-up examinations during 2002-4 (BMES-3). The study was approved by the Human Research Ethics Committee of the University of Sydney and was conducted adhering to the tenets of the Declaration of Helsinki. Signed informed consent was obtained from all the participants at each examination.

Audiological Assessment

Pure-tone audiometry at both visits was performed by audiologists in sound-treated booths, using TDH-39 earphones and Madsen OB822 audiometers (Madsen Electronics, Denmark). Sound-proof rooms were set-up according to International Standards Organization protocol 8253-2. Bilateral hearing impairment was determined as the pure-tone average of audiometric hearing thresholds at 500, 1000, 2000, and 4000 Hz ($PTA_{0.5-4\ kHz}$) in the better ear, defining any hearing loss as $PTA_{0.5-4\ kHz}$ >25 dB HL; mild hearing loss as $PTA_{0.5-4\ kHz}$ >25–40 dB HL; and moderate to severe hearing loss as $PTA_{0.5-4\ kHz}$ >40 dB HL.

Assessment of Visual Impairment

Monocular distance logMAR (logarithm of the minimum angle of resolution) visual acuity was measured with forced-choice procedures using the retroilluminated chart with automatic calibration to 85 cd/m^2 (Vectorvision CSV-100 TM; Vectorvision Inc, Dayton, Ohio) according to the Early Treatment Diabetic Retinopathy Study protocol [23]. This was conducted with habitual correction (presenting visual acuity, with current eyeglasses, if worn) and after subjective refraction (best-corrected visual acuity). For each eye, visual acuity was recorded as the number of letters read correctly from 0 to 70. For the present study, any visual impairment was defined as presenting or best-corrected visual acuity of the better eye less than 39 letters (<20/40). DSI was defined as concurrent visual (either presenting or best-corrected) and hearing impairment, as determined using the above definitions.

Information on Mortality

To identify and confirm persons who died after BMES-2, demographic information including surname, first and second names, sex and date of birth of the examined participants were cross-matched with Australian National Death Index (NDI) data for deaths, to December 2007. A probabilistic record linkage package was used, adopting a multiple pass procedure in which both data sets were grouped based on different characteristics (e.g., date of birth, name, sex) each time. Matches were divided into exact and non-exact. All non-exact matched records were examined manually and accepted if there was only one non-exact matched characteristic that was not critical. Information provided by family members during follow-up was also included if the participant was reported to have died on or before December 2007. The *International Classification of Diseases, Ninth Revision (ICD-9)* [24] and *International Statistical Classification of Diseases, 10th Revision (ICD-10)* [25] cause of death codes were also obtained. The following cause-specific mortality codes were used in our analyses: coronary heart disease (ICD-9:410.0–9, 411.0–8, 412, 414.0–9, and ICD-10: I21.0–9, I22.0–9, I23.0–8, I24.0–9, I25.0–9); stroke (ICD-9:430.0–438.9 and ICD-10: I60.0-I69.9); or cancer (ICD-9:140–208). The primary cause of death (i.e. death from any cause, stroke, coronary heart disease or cancer) was used in statistical modeling. The validity of Australian NDI data has been reported to have high sensitivity and specificity (93.7% and 100.0%, respectively) for all-cause mortality [26]. The census cut-off point for mortality was December 2007 (10-year follow up).

Assessment of Covariates

A face-to-face interview with trained interviewers was conducted, and comprehensive data including information about medical history, hearing, demographic factors, socio-economic characteristics, lifestyle and health risk behaviour such as exercise, and smoking, were obtained from all participants. The medical history included cardiovascular or other systemic disease and associated risk factors, and medications used. A past history of angina, diabetes, myocardial infarction, and stroke was determined by responses to a question: "Has a doctor advised you that you have any of the following conditions?" Cognitive decline was assessed using the mini mental state examination (MMSE) questionnaire [27]. Participants with scores <24 were considered cognitively impaired. Self-rated health was assessed by asking: "For somebody your age, would you say your health is excellent, very good, good, fair, or poor?" Low self-rated health was defined as fair or poor.

Classification of hypertension was based on the 2003 World Health Organization/International Society of Hypertension guidelines [28]. Participants were classified as having hypertension stage 1 if systolic blood pressure was 140 to 159 mm Hg or if diastolic blood pressure was 90 to 99 mm Hg. Participants were classified as having hypertension stage 2 if they were previously diagnosed with hypertension and were using antihypertensive medications, if systolic blood pressure was 160 mm Hg or greater, or if diastolic blood pressure was 100 mm Hg or greater at examination. Body mass index was calculated as weight in kilograms divided by height in meters squared. Disability in walking at baseline was assessed as present if the participant was observed by a trained examiner to have walking difficulties or used walking aids or a wheelchair.

Statistical Analysis

SAS statistical software (SAS Institute, Cary NC) version 9.1 was used for analyses. The association between single sensory impairment and DSI with mortality was examined using Cox regression models to estimate hazard ratios (HR) and 95% confidence intervals (CI). Multivariable regression models were first adjusted for age (entered as a continuous variable) and sex, and then further adjusted for confounders that were found to be significantly associated with mortality i.e. body mass index, systolic blood pressure, current smoking status, poor self-rated health, walking disability, presence of hypertension and/or diabetes, history of cancer, angina, stroke and/or acute myocardial infarction and cognitive impairment. We estimated the proportion surviving using the Kaplan Meier method. Kaplan-Meier survival curves are generated from the fitted Cox model using mean covariate values of age and sex.

Results

Table 1 shows the baseline characteristics of study participants with and without DSI. Those with DSI compared to those without DSI were more likely to be older, male, hypertensive and cognitively impaired, and also to have poorer self-rated health, walking disability, diabetes, stroke, angina, acute myocardial infarction, higher systolic BP and lower BMI (Table 1). We assessed the 10-year mortality risk in participants with presenting visual impairment (bilateral) and hearing impairment (Table 2). Among participants with presenting visual impairment (better eye) and bilateral hearing impairment at baseline, 64% had died 10 years later compared to 11% without any sensory loss, and 26% and 30% with only a vision or hearing loss, respectively. After multivariable adjustment, participants with DSI (i.e. presenting visual impairment and any level of hearing impairment) had a 62% increased risk of dying 10 years later compared to those without any sensory impairment, HR 1.62 (95% CI 1.16–2.26). This association was more marked in participants with both presenting visual impairment and moderate to severe hearing loss, multivariable-adjusted HR 1.84 (95% CI 1.19–2.86). Having a single sensory loss (i.e. either presenting visual impairment or any level of hearing loss) did not significantly increase the risk of mortality over 10 years. Figure 1 shows the 10-year survival of participants by the presence or absence of sensory loss. Persons with DSI had lower survival than those with a single sensory impairment (either presenting vision or hearing loss alone) or without any sensory impairment.

Table 1. Baseline characteristics of Blue Mountains Eye Study participants stratified by the presence of dual sensory impairment (n = 2812).

	Dual sensory impairment[a]		
Mortality risk marker	**No (n = 1865)**	**Yes (n = 947)**	**p-value**
Age, *yrs*	64.2 (7.8)	73.7 (8.4)	<0.0001
Male	745 (40.0)	471 (49.7)	<0.0001
Current smoker	187 (10.1)	86 (9.1)	0.43
Poor self-rated health	313 (16.9)	223 (23.7)	<0.0001
Body mass index, *kg/m²*	27.9 (4.7)	27.2 (4.7)	0.0004
Systolic blood pressure, *mm Hg*	144.2 (21.0)	150.9 (22.3)	<0.0001
Walking disability	54 (2.9)	140 (14.8)	<0.0001
Diabetes	161 (8.6)	128 (13.5)	<0.0001
Hypertension[b]	1377 (74.0)	781 (82.6)	<0.0001
Stroke	52 (2.8)	67 (7.1)	<0.0001
Angina	141 (7.6)	150 (16.1)	<0.0001
Acute myocardial infarction	108 (5.8)	102 (11.0)	<0.0001
Cancer	208 (11.2)	106 (11.3)	0.94
Cognitive impairment[c]	20 (1.1)	59 (6.2)	<0.0001

Data are presented as mean (SD) and n (%), unless otherwise specified.
[a]Any hearing loss (>25 dB HL) and best-corrected visual impairment (<20/40).
[b]Hypertension Stage I -140/90–160/100; Stage II - >160/100 or treated.
[c]Cognitive impairment defined as mini-mental state examination score ≤24.

Non-significant associations were observed between concurrent presenting visual impairment and hearing impairment at baseline with 10-year cause-specific mortality, after multivariable adjustment: coronary heart disease mortality - HR 1.47 (95% CI 0.83–2.58); stroke mortality - HR 1.05 (0.50–2.22); and cancer mortality – HR 1.79 (95% CI 0.99–3.23).

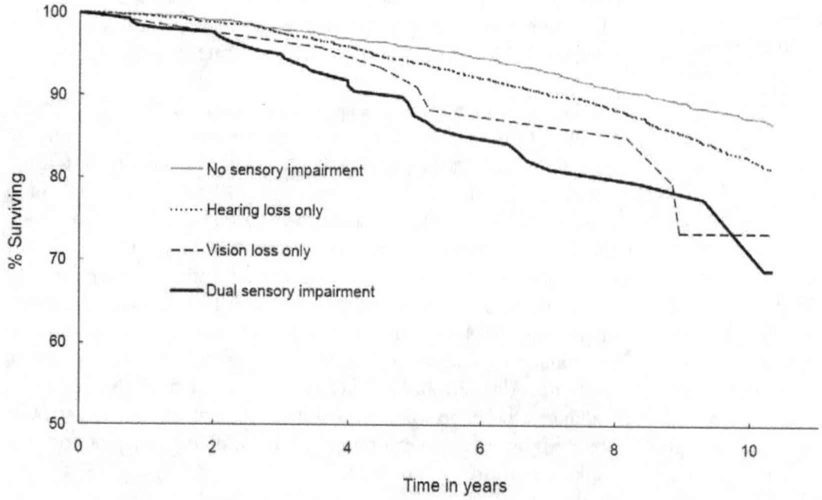

Figure 1. Age-sex adjusted Kaplan-Meier survival curves by presence of sensory impairment (presenting bilateral visual impairment and/or bilateral hearing impairment) among Blue Mountains Eye Study participants aged 55 years and older (n = 2806).

Table 2. All-cause mortality (over 10 years) in participants with bilateral hearing impairment and presenting visual impairment in the Blue Mountains Eye Study from 1997 to 2007 (n = 2806).

			Hazard ratio (95% confidence interval)	
Visual impairment (<20/40)	**Hearing impairment (dB HL)**	**no. of deaths (%)**	**Model 1[a]**	**Model 2[b]**
No visual impairment	≤25 (No hearing loss)	196 (10.9)	1.0 (reference)	1.0 (reference)
	>25 (Any hearing loss)	240 (30.2)	1.35 (1.10–1.65)	1.24 (0.99–1.54)
	>25-≤40 (Mild hearing loss)	153 (27.4)	1.33 (1.06–1.65)	1.27 (1.01–1.61)
	>40 (Moderate-severe hearing loss)	87 (37.0)	1.39 (1.06–1.83)	1.16 (0.87–1.56)
Presenting	≤25 (No hearing loss)	20 (25.6)	1.43 (0.90–1.65)	1.05 (0.61–1.80)
	>25 (Any hearing loss)	83 (63.9)	2.27 (1.70–3.05)	1.62 (1.16–2.26)
	>25-≤40 (Mild hearing loss)	44 (59.5)	2.10 (1.47–2.99)	1.46 (0.98–2.16)
	>40 (Moderate-severe hearing loss)	39 (69.6)	2.53 (1.74–3.68)	1.84 (1.19–2.86)

[a]Adjusted for age and sex.
[b]Further adjusted for body mass index, systolic blood pressure, current smoking status, poor self-rated health, walking disability, presence of hypertension and/or diabetes, history of cancer, angina, stroke and/or acute myocardial infarction and cognitive impairment.

We also assessed the risk of mortality in participants with best-corrected visual impairment (bilateral) and hearing impairment (Table 3). Among participants with best corrected visual impairment and bilateral hearing impairment at baseline, 76% had died 10 years later compared to 11% without any sensory loss, and 40% and 33% with only a vision or hearing loss, respectively. After multivariable adjustment, having both best corrected visual impairment and moderate to severe hearing loss increased the mortality risk by two-fold, when compared to those without any sensory loss. Having any or mild hearing loss (but without best corrected visual impairment) was associated with an increased risk of dying of 29% and 32%, respectively.

Discussion

To our best knowledge, this is the first population-based study to demonstrate that older adults with objectively measured DSI are at an increased risk of death from all causes compared to those without any sensory loss or a single sensory impairment. Specifically, participants with both presenting visual impairment (better eye) and bilateral hearing impairment at baseline had a 62% increased risk of dying 10 years later, independent of age, sex, self-rated health and the presence of known mortality markers. This association with mortality was more marked among older adults with concurrent moderate to severe hearing loss and any presenting or best-corrected vision loss.

Older adults in the BMES with clinically confirmed DSI compared to their counterparts without DSI had a 62% increased risk of total mortality. This finding is relatively similar to the HRs reported in a U.S. study: among men (HR 1.23 [95% CI 1.04–1.46]) and women (HR 1.63 [95% CI 1.37–1.93]) [20]. Also, in the Canadian National Population Health Survey [29], self-reported hearing impairment but not vision impairment were significantly associated with a greater risk of total mortality 12 years later, among 12,375 participants aged 18 and older. In our study, baseline DSI conferred a greater risk of dying 10 years later compared to having only presenting visual impairment or hearing impairment alone. This result suggests a potential interactive effect of DSI on survival, that is, the negative effects of vision are multiplied by the effects from hearing loss [12]. Our finding also concur with previous reports suggesting that the presence of more

Table 3. All-cause mortality (over 10 years) in participants with bilateral hearing impairment and best-corrected visual impairment in the Blue Mountains Eye Study from 1997 to 2007 (n = 2812).

			Hazard ratio (95% confidence interval)	
Visual impairment (<20/40)	**Hearing impairment (dB HL)**	**no. of deaths (%)**	**Model 1[a]**	**Model 2[b]**
No visual impairment	≤25 (No hearing loss)	208 (11.2)	1.0 (reference)	1.0 (reference)
	>25 (Any hearing loss)	290 (32.9)	1.41 (1.16–1.71)	1.29 (1.04–1.59)
	>25-≤40 (Mild hearing loss)	180 (29.6)	1.38 (1.12–1.71)	1.32 (1.06–1.66)
	>40 (Moderate-severe hearing loss)	110 (40.3)	1.46 (1.14–1.89)	1.22 (0.92–1.61)
Best corrected	≤25 (No hearing loss)	8 (40.0)	2.07 (1.01–4.22)	1.80 (0.79–4.12)
	>25 (Any hearing loss)	34 (75.6)	2.60 (1.74–3.90)	1.59 (1.00–2.52)
	>25-≤40 (Mild hearing loss)	17 (68.0)	2.17 (1.28–3.67)	1.20 (0.65–2.22)
	>40 (Moderate-severe hearing loss)	17 (85.0)	3.32 (1.95–5.63)	2.19 (1.20–4.03)

[a]Adjusted for age and sex.
[b]Further adjusted for body mass index, systolic blood pressure, current smoking status, poor self-rated health, walking disability, presence of hypertension and/or diabetes, history of cancer, angina, stroke and/or acute myocardial infarction and cognitive impairment.

than one sensory impairment increases morbidity relative to single sensory impairments [21,30–32].

We documented a gradient effect from the severity of DSI on mortality risk. Specifically, participants with concurrent moderate to severe hearing loss (>40 dB HL) and any visual impairment (<20/40) had a higher risk of dying 10 years later, than those with mild hearing loss (<25–40 dB HL) and any vision loss (particularly those with best-corrected visual impairment). This finding concurs with the US study by Lee et al. [21] which showed that moderate to severe concurrent hearing and vision impairment in women significantly increased their risk of mortality. This is not surprising, as with increasing level of measured hearing impairment the likelihood of communication difficulties also increases [33], which in turn can cause increasing social isolation [34] and also a higher likelihood of experiencing functional disability [13], factors that could negatively impact on life expectancy [35,36].

It is hypothesized that the increased risk of mortality observed in persons with DSI is mediated by factors known to increase the risk of hearing and visual impairment in older adults (e.g., cardiovascular disease, hypertension and diabetes) [20,37,38]. However, in the BMES, a significant reduction in survival was observed in persons with DSI, even after controlling for cardiovascular risk factors (e.g., body mass index, smoking, hypertension) and events (e.g., angina, acute myocardial infarction), which supports findings from the study by Lam et al. [20] Moreover, we did not observe significant associations between DSI with 10-year coronary heart disease or stroke mortality. Therefore, these data together suggest that exposure to vascular risk factors are not likely to be the link between DSI and mortality risk, although, residual confounding from vascular risk factors cannot be fully discounted.

Alternatively, it is speculated that presence of DSI could be a marker for frailty (e.g., handgrip strength, peak expiratory flow), illness or possibly accelerated aging processes [21,39]. Given that frailty is a strong predictor of mortality [40], the association between decreased vision and hearing and increased risk of dying is not unexpected. Additionally, a decline in psychosocial functioning could underlie the relationship between DSI and mortality risk. Visual impairment was shown to be associated with difficulty in performing ADL [41], social isolation [42] and depression [43]. Similarly, impaired hearing has also shown to negatively impact on participation in social activities [44], functional independence [13] and mental health [8]. Other potential mechanisms could be that both hearing and vision impairments are associated with a greater risk of accident and injury [45–48], which in turn could underlie the greater risk of mortality among older adults with DSI. However, we are unable to confirm this hypothesis as there were only around <1% of BMES participants who had died from injury (e.g. falls related) or accident, hence; we did not have sufficient study power to analyze these associations with DSI.

As sensory problems are common experiences within older age groups, they are often overlooked or dismissed [30]. Our study could have potential public health implications, as it suggests that identifying and targeting DSI in older adults could be a potentially useful strategy for preventing a decline in their life expectancy. Specifically, regular assessment of presence of DSI in older persons could lead to earlier detection and facilitation of rehabilitation and therapy that could reduce the negative impacts of DSI. Correction of visual and hearing impairment could improve survival [42,49], hence, strategies including the provision of corrective lenses, hearing aids, assistive devices (e.g., magnifiers, listening devices) and rehabilitative services such as visual, auditory and communication training [21,50] should be encouraged and/or implemented by clinicians in order to promote both longevity and an improved quality of life in their older sensory impaired patient.

The strengths of this study include the use of a representative cohort with a relatively high participation rate, the use of standardized audiometric and vision testing, with measures of sensory function at more than one point in time [51], and ascertainment of mortality and its causes using validated Australian National Death Index data. We previously showed that the door-to-door census which was used as a sampling frame for the BMES is less likely to be subject to selection bias [52]. This evidence together with the high response rate means that our door-to-door census can be regarded as being close to a gold standard as can realistically be achieved [53]. Despite the high internal validity of the BMES, we need to caution about the generalizability of our study findings. The study population is not a random sample of the wider Australian population. However, the findings from this study could be reasonably generalized to the Australian population over the age of 55, as it was previously observed that the demographic characteristics of this sample population are not markedly different from the Australian population apart from a lower proportion of immigrants [52]. Second, while we had robust data on a range of confounders, other unmeasured or unknown factors (e.g., lifestyle or societal factors) could have influenced our study findings. Finally, age was entered into the multivariable model assuming a linear relationship with mortality risk, hence, we cannot disregard the possibility that some of the effects of aging are being picked up by hearing impairment, vision impairment and/or other independent variables (e.g. walking disability).

In summary, we found that the presence of DSI independently predicted an increased risk of mortality in older adults. These findings emphasize to clinicians the importance of recognizing that older adults with concurrent vision and hearing loss are at an increased risk of mortality compared to their non-impaired counterparts or those with only a single sensory impairment. Public health strategies to encourage earlier identification of older adults with DSI and their appropriate referral to rehabilitative services and support could improve life expectancy in this vulnerable population.

Author Contributions

Conceived and designed the experiments: BG PM. Performed the experiments: BG PM JS SRL GB CMM. Analyzed the data: GB. Contributed reagents/materials/analysis tools: PM BG GB. Wrote the paper: BG PM SRL.

References

1. Taylor HR, Keeffe JE, Vu HT, Wang JJ, Rochtchina E, et al. (2005) Vision loss in Australia. Med J Aust 182: 565–568.
2. Gopinath B, Rochtchina E, Wang JJ, Schneider J, Leeder SR, et al. (2009) Prevalence of age-related hearing loss in older adults: Blue Mountains Study. Arch Intern Med 169: 415–416.
3. Schneider JM, Gopinath B, McMahon CM, Leeder SR, Mitchell P, et al. (2011) Dual Sensory Impairment in Older Age. J Aging Health.
4. Chia EM, Mitchell P, Ojaimi E, Rochtchina E, Wang JJ (2006) Assessment of vision-related quality of life in an older population subsample: the blue mountains eye study. Ophthalmic Epidemiol 13: 371–377.
5. Chia EM, Wang JJ, Rochtchina E, Smith W, Cumming RR, et al. (2004) Impact of bilateral visual impairment on health-related quality of life: the Blue

Mountains Eye Study. Invest Ophthalmol Vis Sci 45: 71–76.
6. Tay T, Wang JJ, Lindley R, Chia EM, Landau P, et al. (2007) Sensory impairment, use of community support services, and quality of life in aged care clients. Journal of Aging and Health 19: 229–241.
7. Tay T, Wang JJ, Kifley A, Lindley R, Newall P, et al. (2006) Sensory and cognitive association in older persons: findings from an older Australian population. Gerontology 52: 386–394.
8. Gopinath B, Wang JJ, Schneider J, Burlutsky G, Snowdon J, et al. (2009) Depressive symptoms in older adults with hearing impairments: the Blue Mountains Study. J Am Geriatr Soc 57: 1306–1308.
9. Chia EM, Wang JJ, Rochtchina E, Cumming RR, Newall P, et al. (2007) Hearing impairment and health-related quality of life: the Blue Mountains Hearing Study. Ear Hear 28: 187–195.
10. Gopinath B, Schneider J, Hickson L, McMahon CM, Burlutsky G, et al. (2012) Hearing handicap, rather than measured hearing impairment, predicts poorer quality of life over 10 years in older adults. Maturitas 72: 146–151.
11. Schneider J, Gopinath B, Karpa MJ, McMahon CM, Rochtchina E, et al. (2010) Hearing loss impacts on the use of community and informal supports. Age Ageing 39: 458–464.
12. Schneider JM, Gopinath B, McMahon CM, Leeder SR, Mitchell P, et al. (2011) Dual sensory impairment in older age. J Aging Health 23: 1309–1324.
13. Gopinath B, Schneider J, McMahon CM, Teber E, Leeder SR, et al. (2012) Severity of age-related hearing loss is associated with impaired activities of daily living. Age Ageing 41: 195–200.
14. Karpa MJ, Mitchell P, Beath K, Rochtchina E, Cumming RG, et al. (2009) Direct and indirect effects of visual impairment on mortality risk in older persons. Arch Ophthalmol 127: 1347–1353.
15. Cugati S, Cumming RG, Smith W, Burlutsky G, Mitchell P, et al. (2007) Visual impairment, age-related macular degeneration, cataract, and long-term mortality: the Blue Mountains Eye Study. Arch Ophthalmol 125: 917–924.
16. Freeman EE, Egleston BL, West SK, Bandeen-Roche K, Rubin G (2005) Visual acuity change and mortality in older adults. Invest Ophthalmol Vis Sci 46: 4040–4045.
17. Karpa MJ, Gopinath B, Beath K, Rochtchina E, Cumming RG, et al. (2010) Associations between hearing impairment and mortality risk in older persons: the Blue Mountains Hearing Study. Ann Epidemiol 20: 452–459.
18. Reuben DB, Mui S, Damesyn M, Moore AA, Greendale GA (1999) The prognostic value of sensory impairment in older persons. J Am Geriatr Soc 47: 930–935.
19. Appollonio I, Carabellese C, Magni E, Frattola L, Trabucchi M (1995) Sensory impairments and mortality in an elderly community population: a six-year follow-up study. Age Ageing 24: 30–36.
20. Lam BL, Lee DJ, Gomez-Marin O, Zheng DD, Caban AJ (2006) Concurrent visual and hearing impairment and risk of mortality: the National Health Interview Survey. Arch Ophthalmol 124: 95–101.
21. Lee DJ, Gomez-Marin O, Lam BL, Zheng DD, Arheart KL, et al. (2007) Severity of concurrent visual and hearing impairment and mortality: the 1986–1994 National Health Interview Survey. J Aging Health 19: 382–396.
22. Laforge RG, Spector WD, Sternberg J (1992) The relationship of vision and hearing impairment to one-year mortality and functional decline. Journal of Aging and Health 4: 126–148.
23. Attebo K, Mitchell P, Smith W (1996) Visual acuity and the causes of visual loss in Australia. The Blue Mountains Eye Study. Ophthalmology 103: 357–364.
24. World Health Organization (1977) Manual if the international statistical classification of disease, injuries and causes of death. Vol 1. Geneva, World Health Organization.
25. World Health Organization (1992) International statistical classification of diseases and related health problems. tenth revision[ICD-10]. Geneva, World Health Organization.
26. Magliano D, Liew D, Pater H, Kirby A, Hunt D, et al. (2003) Accuracy of the Australian National Death Index: comparison with adjudicated fatal outcomes among Australian participants in the Long-term Intervention with Pravastatin in Ischaemic Disease (LIPID) study. Aust N Z J Public Health 27: 649–653.
27. Folstein MF, Folstein SE, McHugh PR (1975) "Mini-Mental State": A practical method for grading the cognitive state of patients for the clinician. J Psychiat Res 12: 189–198.
28. World Health Organization (WHO)/International Society of Hypertension (ISH) statement on management of hypertension (2003) J Hypertens 21: 1983–1992.
29. Feeny D, Huguet N, McFarland BH, Kaplan MS, Orpana H, et al. (2012) Hearing, mobility, and pain predict mortality: a longitudinal population-based study. J Clin Epidemiol 65: 764–777.
30. Crews JE, Campbell VA (2004) Vision impairment and hearing loss among community-dwelling older Americans: implications for health and functioning. Am J Public Health 94: 823–829.
31. Carabellese C, Appollonio I, Rozzini R, Bianchetti A, Frisoni GB, et al. (1993) Sensory impairment and quality of life in a community elderly population. J Am Geriatr Soc 41: 401–407.
32. Lee DJ, Lam BL, Gomez-Marin O, Zheng DD, Caban AJ (2005) Concurrent hearing and visual impairment and morbidity in community-residing adults: the National Health Interview Survey, 1986 to 1996. J Aging Health 17: 531–546.
33. Lutman ME, Brown EJ, Coles RR (1987) Self-reported disability and handicap in the population in relation to pure-tone threshold, age, sex and type of hearing loss. Br J Audiol 21: 45–58.
34. Arlinger S (2003) Negative consequences of uncorrected hearing loss–a review. Int J Audiol 42 Suppl 2: 2S17–2S20.
35. Hanson BS, Isacsson SO, Janzon L, Lindell SE (1989) Social network and social support influence mortality in elderly men. The prospective population study of "Men born in 1914," Malmo, Sweden. Am J Epidemiol 130: 100–111.
36. Stessman J, Hammerman-Rozenberg R, Cohen A, Ein-Mor E, Jacobs JM (2009) Physical activity, function, and longevity among the very old. Arch Intern Med 169: 1476–1483.
37. Mitchell P, Gopinath B, McMahon CM, Rochtchina E, Wang JJ, et al. (2009) Relationship of Type 2 diabetes to the prevalence, incidence and progression of age-related hearing loss. Diabet Med 26: 483–488.
38. Gopinath B, Flood VM, McMahon CM, Burlutsky G, Smith W, et al. (2010) The effects of smoking and alcohol consumption on age-related hearing loss: the Blue Mountains Hearing Study. Ear Hear 31: 277–282.
39. Cugati S, Cumming RG, Smith W, Burlutsky G, Mitchell P, et al. (2007) Visual impairment, age-related macular degeneration, cataract, and long-term mortality: the Blue Mountains Eye Study. Arch Ophthalmol 125: 917–924.
40. Fried LP, Tangen CM, Walston J, Newman AB, Hirsch C, et al. (2001) Frailty in older adults: evidence for a phenotype. J Gerontol A Biol Sci Med Sci 56: M146–M156.
41. Keller BK, Morton JL, Thomas VS, Potter JF (1999) The effect of visual and hearing impairments on functional status. J Am Geriatr Soc 47: 1319–1325.
42. Appollonio I, Carabellese C, Frattola L, Trabucchi M (1996) Effects of sensory aids on the quality of life and mortality of elderly people: a multivariate analysis. Age Ageing 25: 89–96.
43. Evans JR, Fletcher AE, Wormald RP (2007) Depression and anxiety in visually impaired older people. Ophthalmology 114: 283–288.
44. Gopinath B, Hickson L, Schneider J, McMahon CM, Burlutsky G, et al. (2012) Hearing-impaired adults are at increased risk of experiencing emotional distress and social engagement restrictions five years later. Age Ageing.
45. Viljanen A, Kaprio J, Pyykko I, Sorri M, Pajala S, et al. (2009) Hearing as a predictor of falls and postural balance in older female twins. J Gerontol A Biol Sci Med Sci 64: 312–317.
46. Woodcock K, Pole JD (2008) Educational attainment, labour force status and injury: a comparison of Canadians with and without deafness and hearing loss. Int J Rehabil Res 31: 297–304.
47. Dhital A, Pey T, Stanford MR (2010) Visual loss and falls: a review. Eye (Lond) 24: 1437–1446.
48. Owsley C, Ball K, McGwin G Jr, Sloane ME, Roenker DL, et al. (1998) Visual processing impairment and risk of motor vehicle crash among older adults. JAMA 279: 1083–1088.
49. Mulrow CD, Aguilar C, Endicott JE, Tuley MR, Velez R, et al. (1990) Quality-of-life changes and hearing impairment. A randomized trial. Ann Intern Med 113: 188–194.
50. Heine C, Browning CJ (2002) Communication and psychosocial consequences of sensory loss in older adults: overview and rehabilitation directions. Disabil Rehabil 24: 763–773.
51. Schneider J, Gopinath B, McMahon C, Teber E, Leeder SR, et al. (2012) Prevalence and 5-year incidence of dual sensory impairment in an older Australian population. Ann Epidemiol 22: 295–301.
52. Cdata91 (1994) Australian Population Census 1991. Canberra.
53. Smith W, Mitchell P, Attebo K, Leeder S (1997) Selection bias from sampling frames: Telephone directory and electoral roll compared with door-to-door population census: Results from the Blue Mountains Eye Study. Aust J Public Health 21: 127–133.

18

The Development of Auditory Skills in Young Children with Mondini Dysplasia after Cochlear Implantation

Xueqing Chen[1], Fei Yan[2], Bo Liu[1], Sha Liu[1], Ying Kong[1], Jun Zheng[1], Yongxin Li[1], Shusheng Gong[1], Demin Han[1☯], Luo Zhang[1*☯]

1 Department of Otolaryngology, Head and Neck Surgery, Beijing Tongren Hospital and Beijing Institute of Otolaryngology, Capital Medical University, Beijing, China,
2 Department of Radiology, Beijing Tongren Hospital, Capital Medical University, Beijing, China

Abstract

The aim of this study is to survey and compare the development of auditory skills in young children with Mondini dysplasia and profoundly-deaf young children with radiologically normal inner ears over a period of 3 years after cochlear implantation. A total of 545 young children (age 7 to 36 months) with prelingual, severe to profound hearing loss participated in this study. All children received cochlear implantation. Based on whether or not there was a Mondini dysplasia as diagnosed with CT scanning, the subjects were divided into 2 groups: (A) 514 young children with radiologically normal inner ears and (B) 31 young children with Mondini dysplasia. The Infant-Toddler Meaningful Auditory Integration Scale (IT-MAIS) was used to assess the children's auditory skills that include vocalization changes, spontaneous alerting to sounds in everyday living environments, and the ability to derive meaning from sounds. The assessment was performed prior to surgery and at 1, 3, 6, 9, 12, 24, and 36 months after implant device switch-on. The mean scores for overall auditory skills were not significantly different between groups A and B at pre-surgery, 1, 12, 24, and 36 months post-surgery, but were significantly different at 3, 6, and 9 months post-surgery. The mean scores for all auditory skills in children with Mondini dysplasia showed significant improvement over time. The mean scores for the three subcategories of auditory skills in children with Mondini dysplasia also showed significant differences at pre-surgery, 1, 3, 6, and 9 months, however, there were no significant differences at 12, 24, and 36 months. Overall, the auditory skills of young children with Mondini dysplasia developed rapidly after cochlear implantation, in a similar manner to that of young children with radiologically normal inner ears. Cochlear implantation is an effective intervention for young children with Mondini dysplasia.

Editor: Manuel S. Malmierca, University of Salamanca- Institute for Neuroscience of Castille and Leon and Medical School, Spain

Funding: This work was funded in part by the capital health research and development of special from the Beijing Municipal Health Bureau (No. 2011-1017-01), the research special fund for public welfare industry of health from the Ministry of Health of the People's Republic of China (No. 201202001), the promotion grant for high-level scientific and technological elites in medical science from the Beijing Municipal Health Bureau (No. 2009-3-29), key projects in basic and clinical research cooperation funds from Capital Medical University No. 12JL12), and the National Natural Science Foundation of China (No. 81371103). The funders had no role in study design, data collection and analysis, decision to publish, or preparation of the manuscript.

Competing Interests: The authors have declared that no competing interests exist.

* Email: dr.luozhang@gmail.com

☯ These authors contributed equally to this work.

Introduction

The development of imaging technology has demonstrated that inner ear malformation is a common cause of congenital hearing loss in children. High-resolution computerized tomography has identified that 20% to 38% sensorineural hearing loss in children is due to cochlear malformations [1–4]. Mondini dysplasia, an inner ear abnormality characterized by the development of an incomplete cochlea, was first reported by Mondini in 1791 [5] based on an autopsy examination of the ears of an 8-year old boy with congenital hearing loss. Subsequent studies involving detailed evaluation using polytomography and histologic techniques have demonstrated that there is incomplete partition resulting in fusion of the middle and apical turns to form a cystic apex, whereas the basal turn of the cochlea appears to be normal [6–8]. Mondini dysplasia is hypothesized to be resulted from an arrest of embryogenesis at approximately the seventh gestational week as a consequence of either genetic defects or external insults [9].

Hearing levels of subjects with Mondini dysplasia may range from normal to profound deafness [8]. When profound hearing loss occurs and conventional amplification is insufficient, cochlear implantation may be an effective intervention [10]. Although patients with Mondini dysplasia were once considered as poor candidates for cochlear implantation, several studies have shown positive results for cochlear implantation in this group of patients in recent years [11–19]. Silverstein and colleagues first implanted a multichannel cochlear implant in a 31-year-old man with Mondini dysplasia [15]. The authors demonstrated that there were only modest improvements in objective results of Iowa test battery that comprised of closed-set tests (i.e., vowel recognition, consonant recognition, and four-choice spondee recognition) and open-set tests (i.e., monosyllabic word recognition, everyday sentence understanding, and sentence understanding without context). This adult patient did show the ability to discriminate pure-tone

Table 1. Demographic and clinical characteristics of young children with radiologically normal inner ears (A) and young children with Mondini dysplasia (B).

	Group A (n=514)	Group B (n=31)
Type of implants		
Nucleus (n(%))	380 (74%)	25 (80%)
Medel (n(%))	52 (10%)	3 (10%)
Clarion (n(%))	82 (16%)	3 (10%)
Gender		
Male (n(%))	324 (63%)	14 (45%)
Female (n(%)	190 (37%)	17 (55%)
Age at implantation (months)		
Mean±SE	21.2±0.3	22.2±1.4
Range	7–36	9–36

frequencies and environmental sounds following the implantation[15]. Subsequent studies have demonstrated that multichannel cochlear implants are useful in both children and adults with Mondini dysplasia [16–19]. Indeed, one study demonstrated that the sound-field thresholds following cochlear implantation of the patients with Mondini dysplasia aged from 6 to 42 years at surgery were in the region of 30–40 dB (A) [16], whereas another study showed that the aided thresholds of the patients aged from 2 to 23 years at implantation were similar to those tested in the control group with normal cochleae [17]. Moreover, cochlear implantation in children with Mondini dysplasia was shown to be successful in improving speech production and perception [18] as well as the development of listening skills [19].

Although several studies have shown a clear benefit of cochlear implantation in patients with Mondini dysplasia, there were relatively few reports of the benefits over a long period. The aim of this study is thus to evaluate the development of auditory skills in young children with Mondini dysplasia within 3 years after cochlear implantation and compare it with that in young children with radiologically normal inner ears.

Materials and Methods

Subjects

A total of 545 young children (338 boys and 207 girls), aged 7 months to 36 months, were enrolled into the study at Beijing Tongren Hospital, Capital Medical University, between the years 1999 and 2012. The young children presented as outpatients with severe to profound hearing loss at the Department of Otolaryngology Head and Neck Surgery and were assessed for cochlear implantation surgery.

Study design

All young children underwent a thorough otorhinolaryngological examination and audiometric tests by experienced audiologists using behavioral audiometry and electrophysiological tests including auditory brainstem response (ABR), distortion product otoacoustic emission (DPOAE), and tympanometry. Following the examinations and tests, all children who were free of any external or middle ear pathology were assessed further for a diagnosis of prelingual, severe to profound hearing loss.

Each child with a diagnosis of prelingual severe to profound hearing loss received high-resolution computed tomography (HRCT) examination, with 1-mm contiguous slice through the temporal bone. Radiologists reviewed the CT images on a clinical picture archiving and communicating system, and examined the temporal bone for the presence of cochlear, vestibular, or semicircular canal abnormalities. The diagnosis of Mondini dysplasia was confirmed based on the presence of a shortened cochlea with only one and a half turns, incomplete interscalar septum or osseous spiral lamina between the middle and apical turns, and a fully developed basal turn. The vestibule and semicircular canals were not required to be abnormal.

Based on the absence or presence of a Mondini dysplasia, the subjects were divided into 2 groups: (A) children with a congenital sensorineural hearing loss despite having a radiologically normal inner ear and (B) children with a Mondini dysplasia. The information of the types of cochlear implant system used in the young children and other demographical information of the two groups are shown in Table 1. Four weeks after surgery the implant switch-on programming session was performed by experienced audiologists. Regular programming, assessment and intensive habilitation were followed-up for each child at specified times over a period of 3 years.

The study protocol was approved by the Ethics Review Committee of Beijing Tongren Hospital and the parents or legal guardians of each child provided written informed consent prior to entry into the study.

Measurements

With a validated translated version of the Infant-Toddler Meaningful Auditory Integration Scale (IT-MAIS) [20], the

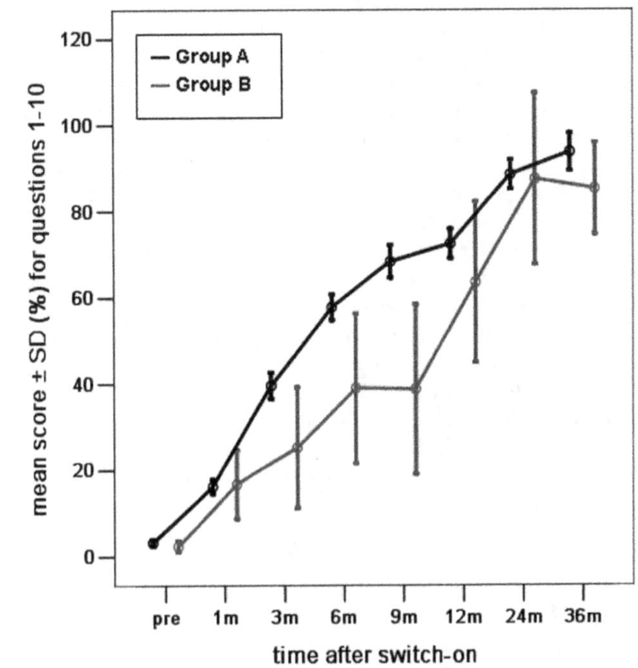

Figure 1. The mean scores for the development of overall auditory skills (questions 1–10) for young children with radiologically normal inner ears (Group A) and young children with Mondini dysplasia (Group B), at different intervals before and after the switch-on programming session over a period of 3 years after cochlear implantation. (score shown as percentage of total score of Questions 1–10/40×100).

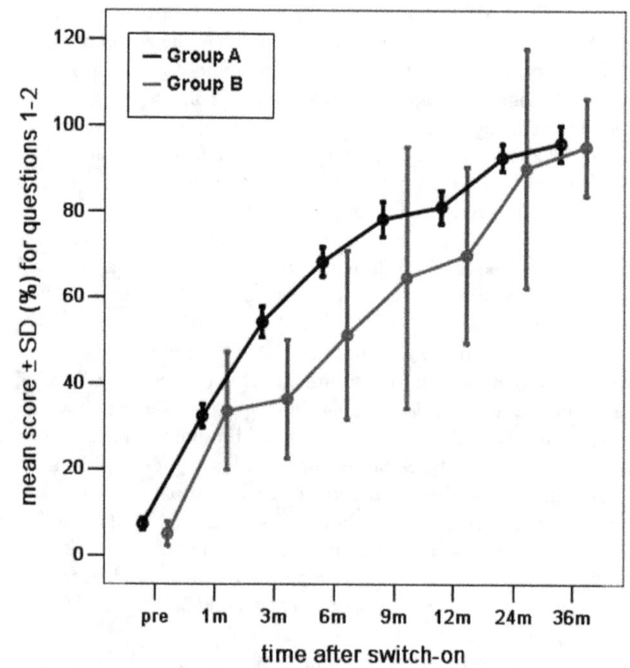

Figure 2. The mean scores for vocalization behaviors (questions 1–2) for young children with radiologically normal inner ears (Group A) and young children with Mondini dysplasia (Group B), at different intervals before and after the switch-on programming session over a period of 3 years after cochlear implantation. (score shown as percentage of total score of Questions 1 and 2/8×100).

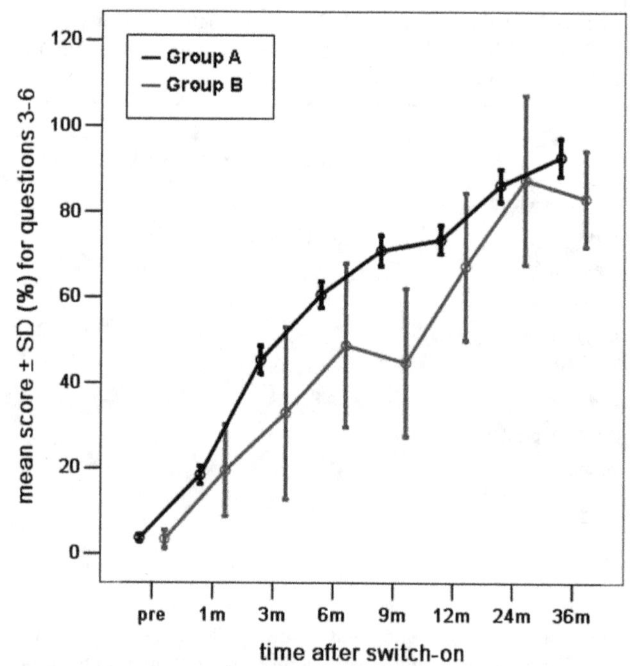

Figure 3. The mean scores for the development of the ability of alerting to sounds (questions 3–6) for young children with radiologically normal inner ears (Group A) and young children with Mondini dysplasia (Group B), at different intervals before and after the switch-on programming session over a period of 3 years after cochlear implantation. (score shown as percentage of total score of Questions 3, 4, 5 and 6/16×100).

auditory skill performance of all young children was evaluated at regular intervals: pre-surgery and at 1, 3, 6, 9, 12, 24, and 36 months after switch-on programming. The IT-MAIS is a 10-question parent questionnaire that inquires about the child's spontaneous auditory behaviors in their daily life environments. The questionnaire assesses three different kinds of auditory skills: (1) vocalization changes with device use (Questions 1 and 2), (2) spontaneous alerting to sounds in everyday living environments (Questions 3 through 6), and (3) the ability to derive meaning from sounds (Questions 7 through 10). Following explanation of the questionnaire and its outcomes to the parents of children with cochlear implants, trained audiologists engaged in face-to-face sessions with the parents to elicit detailed responses to each of the questions in the IT-MAIS. The parents were asked to provide as many examples as possible of their young child's auditory skill related behaviors. The parents' responses were recorded in detail and assigned a score based on the frequency of the occurrence of target responses. Each question was assessed on a scale of 0 to 4 (0 = never, 1 = rarely, 2 = occasionally, 3 = frequently, and 4 = always) [21].

Statistics

Statistical analyses were performed using the SPSS 13.0 statistical software. Arcsine transformation of the percentage data in this study (i.e., $y = 2 \times \sin^{-1}\sqrt{p}$, where p is the percentage score) was performed before the data were subjected to an analysis of variance (ANOVA) [22]. Independent sample t-test was used to determine the significance of any difference in overall auditory development between groups A and B, and also any difference in the unaided pure tone thresholds between the two groups. The significance of differences in the development of the overall and

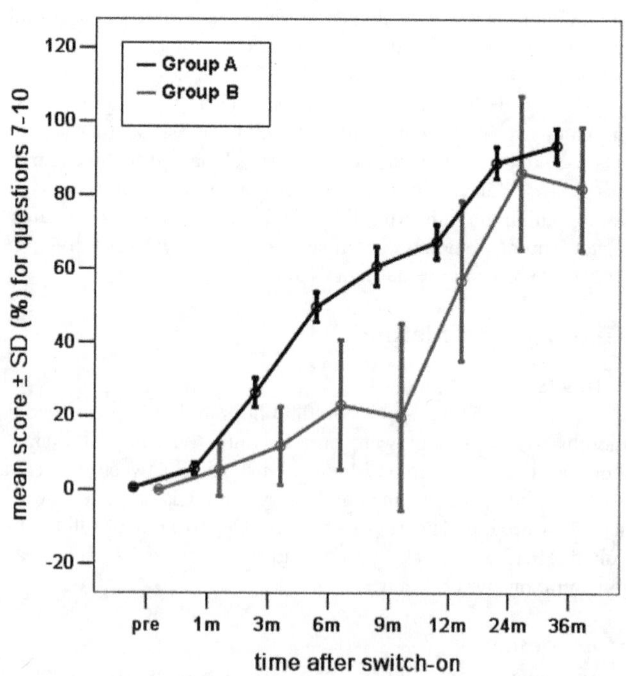

Figure 4. The mean scores for the development of the skill of deriving meaning from sounds (questions 7–10) for young children with radiologically normal inner ears (Group A) and young children with Mondini dysplasia (Group B), at different intervals before and after the switch-on programming session over a period of 3 years after cochlear implantation. (score shown as percentage of total score of Questions 7, 8, 9 and 10/16×100).

Table 2. *P*-values of post-hoc analysis of auditory skills.

Evaluating interval	Overall auditory skills	Vocalization behavior	Alerting to sounds	Deriving meaning from sounds
pre-surgery to 1-month	0.002	0.000	0.020	0.870
pre-surgery to 3-month	0.008	0.001	0.099	0.313
pre-surgery to 6-month	0.002	0.000	0.001	0.218
pre-surgery to 9-month	0.026	0.000	0.005	0.795
pre-surgery to 12-month	0.000	0.000	0.000	0.002
pre-surgery to 24-month	0.010	0.000	0.014	0.019
pre-surgery to 36-month	0.000	0.000	0.000	0.000
1-month to 3-month	0.999	1.000	1.000	0.997
1-month to 6-month	0.314	1.000	0.167	0.772
1-month to 9-month	0.460	0.258	0.180	0.992
1-month to 12-month	0.002	0.003	0.002	0.005
1-month to 24-month	0.013	0.000	0.018	0.008
1-month to 36-month	0.000	0.000	0.000	0.000
3-month to 6-month	0.993	1.000	0.996	1.000
3-month to 9-month	0.995	0.813	1.000	1.000
3-month to 12-month	0.043	0.028	0.194	0.050
3-month to 24-month	0.015	0.000	0.039	0.008
3-month to 36-month	0.000	0.000	0.007	0.000
6-month to 9-month	1.000	1.000	1.000	1.000
6-month to 12-month	0.704	1.000	0.927	0.533
6-month to 24-month	0.061	0.023	0.235	0.016
6-month to 36-month	0.003	0.000	0.067	0.002
9-month to 12-month	0.736	1.000	0.644	0.661
9-month to 24-month	0.074	0.695	0.178	0.034
9-month to 36-month	0.008	0.053	0.019	0.017
12-month to 24-month	0.754	1.000	0.973	0.573
12-month to 36-month	0.481	0.064	0.994	0.470
24-month to 36-month	1.000	1.000	1.000	1.000

A *p*-value of less than 0.05 is considered statistically significant.

three different auditory skills in young children with Mondini dysplasia (group B) were determined using a one-way ANOVA or post-hoc analyses. A *p*-value of less than 0.05 was considered to be statistically significant.

Results

Subject characteristics

The demographic and clinical characteristics of the young children are shown in Table 1. The age at implantation ranged from 7–36 months with a mean age of 21.2±0.3 months. No serious cochlear implant-related or surgery-related complications were observed over the course of the study in any of the children.

Differences in overall auditory development between groups A and B

The mean scores for overall auditory skills were not significantly different between groups A and B at pre-surgery and 1, 12, 24, and 36 months post-implantation surgery, however, there were significant differences at 3, 6, and 9 months post-implantation surgery ($p < 0.05$) (Figure 1).

Next, we evaluated the auditory skills in the three subcategories (Figures 2, 3, 4). The differences in mean scores for the skill of vocalization behavior were not statistically significant between groups A and B at pre-operation and 1, 6, 9, 12, 24, and 36 months post-implantation surgery. Significant differences were observed at 3 months post-implantation surgery ($p < 0.05$) (Figure 2). The mean scores for the skill of alerting to sounds were not significantly different between groups A and B at pre-surgery and 1, 3, 6, 12, and 24 months post-implantation surgery. There was a significant difference at 9, and 36 months post-implantation surgery ($p < 0.05$) (Figure 3). Similarly, the differences in mean scores for the skill of deriving meaning from sounds were not statistically significant between groups A and B at 1, 3, 12, 24, and 36 months post-implantation surgery, but were significant at pre-surgery and 6, and 9 months post-implantation surgery ($p < 0.05$) (Figure 4).

The development of auditory skills in young children with Mondini dysplasia

The mean scores for all auditory skills in young children with Mondini dysplasia showed a significant improvement over time

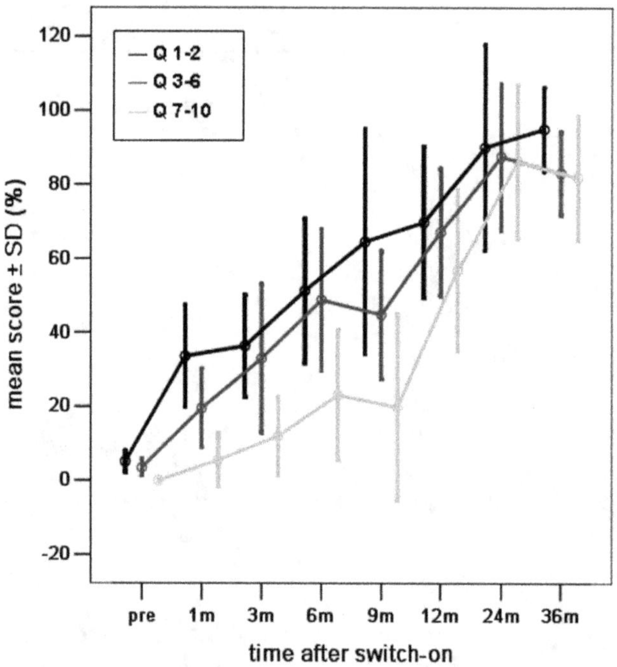

Figure 5. The mean scores for vocalization behaviors (questions 1–2), the ability of alerting to sounds (questions 3–6), and the skill of deriving meaning from sounds (questions 7–10) for young children with Mondini dysplasia (Group B), at different intervals before and after the switch-on programming session over a period of 3 years after cochlear implantation.

(one-way ANOVA, all $p = 0.000$) (Figures 1, 2, 3, 4). The mean scores for all auditory skills increased significantly between pre-surgery interval and each interval post-implantation surgery, as assessed by the post-hoc analyses ($p < 0.05$)(Table 2). However, the scores for the skill of alerting to sounds were not significantly different between pre-surgery and 3 months post implantation surgery. The scores for the skill of deriving meaning from sounds were also not significantly different between pre-surgery and at 1, 3, 6 and 9 months post implantation surgery. The mean scores for all auditory skills increased significantly between 1 month interval and each interval after 9 months ($p < 0.05$). No significant differences were noted for any of the auditory skills between 1 month and at 3, 6, and 9 months post-implantation.

Comparison of scores at time intervals between 3 to 9 months indicated no significant differences for all auditory skills between 3 months and at 6 and 9 months. The differences were statistically significant in the mean scores for all auditory skills between 3 months and those after 9 months ($p < 0.05$), except for the scores between 3 and 12 months interval post implantation surgery for the skills of alerting to sounds and deriving meaning from sounds. No significant differences were found for the scores of all auditory skills between 6 months and at 9, 12, and 24 months, except between 6 and 24 months interval post-implantation surgery for the skills of vocalization behavior and deriving meaning from sounds ($p < 0.05$). The differences were statistically significant in the mean scores for all auditory skills between 6 and 36 months ($p < 0.05$). However, no significant difference was noted for the skill of alerting to sounds during this time interval.

Similarly, comparison of the scores for time intervals between 9 to 36 months showed no significant differences for all auditory skills between 9 months and 12 or 24 months, except for the scores between 9 and 24 months for the skill of deriving meaning from sounds ($p < 0.05$). The mean scores for all auditory skills increased significantly between 9 and 36 months ($p < 0.05$), except for the skill of vocalization behavior during this time interval. No significant differences were noted for the mean scores for all auditory skills between 12 months and any intervals after 12 months. The mean scores for all auditory skills also indicated no significant differences between 24 and 36 months.

The mean scores for the three individual auditory skills in young children with Mondini dysplasia showed significant differences at pre-surgery, 1, 3, 6, and 9 months (all $p < 0.05$), but not at any other study periods 12 months onwards (Figure 5).

The differences in unaided pure tone thresholds between groups A and B

Table 3 shows the mean unaided pure tone thresholds at octave frequencies from 0.25 to 4 kHz for groups A and B before surgery. There were significant differences between the two groups at 2 kHz for either ear and at 1 kHz for the right ear ($p < 0.05$), but not at any other octave frequencies tested.

Discussion

This study showed that the auditory skills of young children with Mondini dysplasia developed rapidly over a period of 3 years after cochlear implantation, in a similar manner to those of young children with radiologically normal inner ears. Otte et al [23] suggested that there are around 36,000 spiral ganglion cells in subjects with a normal cochlea in the first decade of their lives and that at least 10,000 ganglion cells with no less than 3000 located in the apical 10 mm of the organ of Corti are necessary for speech

Table 3. Unaided pure tone thresholds of young children with radiologically normal inner ears (Group A) and young children with Mondini dysplasia (Group B).

	Left ear					**Right ear**				
Frequency(kHz)	0.25	0.5	1	2	4	0.25	0.5	1	2	4
Group A										
Mean (dB HL)	99	105	109	112	113	100	105	109	112	113
SD (dB HL)	13	11	9	10	10	12	12	10	11	11
Group B										
Mean (dB HL)	100	108	104	105	111	98	103	104	104	107
SD (dB HL)	18	12	12	11	11	17	13	12	11	12

discrimination. Other researchers suggested that the spiral ganglion cell is the vital neural element required for electrical stimulation through a cochlear prosthesis [24,25] and that a smaller number of ganglion cells may be necessary when an electrical stimulation is applied, compared to a larger number of ganglion cells being necessary when an acoustic stimulation is presented. Linthicum et al. [26] reported that two cochlear implant users with normal bony cochleae and average scores on auditory testing had only 3,212 and 3,376 surviving spiral ganglion cells, respectively. Another histological study by Schmidt [27] assessing the number of cochlear neuronal cells in ears of 20 subjects with hearing loss caused by developmental defects demonstrated that the numbers of spiral ganglion cells in Mondini dysplasia ranged from 7,677 in one case to 16,110 in another case. Although the minimum number of spiral ganglion cells necessary for response to electrical stimulation has not been ascertained, the number of cells noted in subjects with even severe Mondini dysplasia is probably large enough to trigger neural responses by electrical stimulation from a cochlear implant system [26]. In this context, this may explain why the mean scores of auditory skills were not significantly different between the two groups of subjects investigated in the current study after 1 year of implant use. Alternatively, this lack of a significant difference between the two groups may also be a consequence of similar mean unaided pure tone thresholds at each octave frequency from 0.25 to 4 kHz before cochlear implantation in the young children from both groups; which allowed the children with Mondini dysplasia to develop appropriate auditory skills relative to the young children with radiologically normal inner ears.

Furthermore, as all young children were recommended to attend regular mapping sessions and effective speech and hearing rehabilitation programs after cochlear implantation, these programs might have helped all the young children with Mondini dysplasia develop their auditory skills quite well and at similar rates when compared to the young children with radiologically normal inner ears [28,29]. Previous study has indicated that early implantation provides better opportunity for children with profound hearing loss to acquire communication skills [21]. Tone recognition and production were consistently correlated with age at implantation [30,31]. Pediatric patients should be implanted early to receive maximum benefit from a cochlear implant [30–32]. With the application of universal newborn hearing screening (UNHS) and the development in hearing diagnosis technology, it has become possible to identify children with congenital hearing loss at an early age and thus helped clinicians to diagnose and treat Mondini dysplasia patients more easily by cochlear implant surgery. This has in turn provided children with Mondini dysplasia a better opportunity to be able to develop auditory skills at an early age.

A study by Kim and colleagues [33] has indicated that although children with inner ear malformation receive considerable benefit from cochlear implants over a long period, there may be a slight delay in the development of auditory skills in these children at the early stages after cochlear implantation surgery. Our findings are in accordance with the findings of Kim and colleagues [33] in that we observed a relatively slow development of auditory skills, especially in the first year after cochlear implantation surgery in young children with Mondini dysplasia. Our findings further demonstrated that despite this delayed development in the auditory skills of children with Mondini dysplasia, they catch up with those with radiologically normal inner ears after 1 year of implant use, and show similar overall auditory skills as well as the three individual subcategories of auditory skills within the first two years after cochlear implantation. Our findings are also in accordance with those of Kim and colleagues [33] who demonstrated that the Phonetically Balanced Kindergarten test for phonemes was not statistically significant between children with inner ear malformations and those with radiologically normal inner ears at 2 years after cochlear implantation. Furthermore, the findings from the current study in children with Mondini dysplasia are consistent with our previous findings [32,34] in children with radiologically normal inner ears and large vestibular aqueduct syndrome (LVAS) that development of the three individual subcategories of auditory skills follows a similar pattern. In particular, the improvement of vocalization behavior was superior to the other two subcategories of auditory skills, especially within the first year after cochlear implantation, and the ability of deriving meaning from sounds was the slowest developed skill.

In conclusion, the findings of this study confirm that cochlear implantation is an effective intervention for young children with Mondini dysplasia, when the amplification of optimal hearing aids is insufficient. These findings further indicate that young children with Mondini dysplasia require a slightly longer time to attain appropriate auditory skills than those with radiologically normal inner ears and thus suggest that more attention should be paid to their training during the first year post implantation. Overall, these data provide a basic time-frame for speech and hearing habilitation programs for young children with Mondini dysplasia following cochlear implantation surgery and highlight the importance of early implantation in those children.

Author Contributions

Conceived and designed the experiments: XC FY DH LZ. Performed the experiments: XC FY BL SL YK JZ YL SG DH LZ. Analyzed the data: XC FY BL SL YK JZ YL SG DH LZ. Contributed reagents/materials/analysis tools: XC FY BL SL YK JZ YL SG DH LZ. Wrote the paper: XC FY DH LZ.

References

1. Antonelli PJ, Varela AE, Mancuso AA (1999) Diagnostic yield of high-resolution computed tomography for pediatric sensorineural hearing loss. Laryngoscope 109: 1642–1647.
2. McClay JE, Tandy R, Grundfast K, Choi S, Vezina G, et al. (2002) Major and minor temporal bone abnormalities in children with and without congenital sensorineural hearing loss. Arch Otolaryngol Head Neck Surg 128: 664–671.
3. Mafong DD, Shin EJ, Lalwani AK (2002) Use of laboratory evaluation and radiologic imaging in the diagnostic evaluation of children with sensorineural hearing loss. Laryngoscope 112: 1–7.
4. Wu CC, Chen YS, Chen PJ, Hsu CJ (2005) Common clinical features of children with enlarged vestibular aqueduct and Mondini dysplasia. Laryngoscope 115: 132–137.
5. Mondini C (1791) Anatomica surdi nati sectio: De Bononiensi scientarium et artium instituto atque academia commentarii. Bononiae 7: 419–428.
6. Jensen J (1967) Tomography of the inner ear in deaf children. J Laryngol Otol 81: 27–35.
7. Zheng Y, Schachern PA, Cureoglu S, Mutlu C, Dijalilian H, et al. (2002) The shortened cochlea: its classification and histopathologic features. Int J Pediatr Otorhinolaryngol 63: 29–39.
8. Sennaroglu L, Saatci I (2002) A New Classification for Cochleovestibular Malformations. Laryngoscope 112: 2230–2241.
9. Jackler RK, Luxford WM, House WF (1987) Congenital malformations of the inner ear: a classification based on embryogenesis. Laryngoscope 97: 2–14.
10. Miyamoto RT, Robbins AJ, Myres WA, Pope ML (1986) Cochlear implantation in the Mondini inner ear malformation. Am J Otol 7: 258–261.
11. Phelps PD (1992) Cochlear implants for congenital deformities. J Laryngol Otol 106: 967–970.
12. Janssens S, Govaerts PJ, Casselman J, Van Rompaey W, Van Langenhove A, et al. (1996) The LAURA multichannel cochlear implant in a true Mondini dysplasia. Eur Arch Otorhinolaryngol 253: 301–304.
13. Mangabeira-Albernaz PL (1983) The Mondini dysplasia: from early diagnosis to cochlear implant. Acta Otolaryngol 95: 627–631.

14. Suzuki C, Sando I, Fagan JJ, Kamerer DB, Knisely AS (1998) Histopathological features of a cochlear implant and otogenic meningitis in Mondini dysplasia. Arch Otolaryngol Head Neck Surg 124: 462–466.
15. Silverstein H, Smouha E, Morgan N (1988) Multichannel cochlear implantation in a patient with bilateral Mondini deformities. Am J Otol 9: 451–455.
16. Munro KJ, George CR, Haacke NP (1996) Audiological findings after multichannel cochlear implantation in patients with Mondini dysplasia. Br J Audiol 30: 369–379.
17. Li YX, Han DM, Zhao XT, Chen XQ, Kong Y, et al. (2004) Multi-channel cochlear implants in patients with Mondini malformation. Zhonghua Er Bi Yan Hou Ke Za Zhi 39: 89–92.
18. Kanchanalarp C, Cheewaruangroj W, Kasemsuwan L, Thawin C, Sriwanyong S (2005) Pediatric cochlear implantation: experience in Thai patients. J Med Assoc Thai 88: 484–491.
19. Arnoldner C, Baumgartner WD, Gstoettner W, Egelierler B, Czerny C, et al. (2004) Audiological performance after cochlear implantation in children with inner ear malformations. Int J Pediatr Otorhinolaryngol 68: 457–467.
20. Osberger MJ, Geier L, Zimmerman-Phillips S, Barker MJ (1997) Use of a parent-report scale to assess benefit in children given the Clarion cochlear implant. Am J Otol 18: S79–80.
21. Robbins AM, Koch DB, Osberger MJ, Zimmerman-Phillips S, Kishon-Rabin L (2004) Effect of age at cochlear implantation on auditory skill development in infants and toddlers. Arch Otolaryngol Head Neck Surg 130: 570–574.
22. Studebaker GA (1985) A "rationalized" arcsine transform. J Speech Hear Res 28: 455–462.
23. Otte J, Schuknecht HF, Kerr AG (1978) Ganglion cell populations in normal and pathological human cochleae. Implications for cochlear implantation. Laryngoscope 88: 1231–1246.
24. Clopton BM, Spelman FA, Miller JM (1980) Estimates of essential neural elements for stimulation through cochlear prostheses. Ann Otol RhinolLaryngol Suppl 89: 5–7.
25. Kiang NY, Eddington DK, Delgutte B (1979) Fundamental considerations in designing auditory implants. Acta Otolaryngol 87: 204–218.
26. Linthicum FH, Fayad J, Otto S, Galey FR, House W (1991) Inner ear morphological changes resulting from cochlear implantation. Am J Otol 12: 8–10.
27. Schmidt JM (1985) Cochlear neuronal populations in developmental defects of the inner ear: implications for cochlear implantation. Acta Otolaryngol 99: 14–20.
28. Rance G, Dowell RC (1997) Speech processor programming. In: Clark GM, Cowan RSC, Dowell RC, editors. Cochlear implantation for infants and children: advances. San Diego, California: Singular Publishing Group, Inc. pp.147–170.
29. Barker EJ, Dettman SJ, Dowell RC (1997) Habilitation: infants and young children. In: Clark GM, Cowan RSC, Dowell RC, editors. Cochlear implantation for infants and children: advances. San Diego, California: Singular Publishing Group, Inc. pp.171–190.
30. Han D, Liu B, Zhou N, Chen X, Kong Y, et al. (2009) Lexical tone perception with HiResolution and HiResolution 120 sound-processing strategies in pediatric Mandarin-speaking cochlear implant users. Ear Hear 30: 169–177.
31. Zhou N, Huang J, Chen X, Xu L (2013) Relationship between tone perception and production in prelingually deafened children with cochlear implants. Otol Neurotol 34: 499–506.
32. Chen X, Liu S, Liu B, Mo L, Kong Y, et al. (2010) The effects of age at cochlear implantation and hearing aid trial on auditory performance of Chinese infants. Acta Otolaryngol 130: 263–270.
33. Kim LS, Jeong SW, Huh MJ, Park YD (2006) Cochlear implantation in children with inner ear malformations. Ann Otol Rhinol Laryngol 115: 205–214.
34. Chen X, Liu B, Liu S, Mo L, Liu H, et al. (2011) The development of auditory skills in infants with isolated Large Vestibular Aqueduct Syndrome after cochlear implantation. Int J Pediatr Otorhinolaryngol 75: 943–947.

19

Diet-Induced Obesity Exacerbates Auditory Degeneration via Hypoxia, Inflammation, and Apoptosis Signaling Pathways in CD/1 Mice

Juen-Haur Hwang[1,2,3], **Chuan-Jen Hsu**[4], **Wei-Hsuan Yu**[5], **Tien-Chen Liu**[4*], **Wei-Shiung Yang**[1,6,7*]

1 Graduate Institute of Clinical Medicine, College of Medicine, National Taiwan University, Taipei, Taiwan, **2** Department of Otolaryngology, Buddhist Dalin Tzu-Chi General Hospital, Chiayi, Taiwan, **3** School of Medicine, Tzu Chi University, Hualien, Taiwan, **4** Department of Otolaryngology, National Taiwan University, Hospital, Taipei, Taiwan, **5** Institute of Biochemistry and Molecular Biology, College of Medicine, National Taiwan University, Taipei, Taiwan, **6** Department of Internal Medicine, National Taiwan University, Hospital, Taipei, Taiwan, **7** Research Center for Developmental Biology and Regenerative Medicine, National Taiwan University, Taipei, Taiwan

Abstract

The aim of this study was to investigate the mechanisms of diet-induced obesity on hearing degeneration in CD/1 mice. Sixty 4-week-old male CD/1 mice were randomly and equally divided into 2 groups. For 16 weeks, the diet-induced obesity (DIO) group was fed a high fat diet and the control group was fed a standard diet of 13.43 % kcal fat. The morphometry, biochemistry, auditory brainstem response thresholds, omental fat, and histopathology of the cochlea were compared between the beginning and end of the study (4 vs. 20 weeks old). The results show that the body weight, fasting plasma triglyceride concentrations, and omental fat weight were higher in the DIO group than in the control group at the end of experiment. The auditory brainstem response thresholds at high frequencies were significantly elevated in the DIO group compared to those of the control group. Histology studies showed that, compared to the control group, the DIO group had blood vessels with smaller diameters and thicker walls in the stria vascularis at the middle and basal turns of the cochlea. The cell densities in the spiral ganglion and spiral ligament at the basal turn of the cochlea were significantly lower in the DIO group. Immunohistochemical staining showed that hypoxia-induced factor 1 (HIF-1), tumor necrosis factor alpha (TNF-α), nuclear factor kappa B (NF-κB), caspase 3, poly(ADP-ribose) polymerase-1, and apoptosis inducing factor were all significantly more dense in the spiral ganglion and spiral ligament at the basal turn of cochlea in the DIO group. Our results suggest that diet-induced obesity exacerbates hearing degeneration via increased hypoxia, inflammatory responses, and cell loss in the spiral ganglion and spiral ligament and is associated with the activation of both caspase-dependent and -independent apoptosis signaling pathways in CD/1 mice.

Editor: Guillermo López-Lluch, Universidad Pablo de Olavide, Centro Andaluz de Biología del Desarrollo-CSIC, Spain

Funding: This project was supported by grant DTCRD-98 (2)-03 from the Buddhist Dalin Tzu Chi General Hospital. The funders had no role in study design, data collection and analysis, decision to publish, or preparation of the manuscript.

Competing Interests: The authors have declared that no competing interests exist.

* E-mail: wsyang@ntu.edu.tw (WSY); liuent@ntu.edu.tw (TCL)

Introduction

Obesity-related cardiometabolic disorders are known to be associated with hearing impairment [1-5]. Whether obesity per se could lead to hearing impairment was uncertain until the recent publication of 2 independent studies [6,7]. In a European population-based multicenter study, occupational noise, smoking, and a high body mass index (BMI) were found to be risk factors for hearing impairment [6]. Our own epidemiological study also showed that waist circumference (WC), a measurement of visceral or central obesity, is an independent risk factor for hearing impairment in Taiwanese [7]. However, the detailed mechanisms of obesity-related hearing impairment have seldom been explored. Obesity has been hypothesized to directly impair the function of many organ systems via obesity-related oxidative stress and lipotoxicity [8–10]. Obesity-induced inflammation also results in the infiltration of macrophages and the release of proinflammatory cytokines, which could exacerbate end-organ damage and cell apoptosis in the heart, kidney, pancreas, liver, and skeletal muscle via the caspase-dependent signaling pathway [10]. Lipotoxicity can also lead to cell death via caspase-independent signaling pathways, as demonstrated in pancreatic beta-cell lines [11]. However, no reports have addressed the effects of lipotoxicity and its related apoptosis signaling pathways on the peripheral auditory organ.

In this study, we aimed to address the possible mechanisms of diet-induced obesity (DIO) on hearing impairment in CD/1 mice. The CD/1 mouse strain is particularly well-suited to this type of study because these mice have early onset of hearing impairment, beginning at 4 weeks of age. This feature allowed us to observe the effects of DIO on hearing degeneration earlier in the lifespan of the mice, thus avoiding biochemical insults other than obesity itself [12]. In the cochlea of CD/1 mice, a prominent decline in spiral ganglion (SG) neuron density occurs at a young age. By the age of 6 months, these mice have a severe loss of SG neurons and fibrocytes in spiral ligaments (SL) and the Organ of Corti in the cochlear basal turn [12–14]. The mechanisms of degeneration in the SG may involve hypoxia, oxidative stress damage, increased expression of TNF-α, loss of neuronal protection, and activation of the caspase-dependent cell apoptosis signaling pathway [13]. No studies have investigated caspase-independent apoptosis signaling pathways in the auditory system of CD/1 mice.

We hypothesized that DIO could exacerbate hearing degeneration in CD/1 mice by increasing cochlear hypoxia and inflammation. In addition, a high fat diet might increase cell death in the inner ear through activation of both caspase-dependent and -independent apoptosis signaling pathways.

Results

Table 1 shows that the baseline characteristics of the control and DIO groups were not significantly different at the beginning of the study. ABR thresholds were very similar between the 2 groups, as determined by click sounds using 8 kHz, 16 kHz, and 32 kHz tone bursts.

Table 2 compares the control and DIO groups at the end of the study (20 weeks of age). BW (55.6±8.0 vs. 46.8±6.8 g; Student's t-test, p = 0.0002) and omental fat weight (2.6±0.7 vs. 1.4±1.1 g; Student's t-test, p = 0.0106) were significantly higher in the DIO group than in the control group. Fasting plasma TG was elevated significantly in the DIO group compared to the control group. Fasting HDL and glucose were not significantly different between the 2 groups. Both groups showed elevated ABR thresholds at the end of the study compared to those at the beginning at all frequencies tested. However, the ABR threshold was significantly higher in the DIO group than in the control group at 32 k Hz [98.7±1.0 vs. 92.5±4.6 dB sound pressure level (SPL); Student's t-test, p = 0.0080] and 16kHz sound stimulation (78.3±13.2 vs. 70.5±9.2 dB SPL; Student's t-test, p = 0.0240), and of borderline significance at 8 kHz (69.6±11.5 vs. 64.0±8.5 dB SPL; Student's t-test, p = 0.0637). However, the threshold was not significantly different between the 2 groups as determined by click sound stimulation, which reflects the thresholds around 4 kHz. These findings suggest that diet-induced obesity exacerbated hearing degeneration in CD/1 mice, especially at higher frequencies.

The mean thickness of the SV was not significantly different between the 2 groups at any of the 3 turns (Table 3). However, the mean internal diameter of vessels in the SV was significantly smaller in the DIO group than in the control group at the middle turn (3.9±0.3 vs. 4.8±0.5 μm; Student's t-test, p<0.0001) and the basal turn (3.7±0.5 vs. 4.5±0.5 μm; Student's t-test, p<0.0001). The ratio of the mean vessel wall thickness to its radius in the SV was significantly larger in the DIO group than in the control group at the middle turn (30.2±4.8 % vs. 27.3±5.0 %; Student's t-test, p = 0.0535) and basal turn (31.9±4.2 % vs. 28.3±2.9 %; Student's t-test, p = 0.0004).

The density of SG neurons was significantly lower in the DIO group (9.8±2.5/50 μm^2) than in the control group (12.0±3.6/ 50 μm^2) at the basal turn of the cochlea (Wilcoxon rank-sum test, p = 0.0092), but not at the middle turn or the apex.

The density of fibrocytes in the lower part of the SL was lower of borderline significance in the DIO group (6.5±2.6/50 μm^2) than in the control group (8.6±3.2/50 μm^2) at the basal turn of the cochlea (Wilcoxon rank-sum test, p = 0.0515), but not at the middle turn or the apex.

In the Organ of Corti, IHC and OHCs degenerated mildly at the apex and moderately at the middle and basal turns, but the extent of OHC loss was similar in both groups (Table 3).

Figures 1a and b show a representative radial section of HIF-1α staining in the basal turn of the cochlea. HIF-1α was expressed moderately in SG and OHCs and mildly in SL, SV, and IHC in both groups. Compared to the control group, the DIO group showed significantly increased HIF-1α staining in the SG (65.8±16.7% vs. 50.0±19.7%; Wilcoxon rank-sum test, p = 0.0292) (Figure 1c).

Figures 1d and e show a representative radial section of TNF-α staining in the basal turn of the cochlea. TNF-α was expressed moderately in the SG and SL and mildly in the SV and the Organ of Corti of the cochlea in both groups. Compared to the control group, the DIO group showed significantly increased TNF-α staining in the SG (80.2±17.9% vs. 67.5±21.0%; Wilcoxon rank-sum test, p = 0.0118) (Figure 1f) and the SL (88.6±8.9% vs. 74.6±22.6%; Wilcoxon rank-sum test, p = 0.0374) (Figure 1f).

Figures 1g and h show a representative radial section of NF-κB staining in the basal turn of the cochlea. NF-κB expression was high in the SG, SL, and OHCs, and moderate in the SV and IHC in both groups. Compared to the control group, the DIO group showed significantly increased NF-κB staining in the SG (93.7±6.7% vs. 87.7±12.7%; Wilcoxon rank-sum test, p = 0.0453) (Figure 1i) and the SL (91.5±9.5% vs.81.5±16.4%; Wilcoxon rank-sum test, p = 0.0368) (Figure 1i).

Figures 2a and b show a representative radial section of caspase 3 staining in the basal turn of the cochlea. Caspase 3 was stained intensely in the SG and SL, mildly in the SV, and moderately in the Organ of Corti in both groups. Compared to the control

Table 1. Baseline characteristics of the both groups at the beginning of this study.

Mean±SD	Control group (n = 30)	DIO group (n = 30)	p values*
BW (gm)	28.1±2.4	27.6±3.6	0.6724
Plasma biochemistry			
TG (mg/dl)	83.7±9.3	87.5±11.6	0.6602
HDL-C (mg/dl)	117.1±25.1	122.9±24.4	0.7710
Glucose (mg/dl)	147.0±47.0	128.3±31.1	0.5493
ABR thresholds (dB SPL)			
Click sound	49.3±4.8	52.2±3.8	0.3109
8 kHz tone burst	37.0±8.5	36.3±8.2	0.9041
16 kHz tone burst	47.3±1.5	48.5±5.5	0.6728
32 kHz tone burst	55.2± 4.6	54.5± 3.8	0.7354

Abbreviations: SD: standard deviation; DIO: diet-induced obesity; BW: body weight; TG: triglyceride; HDL-C: high-density lipoprotein cholesterol; ABR: auditory brainstem response.
*Student's t-test.

Table 2. Comparisons of the both groups at the end of this study.

Mean±SD	Control group (n = 30)	DIO group (n = 30)	p values*
BW (gm)	46.8±6.8	55.6±8.0	0.0002
Omentum fat (gm)	1.4±1.1	2.7±0.7	0.0106
Plasma biochemistry			
TG (mg/dl)	83.5±21.3	101.9±27.9	0.0380
HDL-C (mg/dl)	96.5±51.8	90.0±43.2	0.6314
Glucose (mg/dl)	199.0±36.5	197.0±70.0	0.9077
ABR thresholds (dB SPL)			
Click sound	66.6±8.3	70.9±11.9	0.1654
8 kHz tone burst	64.0±8.5	69.6±11.5	0.0637
16 kHz tone burst	70.5±9.2	78.3±13.2	0.0240
32 kHz tone burst	92.5±4.6	98.7±1.0	0.0080

Abbreviations: SD: standard deviation; DIO: diet-induced obesity; BW: body weight; TG: triglyceride; HDL-C: high-density lipoprotein cholesterol; ABR: auditory brainstem response.
*Student's t-test.

group, the DIO group showed increased caspase 3 staining in the SG (93.8±6.6 % vs. 88.6±11.1%; Wilcoxon rank-sum test, p = 0.0635) (Figure 2c) and significantly in the SL (94.7±6.5% vs. 88.3±7.2%; Wilcoxon rank-sum test, p = 0.0009) (Figure 2c).

Figures 2d and e show a representative radial section of PARP-1 staining in the basal turn of the cochlea. PARP-1 was stained intensely in the SG, moderately in the SL and the Organ of Corti, and mildly in the SV of the cochlea in both groups. Compared to the control group, the DIO group showed significantly increased PARP-1staining in the SG (92.8±5.9% vs. 87.8±4.6%; Wilcoxon rank-sum test, p = 0.0030) (Figure 2f) and the SL (66.4±10.6% vs. 59.8±9.2%; Wilcoxon rank-sum test, p = 0.0101) (Figure 2f).

Figures 2g and h show a representative radial section of AIF staining in the basal turn of the cochlea. AIF was stained intensely in the SG and SL and moderately in the SV and the Organ of Corti in both groups. Compared to the control group, the DIO group showed significantly increased AIF staining in the SG (95.7±5.2% vs. 92.5±3.0%; Wilcoxon rank-sum test, p = 0.0050) (Figure 2i) and the SL (97.0±3.9% vs. 94.4±4.5%; Wilcoxon rank-sum test, p = 0.0520) (Figure 2i).

Discussion

This animal study demonstrates that a high fat diet can lead to body weight gain, abdominal fat accumulation, elevated plasma TG, and elevated hearing thresholds (especially at high frequencies) in CD/1 mice. The most notable histological findings resulting from a high fat diet were narrowed blood vessels in the SV, increased inflammatory responses, and increased cell loss in the SG and SL in the basal turn of the cochlea. Furthermore, a high fat diet also resulted in cell death via activation of both caspase-dependent and -independent apoptosis signaling pathways.

Previous studies have shown that genetic susceptibility and environmental factors including noise, ototoxic medication, chemical exposure, tobacco, hormone replacement therapy, diabetes mellitus (DM), hypertension (HTN), dyslipidemia, and socioeconomic status were associated with peripheral hearing dysfunction in humans [16,17]. Recently, BMI [6] and WC [7] were reported to be novel independent risk factors for hearing impairment in humans. The concentration of plasma adiponectin, one of the anti-inflammatory adipocytokines, was also shown to be negatively associated with hearing threshold in humans [18].

Lee et al. [19] reported that *ob/ob* mice, a model for type 2 diabetes and obesity [20], exhibited early sensorineural hearing loss. Vasilyeva et al. [21] reported that the hearing functions of CBA/CaJ mice with type 2 DM (HFD-induced) degenerated more rapidly than those of CBA/CaJ mice with type 1 DM (streptozotocin-induced), even though blood glucose levels were higher in type 1 DM mice. We therefore propose that, in addition to glucotoxicity, obesity itself and its related lipotoxicity might be responsible for hearing impairment.

Previous animal studies and our current study have all shown that a high fat diet can lead to hearing impairment through cochlear microangiopathy, neuropathy, and/or damage to the Organ of Corti [22,23]. Loss of SG cells and degeneration of outer hair cells were observed in the middle and basal turns of the cochlea in *ob/ob* mice [19]. The pathological findings of the current study were similar to those observed in *ob/ob* mice in Lee's study [19]. Their study found that obesity in *ob/ob* mice was caused by leptin deficiency and that hyperglycemia might confound the process of hearing degeneration. In contrast, diet-induced obesity in our study often presented with hyperleptinemia [24], which reflects the actual state that commonly occurs in human obesity [25]. Secondly, plasma TG was only slightly higher in the DIO group than in the control group in our study. Thus, our results were less confounded by plasma glucose concentrations.

Apoptosis is regulated by at least two important signaling pathways: caspase-dependent and caspase-independent. Caspase 3 is the effector in the caspase-dependent apoptosis signaling pathway, whereas PARP-1, AIF, and endonuclease G (EndoG) play key roles in the caspase-independent apoptosis signaling pathway. Oxidative stress or reactive oxidative species can cause DNA damage and activate PARP-1, which enters mitochondria and activates AIF. During apoptosis, AIF is released from the mitochondrial intermembrane space to the cytosol and nucleus, independent of Bid for mitochondrial release, activating EndoG and finally leading to cell death [26]. AIF plays a key role in neurodegenerative diseases [27] and several other disease processes [28,29]. For example, AIF and mitochondrial fusion might play important roles in cerebellar Purkinje cell loss in Harlequin mice [30], seizure-induced neuronal death [31],

Table 3. Observations of cochlear sections by H&E stain in both groups at the end of this study.

Mean±SD	Control	DIO	p value*
SV thickness (μm)			
Apical turn	17.3±2.4	15.4±3.5	0.1015
Middle turn	17.8±2.1	17.7±2.9	0.8898
Basal turn	17.1±3.6	17.2±2.5	0.9519
Internal diameter of vessels in SV(μm)			
Apical turn	4.6±0.6	4.0±0.5	0.0008
Middle turn	4.8±0.5	3.9±0.3	<0.0001
Basal turn	4.5±0.5	3.7±0.5	<0.0001
Vessel wall to radius ratio in SV (%)			
Apical turn	29.6±1.6	30. 1±4.3	0.7683
Middle turn	27.3±5.0	30.2±4.8	0.0535
Basal turn	28.3±2.9	31.9±4.2	0.0004
Cell density of SG (/50 μm^2)			
Apical turn	9.9±3.8	9.6±3.3	0.7691
Middle turn	12.8±3.8	11.6±3.0	0.0915
Basal turn	12.0±3.6	9.8±2.5	0.0092
Cell density of SL (/50 μm^2)			
Apical turn	8.4±3.3	7.4±3.0	0.3110
Middle turn	9.8±3.2	8.2±3.0	0.2941
Basal turn	8.6±3.2	6.5±2.6	0.0515
IHC			
Apical turn	0.6±0.5	0.8±0.4	0.3953
Middle turn	0.6±0.4	0.8±0.3	0.1917
Basal turn	0.5±0.3	0.6±0.3	0.3202
OHCs			
Apical turn	2.0±1.2	2.1±0.8	0.8931
Middle turn	2.1±1.0	2.1±0.6	0.8125
Basal turn	1.2±0.7	0.8±0.8	0.1010

Abbreviations: SD: standard deviation; DIO: diet-induced obesity; SV: stria vascularis; SG: spiral ganglion; SL: spiral ligament; IHC: inner hair cell; OHCs: outer hair cells.
N = 30 for all observations except for the apical turn (n = 14).
*Student's t-test for SV thickness, internal diameter of vessels in SV, and vessel wall to radius ratio in SV. Wilcoxon rank-sum test for other items.

apoptosis of retinal cells in RCS rats [28], and apoptosis of semitendinosus muscle cells in older humans [29].

In fact, both caspase-dependent and -independent apoptotic mitochondrial pathways may be involved in many diseases, including ischemia/reperfusion-related brain damage [26,32], death of dopaminergic neurons in the substantia nigra of Parkinson's disease patients [33], and retinitis pigmentosa [34]. Lipotoxicity could also lead to cell apoptosis via caspase-dependent and -independent signaling pathways in pancreatic beta-cell lines [11].

Riva et al. [13] reported that the mechanisms of cochlear degeneration in CD/1 mice involve hypoxia, increased HIF-1α and oxidative stress, increased expression of TNF-α, and increased cell death in the cochlea. The Schwann cells of the SG were observed to be more vulnerable to free radical damage than were the neurons, and they degenerated more rapidly in CD/1 mice [13]. The signaling pathway responsible for cell apoptosis in the cochlea of CD/1 mice involved the activation of caspase-3 and Bax-mediated apoptosis via p53 protein accumulation [13]. Here, our results show that obesity increased hypoxic (HIF-1α) and inflammatory responses (TNF-α and NF-κB) in the cochlea of CD/1 mice, especially in the SG and SL. Diet-induced obesity also increased apoptosis of inner ear cells via caspase-independent signaling pathways in CD/1 mice.

It may be argued that diet-induced obesity exacerbates hearing dysfunction indirectly via its co-morbidities [1–5]. As mentioned in the introduction, we chose CD/1 mice as the animal model for this study to allow earlier detection of hearing degeneration and to avoid potential interference from other metabolic abnormalities [12]. However, we still cannot entirely exclude these possibilities. Although the fasting plasma glucose and HDL were similar in both groups, lipotoxicity might occur earlier than glucotoxicity in the pathogenesis of diabetic mellitus, as reported in previous studies [35]. Obesity is independently associated with increased risk of CKD in non-diabetic and non-hypertensive adults [36,37]. Central obesity or waist circumference has been reported to independently predict both CKD and end-stage renal diseases [38]. Obesity is also reported to interact with non–insulin-dependent diabetes mellitus in affecting cochlear dysfunction [21,39]. Therefore, we believe that obesity itself might also cause hearing impairment early and directly via lipotoxicity.

There are some limitations in this study. While the mice in the control group were fed a standard diet, some of them became overweight at the end of the study, possibly confounding the results. A lean control group is needed to determine the extent to which auditory degeneration is truly influenced by weight gain. Another limitation of the study is that the control and DIO groups were not consuming the same diet. It is difficult to determine whether the observed differences in ABR and histopathology are due to weight gain or the intake of dietary fat.

In conclusion, diet-induced obesity could exacerbate the hearing impairment observed in CD/1 mice. The most notable histological findings were narrowed blood vessels in the SV, increased inflammatory responses, and increased cell loss in the SG and SL (especially in the basal turn of the cochlea) in CD/1 mice. A high fat diet might increase the death of inner ear cells by activating both caspase-dependent and caspase-independent apoptosis signaling pathways.

Materials and Methods

Animals

Sixty 4-week-old male CD/1 mice (BioLASCO Taiwan Co., Ltd.) with normal external and middle ear parameters were used in these experiments. The mice had hearing thresholds≤50 decibel sound pressure level (dB SPL) as determined by sound stimulation using 8 kHz tone bursts.

The mice were randomly divided into two groups at the age of 4 weeks. For 16 weeks, the "DIO" group was fed the AIN-93G modified diet to provide 60% of the calories from fat (DIO Series Diets: D12492, Research Diets Company, NJ, U.S.A.) and the "control" group was fed the AIN-93G standard diet, which provides 13.43 % of the calories from fat (Fwusow Industry Co., Ltd, Taiwan).

Animals were housed with 5 mice per cage in a temperature-controlled room on a constant 12 hr light/dark cycle. Food and tap water were available freely throughout the experiments. The Institutional Animal Care and Use Committee of Buddhist Dalin Tzu Chi General hospital approved the protocol used in this study.

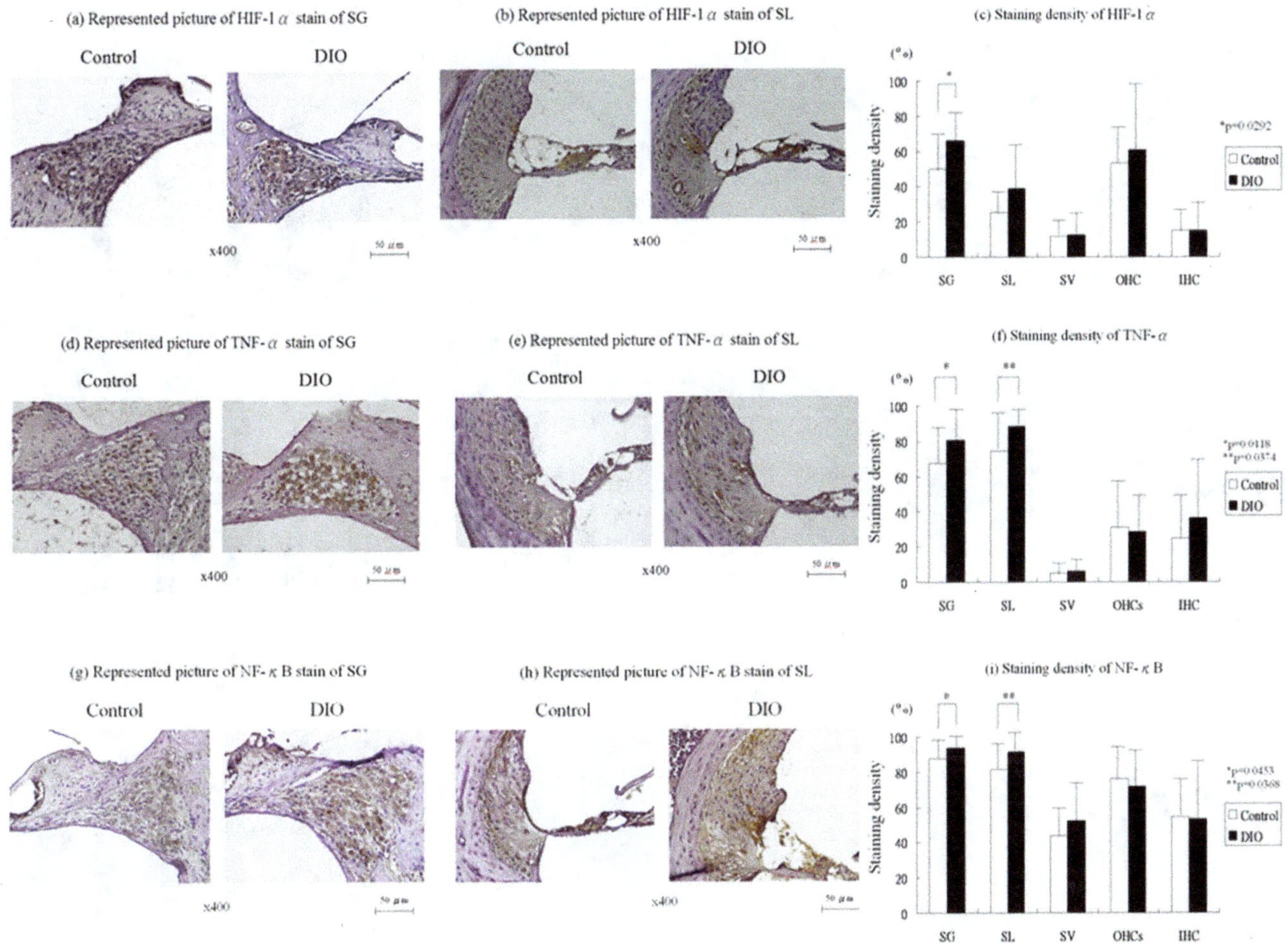

Figure 1. Immunohistochemical studies of cochlea. Representative radial section of hypoxia-induced factor (HIF) 1-α staining in the cochlear basal turn (a,b). The intensity of HIF-1α stain was significantly greater in the DIO group than in the control group in the SG and SL (c). Representative radial section of TNF-α stain in the cochlear basal turn (d,e). The intensity of tumor necrosis factor (TNF)-α stain was significantly tenser in the DIO group than in the control group in SG and SL (f). Representative radial section of NF-κB stain in the cochlear basal turn (g,h). The intensity of nuclear factor kappaB (NF-κB) stain was significantly greater in the DIO group than in the control group in SG and SL (i).

Body weight, plasma biochemistry and auditory brainstem responses (ABR)

Body weight (BW), plasma biochemistry, and ABR were measured at the beginning (at 4 weeks old) and end of the study (at 20 weeks old) under general anesthesia by intraperitoneal injection of pentobarbital (35 mg/kg).

ABR was conducted in a double-walled, soundproof booth. Click sounds and tone bursts (8 kHz, 16 kHz, and 32 kHz) were delivered sequentially via earphones (Telephonics Corp., Farmingdale, NY). Hearing thresholds of these four stimuli were determined by the presence of ABR waves (Intelligent Hearing Systems, Miami, FL).

After an overnight fast, blood samples (about 1.0 ml) were obtained by medial canthus puncture, and the blood was placed in heparin-coated capillary tubes. The plasma was retrieved immediately after centrifugation and was sent for biochemical analysis. Plasma glucose, triglyceride (TG), and high density lipoprotein (HDL) concentrations were measured by hexokinase-glucose-6-phosphate dehydrogenase method, enzymatic method, and homogeneous method using SIEMENS Dimension RxL Max. Chemistry Ananlyzer (SIEMENS), respectively.

Omental fat weight and histology of the cochlea

At the end of the study, omental fat was excised for weight measurements under general anesthesia with intraperitoneal injection of pentobarbital (35 mg/kg).

Animals were intracardially perfused with 2.5% glutaraldehyde and 4% paraformaldehyde in phosphate buffered saline (PBS: NaCl, 150 mM; KH2PO4, 2 mM; Na2HPO4 2H2O, 8 mM, pH 7.4) before being euthanized. The temporal bones were removed, and the cochlea was perfused with the above fixative through the oval and round windows to an outlet in the apex. After 24-hr post-fixation in the same fixative at 4°C, the temporal bones were decalcified in 10% EDTA solution, 4% paraformaldehyde, and 2.5% glutaraldehyde in PBS (pH 7.4) for 1 week at room temperature. The temporal bones were then rinsed in PBS, dehydrated through a graded series of alcohol and xylene, and embedded in paraffin. Embedded cochleae were sectioned at 5 μm thickness and the cochlear structures were observed at the mid-modiolar level using a light microscope.

Hematoxylin and Eosin (H & E) staining. The density of SG neurons and fibrocytes in the lower part of the SL within a central region of 50×50 μm^2 were measured under ×400 magnification. The thickness of the middle part of the stria

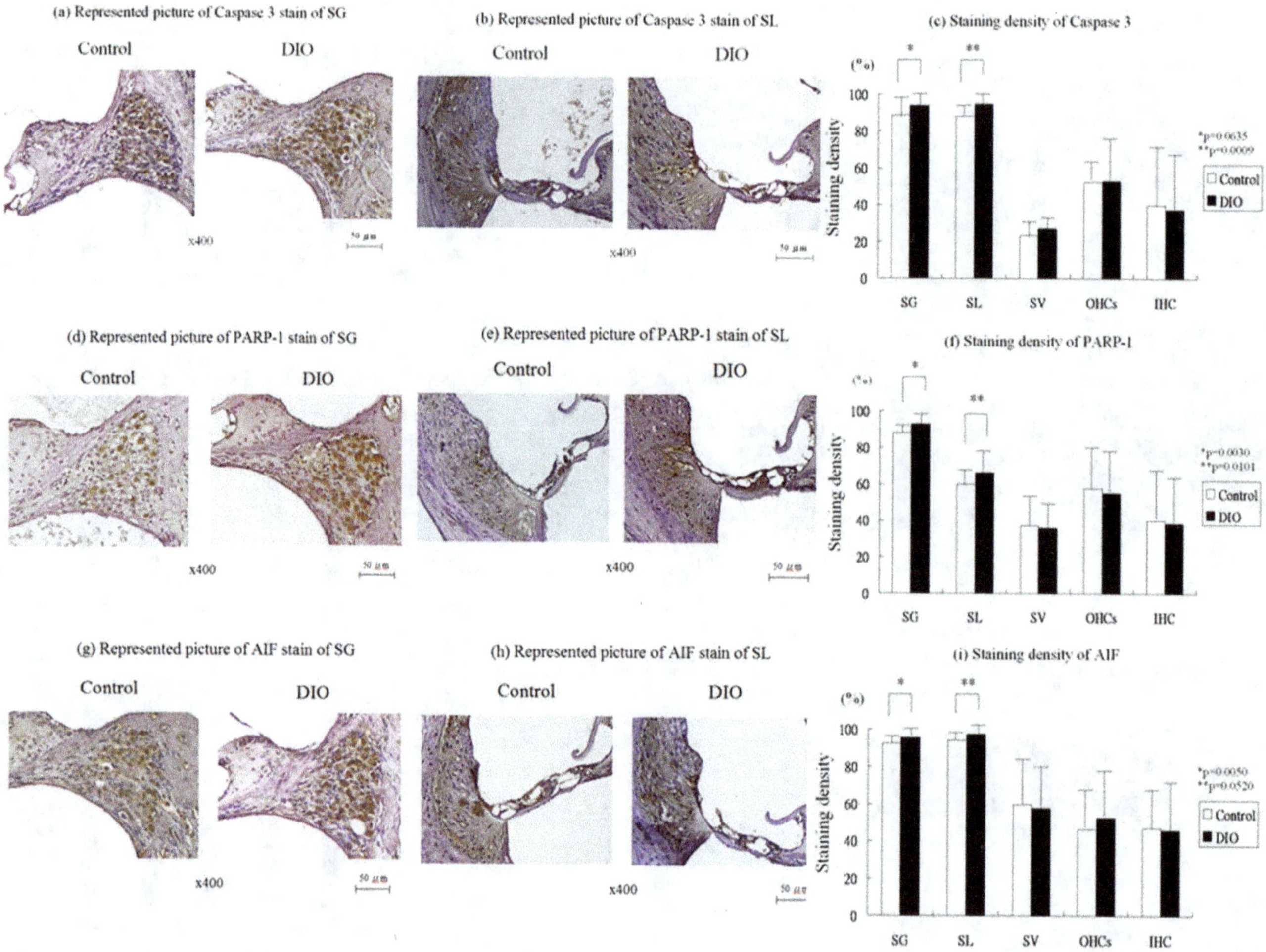

Figure 2. Immunohistochemical studies of cochlea. Representative radial section of caspase 3 staining in the cochlear basal turn (a,b). The intensity of caspase 3 stain was significantly tenser in the DIO group than in the control group in SG and SL (c). Representative radial section of poly(ADP-ribose) polymerase-1 (PARP-1) stain in the cochlear basal turn (d,e). The intensity of PARP-1 stain was significantly greater in the DIO group than in the control group in SG and SL (f). Representative radial section of apoptosis inducing factor (AIF) stain in the cochlear basal turn (g,h). The intensity of AIF stain was significantly tenser in the DIO group than in the control group in SG and SL (i).

vascularis (SV), the mean internal diameter, and the vessel wall to radius ratio of the SV vessels in the SV were calculated under ×400 magnification. The morphology and numbers of outer and inner hair cells in the Organ of Corti were observed under ×400 magnification.

The above features were observed in two adjacent cochlear sections at the same mid-modiolar level and averaged for each mouse.

Immunohistochemical staining. The sections were heat-treated at 95°C in 10 mM sodium citrate buffer for 20 min, incubated in 3% H_2O_2 for 10 min at room temperature, and blocked in 5% skim milk to prevent non-specific labeling. The specimens were then incubated overnight at 4°C with one of the following primary antibodies: mouse monoclonal anti-hypoxia-induced factor (HIF) 1-α (1:250 dilution) (Abcam plc, Cambridge, U.K.), rabbit polyclonal anti-tumor necrosis factor (TNF)-α (1:500 dilution) (Abbiotec, LLC, San Diego, U.S.A.), rabbit polyclonal anti-nuclear factor kappaB (NF-κB) p65 (1:1000 dilution) (Abcam plc, Cambridge, U.K.), rabbit anti-caspase 3 (1:500 dilution) (R&D systems, Inc., U.S.A.), rabbit monoclonal anti-poly(ADP-ribose) polymerase-1 (PARP-1) (1:500 dilution) (Abcam plc, Cambridge, U.K.), or rabbit anti-apoptosis inducing factor (AIF) (1:1000 dilution) (R&D systems, Inc., U.S.A.). Slides were washed in PBS three times, exposed to a secondary antibody for 1 h at room temperature, and stained using the DAB staining kit (R&D systems, Inc., U.S.A.) according to the manufacturer's protocol. Slides were dehydrated, mounted, and observed through a light microscope. The images were acquired using a CCD camera (Dage-MTI Inc, Michigan City, Ind) connected to a personal computer and analyzed using image analysis software (Image-Pro Plus, version 6.0; Media Cybernetics, Silver Springs, MD).

The structures in question were observed in two adjacent cochlear sections at the same mid-modiolar level and averaged for each mouse. Stained regions were quantified as the percentage of the entire target area [15].

Statistical analysis

The data were presented as means±standard deviation (SD) unless indicated otherwise. BW, biochemistry, omental fat weight, ABR thresholds, and histological findings were compared between the two study groups using the Student's t-test if the data show a normal distribution or Wilcoxon rank-sum test if the data did not show a normal distribution. All analyses were performed using

STATA 10.0 software (Stata Corp, L.P., College Station, TX). P values<0.05 were considered statistically significant.

Author Contributions

Conceived and designed the experiments: JHH. Performed the experiments: JHH. Analyzed the data: JHH. Contributed reagents/materials/analysis tools: CJH WHY TCL WSY. Wrote the paper: JHH.

References

1. Evans MB, Tonini R, Shope CD, Oghalai JS, Jerger JF, et al. (2006) Dyslipidemia and auditory function. Otol Neurotol. 27: 609–614.
2. Frisina ST, Mapes F, Kim S, Frisina DR, Frisina RD (2006) Characterization of hearing loss in aged type II diabetics. Hear Res. 211: 103–113.
3. Friedland DR, Cederberg C, Tarima S (2009) Audiometric pattern as a predictor of cardiovascular status: development of a model for assessment of risk. *Laryngoscope* 119: 473–486.
4. Hwang JH, Chen JC, Hsu CJ, Liu TC (2011) Association of obstructive sleep apnea and auditory dysfunctions in older subjects. *Otolaryngol Head Neck Surg* 144: 114–119.
5. Hwang JH, Ho HC, Hsu MC, Chen JC (2011) Effect of transient ischemic attack on hearing thresholds of older subjects. *Audiol Neurotol EXTRA* 1: 1–8.
6. Fransen E, Topsakal V, Hendrickx JJ, Van Laer L, Huyghe JR, et al. (2008) Occupational Noise, Smoking, and a High Body Mass Index are Risk Factors for Age-related Hearing Impairment and Moderate Alcohol Consumption is Protective: A European Population-based Multicenter Study. *J Assoc Res Otolaryngol.* 9: 264–276.
7. Hwang JH, Wu CC, Hsu CJ, Liu TC, Yang WS (2009) Association of central obesity with the severity and audiometric configurations of age-related hearing impairment. *Obesity* 17:1796–1801.
8. Jackson AW, Lee DC, Sui X, Morrow JR Jr, Church TS, et al. (2010) Muscular Strength Is Inversely Related to Prevalence and Incidence of Obesity in Adult Men. *Obesity* 18: 1988–1995.
9. Kabrhel C, Varraso R, Goldhaber SZ, Rimm EB, Camargo CA (2009) Prospective Study of BMI and the Risk of Pulmonary Embolism in Women. *Obesity* 17: 2040–2046.
10. Schaffer JE (2003) Lipotoxicity: when tissues overeat. *Curr Opin Lipidol.* 14: 281–287.
11. Maestre I, Jordán J, Calvo S, Reig JA, Ceña V, et al. (2003) Mitochondrial dysfunction is involved in apoptosis induced by serum withdrawal and fatty acids in the beta-cell line INS-1. *Endocrinology* 144: 335–345.
12. Shone G, Raphael Y, Miller JM (1991) Hereditary deafness occurring in cd/1 mice. *Hear Res.* 57: 153–156.
13. Riva C, Donadieu E, Magnan J, Lavieille JP (2007) Age-related hearing loss in CD/1 mice is associated to ROS formation and HIF target proteins up-regulation in the cochlea. *Exp Gerontol.* 42: 327–336.
14. Wu T, Marcus DC (2003) Age-related changes in cochlear endolymphatic potassium and potential in CD-1 and CBA/CaJ mice. *J Assoc Res Otolaryngol.* 4: 353–362.
15. Lin YS, Chen CM, Soong BW, Wu YR, Chen HM, et al. (2011) Dysregulated brain creatine kinase is associated with hearing impairment in mouse models of Huntington disease. *J CLIN INVEST.* 121: 1519–1523.
16. Lin YH, Wu CC, Hsu CJ, Hwang JH, Liu TC (2011) The grainyhead-like 2 gene (GRHL2) single nucleotide polymorphism is not associated with age-related hearing impairment in Han Chinese. *Laryngoscope.* 121(6): 1303–1307.
17. Van Eyken E, Van Camp G, Van Laer L (2007) The complexity of age-related hearing impairment: contributing environmental and genetic factors. *Audiol Neurootol* 12: 345–358.
18. Hwang JH, Hsu CJ, Liu TC, Yang WS (2011) Association of plasma adiponectin levels with hearing thresholds in adults. *Clin Endocrinol (Oxf).* 75: 614–620.
19. Lee HS, Kim KR, Chung WH, Cho YS, Hong SH (2008) Early sensorineural hearing loss in ob/ob mouse, an animal model of type 2 diabetes. *Clin Exp Otorhinolaryngol.* 1: 211–216.
20. Lindstrom P (2007) The physiology of obese-hyperglycemic mice [ob/ob mice]. *Scientific World Journal.* 7: 666–685.
21. Vasilyeva ON, Frisina ST, Zhu X, Walton JP, Frisina RD (2009) Interactions of hearing loss and Diabetes Mellitus in the middle age CBA/CaJ mouse model of presbycusis. *Hear Res.* 249(1–2): 44–53.
22. Hidaka T (1997) Scanning and transmission electron microscopic observations of the inner ear of hamsters with hyperlipidemia. *Nippon Jibiinkoka Gakkai Kaiho.* 100: 900–908. [Article in Japanese]
23. Sikora MA, Morizono T, Ward WD, Paparella MM, Leslie K (1986) Diet-induced hyperlipidemia and auditory dysfunction. *Acta Otolaryngol.* 102: 372–381.
24. Nicholson A, Reifsnyder PC, Malcolm RD, Lucas CA, MacGregor GR, et al. (2010) Diet-induced obesity in two C57BL/6 substrains with intact or mutant nicotinamide nucleotide transhydrogenase (Nnt) gene. *Obesity* 18: 1902–1905.
25. Madsen AN, Hansen G, Paulsen SJ, Lykkegaard K, Tang-Christensen M, et al. (2010) Long-term characterization of the diet-induced obese and diet-resistant rat model: a polygenetic rat model mimicking the human obesity syndrome. *J Endocrinol.* 206: 287–296.
26. Cho BB, Toledo-Pereyra LH (2008) Caspase-independent programmed cell death following ischemic stroke. *J Invest Surg.* 21: 141–147.
27. Yu SW, Wang H, Poitras MF, Coombs C, Bowers WJ, et al. (2000) Mediation of poly(ADP-ribose) polymerase-1-dependent cell death by apoptosis-inducing factor. *Science* 297: 259–263.
28. Mizukoshi S, Nakazawa M, Sato K, Ozaki T, Metoki T, et al. (2010) Activation of mitochondrial calpain and release of apoptosis-inducing factor from mitochondria in RCS rat retinal degeneration. *Exp Eye Res.* 91: 353–361.
29. Park SY, Kim HY, Lee JH, Yoon KH, Chang MS, et al. (2010) The age-dependent induction of apoptosis-inducing factor (AIF) in the human semitendinosus skeletal muscle. *Cell Mol Biol Lett.* 15: 1–12.
30. Chung SH, Calafiore M, Plane JM, Pleasure DE, Deng W (2011) Apoptosis inducing factor deficiency causes reduced mitofusion 1 expression and patterned Purkinje cell degeneration. *Neurobiol Dis.* 41: 445–457.
31. Engel T, Caballero-Caballero A, Schindler CK, Plesnila N, Strasser A, et al. (2010) BH3-only protein Bid is dispensable for seizure-induced neuronal death and the associated nuclear accumulation of apoptosis-inducing factor. *J Neurochem.* 115: 92–101.
32. Nakka VP, Gusain A, Mehta SL, Raghubir R (2008) Molecular mechanisms of apoptosis in cerebral ischemia: multiple neuroprotective opportunities. *Mol Neurobiol.* 37: 7–38.
33. Schulz JB (2006) Anti-apoptotic gene therapy in Parkinson's disease. *J Neural Transm Suppl.* 70: 467–476.
34. Cottet S, Schorderet DF (2009) Mechanisms of apoptosis in retinitis pigmentosa. *Curr Mol Med.* 9: 375–383.
35. Mittra S, Bansal VS, Bhatnagar PK (2008) From a glucocentric to a lipocentric approach towards metabolic syndrome. *Drug Discov Today.* 13: 211–218.
36. Cohen AH (1975) Massive obesity and the kidney. A morphologic and statistical study. *Am J Pathol* 81: 117–130.
37. Reynolds K, Gu D, Muntner P, Chen J, Wu X, et al. (2007) Body mass index and risk of ESRD in China. *Am J Kidney Dis* 50: 754–764.
38. Chou CL, Fang TC (2010) Incidental chronic kidney disease in metabolic syndrome. *Tzu Chi Med J* 22: 11–17.
39. McQueen CT, Baxter A, Smith TL, Raynor E, Yoon SM, et al. (1999) Non-insulin-dependent diabetic microangiopathy in the inner ear. *J Laryngol Otol.* 113: 13–18.

20

Differences in the Pathogenicity of the p.H723R Mutation of the Common Deafness-Associated *SLC26A4* Gene in Humans and Mice

Ying-Chang Lu[1,2]⁹, Chen-Chi Wu[2,3]⁹, Ting-Hua Yang[2], Yin-Hung Lin[2], I-Shing Yu[4], Shu-Wha Lin[4], Qing Chang[5], Xi Lin[5], Jau-Min Wong[1], Chuan-Jen Hsu[2,6]*

1 Institute of Biomedical Engineering, National Taiwan University, Taipei, Taiwan, **2** Department of Otolaryngology, National Taiwan University Hospital, Taipei, Taiwan, **3** Department of Medical Genetics, National Taiwan University Hospital, Taipei, Taiwan, **4** Transgenic Mouse Models Core (TMMC), Division of Genomic Medicine, Research Center For Medical Excellence, National Taiwan University, Taipei, Taiwan, **5** Department of Otolaryngology, Emory University School of Medicine, Atlanta, Georgia, United States of America, **6** Department of Otolaryngology, College of Medicine, National Taiwan University, Taipei, Taiwan

Abstract

Mutations in the *SLC26A4* gene are a common cause of human hereditary hearing impairment worldwide. Previous studies have demonstrated that different *SLC26A4* mutations have different pathogenetic mechanisms. By using a genotype-driven approach, we established a knock-in mouse model (i.e., $Slc26a4^{tm2Dontuh/tm2Dontuh}$ mice) homozygous for the common p.H723R mutation in the East Asian population. To verify the pathogenicity of the p.H723R allele in mice, we further generated mice with compound heterozygous mutations (i.e., $Slc26a4^{tm1Dontuh/tm2Dontuh}$) by intercrossing $Slc26a4^{+/tm2Dontuh}$ mice with $Slc26a4^{tm1Dontuh/tm1Dontuh}$ mice, which segregated the c.919-2A>G mutation with an abolished *Slc26a4* function. Mice were then subjected to audiologic assessments, a battery of vestibular evaluations, inner ear morphological studies, and noise exposure experiments. The results were unexpected; both $Slc26a4^{tm2Dontuh/tm2Dontuh}$ and $Slc26a4^{tm1Dontuh/tm2Dontuh}$ mice showed normal audiovestibular phenotypes and inner ear morphology, and they did not show significantly higher shifts in hearing thresholds after noise exposure than the wild-type mice. The results indicated not only the p.H723R allele was non-pathogenic in mice, but also a single p.H723R allele was sufficient to maintain normal inner ear physiology in heterozygous compound mice. There might be discrepancies in the pathogenicity of specific *SLC26A4* mutations in humans and mice; therefore, precautions should be taken when extrapolating the results of animal studies to humans.

Editor: Mark S. Shapiro, University of Texas Health Science Center, United States of America

Funding: This study was supported by research grants from the National Health Research Institute (NHRI-EX101-10147PI), National Science Council of the Executive Yuan of the Republic of China (NSC-99-2314-B-002-056-MY3), and National Taiwan University Hospital (NTUH-100-001597). The funders had no role in study design, data collection and analysis, decision to publish, or preparation of the manuscript.

Competing Interests: The authors have declared that no competing interests exist.

* E-mail: cjhsu@ntu.edu.tw

⁹ These authors contributed equally to this work.

Introduction

Mutations in the *SLC26A4* (*PDS*, GeneID: 5172) gene are the second most frequent cause of human hereditary hearing impairment worldwide, next to mutations in the *GJB2* (GeneID: 2706) gene [1]. In some populations, *SLC26A4* mutations can be identified in approximately 13–14% of deaf patients [2]. *SLC26A4* encodes pendrin, an iodide/chloride/bicarbonate transporter expressed in the inner ear [3], thyroid [4], kidney [5,6], salivary duct [7], and respiratory tract [8]. Recessive *SLC26A4* mutations contribute to both Pendred syndrome (PS; MIM #274600) [9] and nonsyndromic hearing loss (DFNB4; MIM #600791) [10], which share the phenotypes of sensorineural hearing impairment (SNHI) accompanied by an enlarged vestibular aqueduct (EVA; MIM 603545) and/or incomplete partition of the cochlea (i.e., Mondini dysplasia), although the phenotype of PS also includes goiter. To date, more than 100 *SLC26A4* mutations have been identified (Pendred/BOR Homepage; www.healthcare.uiowa.edu/labs/pendredandbor). Previous reports have described that different *SLC26A4* genotypes were correlated with distinct clinical phenotypes, and patients with PS are more likely to have 2 *SLC26A4* mutant alleles than those with DFNB4 [11,12]. Many affected patients suffer from progressive or fluctuating hearing loss [13], implying that the natural course can be halted with preventive or therapeutic measures if the pathogenetic mechanisms of *SLC26A4* mutations are better elucidated.

In recent years, the understanding of the pathogenesis of DFNB4 and PS has been accelerated by various mouse models with mutations in the *Slc26a4* (GeneID: 23985) gene. Certain mouse models revealed congenital profound hearing loss, including the knock-out $Slc26a4^{-/-}$ mice [14], the $Slc26a4^{loop/loop}$ mice with the p.S408F mutation [15], and the $Slc26a4^{tm1Dontuh/tm1Dontuh}$ mice with the c.919-A>G mutation that we previously reported [16]. The conditional knock-out Tg[E];Tg[R];$Slc26a4^{\Delta/\Delta}$ mice demonstrated hearing loss of various severity dependent on the time of *Slc26a4* expression, with doxycycline initiation at E18.5 resulting in partial hearing loss [17]. These mouse models have provided excellent insight into the pathogenesis; however, 2 basic problems might hurdle the bench-to-bedside translation. First, similar to their human counterparts, mice with different mutations, to some extent, demonstrated different phenotypes, indicating that the pathology associated with each distinct mutation is different. Second, to date, no mouse model that can perfectly simulate the progressive or fluctuating hearing loss in humans has been reported. Investigating mice with other *Slc26a4* mutations might tackle these problems. Accordingly, in this study, we generated a knock-in mouse model with the p.H723R (c.2168A>G) mutation, a common *SLC26A4* mutation in the East Asian population [18–22], and then, we characterized the associated audiovestibular phenotypes as well as the inner ear pathology.

Materials and Methods

Construction of Slc26a4$^{tm2Dontuh/tm2Dontuh}$ Knock-in Mice

The mutation gene-targeting vector was constructed using a recombineering approach previously developed by Dr. Copeland's group [23,24]. From the bMQ323G13 BAC clone (Sanger Institute, Cambridge, UK), we subcloned a 12.8-kb fragment spanning introns 17–21 of *Slc26a4* into the PL253 plasmid (Fig. 1A). The subcloned genomic 12.8-kb region was modified in a subsequent targeting round by inserting the neomycin (*neo*) cassette from the PL452 plasmid and creating the c.2168A>G mutation in exon 19. The targeting vector was then linearized by *Not*I digestion and electroporated into R1 embryonic stem (ES) cells. G418 (240 μg/mL) and ganciclovir (2 μM) double-resistant clones were analyzed by Southern blot hybridization (Fig. 1B).

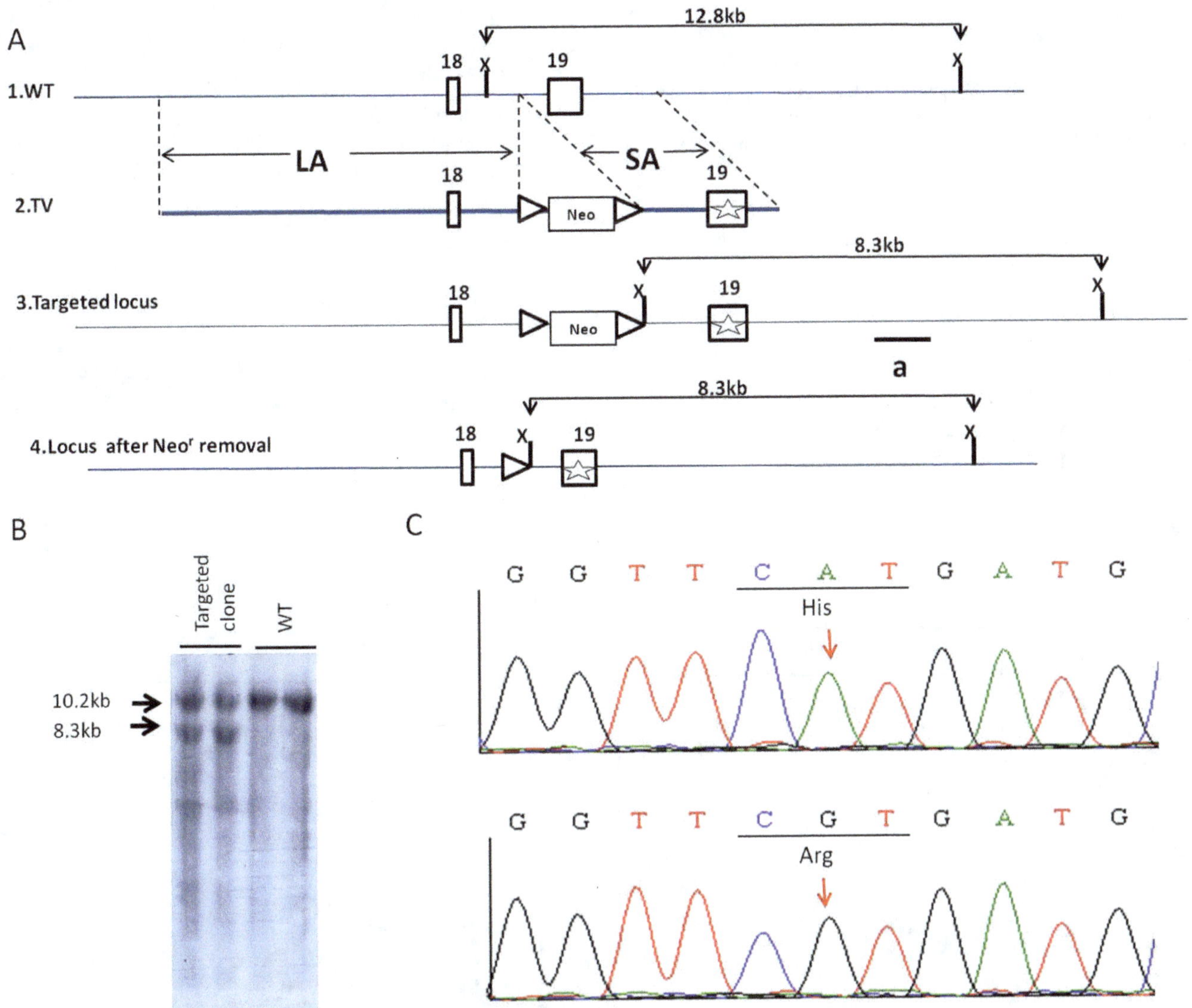

Figure 1. Generation of mice with the *Slc26a4* p.H723R mutation. (A) Targeting scheme. A BAC clone (clone no. bMQ-323G13 Geneservice™) from the 129S7/AB2.2 BAC library containing the mouse *Slc26a4* genomic region was used to construct the targeting vector. (1) Restriction map of the wild-type genomic mouse *Slc26a4* locus. The expected size of the *Xba*I restriction fragment was 12.8 kb. (2) Targeting vector (TV) construction. The *loxP*-flanked neomycin resistance gene (*neo*) was used as a selection marker during embryonic stem (ES) cell culture. The c.2168 A>G mutation in exon 19 is labeled with a star. (3–4) The targeted locus was introduced, and then, the *neo* cassette was removed. LA, long arm; SA, short arm. (B) Southern blot analysis of ES cell clones. Genomic DNA from 2 targeted and 2 wild-type clones were digested with *Xba*I and hybridized with the probe to verify the targeting event. (C) DNA sequencing of *Slc26a4*$^{+/+}$ and *Slc26a4*$^{tm2Dontuh/tm2Dontuh}$ mice. The electrophoretogram shows the p.H723R mutation. The A to G mutation (arrow) at position 2168 led to the replacement of a histidine (His, H) residue at position 723 with arginine (Arg, R).

The retained *neo* cassette flanked by *loxP* sites was excised *in vivo* by transfecting the targeted clone with plasmid transiently expressing the Cre recombinase. Established ES clones were then identified by polymerase chain reaction (PCR) screening and subsequently injected into C57BL/6 blastocysts to produce chimeras. After germline transmission of the targeted mutation allele, we produced the congenic $Slc26a4^{+/tm2Dontuh}$ mouse line used in this study by repeated backcrossing into the C57BL/6 inbred strain for 6–10 generations, after which mice homozygous for the mutation (i.e., $Slc26a4^{tm2Dontuh/tm2Dontuh}$) were obtained by intercrossing heterozygous mice (i.e., $Slc26a4^{+/tm2Dontuh}$) (Fig. 1C). Reverse transcription-PCR (RT-PCR) of mRNA of inner ear extract followed by direct sequencing also indicated a pure non-chimeric genetic background without unintentionally wild-type *Slc26a4* expression in $Slc26a4^{tm2-Dontuh/tm2Dontuh}$ mice. Corresponding to the human genotypes, mice with compound heterozygous mutations for p.H723R and c.919-2A>G (i.e., $Slc26a4^{tm1Dontuh/tm2Dontuh}$) were also generated by intercrossing heterozygous $Slc26a4^{+/tm2Dontuh}$ mice with $Slc26a4^{tm1-Dontuh/tm1Dntuh}$ mice. All animal experiments were carried out in accordance with animal welfare guidelines and approved by the Institutional Animal Care and Use Committee (IACUC) of National Taiwan University College of Medicine (approval no. 20110123).

Audiological and Vestibular Evaluations

For audiological evaluations, the mice were anesthetized with sodium pentobarbital (35 mg/kg) delivered intraperitoneally and placed in a head-holder within an acoustically and electrically insulated and grounded test room. We used an evoked potential detection system (Smart EP 3.90; Intelligent Hearing Systems, Miami, FL, USA) to measure the thresholds of the auditory brainstem response (ABR) in mice. Click sounds, as well as 8, 16, and 32 kHz tone bursts at varying intensity, were generated to evoke ABRs in mice. The response signals were recorded with subcutaneous needle electrodes. The active electrodes were inserted into the vertex and the ipsilateral retro-auricular region with a ground electrode on the back of the mice.

For vestibular evaluations, mice were subjected to a battery of tests, including observation of their circling behavior and head tilting (performed at 3 weeks of age), reaching test, swimming test, gripping test, and a rotarod test (all performed at 8 weeks of age). The methodology of each vestibular test is described in details in our previous study [16].

Inner Ear Morphology Studies

Tissues from the inner ears of mice were subjected to hematoxylin and eosin (H&E) staining, and the morphology of

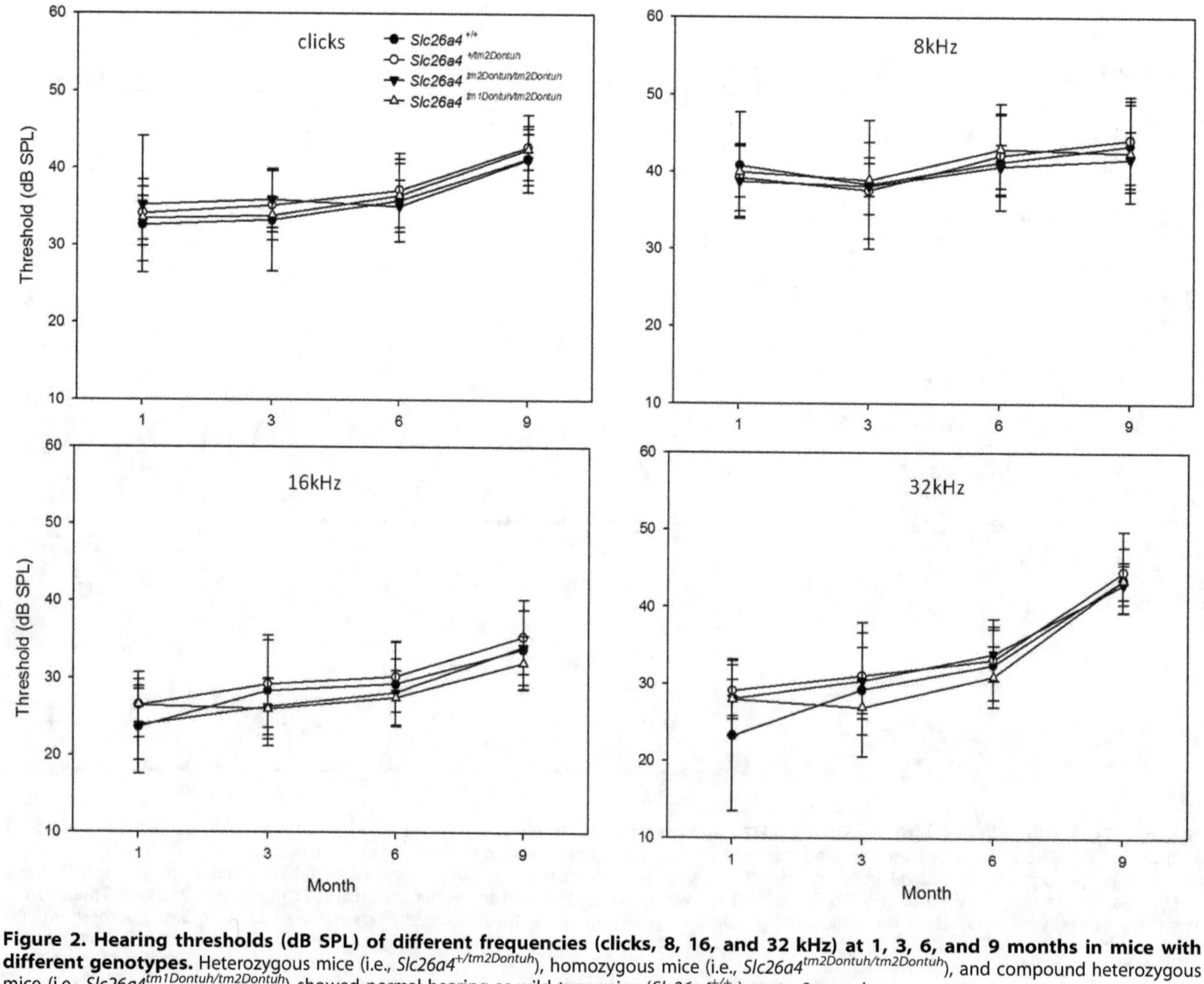

Figure 2. Hearing thresholds (dB SPL) of different frequencies (clicks, 8, 16, and 32 kHz) at 1, 3, 6, and 9 months in mice with different genotypes. Heterozygous mice (i.e., $Slc26a4^{+/tm2Dontuh}$), homozygous mice (i.e., $Slc26a4^{tm2Dontuh/tm2Dontuh}$), and compound heterozygous mice (i.e., $Slc26a4^{tm1Dontuh/tm2Dontuh}$) showed normal hearing as wild type mice ($Slc26a4^{+/+}$) up to 9 months.

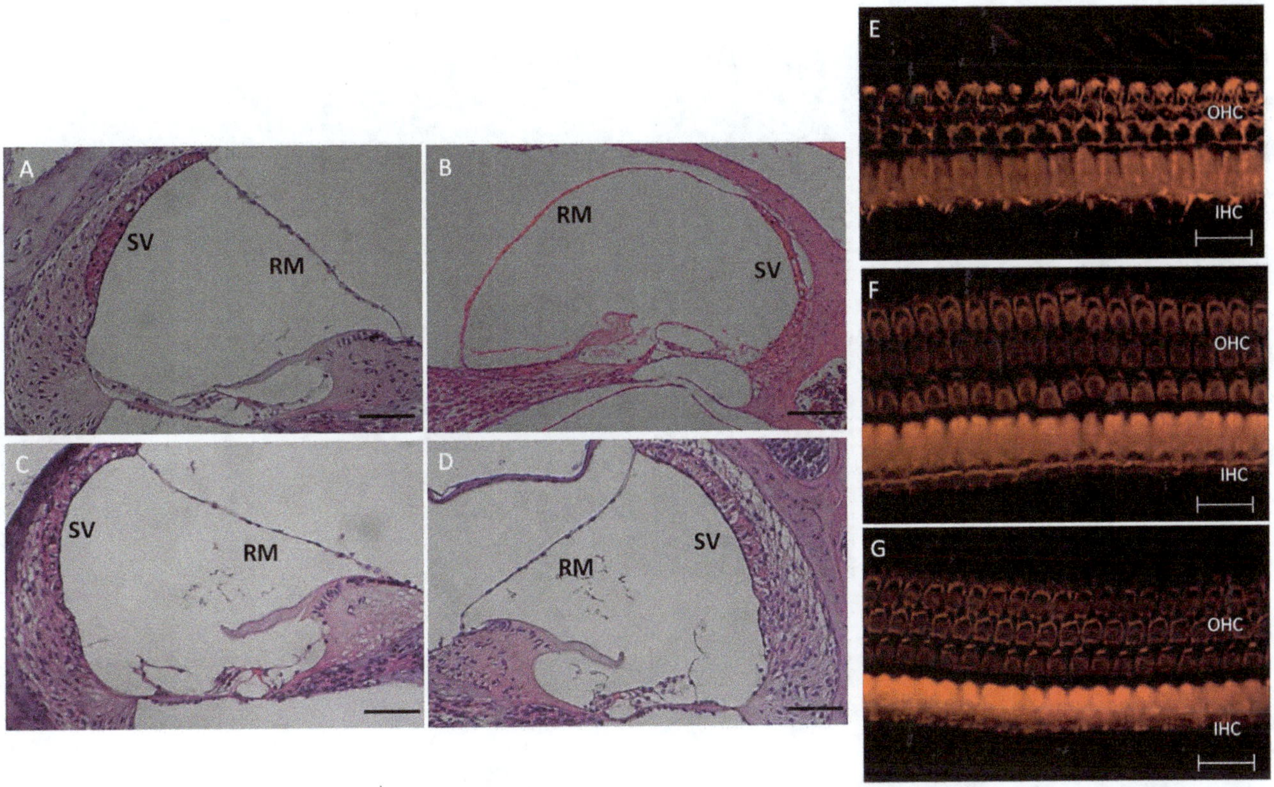

Figure 3. Comparison of Cochlear morphology in mice with different genotypes at P60. Compared with cochlear morphology in *Slc26a4*$^{+/+}$ mice (A), severe endolymphatic hydrops (dilatation of scala media) and a significant atrophy of the stria vascularis (B), as well as degenerated hair cells (E), were observed in *Slc26a4*$^{tm1Dontuh/tm1Dontuh}$ mice. In contrast, normal cochlear morphology was revealed in both *Slc26a4*$^{tm2Dontuh/tm2Dontuh}$ mice (C) and *Slc26a4*$^{tm1Dontuh/tm2Dontuh}$ mice (D). No degeneration of cochlear hair cells at the basal turn was observed in *Slc26a4*$^{tm2Dontuh/tm2Dontuh}$ mice (F) and *Slc26a4*$^{tm1Dontuh/tm2Dontuh}$ mice (G). IHC: inner hair cells; OHC: outer hair cells; RM: Reissner's membrane; SV: stria vascularis; A, B, C, D: hematoxylin and eosin (H&E) staining; E, F, G: fluorescence confocal microscopy; Bar = 150 μm (A–D) and 20 μm (E–G).

each sample was examined with a Leica optical microscope. For both light microscopy and scanning electron microscopy (SEM) studies, inner ears from adult mice were fixed by perilymphatic perfusion with 4% paraformaldehyde (PFA) in phosphate-buffered saline (PBS) through round and oval windows and a small fenestra in the apex of the cochlear bony capsule. Specimens were subsequently rinsed in PBS buffer and decalcified in 4% PFA with 0.35 M EDTA at 4°C for 1 week. For light microscopy studies, the samples were dehydrated and embedded in paraffin. Subsequently, serial sections (7 μm) were stained with H&E. For SEM studies, the samples were dehydrated in ethanol, critical-point dried, gold sputter coated, and then examined in a field emission scanning electron microscope (S-4500; Hitachi, Tokyo, Japan).

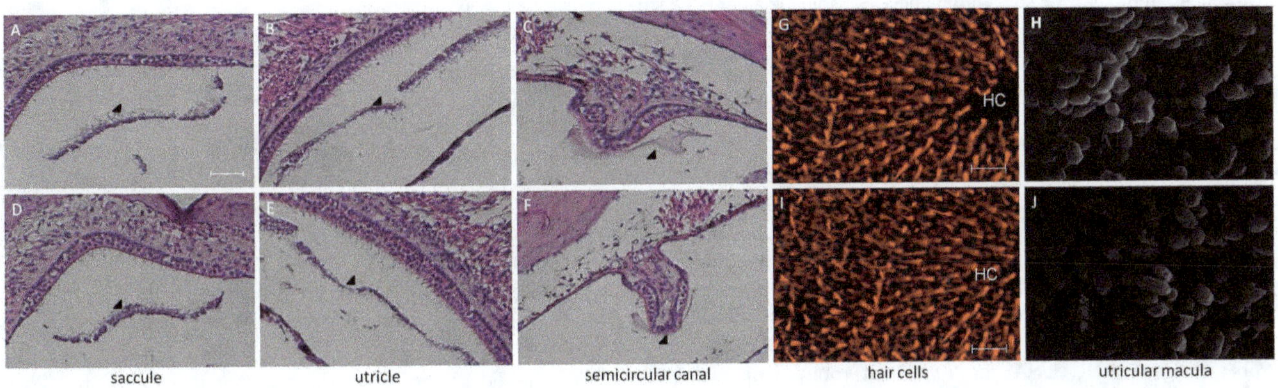

Figure 4. Comparison of Vestibular morphology in mice with different genotypes at P60 (*Slc26a4*$^{tm2Dontuh/tm2Dontuh}$ mice: A, B, C, G, H; *Slc26a4*$^{tm1Dontuh/tm2Dontuh}$ mice: D, E, F, I, J). Normal morphological findings and amount of otoconia in the vestibule (arrowhead) are shown in both mice (A, B, C, D, E, F). No degeneration of vestibular hair cells in both mice is observed by fluorescence confocal microscopy (G, H). Scanning electron microscopic findings show normal otoconia at the utricle in both mice (I, J). Bar = 50 μm (A–F) and 10 μm (G–H).

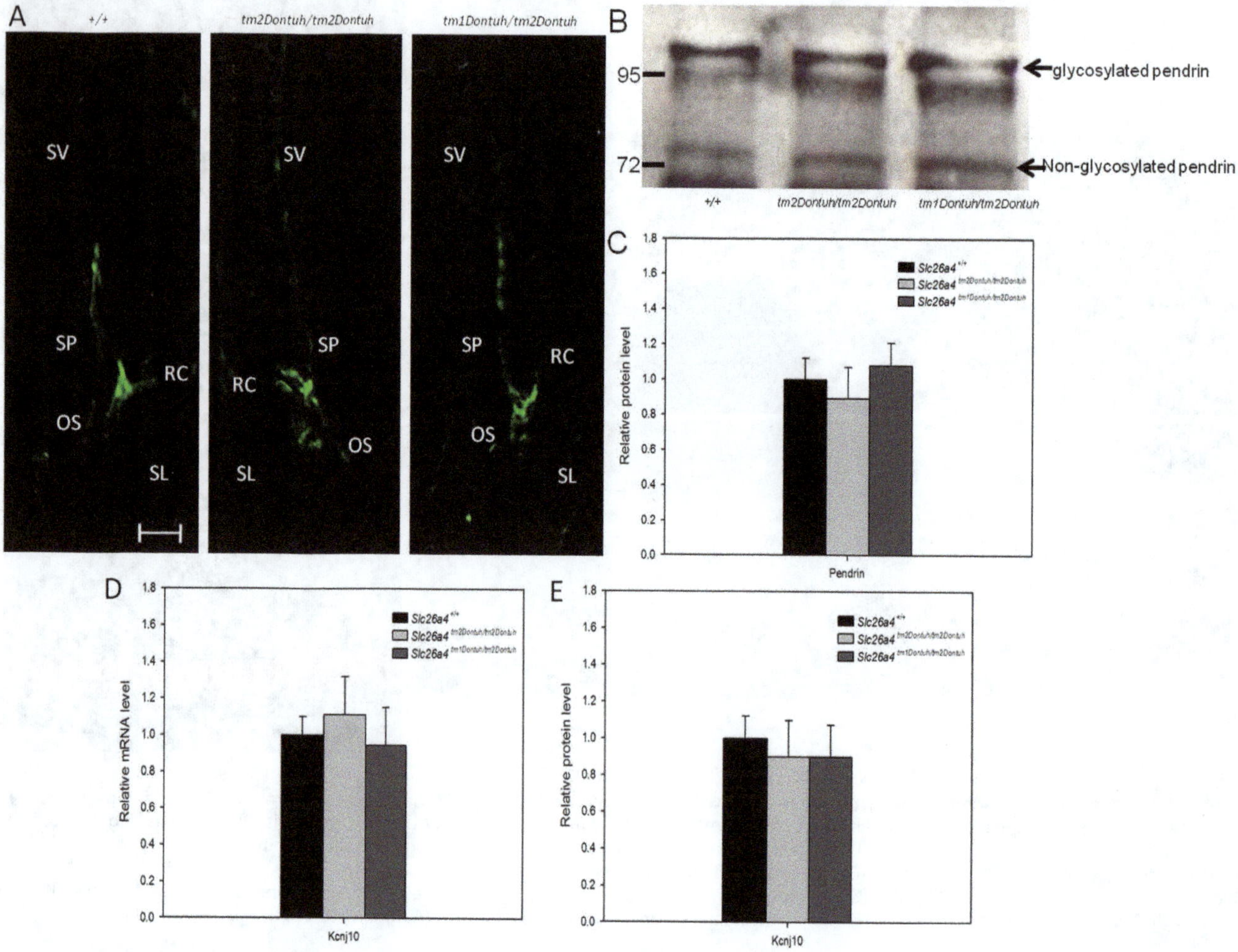

Figure 5. Expression of pendrin and *Kcnj10*. (A) Pendrin is normally distributed in the spiral prominence and root cells (stained in green) in *Slc26a4*$^{+/+}$ (left), *Slc26a4*$^{tm2Dontuh/tm2Dontuh}$ (middle), and *Slc26a4*$^{tm1Dontuh/tm2Dontuh}$ mice (right), indicating that the expression of pendrin is not affected by the p.H723R mutation in mice. (B) Immunoblotting of pendrin expression at P42. Both *Slc26a4*$^{tm2Dontuh/tm2Dontuh}$ and *Slc26a4*$^{tm1Dontuh/tm2Dontuh}$ mice expressed pendrin of molecular weight comparable to the wild-type mice, indicating that the glycosylation process remained unaffected in the p.H723R-pendrin. (C) Quantification of pendrin protein expression at P42. The expression levels of pendrin in *Slc26a4*$^{tm2Dontuh/tm2Dontuh}$ mice and *Slc26a4*$^{tm1Dontuh/tm2Dontuh}$ mice were 0.89±0.18 and 1.08±0.13, showing no significant difference as compared with 1.00±0.11 in *Slc26a4*$^{+/+}$ mice (mean percentage ± SE, n = 3). (D) Quantification of mRNA expression of *Kcnj10* at P15 by real-time PCR. *Slc26a4*$^{tm2Dontuh/tm2Dontuh}$ mice and *Slc26a4*$^{tm1Dontuh/tm2Dontuh}$ mice did not show significantly different mRNA levels of *Kcnj10* as compared with *Slc26a4*$^{+/+}$ mice. (E) Quantification of Kcnj10 protein expression at P15 by western blotting. The expression levels of Kcnj10 protein in *Slc26a4*$^{tm2Dontuh/tm2Dontuh}$ mice and *Slc26a4*$^{tm1Dontuh/tm2Dontuh}$ mice were 0.90±0.19 and 0.90±0.17, showing no significant difference as compared with 1.00±0.12 in *Slc26a4*$^{+/+}$ mice (mean percentage ± SE, n = 3). RC: root cells; SP: spiral prominence; SL: spiral ligament; SV: stria vascularis; Bar = 20 μm.

Whole-mount studies of mouse inner ear specimens were performed as previously described [25] with some minor modifications. Briefly, after perfusion with 4% PFA, the cochleae were postfixed in the same solution for 2 h at room temperature and washed in PBS. The samples were permeabilized in 1% Triton X-100 for 30 min and washed with PBS, followed by overnight incubation at 4°C in the blocking solution. The tissues were then stained with rhodamine-phalloidin (1:100 dilution; Molecular Probes, Eugene, OR, USA). After washing in PBS, the tissues were mounted using the ProLong Antifade kit (Molecular Probes, Eugene, OR, USA) for 20 min at room temperature. Images of the tissues were obtained using a laser scanning confocal microscope (Zeiss LSM 510; Germany).

Expression of Pendrin

For pendrin expression experiments, we prepared tissue sections from the inner ears of *Slc26a4*$^{tm1Dontuh/tm2Dontuh}$ and *Slc26a4*$^{tm2Dontuh/tm2Dontuh}$ mice. Tissue sections mounted on silane-coated glass slides were then deparaffinized in xylene and rehydrated in ethanol. After antigen heat retrieval (500 W microwave oven, in 10 mM citric buffer, pH 6.0, for 20 min), the slides were incubated overnight at 4°C with primary antibodies in PBS and Tween (PBST) (rabbit anti-pendrin, 1:100 [H195]; mouse anti-Myosin VIIa, 1:100 [C-5]; Santa Cruz Biotechnology, Santa Cruz, CA, USA). The slides were then washed and incubated for 1 h at 25°C with appropriate secondary antibodies at a 1:1000 dilution in PBST. After incubation, the slides were washed with PBST and mounted with the ProLong Antifade kit at 25°C. Images were obtained using a laser scanning confocal microscope (Zeiss LSM 510; Germany).

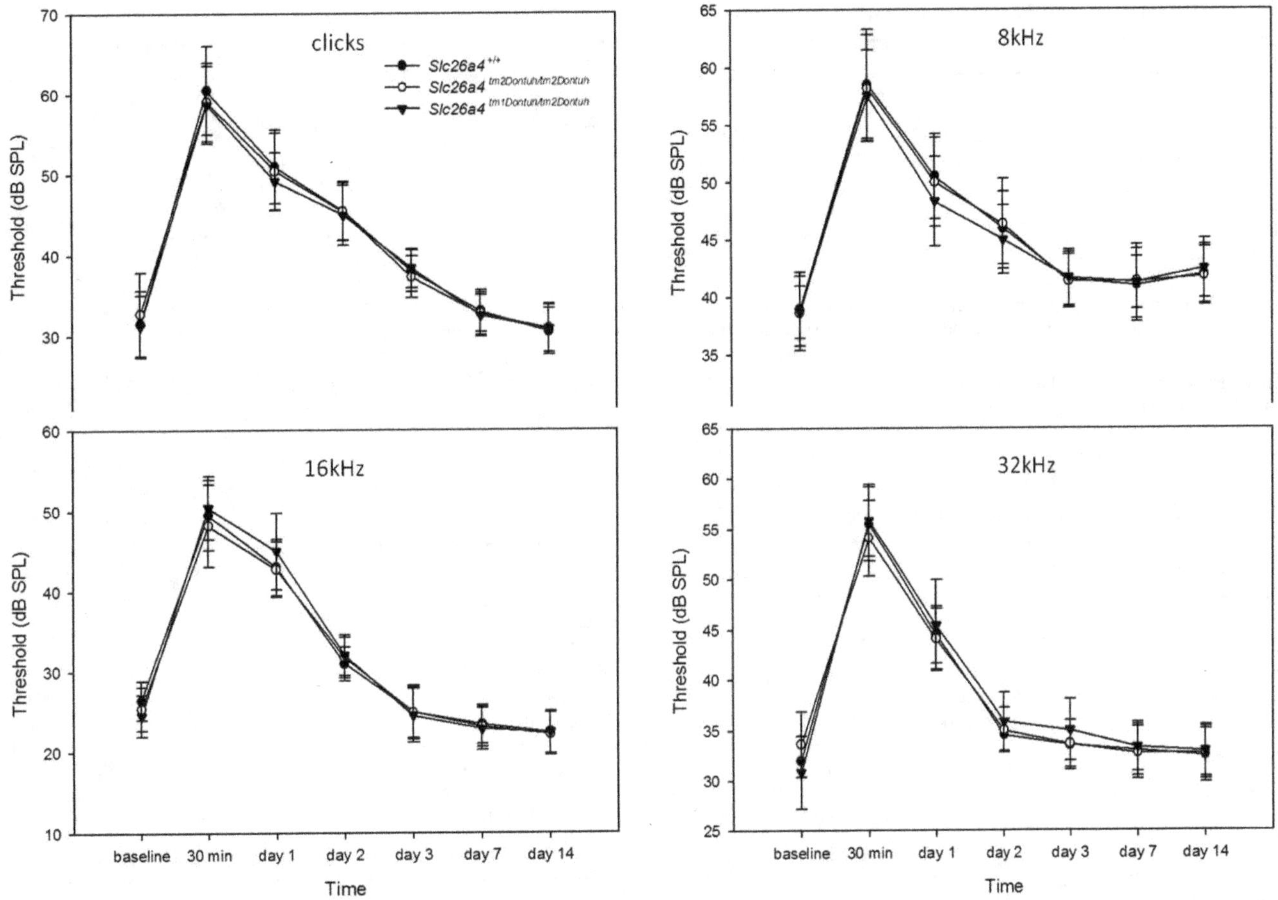

Figure 6. Chronological change of hearing thresholds (dB SPL) of different frequencies (clicks, 8, 16, and 32 kHz) in mice with different genotypes. Neither *Slc26a4*$^{tm2Dontuh/tm2Dontuh}$ mice nor *Slc26a4*$^{tm1Dontuh/tm2Dontuh}$ mice had a significantly higher shift in hearing thresholds at any of the frequencies at 30 min or at day 1, 2, 3, 7, and 14 after noise exposure as compared with *Slc26a4*$^{+/+}$ mice.

Real-time PCR

Total RNA was purified using Trizol reagent (Invitrogen, CA, USA) according to the manufacturer's protocol and stored at −80°C until further use. Total RNA was treated with DNase and then reverse transcribed into first-strand cDNA in a 20-μL reaction volume using SuperScript III Reverse Transcriptase (Invitrogen, CA, USA). Quantitative real-time reverse transcription (RT)-PCR assays of *Kcnj10* cDNA were performed using a gene-specific double fluorescently labeled TaqMan probe in an ABI Prism 7900 Sequence Detection System (Applied Biosystems) in accordance with the manufacturer's recommendations. The relative mRNA expression level was determined by the $2^{-\Delta\Delta C_t}$ analysis method, and calculations were performed using the software provided by the manufacturer (Applied Biosystems). Specimens from 5 mice were collected for each experiment, and the experiments were performed in triplicates and averaged. The average mRNA expression level in wild-type mice was normalized to 1 as the control.

Western Blot Analysis

Protein extracts of the inner ear were homogenized in RIPA buffer (Millipore, MO, USA). Equal amounts of proteins were supplemented with dithiothreitol, heated for 5 min at 95°C, separated by SDS gel electrophoresis, and then transferred to a PVDF membrane (Amersham Pharmacia Biotech, Little Chalfont, UK) by semi-dry electroblotting. The PVDF membranes were developed with an enhanced chemiluminescence western blot detection kit (Pierce SuperSignal® West Dura, Rockford, IL, USA) and exposed to Lumi-Film chemiluminescent detection films (Roche Diagnostics, Mannheim, Germany). The specimens were collected from 5 mice for each experiment, and the experiments were performed in triplicates and averaged. The average protein expression level in wild-type mice was normalized to 1 as the control.

Noise Exposure Experiments

For the noise exposure experiments, 10 mice of each genotype were exposed for 3 h to octave-band noise with a peak at 4 kHz, 115 dB SPL. The noise room was fitted with a speaker (model NO. 1700–2002, GSI) driven by a noise generator (GSI-61; Grason-Stadler, Inc.) and a power amplifier (5507-Power; TECHRON). ABR thresholds (dB SPL) in mice at different frequencies (click, 8 kHz, 16 kHz, and 32 kHz) were then recorded at 30 min and at day 1, 2, 3, 7, and 14 after noise exposure.

Thyroid and Renal Serum Biochemistry

Terminal blood samples were obtained from mice at postnatal day 15 to compare the early postnatal T4 surge [26], as well as at 2 and 6 months of age to monitor the long-term thyroid and renal

Table 1. Comparison of phenotypes among mouse strains segregating different Slc26a4 mutations.

	Slc26a4$^{-/-}$	*Slc26a4*$^{loop/loop}$	*Slc26a4*$^{tm1Dontuh/tm1Dontuh}$	Tg[E];Tg[R];*Slc26a4*$^{\Delta/\Delta}$	*Slc26a4*$^{tm2Dontuh/tm2Dontuh}$
Audiological phenotypes	Profound hearing loss (>100 dB SPL)	Profound hearing loss (>100 dB SPL)	Profound hearing loss (>120 dB SPL)	Hearing levels depend on the time of *Slc26a4* expression. Doxycycline initiation at E18.5 (IE 18.5) results in partial hearing loss.	Normal
Vestibular phenotypes	Vestibular deficits, including head-tilting and circling	Variable vestibular deficits, including circling and tilted body.	46% of mice with head-tilting and circling.	ND	Normal
Inner Ear Morphology Vestibular aqueduct	Enlarged	ND	Enlarged	Sizes depend on the time of *Slc26a4* expression. Significantly enlarged in IE18.5 mice.	Normal
Scala media	Enlarged	ND	Enlarged	Not enlarged (IE18.5)	Normal
Cochlear hair cells	Severe degeneration of inner and outer hair cells by P30.	ND	Severe degeneration of inner and outer hair cells at 6 wks.	Functionally intact at P25 to P35 (IE18.5)	Normal
Vestibular hair cells	Severe degeneration of vestibular hair cells by P30.	Normal morphology of vestibular hair cells at 2 m.	Loss and degeneration of utricular hair cells correlated to the vestibular phenotypes	ND	Normal
Otoconia	Almost complete absence of otoconia with occasional presence of giant otoconia.	Giant otoconia in the utricle from P0 to 10 m; gradual change in otoconia composition to calcium oxalate in the saccule from P0 to 10 m; ectopic otoconia in the semicircular canal.	Decreased amount of otoconia in the saccule and utricle, formation of giant otoconia in the saccule and utricle, and ectopic distribution of otoconia into the semicircular canal	ND	Normal

ND, not described.
Slc26a4$^{loop/loop}$: mice homozygous for the p.S408F mutation.

profiles. Total T4 was measured in undiluted serum (25 μL) by RIA (Diagnostic Products Corp., Los Angeles, CA, USA). Thyroid-stimulating hormone (TSH), Blood urea nitrogen (BUN) and serum creatinine (CREA) were measured by the research services of National Taiwan University Hospital.

Results

Audiological and Vestibular Phenotypes

Wild-type mice (i.e., *Slc26a4*$^{+/+}$), heterozygous mice (i.e., *Slc26a4*$^{+/tm2Dontuh}$), and homozygous mice (i.e., *Slc26a4*$^{tm2Dontuh/tm2Dontuh}$) (n = 10 each) were subjected to audiological evaluations at 1, 3, 6, and 9 months. Both *Slc26a4*$^{+/tm2Dontuh}$ and *Slc26a4*$^{tm2Dontuh/tm2Dontuh}$ mice had normal hearing up to 9 months (Fig. 2), indicating that the p.H723R allele does not lead to deafness in mice. To verify the pathogenicity of the p.H723R allele in mice, we further generated mice with compound heterozygous mutations (i.e., *Slc26a4*$^{tm1Dontuh/tm2Dontuh}$) by intercrossing *Slc26a4*$^{+/tm2Dontuh}$ mice with *Slc26a4*$^{tm1Dontuh/tm1Dontuh}$ mice, which segregated the c.919-2A>G mutation with an abolished function [16]. Similar to the mice heterozygous for the c.919-2A>G mutation (i.e., *Slc26a4*$^{+/tm1Dontuh}$), *Slc26a4*$^{tm1Dontuh/tm2Dontuh}$ mice (n = 10) had normal hearing up to 9 months; this finding confirmed that the p.H723R allele was not pathogenic and a single p.H723R allele was sufficient to maintain normal hearing in mice.

A total of 60 mice, including *Slc26a4*$^{+/+}$ mice, *Slc26a4*$^{+/tm2Dontuh}$ mice, *Slc26a4*$^{tm2Dontuh/tm2Dontuh}$ mice, and *Slc26a4*$^{tm1Dontuh/tm2Dontuh}$ mice (n = 15 each), were subjected to vestibular evaluations (Table S1). Similar to the normal audiological phenotypes, neither heterozygous mice (i.e., *Slc26a4*$^{+/tm2Dontuh}$) nor homozygous mice (i.e., *Slc26a4*$^{tm2Dontuh/tm2Dontuh}$) showed vestibular deficits such as head tilting and circling behavior, and both groups performed normally on reaching, swimming, gripping, and rotarod tests. Similarly, compound heterozygous mice (i.e., *Slc26a4*$^{tm1Dontuh/tm2Dontuh}$) also did not show vestibular deficits, indicating that a single p.H723R allele was sufficient to maintain normal vestibular function in mice.

Cochlear Morphology

Cochlear morphology was investigated in homozygous mice (i.e., *Slc26a4*$^{tm2Dontuh/tm2Dontuh}$) and compound heterozygous mice (i.e., *Slc26a4*$^{tm1Dontuh/tm2Dontuh}$). The cochlear morphologies of wild-type mice and the profoundly deaf *Slc26a4*$^{tm1Dontuh/tm1Dontuh}$ mice were also compared. Abnormal morphological findings in *Slc26a4*$^{tm1Dontuh/tm1Dontuh}$ mice, such as severe endolymphatic hydrops with dilatation of the scala media (Fig. 3B), significant atrophy of the stria vascularis (Fig. 3B), and degeneration of the cochlear hair cells (Fig. 3E), were not observed in *Slc26a4*$^{tm2Dontuh/tm2Dontuh}$ mice (Fig. 3C and 3F) and *Slc26a4*$^{tm1Dontuh/tm2Dontuh}$ mice (Fig. 3D and 3G).

Vestibular Morphology

The vestibular morphology was investigated in homozygous mice (i.e., *Slc26a4*$^{tm2Dontuh/tm2Dontuh}$) (Fig. 4A, 4B, and 4C) and compound heterozygous mice (i.e., *Slc26a4*$^{tm1Dontuh/tm2Dontuh}$) (Fig. 4D, 4E, and 4F). Both mice showed normal morphological findings and amount of otoconia in the vestibule. Fluorescence confocal microscopy revealed that vestibular hair cells in *Slc26a4*$^{tm2Dontuh/tm2Dontuh}$ mice and *Slc26a4*$^{tm1Dontuh/tm2Dontuh}$ mice were not degenerated (Fig. 4G and 4I). SEM revealed normal otoconia at the utricle in *Slc26a4*$^{tm2Dontuh/tm2Dontuh}$ mice and *Slc26a4*$^{tm1Dontuh/tm2Dontuh}$ mice (Fig. 4H and 4J).

Immunolocalization and Expression of Pendrin

We then investigated the expression of pendrin in the cochlea of *Slc26a4*$^{tm2Dontuh/tm2Dontuh}$ mice and *Slc26a4*$^{tm1Dontuh/tm2Dontuh}$ mice (Fig. 5A) by immunolocalization. In both strains of mice, pendrin was normally distributed in the spiral prominence and root cells, indicating that the expression of pendrin was not affected by the p.H723R mutation in mice. Compared with the wild-type mice, no significant difference in the molecular weight (Fig. 5B) or the expression level (Fig. 5C) of pendrin were observed in *Slc26a4*$^{tm2Dontuh/tm2Dontuh}$ mice and *Slc26a4*$^{tm1Dontuh/tm2Dontuh}$ mice by western blotting analyses.

Kcnj10 Expression

We then investigated the expression of *Kcnj10* (GeneID: 16513) in *Slc26a4*$^{+/+}$mice, *Slc26a4*$^{tm2Dontuh/tm2Dontuh}$ mice, and *Slc26a4*$^{tm1Dontuh/tm2Dontuh}$ mice by real-time PCR (for mRNA expression) and western blotting (for protein expression) analyses. It has been demonstrated that *Slc26a4*-depleted mice showed decreased *Kcnj10* expression, which contributes to the failure of endocochlear potential generation [27]. *KCNJ10* (GeneID: 3766) mutations have been observed in EVA patients via digenic inheritance with *SLC26A4* mutations [28]. In this study, the stria vascularis of P15 mouse cochleae from *Slc26a4*$^{+/+}$ mice, *Slc26a4*$^{tm2Dontuh/tm2Dontuh}$ mice, and *Slc26a4*$^{tm1Dontuh/tm2Dontuh}$ mice were isolated by microdissection, and total RNA and protein extracted from these tissue fractions were used for real-time PCR and quantitative immunoblot analyses. Compared with the wild-type mice, no significant differences in the mRNA (Fig. 5D) or protein levels of Kcnj10 (Fig. 5E) were observed in *Slc26a4*$^{tm2Dontuh/tm2Dontuh}$ mice and *Slc26a4*$^{tm1Dontuh/tm2Dontuh}$ mice.

Noise Exposure Experiments

We then attempted to induce audiologic phenotypes in transgenic mice with noise exposure [29]. Neither *Slc26a4*$^{tm2Dontuh/tm2Dontuh}$ mice nor *Slc26a4*$^{tm1Dontuh/tm2Dontuh}$ mice showed a significantly higher shift in hearing thresholds at all frequencies 30 min and at day 1, 2, 3, 7, and 14 after noise exposure than *Slc26a4*$^{+/+}$ mice (Fig. 6); this finding confirmed their normal audiologic phenotypes.

Thyroid and Renal Profiles

Goiter was not observed in *Slc26a4*$^{+/+}$ mice, *Slc26a4*$^{tm2Dontuh/tm2Dontuh}$ mice, and *Slc26a4*$^{tm1Dontuh/tm2Dontuh}$ mice (n = 5 each) until the mice were 6-months old. Blood chemistry, including total T4, TSH, BUN, and CREA, were all within normal limits at postnatal day 15, 2 and 6 months (Table S2).

Discussion

In this study, we generated a knock-in mouse model, denoted as *Slc26a4*$^{tm2Dontuh/tm2Dontuh}$ mice, which segregates the common deafness-associated p.H723R mutation in humans. The p.H723R mutation was found in both nonsyndromic EVA and PS families [18,30]. This missense mutation was the most prevalent *SLC26A4* mutation among the Japanese [18] and Koreans [19], and the second most prevalent *SLC26A4* mutation among the Han Chinese [20,21]. Recent reports indicated that the p.H723R mutation arose from a common ancestor and was not a mutational hot spot [31]. The pathogenicity of the p.H723R mutation in humans was confirmed by several lines of evidence supporting the fact that p.H723R co-segregated with the phenotypes in the affected families, the prevalence of p.H723R was low in the control populations, and the p.H723 amino acid residue was evolutionally conserved [18]. Moreover, in human cell lines, the p.H723R has been related to trafficking/folding/glycosylation defects of the pendrin protein. In transfected HEK293 cells and HeLa cells, p.H723R caused protein retention in endoplasmic reticulum and abolished complex glycosylation of pendrin, and the defects in protein processing could be restored considerably by low temperature incubation or treatment with sodium butyrate [32]. Further study revealed the folding defect in the p.H723R-pendrin, and treatment of salicylate, which functioned as a pharmacological chaperone, could restore normal protein localization and anion exchange activity [33].

Interestingly, as shown in the present study, both heterozygous mice (i.e., *Slc26a4*$^{+/tm2Dontuh}$) and homozygous mice (i.e., *Slc26a4*$^{tm2Dontuh/tm2Dontuh}$) with the knock-in p.H723R mutation had normal audiovestibular phenotypes, including normal hearing thresholds up to 9 months, excellent balancing ability, and an intact cochlear and vestibular morphology. There are several possibilities why the p.H723R mutation did not lead to the expected abnormal phenotype in mice. The first possibility is that the abnormal phenotype was present but not yet discovered or that the abnormal phenotype will become evident only under certain environmental conditions [34]. Although this possibility could not be completely ruled out by the results of this study, it was largely weakened after an exhaustive investigation of the audiovestibular phenotypes, including examination of hearing levels up to 9 months, a battery of vestibular tests, comprehensive inner ear morphological studies, and noise exposure experiments. The second possibility is that the phenotypic effects of the p.H723R mutation are influenced by the genetic background of the mice [35]. This was also unlikely; as in our previous study, we generated a knock-in *Slc26a4* mouse model with abnormal audiovestibular phenotypes by using the same C57BL/6 strain. Another possibility, which became the most likely scenario for our study after the former 2 possibilities were refuted, is that, there are, in fact, no abnormal phenotypes.

In particular, the absence of abnormal audiovestibular phenotypes in homozygous mice alone is not sufficient to exclude the pathogenicity of p.H723R in mice because the function of the *Slc26a4* p.H723R mutation might be only partially defective, and even harboring 2 p.H723R alleles might still maintain adequate *Slc26a4* function. To elucidate the pathogenicity of the p.H723R allele, we further generated mice with compound heterozygous mutations (i.e., *Slc26a4*$^{tm1Dontuh/tm2Dontuh}$) by intercrossing *Slc26a4*$^{+/tm2Dontuh}$ mice with *Slc26a4*$^{tm1Dontuh/tm1Dontuh}$ mice, which segregated the c.919-2A>G mutation with abolished function. Mice that were compound heterozygous for p.H723R and c.919-2A>G (i.e., *Slc26a4*$^{tm1Dontuh/tm2Dontuh}$) had normal audiovestibular phenotypes, indicating that a single p.H723R allele was sufficient to maintain normal inner ear physiology. Moreover, the expression of the downstream *Kcnj10* gene, which diminished at P10–P15 following oxidative stress in *Slc26a4*$^{-/-}$ mice [36], was not compromised in *Slc26a4*$^{tm2Dontuh/tm2Dontuh}$ mice and *Slc26a4*$^{tm1Dontuh/tm2Dontuh}$ mice. These findings indicate that the p.H723R allele is neither pathogenic in mice nor is a mutation with partially ablated function.

As shown in Figure 5, both *Slc26a4*$^{tm2Dontuh/tm2Dontuh}$ and *Slc26a4*$^{tm1Dontuh/tm2Dontuh}$ mice expressed pendrin of molecular weight and expression level comparable to the wild-type mice, indicating that the trafficking/glycosylation process remained unaffected in the murine p.H723R-pendrin. The difference in the intactness of the trafficking/glycosylation process might contribute to the variation in the pathogenicity of p.H723R between mice and humans. We further analyzed the amino-acid sequences of human and mouse pendrin using ConSeq (http://conseq.tau.ac.il/), a website server predicting biologically important residues in protein [37]. Possibly the intact trafficking/glycosylation process of p.H723R in mice might be attributed to a different alignment of amino acid residues in the vicinity, as well as the embedded location of p.H723 in the pendrin (Fig. S1).

Four other mouse models with *Slc26a4* mutations have been reported: knock-out *Slc26a4*$^{-/-}$ mice [14], *Slc26a4*^{loop} mice with the p.S408F mutation generated by ENU mutagenesis [15], *Slc26a4*^{tm1Dontuh} knock-in mice with the common East Asian c.919-2A>G mutation [16], and conditional knock-out Tg[E];Tg[R];*Slc26a4*$^{\Delta/\Delta}$mice [17] (Table 1). *Slc26a4*$^{-/-}$mice are profoundly deaf with significant vestibular deficits and have EVA and scala media, mimicking the phenotypes in humans [14]. Subsequent research on *Slc26a4*^{loop} mice [15] and *Slc26a4*$^{tm1Dontuh/tm1Dontuh}$ mice [16] reported similar auditory and vestibular characteristics, complementing the studies on *Slc26a4*$^{-/-}$mice. To better simulate the less severe audiological phenotype in humans, Choi et al. generated a binary transgenic mouse line in which *Slc26a4* expression could be induced with doxycycline. The authors identified that the E16.5 to P2 was the critical interval in which pendrin was required for acquisition of normal hearing, and demonstrated that doxycycline initiation at E18.5 or discontinuation at E17.5 resulted in partial hearing loss, instead of the profound hearing loss observed in the knock-out *Slc26a4*$^{-/-}$ mice [17]. In contrast, *Slc26a4*$^{tm2Dontuh/tm2Dontuh}$ mice examined in this study had normal audiovestibular phenotypes, representing a distinct and unique mouse strain compared with the other mouse models reported in the literature.

Among humans, patients with PS are more likely to have 2 *SLC26A4* mutant alleles than those with nonsyndromic EVA [11,12]. Moreover, the number of *SLC26A4* mutant alleles is significantly correlated with the severity of hearing loss in individuals with EVA [38,39]. However, because of its diverse mutation spectrum, it is difficult to delineate the phenotypes associated with a specific *SLC26A4* mutation in humans. Consequently, determining the pathogenetic mechanisms of each specific *SLC26A4* mutation largely relies on functional studies performed in *Xenopus* oocytes [40] or cell lines [41,42]. The observation that mice with distinct *Slc26a4* mutations have different phenotypes indicates that transgenic mice may serve as appropriate, direct models to investigate corresponding *SLC26A4* mutations in humans.

In conclusion, using a genotype-driven approach, we generated a knock-in mouse model segregating the common deafness-associated *SLC26A4* p.H723R mutation in humans. To our surprise, mice with the *Slc26a4* p.H723R mutation had a normal audiovestibular phenotype and inner ear morphology. Because there might be differences in the pathogenicity of specific *SLC26A4* mutations in humans and mice, precaution should be taken when extrapolating the results of animal studies to humans.

Supporting Information

Figure S1 **Alignment of amino-acid sequences of human and mouse pendrin.** The amino-acid sequence (a.a. 651–780) of human pendrin (hum-pendrin) was aligned in relative to the sequence of the mouse pendrin (mse-pendrin) using Conseq. Arrows indicate the p.H723 position. The p.H723 is a highly conserved but buried amino acid residue. Different alignments of amino acid residues in the vicinity of p.H723 and the embedded location of p.H723 in the pendrin might contribute to the variation in the pathogenicity of p.H723R between mice and humans. The first row below the sequence lists the predicted burial status of the site (b, buried; e, exposed). The second row indicates residues predicted to be structurally (s) and functionally (f) important.

Table S1 Comparison of vestibular features according to the genotypes and the circling behavior.

Table S2 Blood chemistry of *Slc26a4* male mice at postnatal day 15, 2 and 6 months of age.

Acknowledgments

We thank the staff of the Eighth Core Lab, Department of Medical Research, National Taiwan University Hospital for technical support in performing functional genetic studies. We are also grateful to the Transgenic Mouse Model Core Facility of the National Core Facility Program for Biotechnology, National Science Council and the Gene Knockout Mouse Core Laboratory of National Taiwan University Center of Genomic Medicine for the generation of the transgenic mice.

Author Contributions

Conceived and designed the experiments: YCL CCW CJH. Performed the experiments: YCL THY YHL. Analyzed the data: YCL CCW JMW. Contributed reagents/materials/analysis tools: ISY SWL QC XL. Wrote the paper: YCL CCW CJH.

References

1. Hilgert N, Smith RJ, Van Camp G (2009) Forty-six genes causing nonsyndromic hearing impairment: Which ones should be analyzed in DNA diagnostics? Mutat Res 681: 189–196.
2. Wu CC, Chen PJ, Chiu YH, Lu YC, Wu MC, et al. (2008) Prospective mutation screening of three common deafness genes in a large Taiwanese Cohort with idiopathic bilateral sensorineural hearing impairment reveals a difference in the results between families from hospitals and those from rehabilitation facilities. Audiol Neurootol 13: 172–181.
3. Everett LA, Morsli H, Wu DK, Green ED (1999) Expression pattern of the mouse ortholog of the Pendred's syndrome gene (Pds) suggests a key role for pendrin in the inner ear. Proc Natl Acad Sci U S A 96: 9727–9732.
4. Royaux IE, Suzuki K, Mori A, Katoh R, Everett LA, et al. (2000) Pendrin, the protein encoded by the Pendred syndrome gene (PDS), is an apical porter of iodide in the thyroid and is regulated by thyroglobulin in FRTL-5 cells. Endocrinology 141: 839–845.
5. Royaux IE, Karniski LP, Everett LA, Knepper MA, Green ED, et al. (2001) Pendrin, encoded by the Pendred syndrome gene, resides in the apical region of renal intercalated cells and mediates bicarbonate secretion. Proc Natl Acad Sci U S A 98: 4221–4226.
6. Soleimani M, Greeley T, Petrovic S, Wang ZH, Amlal H, et al. (2001) Pendrin: an apical Cl(−)/OH(−)/HCO(3)(−) exchanger in the kidney cortex. Am J Physiol Renal Physiol 280: F356–364.
7. Shcheynikov N, Yang DK, Wang YX, Zeng WZ, Karniski LP, et al. (2008) The Slc26a4 transporter functions as an electroneutral Cl(−)/I(−)/HCO(3)(−) exchanger: role of Slc26a4 and Slc26a6 in I(−) and HCO(3)(−) secretion and in regulation of CFTR in the parotid duct. J Physiol 586: 3813–3824.
8. Nakao I, Kanaji S, Ohta S, Matsushita H, Arima K, et al. (2008) Identification of pendrin as a common mediator for mucus production in bronchial asthma and chronic obstructive pulmonary disease. J Immunol 180: 6262–6269.
9. Everett LA, Glaser B, Beck JC, Idol JR, Buchs A, et al. (1997) Pendred syndrome is caused by mutations in a putative sulphate transporter gene (PDS). Nat Genet 17: 411–422.
10. Li XC, Everett LA, Lalwani AK, Desmukh D, Friedman TB, et al. (1998) A mutation in PDS causes non-syndromic recessive deafness. Nat Genet 18: 215–217.
11. Pryor SP, Madeo AC, Reynolds JC, Sarlis NJ, Arnos KS, et al. (2005) SLC26A4/PDS genotype-phenotype correlation in hearing loss with enlargement of the vestibular aqueduct (EVA): evidence that Pendred syndrome and

non-syndromic EVA are distinct clinical and genetic entities. J Med Genet 42: 159–165.
12. Azaiez H, Yang T, Prasad S, Sorensen JL, Nishimura CJ, et al. (2007) Genotype-phenotype correlations for SLC26A4-related deafness. Hum Genet 122: 451–457.
13. Mori T, Westerberg BD, Atashband S, Kozak FK (2008) Natural history of hearing loss in children with enlarged vestibular aqueduct syndrome. J Otolaryngol Head Neck Surg 37: 112–118.
14. Everett LA, Belyantseva IA, Noben-Trauth K, Cantos R, Chen A, et al. (2001) Targeted disruption of mouse Pds provides insight about the inner-ear defects encountered in Pendred syndrome. Hum Mol Genet 10: 153–161.
15. Dror AA, Politi Y, Shahin H, Lenz DR, Dossena S, et al. (2010) Calcium oxalate stone formation in the inner ear as a result of an Slc26a4 mutation. J Biol Chem 28: 21724–21735.
16. Lu YC, Wu CC, Shen WS, Yang TH, Yeh TH, et al. (2011) Establishment of a knock-in mouse model with the SLC26A4 c.919–2A>G mutation and characterization of its pathology. PLoS One 6: e22150.
17. Choi BY, Kim HM, Ito T, Lee KY, Li XM, et al. (2011) Mouse model of enlarged vestibular aqueducts defines temporal requirement of Slc26a4 expression for hearing acquisition. J Clin Invest 121: 4516–4525.
18. Tsukamoto K, Suzuki H, Harada D, Namba A, Abe S, et al. (2003) Distribution and frequencies of PDS (SLC26A4) mutations in Pendred syndrome and nonsyndromic hearing loss associated with enlarged vestibular aqueduct: a unique spectrum of mutations in Japanese. Eur J Hum Genet 11: 916–922.
19. Park HJ, Lee SJ, Jin HS, Lee JO, Go SH, et al. (2005) Genetic basis of hearing loss associated with enlarged vestibular aqueducts in Koreans. Clin Genet 67: 160–165.
20. Wu CC, Yeh TH, Chen PJ, Hsu CJ (2005) Prevalent SLC26A4 mutations in patients with enlarged vestibular aqueduct and/or Mondini dysplasia: a unique spectrum of mutations in Taiwan, including a frequent founder mutation. Laryngoscope 115: 1060–1064.
21. Wang QJ, Zhao YL, Rao SQ, Guo YF, Yuan H, et al. (2007) A distinct spectrum of SLC26A4 mutations in patients with enlarged vestibular aqueduct in China. Clin Genet 72: 245–254.
22. Yuan Y, Guo W, Tang J, Zhang G, Wang G, et al. (2012) Molecular epidemiology and functional assessment of novel allelic variants of *SLC26A4* in non-syndromic hearing loss patients with enlarged vestibular aqueduct in China. PLoS One 7: e49984.
23. Lee EC, Yu D, Martinez de Velasco J, Tessarollo L, Swing DA, et al. (2001) A highly efficient Escherichia coli-based chromosome engineering system adapted for recombinogenic targeting and subcloning of BAC DNA. Genomics 73: 56–65.
24. Su KY, Chien WL, Fu WM, Yu IS, Huang HP, et al. (2007) Mice deficient in collapsin response mediator protein-1 exhibit impaired long-term potentiation and impaired spatial learning and memory. J Neurosci 27: 2513–2524.
25. Belyantseva IA, Adler HJ, Curi R, Frolenkov GI, Kachar B (2000) Expression and localization of prestin and the sugar transporter GLUT-5 during development of electromotility in cochlear outer hair cells. J Neurosci 20: RC116.
26. Wangemann P, Kim HM, Billings S, Nakaya K, Li X, et al. (2009) Developmental delays consistent with cochlear hypothyroidism contribute to failure to develop hearing in mice lacking Slc26a4/pendrin expression. Am J Physiol Renal Physiol 297: F1435–1447.
27. Wangemann P, Itza EM, Albrecht B, Wu T, Jabba SV, et al. (2004) Loss of KCNJ10 protein expression abolishes endocochlear potential and causes deafness in Pendred syndrome mouse model. BMC Med 2: 30.
28. Yang T, Gurrola JG II, Wu H, Chiu SM, Wangemann P, et al. (2009) Mutations of KCNJ10 together with mutations of SLC26A4 cause digenic nonsyndromic hearing loss associated with enlarged vestibular aqueduct syndrome. Am J Hum Genet 84: 651–657.
29. Ohlemiller KK, Gagnon PM (2007) Genetic dependence of cochlear cells and structures injured by noise. Hear Res 224: 34–50.
30. Sugiura M, Sato E, Nakashima T, Sugiura J, Furuhashi A, et al. (2005) Long-term follow-up in patients with Pendred syndrome: vestibular, auditory and other phenotypes. Eur Arch Otorhinolaryngol 262: 737–743.
31. Park HJ, Shaukat S, Liu XZ, Hahn SH, Naz S, et al. (2003) Origins and frequencies of SLC26A4 (PDS) mutations in east and south Asians: global implications for the epidemiology of deafness. J Med Genet 40: 242–248.
32. Yoon JS, Park HJ, Yoo SY, Namkung W, Jo MJ, et al. (2008) Heterogeneity in the processing defect of SLC26A4 mutants. J Med Genet 45: 411–419.
33. Ishihara K, Okuyama S, Kumano S, Iida K, Hamana H, et al. (2010) Salicylate restores transport function and anion exchanger activity of missense pendrin mutations. Hear Res 270: 110–118.
34. Barbaric I, Miller G, Dear TN (2007) Appearances can be deceiving: phenotypes of knockout mice. Brief Funct Genomic Proteomic 6: 91–103.
35. Pearson H (2002) Surviving a knockout blow. Nature 415: 8–9.
36. Singh R, Wangemann P (2008) Free radical stress-mediated loss of Kcnj10 protein expression in stria vascularis contributes to deafness in Pendred syndrome mouse model. Am J Physiol Renal Physiol 294: F139–148.
37. Berezin C, Glaser F, Rosenberg J, Paz I, Pupko T, et al. (2004) ConSeq: the identification of functionally and structurally important residues in protein sequences. Bioinformatics 20: 1322–1324.
38. King KA, Choi BY, Zalewski C, Madeo AC, Manichaikul A, et al. (2010) SLC26A4 genotype, but not cochlear radiologic structure, is correlated with hearing loss in ears with an enlarged vestibular aqueduct. Laryngoscope 120: 384–389.
39. Albert S, Blons H, Jonard L, Feldmann D, Chauvin P, et al. (2006) SLC26A4 gene is frequently involved in nonsyndromic hearing impairment with enlarged vestibular aqueduct in Caucasian populations. Eur J Hum Genet 14: 773–779.
40. Scott DA, Wang R, Kreman TM, Andrews M, McDonald JM, et al. (2000) Functional differences of the PDS gene product are associated with phenotypic variation in patients with Pendred syndrome and non-syndromic hearing loss (DFNB4). Hum Mol Genet 9: 1709–1715.
41. Taylor JP, Metcalfe RA, Watson PF, Weetman AP, Trembath RC (2002) Mutations of the PDS gene, encoding pendrin, are associated with protein mislocalization and loss of iodide efflux: implications for thyroid dysfunction in Pendred syndrome. J Clin Endocrinol Metab 87: 1778–1784.
42. Choi BY, Stewart AK, Madeo AC, Pryor SP, Lenhard S, et al. (2009) Hypo-functional SLC26A4 variants associated with nonsyndromic hearing loss and enlargement of the vestibular aqueduct: genotype-phenotype correlation or coincidental polymorphisms? Hum Mutat 30: 599–608.

21

Molecular Genetics of the Usher Syndrome in Lebanon: Identification of 11 Novel Protein Truncating Mutations by Whole Exome Sequencing

Ramesh Reddy[1], Somayyeh Fahiminiya[2], Elie El Zir[3], Ahmad Mansour[4], Andre Megarbane[5], Jacek Majewski[2], Rima Slim[1]*

1 Departments of Human Genetics and Obstetrics-Gynecology, McGill University Health Centre, Montreal, Canada, 2 McGill University and Genome Quebec Innovation Centre and Department of Human Genetics, Montreal, Canada, 3 Department of Otorhinolaryngology, Hôpital Sacré-Coeur, Baabda, Lebanon, 4 Department of Ophthalmology, American University of Beirut, Beirut, Lebanon, 5 Unité de génétique médicale, Faculté de médecine, Université Saint Joseph, Beirut, Lebanon

Abstract

Background: Usher syndrome (USH) is a genetically heterogeneous condition with ten disease-causing genes. The spectrum of genes and mutations causing USH in the Lebanese and Middle Eastern populations has not been described. Consequently, diagnostic approaches designed to screen for previously reported mutations were unlikely to identify the mutations in 11 unrelated families, eight of Lebanese and three of Middle Eastern origins. In addition, six of the ten USH genes consist of more than 20 exons, each, which made mutational analysis by Sanger sequencing of PCR-amplified exons from genomic DNA tedious and costly. The study was aimed at the identification of USH causing genes and mutations in 11 unrelated families with USH type I or II.

Methods: Whole exome sequencing followed by expanded familial validation by Sanger sequencing.

Results: We identified disease-causing mutations in all the analyzed patients in four USH genes, *MYO7A*, *USH2A*, *GPR98* and *CDH23*. Eleven of the mutations were novel and protein truncating, including a complex rearrangement in *GPR98*.

Conclusion: Our data highlight the genetic diversity of Usher syndrome in the Lebanese population and the time and cost-effectiveness of whole exome sequencing approach for mutation analysis of genetically heterogeneous conditions caused by large genes.

Editor: Alfred S. Lewin, University of Florida, United States of America

Funding: This work was supported by a grant from the Canadian Institutes of Health Research (86546). The funders had no role in study design, data collection and analysis, decision to publish, or preparation of the manuscript.

Competing Interests: The authors have declared that no competing interests exist.

* Email: rima.slim@muhc.mcgill.ca

Introduction

Usher syndrome (USH) is a group of recessive inherited disorders characterized by neurosensory deafness and progressive vision loss, with or without vestibular dysfunction [1]. USH affects around one in 20,000 individuals and accounts for approximately 50% of all the deaf-blindness cases [2]. Usher syndrome can be clinically classified into three types, USH1, USH2 and USH3 [3]. USH1 is the most severe type of the three with profound congenital deafness, vestibular dysfunction and prepubertal progressive retinitis pigmentosa (RP). USH2 is characterized by moderate to severe congenital deafness and post pubertal onset of RP. USH3 is characterized by progressive hearing loss, retinitis pigmentosa and variable vestibular dysfunction. USH2 is the most common type of USH and accounts for 50–65% of all USH cases [3,4]. USH1 accounts for 10–35% of all USH cases [3,4] while USH3 is rare and accounts for 2–5% of USH cases in several populations with the exception of the Finnish and Ashkenazi populations where USH3 accounts for 40% of all USH cases [3,4].

To date, there are 10 genes known to cause USH (http://hereditaryhearingloss.org). Mutations in 6 genes, *MYO7A* [5], *USH1C* [6], *CDH23* [7], *PCDH15* [8], *USH1G* [9], and *CIB2* [10] have been found causative of USH1. *MYO7A* is the major gene responsible for USH1 and mutations in *MYO7A* alone account for 70% of USH1. *CDH23* is the second commonly mutated gene and mutations in *MYO7A* and *CDH23* together account for 80% of USH1 [11,12]. Mutations in three genes, *USH2A* [*13*], *GPR98* [*14*], and *DFNB31/WHRN* [*15*] have been identified as disease-causing for USH2. *USH2A* is the most frequently mutated gene in USH2 patients and mutations in *USH2A* alone account for 85% of USH2 while mutations in *GPR98* account for 6% of USH2 in the French and other Caucasian populations [16,17]. Mutations in one gene *CLRN1* are found causative for USH3 [18]. Digenic inheritance in USH has been reported with mutations in *GPR98* and *PDZD7* [19] in USH2 patients and with mutations in *CDH23* and *PCDH15* [20] or *MYO7A* and *PCDH15* [21] in USH1 patients. In addition, mutations in *MYO7A, USH1C, DFNB31, CIB2, CDH23* and *PCDH15* were also reported in non-syndromic deafness without retinal degeneration [22,23] and mutations in *USH2A* and *CLRN1* have been reported in patients with isolated RP or retinal dystrophies and no deafness [24–26].

The spectrum of genes and mutations that cause Usher syndrome in the Lebanese and Middle Eastern populations is not known. To date, only two Lebanese USH families, one with a mutation in *USH1C* and one with a mutation in *CLRN1*, have been reported [6,27]. In this study, we describe the use of whole exome sequencing (WES) to identify Usher causing mutations in 11 unrelated families from Lebanon and the Middle East, of which one was linked to USH1B, three linked to USH2A, and two had weak linkage, with lod score of less than 2, to USH2A in a previous study performed before the identification of the USH1B and USH2A associated genes [28,29]. Because some of the families did not have a conclusive linkage to known loci and the genetic causes of Usher syndrome in these populations have not been well studied, we favored the use of WES instead of a targeted sequencing approach. We report the identification of 11 novel protein-truncating mutations in four Usher genes in the 11 families. Our data demonstrate the advantage of WES over traditional approaches for DNA diagnosis of genetically heterogeneous disorders caused by mutations in large genes.

Materials and Methods

Patient Recruitment

This study adhered to the tenets of the Declaration of Helsinki. The study was approved by the Institutional Review Board of the American University of Beirut. Verbal consents were obtained from all enrolled subjects according to the recommendations of the Institutional Review Board of the American University of Beirut that were in place between 1994–1998 and before the implementation of written consent forms. The verbal consents of the subjects were witnessed by at least three study participants. Patients have been clinically evaluated according to the criteria recommended by the Usher Syndrome Consortium [30]. Comprehensive ophthalmic examinations, including routine eye tests, perimetry and electroretinography (ERG) were carried out for each patient (Figure 1). Auditory function of affected subjects was assessed by pure tone audiometry, speech-audiometry, and tympanometry. Hearing impairment was classified as mild (20–40 dB), moderate (41–70 dB), severe (71–95 dB), or profound (>95 dB). Electronystagmography was used to assess spontaneous and positional nystagmus (saccades and pursuit). A standard caloric test (30°C and 44°C) was performed using an ICS caloric irrigation system and observation of the nystagmus using Frenzel's glasses. Detailed family history was obtained through personal interviews with patients and their relatives (Figures S1 and S2). Peripheral blood samples were collected from all available family members for DNA extraction.

Clinical classification and linkage analysis

Based on the clinical evaluations of the 11 studied patients, 4 were classified as USH1 and 7 were classified as USH2 (Table 1). Linkage analysis with microsatellite markers surrounding the USH1B locus on 11q13.5 and USH2A on 1q41 were previously reported on six families [28,29]. Five families were attributed to USH2A and 1 family to USH1B locus.

Exome capture and sequencing

Exome sequencing was carried out at the McGill University and Genome Quebec Innovation Centre, Montreal, Canada as previously detailed [31,32]. In brief, whole exome was captured using the SureSelect Human All Exon Kit version 5 (Agilent Technologies, Inc., Santa Clara, CA) on 3 µg of genomic DNA from all the probands of 11 families. Sequencing was carried out with pair end 100 base reads on the Illumina Hiseq2000 sequencer. The reads were aligned to the human reference genome (hg19) using BWA (v. 0.5.9) [33]. The whole exome coverage at 30X resolution in the 11 patient samples was above 95% (data not shown). A mean coverage of 133X was obtained for all consensus coding sequence (CCDS) exons using the Genome Analysis Toolkit (GATK)[34]. Variants were called and annotated using the SAMTools (v. 0.1.17) [35] and ANNOVAR [36], respectively. To remove systematic false positives, as well as common polymorphisms, the lists of variants were filtered against >1000 of individual in-house exomes. Additionally, the variants with an allele frequency >5% in either the 1000 genomes database (http://www.1000genomes.org) or the NHLBI exomes (v.0.0.14, June 20, 2012) were filtered out. Also, we looked for copy number variants (CNVs) in our patient samples using FishingCNV software [37]. Finally, to focus on likely disease-causing variants, we prioritized frameshift, indel, nonsense, missense and canonical splice site variants for further analysis. Additional analyses such as the identification of regions of homozygosity were performed using custom PERL scripts.

Sanger sequencing validation of identified mutations and bioinformatics analysis

Primers were designed to amplify the fragments containing the mutations using primer 3 software [38]. Sequence analysis was performed using DNASTAR [39] and the sequences were compared to their respective reference sequences (NM_000260.3 for *MYO7A*; NM_206933.2 for *USH2A*; NM_001171933.1 for *CDH23*; and NM_032119.3 for *GPR98*). DNA mutation numbering is based on cDNA sequence with a 'c.' symbol before the number and uses the A of the ATG translation initiation start site as nucleotide 1. Protein numbering starts from the initiation codon. Mutations nomenclatures were checked using Mutalyzer [40]. The amino acid and nucleotide residue conservations across species were examined using NCBI BLAST (http://www.ncbi.nlm.nih.gov/BLAST/). Splice site prediction was performed using the following online available prediction tools, NetGene2 (http://www.cbs.dtu.dk/services/NetGene2), HSF (http://www.umd.be/HSF/), BDGP (http://www.fruitfly.org/seq_tools/splice.html), GENSCAN (http://genes.mit.edu/GENSCAN.html). The possible pathogenic effect of protein-coding variants was examined using two prediction tools, SIFT (http://sift.jcvi.org/) and Polyphen-2 (http://genetics.bwh.harvard.edu/pph2/).

Results

WES was performed on one affected member from each of 11 unrelated families. Of these 11 families, four were diagnosed clinically with USH1 and one had linkage to the region containing *MYO7A* [29] (Tables 1 and S1). The remaining 7 families were diagnosed with USH2 and three of them had a conclusive linkage to 1q41 [28] (Tables 1 and S2). The average coverage of the 10 known Usher genes was around 96% in the 11 patients studied (Figure 2A, Table S3). Analysis of the exome sequencing data identified 12 different mutations in (i) two USH1 genes, *MYO7A* and *CDH23*; (ii) two USH2 genes, *USH2A* and *GPR98* (Table 1); and (iii) no mutations in any other USH gene suggesting

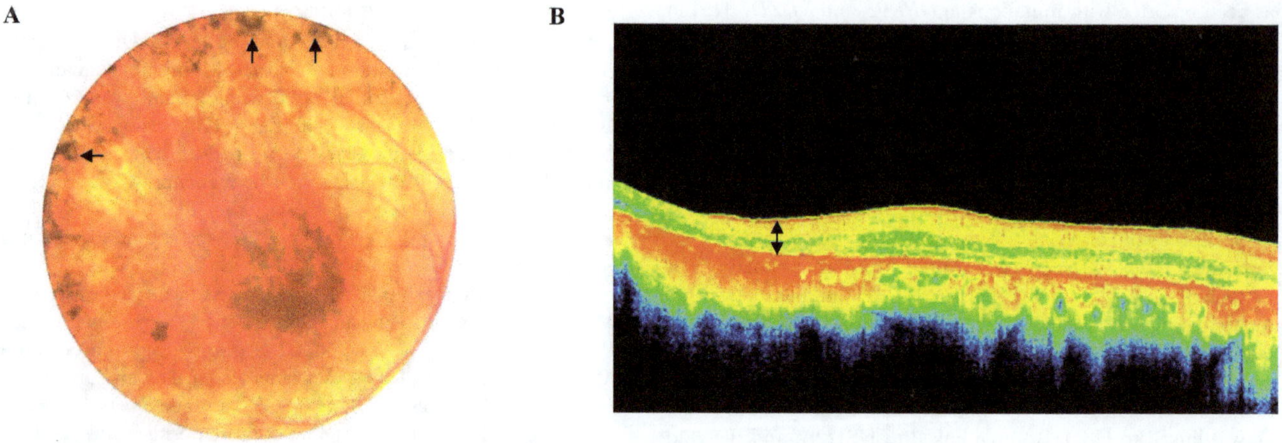

Figure 1. Clinical examination. A. Posterior pole of the right eye of patient USHLB13-II.3 showing atrophy of the retina and choroid with pigment spicules (arrows) anterior to the arcades. **B.** Spectral domain optical coherence tomography of the right eye of the same patient showing significant thinning of the retina (space delineated by double arrow) compared to normal controls.

monogenic inheritance of the disease. Of the 12 identified mutations, three were in *MYO7A*, one in *CDH23*, six in *USH2A*, and two in *GPR98* (Table 1 and Figure S3). One of the 12 mutations was a previously reported missense, p.G955S, in *MYO7A*, and 11 are novel.

The 11 novel mutations included five nonsense in *MYO7A*, *CDH23*, and *USH2A*; four frameshifts in *USH2A* and *GPR98*; a large rearrangement deleting 14,042 bp including exon 83 of *GPR98* and inserting 17 bp; and a missense mutation, R2894K (c.8681 G>A), in *USH2A*. In the latter, the Arginine residue at amino acid position 2894 is highly conserved from Human to Xenopus (Figure 2B) and lies in the Fibronectin-15 domain of the protein and consequently its substitution could have a potential effect on the structure and function of the protein. The effect of this substitution was also predicted to be damaging by polyphen and SIFT prediction programmes [41,42]. In addition, because this missense is caused by a DNA change affecting the first nucleotide of exon 43 that could potentially affect the gene splicing, we used five *in silico* splice prediction programmes to assess its impact. We found that three programmes, BDGP [43], MaxEntscan [44], and NetGene2 [45], predicted the same abnormal splicing affecting the splice acceptor site of exon 43 of *USH2A* and leading to its skipping from the RNA. This would result in a frameshift and premature protein truncation and is an additional argument in favour of the pathogenicity of this DNA change.

To define the rearrangement around exon 83 of *GPR98* identified by exome sequencing, we used primer walking, regular and long range PCR amplification on DNA from affected and unaffected members of USHLB2. This analysis led us to amplify a 5.5 kb PCR fragment containing the deletion flanking regions (Figure 2C, 2D). DNA sequencing of this fragment revealed that the rearrangement consists of a 14,042 bp deletion and of a 17 bp insertion (Figure 2C). The use of RepeatMasker (www.repeatmasker.org) revealed the presence of an AluSC8 repeat on the proximal breakpoint of the deletion in intron 82 (Figure 2C). Comparing the 17 bp insertion with databases revealed its presence at several genomic loci, but the 17 bp did not map to any known repetitive elements.

All the identified mutations were confirmed in the patients and their extended families using Sanger sequencing and all segregated with the disease phenotype (Tables S2 and S3). The 11 identified novel mutations were not found in the LOVD Usher database (https://grenada.lumc.nl/LOVD2/Usher_montpellier/USHbases.html), the deafness variation database (http://deafnessvariationdatabase.com/), or in any of the control populations listed on the exome variant server database (EVS, http://evs.gs.washington.edu/EVS/), the genome variant database (1000 genomes, http://www.1000genomes.org/), and dbSNP (http://www.ncbi.nlm.nih.gov/snp). Altogether, these arguments demonstrate the pathogenicity of the 12 identified mutations and their causation of USH.

Discussion

With the advent of WES, finding mutations in genetically heterogeneous Mendelian disorders has become fast and feasible. Recent studies have demonstrated that mutation detection rate using WES in patients with USH1 and USH2 is more than 90% and suggested the usefulness of this approach for routine molecular diagnosis of USH [17,46]. In our study, we identified the causative genes and mutations in all the 11 families we analyzed, which corroborate previous observations in the field.

To identify USH genes and mutations in 11 USH families from Lebanon and the Middle East, from which only two families with USH syndrome had been characterized at the mutation level, we performed WES on 11 probands and identified disease-causing mutations in all of them. These patients had 12 different mutations, of which 11 are novel and lead to protein truncations. To date and including this study, mutations in 11 Lebanese families clinically with USH, four with USH1, six with USH2, and one with USH3, have been reported [6,27]. Among the four USH1 families, four different genes, three responsible for USH1, *USH1C* [6], MYO7A, and *CDH23*, and one responsible for USH3, *CLRN1* [27], were found mutated, one in each family. Among the six USH2 families, two genes, *USH2A* and *GPR98*, were found mutated in four and two families, respectively (Figure 3). The remaining family was originally diagnosed as USH3, but the diagnosis was revised to PHARC (a neurodegenerative disease characterized by polyneuropathy, hearing loss, ataxia, retinitis pigmentosa, and early-onset cataract) after the identification of a homozygous mutation in *ABHD12* and clinical re-evaluation [47]. Our current and previous data on the 11 Lebanese families indicate that *USH2A* mutations (40%) are the most frequent cause of USH in the Lebanese population, followed

Table 1. Summary of the identified mutations in the four Usher genes.

Family	Ethnicity	Linkage	Proband	Gene	Mutation		Status	Reported
					cDNA	protein		
Usher Type 1								
USHEG5	Egyptian	no linkage data	II-1	*MYO7A*	c.2863G>A	p.G955S	Hom	Reported
USHJO9	Jordanian	linked to 11q13.5 [28]	III-2	*MYO7A*	c.462C>A	p.C154*	Hom	Novel
USHLB12	Lebanese	no linkage data	II-2	*MYO7A*	c.834C>A	p.Y278*	Hom	Novel
USHLB14	Lebanese	no linkage data	II-1	*CDH23*	c.8803C>T	p.R2935*	Hom	Novel
Usher Type 2								
USHLB1	Lebanese	linked to 1q [29]	III-3	*USH2A*	c.11907delA	p.A3970Lfs*14	Hom	Novel
USHLB6	Lebanese	linked to 1q [29]	II-2	*USH2A*	c.531_532insA	p.T178Nfs*4	Hom	Novel
USHLB8	Lebanese	linked to 1q [29]	II-1	*USH2A*	c.14031_14032insA	p.A4678Sfs*5	Hom	Novel
USHLB13	Lebanese	no linkage data	II-1	*USH2A*	c.4707T>G	p.Y1569*	Het	Novel
				USH2A	c.14424C>A	p.C4808*	Het	Novel
USHJO10	Jordanian	no linkage data	III-1	*USH2A*	c.8681G>A	p.R2894K/p.R2853Ifs*5	Hom	Novel
USHLB2	Lebanese	weak linkage	III-2	*GPR98*	c.17756-2239_17856+11702delins17bp	p.G5919Nfs*15	Hom	Novel
USHLB11	Lebanese	weak linkage	II-4	*GPR98*	c.16040delA	p.D5347Vfs*22	Hom	Novel

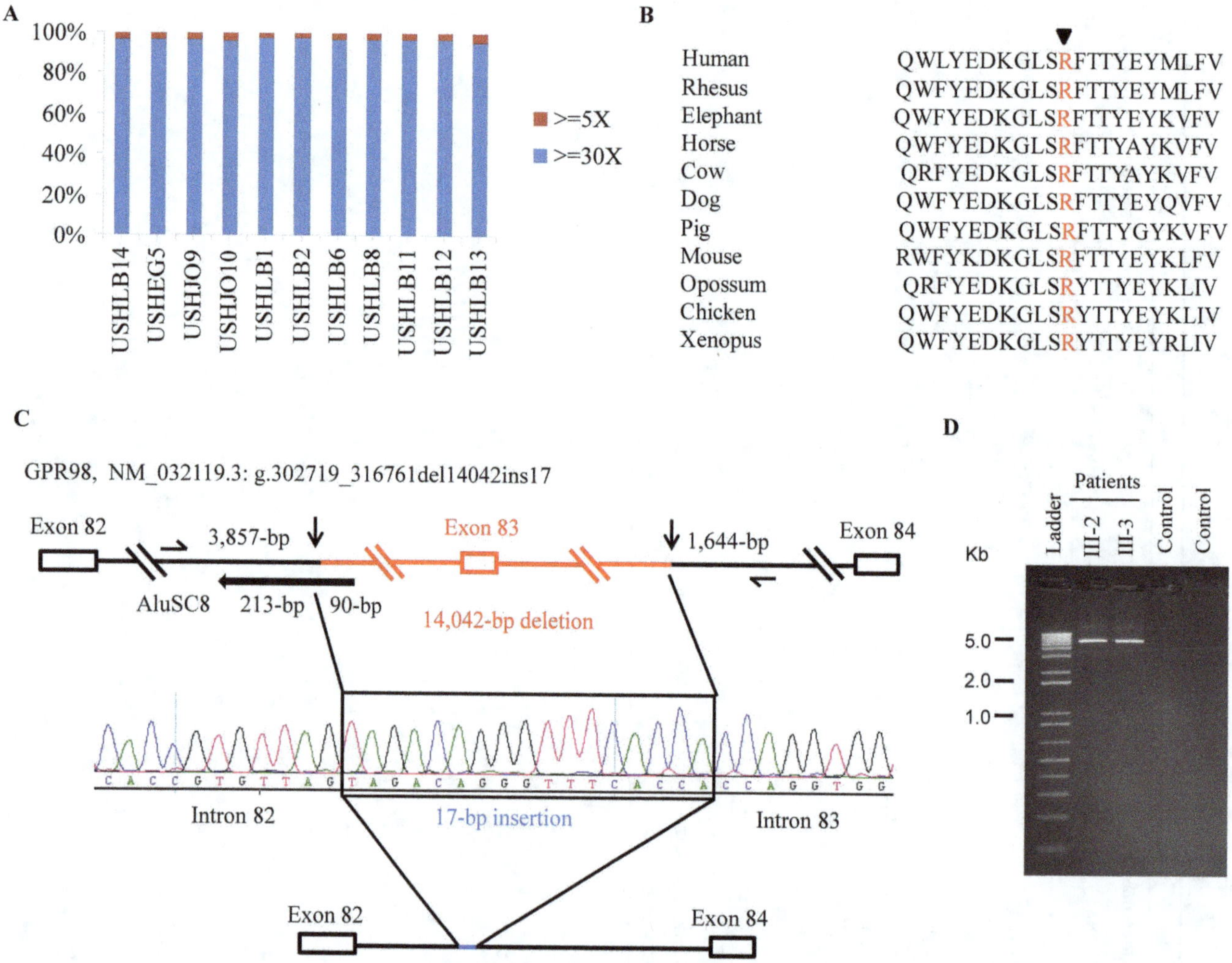

Figure 2. Exome sequencing coverage, conservation of one mutation in *USH2A*, and diagram of the 14,042 bp deletion in *GPR98*. A. Image showing the coverage of the reads at >30X and >5X of the 10 Usher genes in the 11 patients studied using whole exome sequencing. **B.** Conservation of the Arginine (R) at amino acid 2894 in USH2A in different species is shown. **C.** Diagram of the rearrangement deleting exon 83 of *GPR98* in family USHLB2. Arrows indicate the proximal and distal breakpoints of the 14,042 bp deletion. Horizontal arrow shows the AluSC8 repeat overlapping the proximal breakpoint. The 17 bp insertion is shown in a rectangle between the flanking sequences. Primers used for amplifying the 5.5 kb fragment are shown. **D.** Shows the 5.5 kb fragment amplified in the two patients III-2 and III-3 from family USHLB2. The fragment was not amplified in the two control samples due to its large size.

by *GPR98* mutations (20%) while mutations in all the other USH genes seem to be rarer (Figure 3). Analyzing more families from the Lebanese population will help validating our observation on a larger cohort and drawing stronger conclusions about the spectrum of genes and mutations underlying Usher syndrome in Lebanon.

In *GPR98*, we identified a complex rearrangement resulting in the deletion of a 14,042 bp fragment including exon 83 and the insertion of 17 bp. The presence of an AluSC8 repeat on the proximal side of the deletion indicates a possible non-homologous end joining (NHEJ) at its origin. We note that NHEJ-mediated large deletions have been reported in many diseases [48]. In *GPR98*, another large deletion of 136,017 bp had been reported [49] and to our knowledge, the 14,042 bp deletion, reported in this study, is the second large deletion in this gene.

Recently, targeted sequencing approaches aiming at enriching for a subset of Usher genes or related conditions have been used as an alternative to classical methods for molecular diagnosis of Usher syndrome mutations and yielded high rates of mutation detection (70–80%) [17,50,51]. Despite the fact that mutation detection rates in these studies cannot be compared with those obtained in our study since some of our patients had linkage to known USH loci, our analysis indicates that WES is equally efficient and yield equivalent mutation detection rate. In addition, WES will allow not only detecting mutations in known genes, but will identify new genes responsible for Usher syndrome in patients who are negative for mutations in the known genes. The high rate of identified novel mutations in our cohort can be attributed to the large sizes of USH genes, their known high rate of private mutations, the lack of previous mutation analysis on Lebanese patients with USH, and the genetic and allelic heterogeneity of USH in Lebanon, which was unexpected because of the small size of the population and its known high rate of consanguinity.

In conclusion, our study highlights the genetic diversity in the causation of USH in the Lebanese population and reiterates the usefulness and efficiency of WES over traditional approaches for

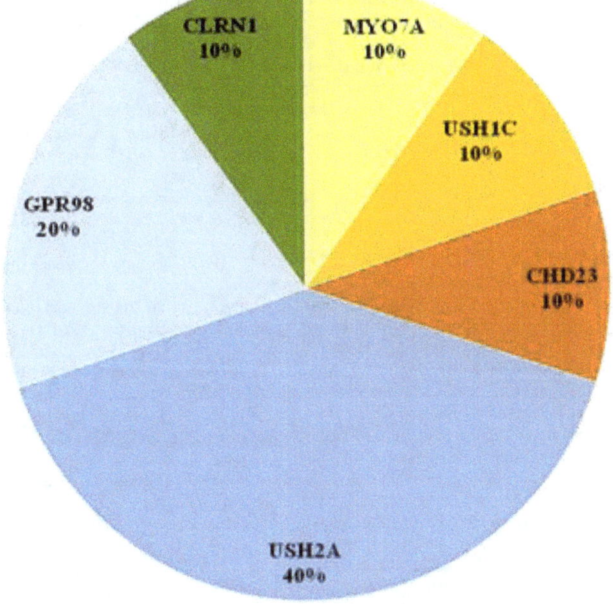

Figure 3. Distribution of mutated genes in ten Lebanese families with USH. Among these ten families, eight are described in this study.

molecular diagnosis of USH. Identification of 11 novel causative mutations for USH in Lebanon adds to the existing causative alleles of USH and genotyping these alleles would be helpful as a first screen in diagnosis of USH patients in Lebanon.

Supporting Information

Figure S1 Pedigrees of the Usher syndrome type 1 families analyzed in this study.

Figure S2 Pedigrees of the Usher syndrome type 2 families analyzed in this study.

Figure S3 Chromatograms of the patients with *MYO7A*, *GPR98*, *USH2A* and *CDH23* mutations.

Table S1 Segregation of the identified mutations in the analyzed USH1 families.

Table S2 Segregation of the identified mutations in the analyzed USH2 families.

Table S3 Sequence coverage of the 10 Usher genes in whole exome sequencing.

Acknowledgments

We thank patients and their family members involved in this study. We also acknowledge the use of the McGill University and Genome Quebec Innovation Centre Facility for exome and Sanger sequencing.

Author Contributions

Conceived and designed the experiments: RR RS. Performed the experiments: RR. Analyzed the data: SF JM RR RS. Contributed reagents/materials/analysis tools: EEZ A. Mansour A. Megabane. Contributed to the writing of the manuscript: RR RS.

References

1. Vernon M (1969) Usher's syndrome—deafness and progressive blindness. Clinical cases, prevention, theory and literature survey. J Chronic Dis 22: 133–151.
2. Boughman JA, Vernon M, Shaver KA (1983) Usher syndrome: definition and estimate of prevalence from two high-risk populations. J Chronic Dis 36: 595–603.
3. Millan JM, Aller E, Jaijo T, Blanco-Kelly F, Gimenez-Pardo A, et al. (2011) An update on the genetics of usher syndrome. J Ophthalmol 2011: 417217.
4. Spandau UH, Rohrschneider K (2002) Prevalence and geographical distribution of Usher syndrome in Germany. Graefes Arch Clin Exp Ophthalmol 240: 495–498.
5. Weil D, Blanchard S, Kaplan J, Guilford P, Gibson F, et al. (1995) Defective myosin VIIA gene responsible for Usher syndrome type 1B. Nature 374: 60–61.
6. Verpy E, Leibovici M, Zwaenepoel I, Liu XZ, Gal A, et al. (2000) A defect in harmonin, a PDZ domain-containing protein expressed in the inner ear sensory hair cells, underlies Usher syndrome type 1C. Nat Genet 26: 51–55.
7. Bolz H, von Brederlow B, Ramirez A, Bryda EC, Kutsche K, et al. (2001) Mutation of CDH23, encoding a new member of the cadherin gene family, causes Usher syndrome type 1D. Nat Genet 27: 108–112.
8. Ahmed ZM, Riazuddin S, Bernstein SL, Ahmed Z, Khan S, et al. (2001) Mutations of the protocadherin gene PCDH15 cause Usher syndrome type 1F. Am J Hum Genet 69: 25–34.
9. Weil D, El-Amraoui A, Masmoudi S, Mustapha M, Kikkawa Y, et al. (2003) Usher syndrome type I G (USH1G) is caused by mutations in the gene encoding SANS, a protein that associates with the USH1C protein, harmonin. Hum Mol Genet 12: 463–471.
10. Riazuddin S, Belyantseva IA, Giese AP, Lee K, Indzhykulian AA, et al. (2012) Alterations of the CIB2 calcium- and integrin-binding protein cause Usher syndrome type 1J and nonsyndromic deafness DFNB48. Nat Genet 44: 1265–1271.
11. Ouyang XM, Yan D, Du LL, Hejtmancik JF, Jacobson SG, et al. (2005) Characterization of Usher syndrome type I gene mutations in an Usher syndrome patient population. Hum Genet 116: 292–299.
12. Nakanishi H, Ohtsubo M, Iwasaki S, Hotta Y, Takizawa Y, et al. (2010) Mutation analysis of the MYO7A and CDH23 genes in Japanese patients with Usher syndrome type 1. J Hum Genet 55: 796–800.
13. Eudy JD, Weston MD, Yao S, Hoover DM, Rehm HL, et al. (1998) Mutation of a gene encoding a protein with extracellular matrix motifs in Usher syndrome type IIa. Science 280: 1753–1757.
14. Weston MD, Luijendijk MW, Humphrey KD, Moller C, Kimberling WJ (2004) Mutations in the VLGR1 gene implicate G-protein signaling in the pathogenesis of Usher syndrome type II. Am J Hum Genet 74: 357–366.
15. Ebermann I, Scholl HP, Charbel Issa P, Becirovic E, Lamprecht J, et al. (2007) A novel gene for Usher syndrome type 2: mutations in the long isoform of whirlin are associated with retinitis pigmentosa and sensorineural hearing loss. Hum Genet 121: 203–211.
16. Le Quesne Stabej P, Saihan Z, Rangesh N, Steele-Stallard HB, Ambrose J, et al. (2012) Comprehensive sequence analysis of nine Usher syndrome genes in the UK National Collaborative Usher Study. J Med Genet 49: 27–36.
17. Besnard T, Vache C, Baux D, Larrieu L, Abadie C, et al. (2012) Non-USH2A mutations in USH2 patients. Hum Mutat 33: 504–510.
18. Joensuu T, Hamalainen R, Yuan B, Johnson C, Tegelberg S, et al. (2001) Mutations in a novel gene with transmembrane domains underlie Usher syndrome type 3. Am J Hum Genet 69: 673–684.
19. Ebermann I, Phillips JB, Liebau MC, Koenekoop RK, Schermer B, et al. (2010) PDZD7 is a modifier of retinal disease and a contributor to digenic Usher syndrome. J Clin Invest 120: 1812–1823.
20. Zheng QY, Yan D, Ouyang XM, Du LL, Yu H, et al. (2005) Digenic inheritance of deafness caused by mutations in genes encoding cadherin 23 and protocadherin 15 in mice and humans. Hum Mol Genet 14: 103–111.
21. Yoshimura H, Iwasaki S, Nishio SY, Kumakawa K, Tono T, et al. (2014) Massively parallel DNA sequencing facilitates diagnosis of patients with Usher syndrome type 1. PLoS One 9: e90688.
22. Ganapathy A, Pandey N, Srisailapathy CR, Jalvi R, Malhotra V, et al. (2014) Non-syndromic hearing impairment in India: high allelic heterogeneity among mutations in TMPRSS3, TMC1, USHIC, CDH23 and TMIE. PLoS One 9: e84773.
23. Di Leva F, D'Adamo P, Cubellis MV, D'Eustacchio A, Errichiello M, et al. (2006) Identification of a novel mutation in the myosin VIIA motor domain in a family with autosomal dominant hearing loss (DFNA11). Audiol Neurootol 11: 157–164.
24. Mendez-Vidal C, Gonzalez-Del Pozo M, Vela-Boza A, Santoyo-Lopez J, Lopez-Domingo FJ, et al. (2013) Whole-exome sequencing identifies novel compound

heterozygous mutations in USH2A in Spanish patients with autosomal recessive retinitis pigmentosa. Mol Vis 19: 2187–2195.
25. Khan MI, Kersten FF, Azam M, Collin RW, Hussain A, et al. (2011) CLRN1 mutations cause nonsyndromic retinitis pigmentosa. Ophthalmology 118: 1444–1448.
26. Glockle N, Kohl S, Mohr J, Scheurenbrand T, Sprecher A, et al. (2014) Panel-based next generation sequencing as a reliable and efficient technique to detect mutations in unselected patients with retinal dystrophies. Eur J Hum Genet 22: 99–104.
27. Akoury E, El Zir E, Mansour A, Megarbane A, Majewski J, et al. (2011) A novel 5-bp deletion in Clarin 1 in a family with Usher syndrome. Ophthalmic Genet 32: 245–249.
28. Saouda M, Mansour A, Bou Moglabey Y, El Zir E, Mustapha M, et al. (1998) The Usher syndrome in the Lebanese population and further refinement of the USH2A candidate region. Hum Genet 103: 193–198.
29. Mouglabey YB, Nimri S, Sayegh F, El Zir E, Slim R (1998) Map refinement of the Usher syndrome type 1B gene, MYO7A, relative to 11q13.5 microsatellite markers. Clin Genet 54: 155–158.
30. Smith RJ, Berlin CI, Hejtmancik JF, Keats BJ, Kimberling WJ, et al. (1994) Clinical diagnosis of the Usher syndromes. Usher Syndrome Consortium. Am J Med Genet 50: 32–38.
31. Fahiminiya S, Majewski J, Roughley P, Roschger P, Klaushofer K, et al. (2013) Whole-exome sequencing reveals a heterozygous LRP5 mutation in a 6-year-old boy with vertebral compression fractures and low trabecular bone density. Bone 57: 41–46.
32. Fahiminiya S, Majewski J, Al-Jallad H, Moffatt P, Mort J, et al. (2014) Osteoporosis Caused by Mutations in PLS3 - Clinical and Bone Tissue Characteristics. J Bone Miner Res.
33. Li H, Durbin R (2009) Fast and accurate short read alignment with Burrows-Wheeler transform. Bioinformatics 25: 1754–1760.
34. McKenna A, Hanna M, Banks E, Sivachenko A, Cibulskis K, et al. (2010) The Genome Analysis Toolkit: a MapReduce framework for analyzing next-generation DNA sequencing data. Genome Res 20: 1297–1303.
35. Li H, Handsaker B, Wysoker A, Fennell T, Ruan J, et al. (2009) The Sequence Alignment/Map format and SAMtools. Bioinformatics 25: 2078–2079.
36. Wang K, Li M, Hakonarson H (2010) ANNOVAR: functional annotation of genetic variants from high-throughput sequencing data. Nucleic Acids Res 38: e164.
37. Shi Y, Majewski J (2013) FishingCNV: a graphical software package for detecting rare copy number variations in exome-sequencing data. Bioinformatics 29: 1461–1462.
38. Untergasser A, Cutcutache I, Koressaar T, Ye J, Faircloth BC, et al. (2012) Primer3–new capabilities and interfaces. Nucleic Acids Res 40: e115.
39. Burland TG (2000) DNASTAR's Lasergene sequence analysis software. Methods Mol Biol 132: 71–91.
40. Wildeman M, van Ophuizen E, den Dunnen JT, Taschner PE (2008) Improving sequence variant descriptions in mutation databases and literature using the Mutalyzer sequence variation nomenclature checker. Hum Mutat 29: 6–13.
41. Adzhubei IA, Schmidt S, Peshkin L, Ramensky VE, Gerasimova A, et al. (2010) A method and server for predicting damaging missense mutations. Nat Methods 7: 248–249.
42. Kumar P, Henikoff S, Ng PC (2009) Predicting the effects of coding non-synonymous variants on protein function using the SIFT algorithm. Nat Protoc 4: 1073–1081.
43. Reese MG, Eeckman FH, Kulp D, Haussler D (1997) Improved splice site detection in Genie. J Comput Biol 4: 311–323.
44. Eng L, Coutinho G, Nahas S, Yeo G, Tanouye R, et al. (2004) Nonclassical splicing mutations in the coding and noncoding regions of the ATM Gene: maximum entropy estimates of splice junction strengths. Hum Mutat 23: 67–76.
45. Hebsgaard SM, Korning PG, Tolstrup N, Engelbrecht J, Rouze P, et al. (1996) Splice site prediction in Arabidopsis thaliana pre-mRNA by combining local and global sequence information. Nucleic Acids Res 24: 3439–3452.
46. Roux AF, Faugere V, Le Guedard S, Pallares-Ruiz N, Vielle A, et al. (2006) Survey of the frequency of USH1 gene mutations in a cohort of Usher patients shows the importance of cadherin 23 and protocadherin 15 genes and establishes a detection rate of above 90%. J Med Genet 43: 763–768.
47. Eisenberger T, Slim R, Mansour A, Nauck M, Nurnberg G, et al. (2012) Targeted next-generation sequencing identifies a homozygous nonsense mutation in ABHD12, the gene underlying PHARC, in a family clinically diagnosed with Usher syndrome type 3. Orphanet J Rare Dis 7: 59.
48. Deininger PL, Batzer MA (1999) Alu repeats and human disease. Mol Genet Metab 67: 183–193.
49. Hilgert N, Kahrizi K, Dieltjens N, Bazazzadegan N, Najmabadi H, et al. (2009) A large deletion in GPR98 causes type IIC Usher syndrome in male and female members of an Iranian family. J Med Genet 46: 272–276.
50. Huang XF, Xiang P, Chen J, Xing DJ, Huang N, et al. (2013) Targeted exome sequencing identified novel USH2A mutations in Usher syndrome families. PLoS One 8: e63832.
51. Besnard T, Garcia-Garcia G, Baux D, Vache C, Faugere V, et al. (2014) Experience of targeted Usher exome sequencing as a clinical test. Mol Genet Genomic Med 2: 30–43.

22

Aminoglycoside-Induced Hair Cell Death of Inner Ear Organs Causes Functional Deficits in Adult Zebrafish (*Danio rerio*)

Phillip M. Uribe[1], Huifang Sun[2], Kevin Wang[1], James D. Asuncion[1], Qi Wang[3], Chien-Wei Chen[1], Peter S. Steyger[3], Michael E. Smith[2], Jonathan I. Matsui[1]*

1 Department of Neuroscience, Pomona College, Claremont, California, United States of America, **2** Department of Biology and Biotechnology Center, Western Kentucky University, Bowling Green, Kentucky, United States of America, **3** Oregon Hearing Research Center, Department of Otolaryngology, Oregon Health & Science University, Portland, Oregon, United States of America

Abstract

Aminoglycoside antibiotics, like gentamicin, kill inner ear sensory hair cells in a variety of species including chickens, mice, and humans. The zebrafish (*Danio rerio*) has been used to study hair cell cytotoxicity in the lateral line organs of larval and adult animals. Little is known about whether aminoglycosides kill the hair cells within the inner ear of adult zebrafish. We report here the ototoxic effects of gentamicin on hair cells in the saccule, the putative hearing organ, and utricle of zebrafish. First, adult zebrafish received a single 30 mg/kg intraperitoneal injection of fluorescently-tagged gentamicin (GTTR) to determine the distribution of gentamicin within inner ear sensory epithelia. After 4 hours, GTTR was observed in hair cells throughout the saccular and utricular sensory epithelia. To assess the ototoxic effects of gentamicin, adult zebrafish received a single 250 mg/kg *intraperitoneal* injection of gentamicin and, 24 hours later, auditory evoked potential recordings (AEPs) revealed significant shifts in auditory thresholds compared to untreated controls. Zebrafish were then euthanized, the inner ear fixed, and labeled for apoptotic cells (TUNEL reaction), and the stereociliary bundles of hair cells labeled with fluorescently-tagged phalloidin. Whole mounts of the saccule and utricle were imaged and cells counted. There were significantly more TUNEL-labeled cells found in both organs 4 hours after gentamicin injection compared to vehicle-injected controls. As expected, significantly fewer hair cell bundles were found along the rostral-caudal axis of the saccule and in the extrastriolar and striolar regions of the utricle in gentamicin-treated animals compared to untreated controls. Therefore, as in other species, gentamicin causes significant inner ear sensory hair cell death and auditory dysfunction in zebrafish.

Editor: Bruce Riley, Texas A&M University, United States of America

Funding: This project was supported by a Pomona College SURP (KW), A Rose Hills Foundation Summer Science and Engineering Research Fellowship (CWC), and National Institutes of Health grants DC04555 (PSS), P20RR16481 and P20GM103436-12 (MES), and DC010998 (JIM). The funders had no role in study design, data collection and analysis, decision to publish, or preparation of the manuscript.

* E-mail: Jonathan.Matsui@pomona.edu

Introduction

Sensory hair cells are mechanoreceptors within the inner ear that transduce sound and head movements into neural signals making them essential for hearing and balance [1,2,3]. Loss of these receptors from excessive noise, ototoxic pharmaceutical agents, and aging can lead to permanent hearing loss and vestibular deficits in humans. Aminoglycoside antibiotics, like gentamicin, are a class of commonly-prescribed and essential antibiotics used to treat severe gram-negative bacterial infections, but they can cause permanent loss of sensory hair cells in humans and other mammals [4].

Zebrafish (*Danio rerio*) have become an established animal model to study sensory hair cell death [5,6,7,8,9,10,11,12,13,14,15,16,17,18,19,20]. While zebrafish do not have a dedicated auditory organ like the mammalian cochlea, they have otolithic vestibular organs such as the saccule and utricle that are similar to mammalian vestibular organs. The zebrafish saccule, as in other teleosts, is thought to process auditory information [21,22]. Zebrafish can detect auditory frequencies between 100 Hz and 4000 Hz [23,24], and also have a lateral line system that detects changes in water flow and is composed of neuromasts along the fish's head and body [7,25,26]. Each neuromast contains sensory hair cells and non-sensory supporting cells that project into the aquatic environment making it very convenient to study the effects of drugs on sensory hair cells *in vivo*.

The vast majority of sensory hair cell death studies in zebrafish have focused on lateral line neuromasts of larvae [6,7,8,9,10,11,12,13,14,15,16,17,18,19,20]. One recent study investigated the regeneration of lateral line hair cells in adult zebrafish [26] and other studies investigated the effect of loud sound on supporting cell proliferation in the saccule of adult zebrafish [27,28,29]. The effect of aminoglycosides on the sensory hair cells within the inner ear of zebrafish has yet to be reported.

The purpose of this study was to establish the extent of hair cell death in the zebrafish inner ear, specifically in the saccule and utricle, following systemic aminoglycoside administration. Our goal was to reliably cause a lesion and assess the extent of the resulting hearing loss by measuring auditory evoked potentials (AEPs). This type of recording is routinely used in humans to assess hearing performance and has been successfully applied in zebrafish [23,24]. We found that gentamicin induced the loss of sensory hair cells across the entire saccule and utricle of adult zebrafish and this was accompanied by shifts in auditory thresholds.

Materials and Methods

Experimental Animals

Transgenic TG (Brn3c:GAP43-GFP)^{s356t} fish on the TL background (AKA Brn3c-GFP zebrafish (*Danio rerio*), a gift from Dr. Herwig Baier, University of California, San Francisco) [20,30,31], or wildtype zebrafish obtained from commercial suppliers were used for these experiments. Zebrafish were maintained on a 14 hour light/10 hour dark cycle using standard procedures [32]. This study was designed based on the recommendations in the Guide for the Care and Use of Laboratory Animals issued by the National Institutes of Health. The Institutional Animal Care and Use Committees of Western Kentucky University (Animal Welfare Assurance #A3558-01) and Pomona College (Animal Welfare Assurance #A3605-01) approved these experiments.

Drug Administration

Adult Brn3c-GFP transgenic zebrafish were anaesthetized with MS-222 (tricaine methanosulfonate; Sigma-Aldrich Corporation, St. Louis, MO), weighed, and given either a single intraperitoneal injection of 30 mg/kg Texas-Red conjugated gentamicin (GTTR; [33]), 250 mg/kg gentamicin sulfate (Sigma), 30 mg/kg unconjugated Texas Red (Life Technologies, Carlsbad, CA), or phosphate-buffered saline (PBS; Sigma) using a micro-injector (World Precision Instruments, Sarasota, FL) [34]. The fish were placed into individual tanks and allowed to recover in the fish facility for 4 or 24 hours before being euthanized, decapitated, and the heads fixed in 4% paraformaldehyde (Sigma) overnight at 4°C. The heads were rinsed three times in PBS for ten minutes each. Saccules and utricles were isolated using microsurgical tools (Fine Science Tools, Foster City, CA) under a Nikon or Leica dissecting microscope [35].

To determine cellular localization of GTTR, isolated organs were permeabilized with 0.1% Triton X-100 (Sigma) in PBS (PBST) for 30 minutes and then incubated with the cyanine monomeric dye TO-PRO-3 (1:1000 in PBST; Life Technologies) for 2–3 hours. TO-PRO-3 binds to DNA and fluorescently labels nuclei. The organs were rinsed with PBS, mounted onto glass slides in Vectashield (Vector Labs, Burlingame, CA), and cover-slipped. Four designated regions of the saccule (5%, 25%, 50%, and 75% along the rostral-caudal length of the organ; Fig. 1), or the extrastriolar and striolar regions of the utricle (Fig. 2), were imaged [27,28]. Images were acquired using a Nikon C1 confocal microscope (Nikon Instruments Inc., Melville, NY). Single images and *z*-series stacks were manipulated with EZ-C1 software (Nikon Instruments).

Auditory Evoked Potentials (AEP)

Twelve zebrafish ranging from 2.9–3.9 cm standard length and 303–731 mg wet mass were used (6 for control; 6 for gentamicin treatment) to measure the effect of systemic gentamicin administration on AEP's. AEP is a non-invasive method of measuring neural responses to auditory stimuli in fish and other vertebrates [36,37]. Each fish was anaesthetized with MS-222, restrained in a mesh sling, and suspended under water in a 19-L plastic vessel. Each fish was suspended so that the top of the head was approximately 6 cm below the surface of the water and 22 cm above the underwater speaker.

Stainless steel subdermal electrodes (27 gauge; Rochester Electro-Medical, Inc., Tampa, FL) were used to record AEPs. A reference electrode was inserted approximately 2 mm subdermally into the medial dorsal surface of the head between the anterior portion of the eyes while a recording electrode was placed 2 mm into the dorsal midline surface of the fish approximately halfway between the anterior insertion of the dorsal fin and the posterior edge of the operculae, directly over the brainstem. A ground electrode was placed in the tail musculature of the fish.

Sound stimuli were presented and AEP waveforms collected using SigGen and BioSig software running on a TDT physiology apparatus (Tucker-Davis Technologies Inc., Alachua, FL). Sounds were computer generated via TDT software and passed through a P1000 power amplifier (Hafler, Tempe, AZ) connected to a University Sound UW-30 underwater speaker (Electro-Voice, Burnsville, MN). Tone bursts were 15, 10, and 5 ms in total duration for 0.1 and 0.25, 4 and 6, and 0.8–4 kHz tones, respectively. Each tone pip had a 2 ms rise and fall time and were gated through a Hanning window similar to the conditions of other AEP studies [38,39,40]. Responses to each tone burst at each SPL were collected using the BioSig software package, with 400 responses averaged for each presentation. Auditory thresholds were determined at 10 frequencies for each fish (0.1, 0.25, 0.4, 0.6, 0.8, 1, 1.5, 2, 3, and 4 kHz). The SPLs of each presented frequency were confirmed using a calibrated underwater hydrophone (calibration sensitivity of −195 dB re 1 V/μPa; ±3 dB, 0.02–10 kHz, omnidirectional, GRAS Type 10CT, Denmark), placed in the same location where fish were held during AEP recording. Auditory thresholds were determined by visual inspection of AEP as in previous studies [38,39]. Separate one-way ANOVAs were calculated for each frequency (i.e., 100 Hz control vs. 100 Hz gentamicin-treated fish) using MS Excel (Microsoft, Redmond, WA).

TUNEL Labeling

To assess relative levels of cell death, isolated organs were processed for Terminal dUTP Nick-End-Labeling (TUNEL) using a previously published protocol [41] to label cells with DNA fragmentation indicative of apoptotic cells. Fish received either an injection of buffer or gentamicin and were allowed to recover for 4 or 24 hours. Fixed organs were permeabilized with proteinase K (10 μg/mL) for 40 minutes at room temperature. The samples were then refixed in 4% paraformaldehyde for 20 minutes and then rinsed with PBS three times for 10 minutes each. The saccules and utricles were processed using an ApopTag Fluorescein *In Situ* Apoptosis Detection kit (Chemicon/EMD Millipore, Billerica, MA) according to manufacturer directions. For each whole-mounted endorgan, images were taken with a Zeiss Axioplan 2 (Carl Zeiss Microscopy, Germany) epifluorescence microscope at 10X and 100X objective magnification and all TUNEL-labeled cells were counted manually. One-way ANOVAs (SYSTAT 13; Systat Software Inc., Chicago, IL) were used to test for differences in numbers of TUNEL-labeled cells between gentamicin-treated animals and buffer-injected controls for each labeled endorgan.

Hair Cell Stereociliary Bundle Counts and Analysis

Fixed, excised saccules and utricles were rinsed with PBS three times for 10 minutes each at room temperature. Isolated organs

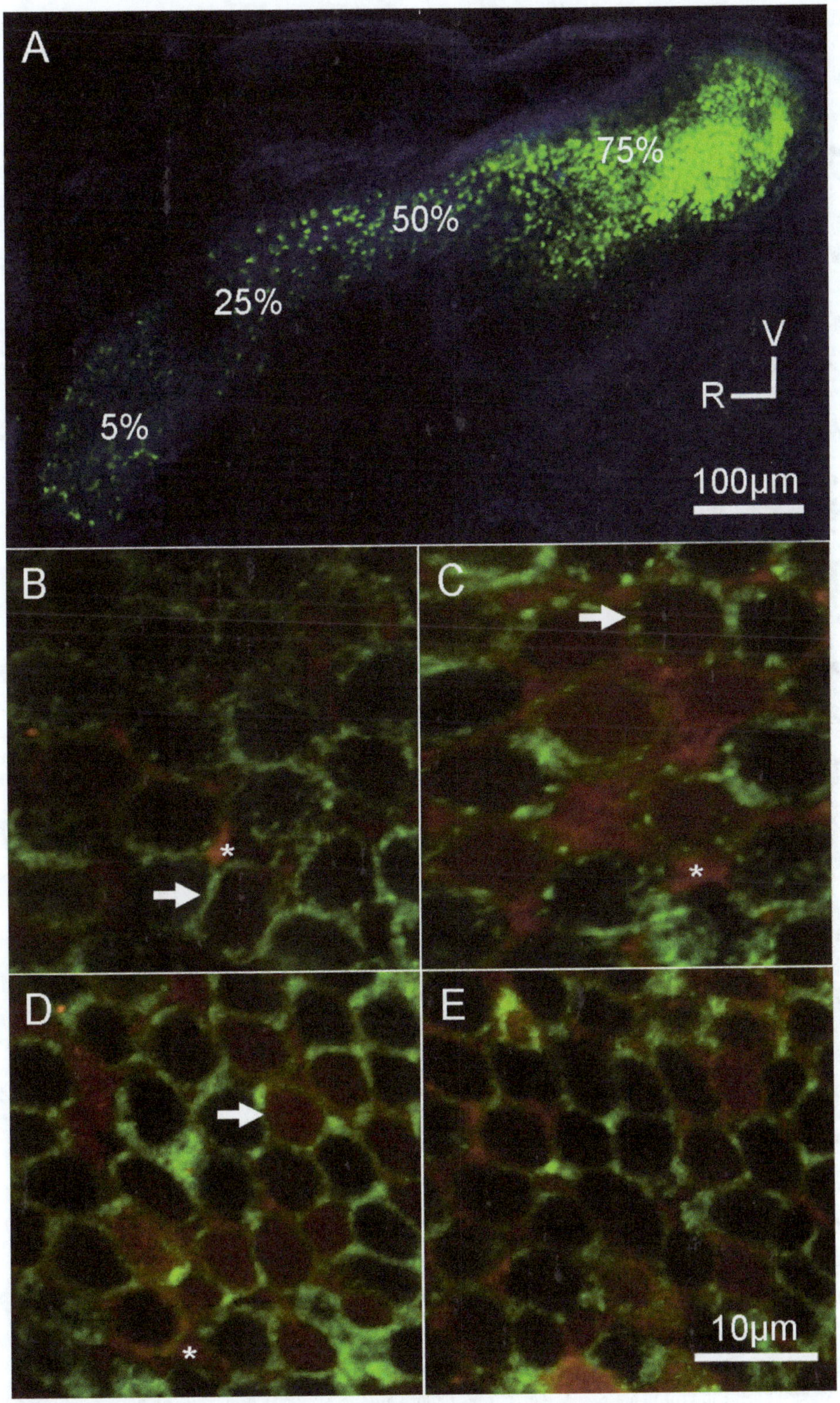

Figure 1. Gentamicin localizes to saccular hair cells. Adult Brn3c-GFP zebrafish received an intraperitoneal injection of Texas Red-conjugated gentamicin (GTTR; 30 mg/kg) and allowed to recover for 4 hours. (A) Low magnification image of the saccule. GFP-labeled hair cells (green) are located along the length of the organ. V = ventral, R = rostral. High magnification images (B–E) are single optical slices from individual *z*-stacks taken at (B) 5%, (C) 25%, (D) 50%, and (E) 75% along the length of the saccule from the rostral end (see A). GTTR fluorescence (red) was localized to hair cells (D, white arrows) and supporting cells (white asterisks) throughout the sensory epithelium. GFP fluorescence (green) is localized to the cell membrane region of hair cells. The *z*-stack slices are taken mid-way into the cell to show the localization patterns, thus neither hair cell nuclei nor stereociliary bundles are visible.

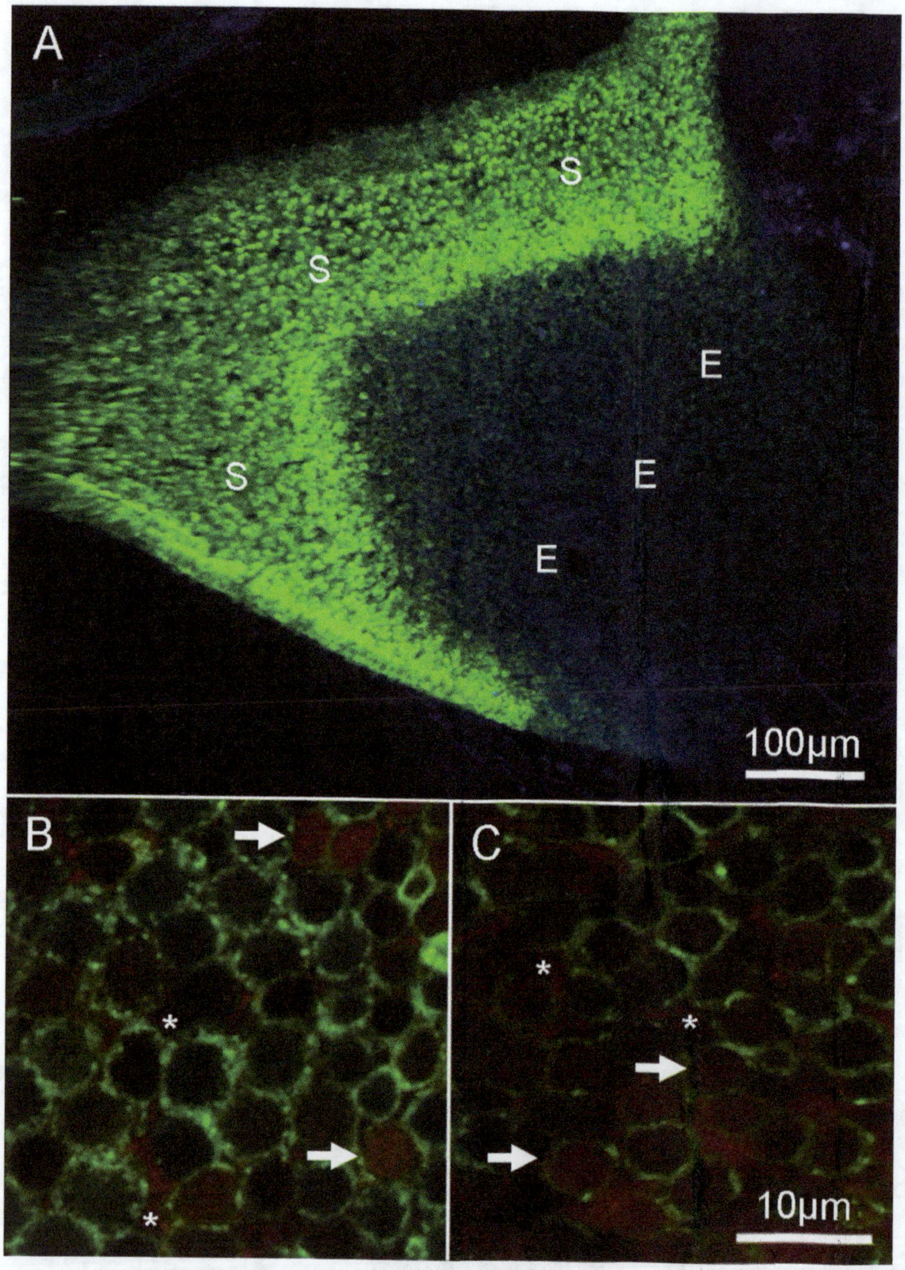

Figure 2. Gentamicin localizes to utricular hair cells. Adult Brn3c-GFP zebrafish received an intraperitoneal injection of GTTR (30 mg/kg) and allowed to recover for 4 hours. (A) Low magnification image of the utricle. GFP-labeled hair cells (green) are located throughout the organ. The striolar region (S) and extrastriolar region (E) are highlighted. High magnification images (B, C) are single optical slices from individual *z*-stacks from (B) striolar and (C) extrastriolar regions. GTTR fluorescence (red) was localized to hair cells (white arrows) and supporting cells (white asterisks) throughout the sensory epitheilum. GFP fluorescence (green) is localized to the cell membrane region of hair cells. The slices are taken mid-way through the cell to show the localization patterns, thus, neither hair cell nuclei nor stereociliary bundles are visible.

were permeabilized with 0.1% PBST for 30 minutes. The stereociliary bundles were labeled with Alexa Fluor 488-conjugated phalloidin (1:100; Life Technologies) in the dark for two hours at room temperature to visualize filamentous actin (F-actin) that are abundant in stereociliary bundles and cuticular plates. After incubation, endorgans were placed on glass slides mounted with Prolong Gold antifade reagent with 4′,6-diamidino-2-phenylindole (DAPI; Life Technologies) to label nuclei and then cover-slipped.

Low (20X objective) and high (100X objective) power images of the saccule were viewed under the FITC filter of a Zeiss Axioplan 2 epifluorescence microscope and were imaged using an AxioCam MRm camera, with image contrast adjusted for easy quantification of phalloidin-labeled hair cell stereociliary bundles. Five designated regions of the saccule (5%, 25%, 50%, 75%, and 95% along the rostral-caudal length of the organ) were imaged [27,28] to determine rostral-caudal shifts in saccular hair cell bundle density, as used previously [23,40]. These locations were chosen as they represent a wide range in hair cell densities [27] and sensitivity to varying frequencies along the rostral-caudal axis of the zebrafish saccule [42]. At each location, images were cropped to a 30 μm×30 μm box using ImageJ (National Institutes of Health, Bethesda, MD) and cell counts performed.

Whole-mounts of utricles were visualized on a Nikon Eclipse Ni Fluorescence Microscope (Nikon Instruments) using a 60X objective and video images were obtained using a Nikon DS-Qi1 Cooled CCD camera and NIS Elements software. Cell counts were made using NIS Elements by placing a 5,000 μm^2 box on the screen and using the cell counter feature. Phalloidin-labeled cells were counted from three boxes of the extrastriolar region and three boxes distributed along the striolar region of each utricle. Care was taken to avoid the lateral regions of sensory epithelia that contain immature hair cells [43,44,45,46] that are more resistant to aminoglycoside toxicity [9] or areas of potential dissection damage. Cell counts from the three boxes were averaged to obtain an estimate of the number of surviving hair bundles/5,000 μm^2 for the striolar and extrastriolar regions of each specimen.

Quantitative data were subjected to either a two-tailed t-test assuming unequal variance (MS Excel) or One-way ANOVA (VassarStats, Vassar College, Poughkeepsie, NY). Post-hoc comparisons, when appropriate, used the Tukey-HSD test.

Results

Localization of Gentamicin in the Inner Ear

Gentamicin kills inner ear sensory hair cells in a variety of adult fish [47,48,49,50,51], yet no studies have reported its effects on sensory hair cells in the inner ear of adult zebrafish. In order to determine if gentamicin can reach the inner ear organs, adult Brn3c-GFP transgenic zebrafish were given a single intraperitoneal injection of Texas Red-conjugated gentamicin (GTTR) and allowed to recover for 4 hours. These zebrafish express green fluorescent protein (GFP) in the cell membranes of sensory hair cells [20,30,31]. The zebrafish were then sacrificed, the head fixed and the inner ear organs were dissected, mounted, and imaged. We focused on the saccule since it is thought to be the putative "auditory" organ in the zebrafish [21,22,23,24]. Four designated regions of the saccule (5%, 25%, 50%, and 75% along the rostral-caudal length of the organ) were imaged (Fig. 1A) [27,28] since they represent a wide range in hair cell density [27] and sensitivity to frequency [42]. We found GTTR fluorescence localized in GFP-labeled hair cells and supporting cells in all regions of the saccule (Fig 1B–E; $n=6$ animals). We also found GTTR-labeled hair cells and supporting cells in the utricle (Fig. 2A) in both striolar (Fig. 2B) and extra-striolar regions (Fig. 2C). As a control experiment, zebrafish injected with unconjugated Texas Red, and examined in the same manner, had negligible levels of Texas Red fluorescence in saccular or utricular hair cells ($n=8$; data not shown).

Gentamicin Affects Zebrafish Swimming Behaviors

In order to assess hair cell death following gentamicin treatment, adult zebrafish received a single 250 mg/kg intraperitoneal injection of gentamicin before being placed into individual tanks to recover for 4 or 24 hours. A preliminary study using transgenic Brn3c-GFP zebrafish showed that a single 250 mg/kg injection of gentamicin resulted in a 50% decrease in hair cells in specific regions of the saccule, and lower concentrations were less toxic (data not shown). Roughly 25% of the gentamicin-injected animals that received 250 mg/kg experienced systemic toxicity and typically died within 30 minutes of injection. Of the fish surviving the first 30 minute post-injection period less than 5% died before being euthanized at the 4 hour or 24 hour time points. All surviving fish were euthanized at either the 4 or 24-hour time point and long-term health effects of acute gentamicin injection were not assessed. Additionally, preliminary trials of serial injections, given once daily, either did not show significant toxicity at lower gentamicin concentrations or resulted in a fatality rate over 50% at higher doses (>50 mg/kg). In those that died there was a noticeable loss of vestibular function with many fish swimming upside down or lying prone on their side prior to death. Gill movement was also sporadic indicative of systemic changes in respiration. Doses >250 mg/kg were fatal to over 50% of injected animals. Therefore, we chose to use 250 mg/kg to induce ototoxic lesions, with lower levels of mortality. Zebrafish that survived treatment had some vestibular deficits. Within minutes after injection, fish were observed swimming off of level horizontal axis with a positive pitch that was maintained until the end of the experiment.

Effects of Gentamicin on Auditory Thresholds

Auditory evoked potentials (AEPs) were recorded from untreated (wildtype) and gentamicin-treated animals. When we tried to record AEPs using the Brn3c-GFP transgenic zebrafish, the untreated control transgenic zebrafish had significant auditory threshold shifts compared to wildtype zebrafish (data not shown); therefore we used wildtype zebrafish for the remaining experiments. AEPs acquired from wildtype animals had stereotypic waveforms that emerged within 10 ms of the onset of the stimulus (Fig. 3A) similar to previous data for adult zebrafish [23,24]. Audiograms were constructed by identifying the auditory thresholds (black arrow; Fig. 3A) in the gentamicin-treated and untreated control animals (Fig. 3B). There was a significant ($p<0.05$) threshold shift in wildtype zebrafish treated with gentamicin at every frequency tested except for 1500 Hz ($n=6$ animals for each treatment group) 24 hours post-injection. This is likely due to the higher variability in AEPs from gentamicin-treated animals at this frequency.

Cytotoxicity Analyses

In order to determine whether sensory hair cells died following gentamicin treatment, wildtype fish injected with gentamicin were allowed to recover for 4 or 24 hours. Some fish were injected with buffer and allowed to recover for 4 hours and served as controls. At the specified time, fish were fixed and processed for TUNEL labeling. Apoptotic cells can be detected by enzymatically labeling (TUNEL-labeling) the free 3′-OH termini of fragmented DNA with modified nucleotides (green cells; Figures 4 and 5). There was a significant increase in the number of TUNEL-labeled saccular (Fig. 4I; $n=9$–12; $p<0.05$) and utricular cells (Fig. 5C; $n=12$; $p<0.001$) 4 hours after gentamicin was administered compared to buffer-injected controls; this increase in the number of TUNEL-labeled cells was maintained 24 hours after gentamicin injection in the utricle (Fig. 5C; $n=9$; $p<0.05$) although this was not statistically different from controls in the saccule (Fig. 4I; $n=9$; $p=0.11$).

In order to determine if gentamicin treatment resulted in fewer sensory hair cells, actin filaments in the saccular and utricular hair cell stereociliary bundles in control and gentamicin-treated animals were specifically labeled with fluorescently-tagged phalloidin. There was a noticeable difference in the number of stereociliary bundles 24 hours after injection with 250 mg/kg gentamicin (Fig. 6F–J) compared to untreated controls (Fig. 6A–E). Hair bundle densities were significantly lower ($p<0.05$ to $p<0.001$) in gentamicin-treated saccules in every area sampled across the rostral-caudal axis (Fig. 6K, $n=6$–12 per sample area per treatment group) 24 hours after of treatment.

Fewer sensory hair bundles were also identified in the utricle after gentamicin treatment. Phalloidin-labeled bundles in both the

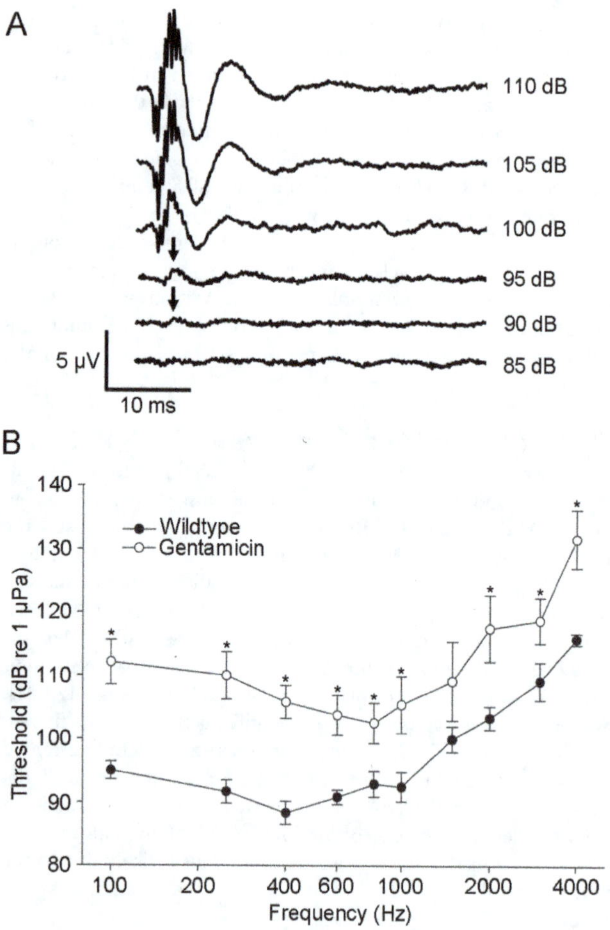

Figure 3. Gentamicin treatment causes auditory threshold shifts following 24 hours of treatment. (A) Electrophysiological recordings of auditory evoked potentials (AEPs) measured at a test frequency of 1000 Hz. Stimulus intensity was decreased from 110 dB to 85 dB in 5 dB steps. The AEPs emerge as a series of peaks (black arrows). In this example, the auditory threshold, as judged by visual inspection, is 90 dB (re: 1 µPa). (B) Auditory thresholds were used to construct audiograms to compare auditory function in treated and control fish. There was a significant auditory threshold shift (*$p<0.05$) at almost every frequency tested in gentamicin-treated fish when compared to untreated controls. n = 6 animals per treatment.

striolar and extrastriolar regions were quantified and expressed as the mean number of stereocilia bundles/5000 $\mu m^2 \pm$ SD. Phalloidin-labeled bundles were counted from three regions in the central extrastriolar zone of each utricle and three regions throughout the striola (Fig. 2A). Hair bundle densities were greater in the striola (63.6±6.4; n = 7) than in extrastriolar regions (43.0±7.3; n = 7) of untreated control zebrafish. Four hours after 250 mg/kg gentamicin injection, there was a significant decrease in the number of stereociliary bundles ($p<0.001$) in both striolar region (49.1±10.1; n = 7) and the extrastriolar region (33.3±7.5; n = 8) compared to untreated controls. Twenty-four hours after the administration of gentamicin, there was still a significant decrease ($p<0.001$) in the number of stereociliary bundles in both striolar (51.9±6.5; n = 10) and extrastriolar regions (28.6±7.2; n = 10) compared to controls. While there were fewer stereociliary bundles in the extrastriolar region after 24 hours of treatment, there was no statistical difference between the two different time points ($p>0.5$).

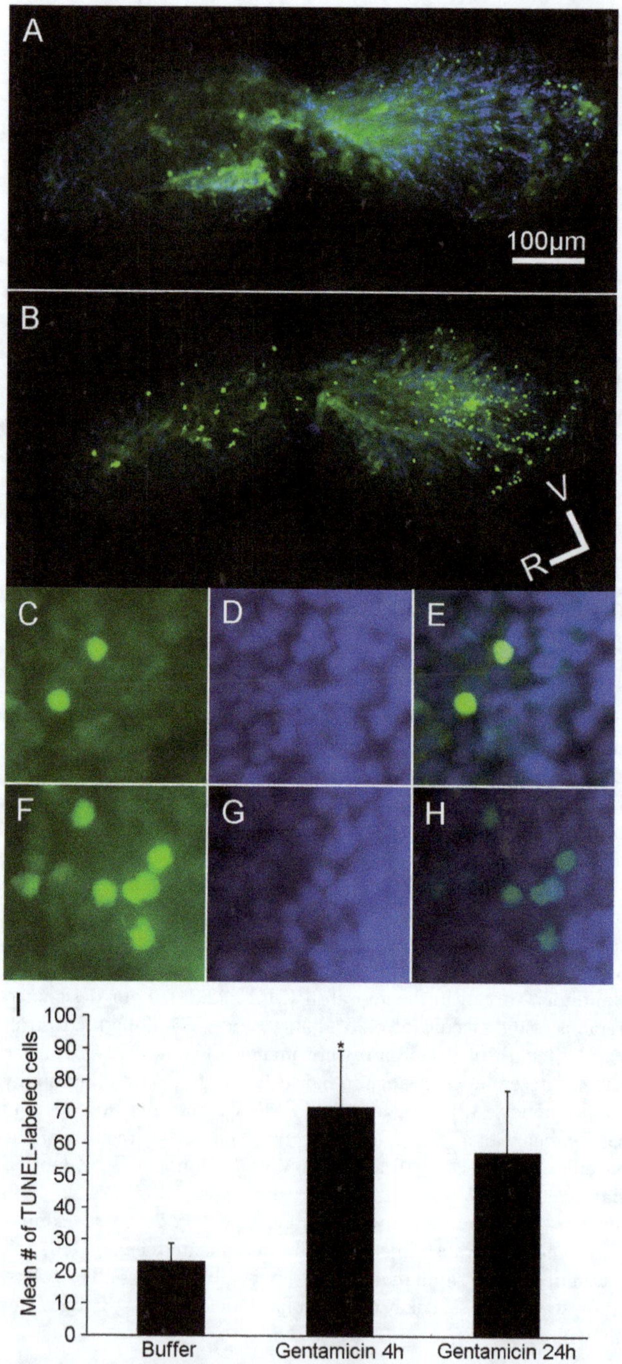

Figure 4. Gentamicin treatment increases the numbers of TUNEL-labeled cells in the adult saccule. Adult wildtype zebrafish received either a single intraperitoneal injection of (A, C, D, E) buffer or (B, F, G, H) 250 mg/kg gentamicin and allowed to recover for either 4 or 24 hours (4 hour data is shown). Fixed saccules were processed using a TUNEL-kit to label apoptotic cells (green cells; A, B, C, E, F, H) and co-labeled with DAPI (blue cells; A, B, D, E, G, H). (A-B) Low power and (C–H) high power images of the saccule reveals few TUNEL-labeled cells scattered throughout the saccule of a buffer-treated animal (A, C, E) but more TUNEL-labeling in a gentamicin-treated animal (B, F, H). (I) Mean number of TUNEL-labeled cells (± SD) in the saccules of buffer- or gentamicin-injected zebrafish. *$p<0.05$; n = 9–12; V = ventral, R = rostral.

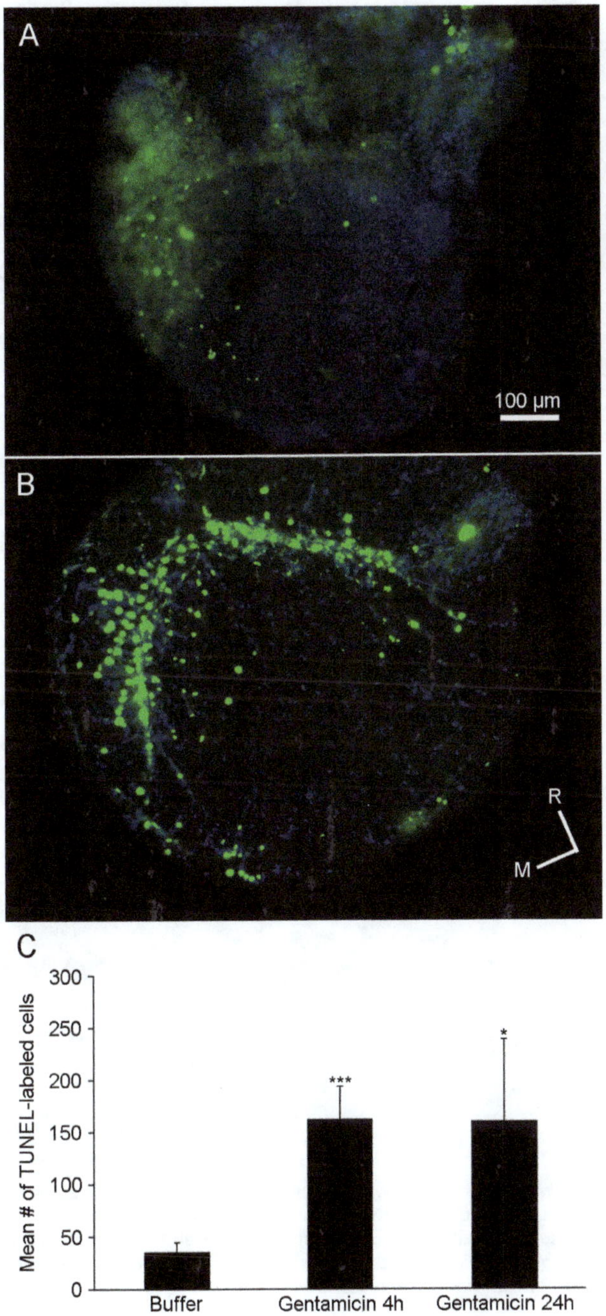

Figure 5. Gentamicin treatment increases the numbers of TUNEL-labeled cells in the adult utricle. Adult wildtype zebrafish received either a single intraperitoneal injection of (A) buffer or (B) 250 mg/kg gentamicin and allowed to recover for either 4 or 24 hours (4 hour data is shown). Fixed utricles were processed using a TUNEL-kit to label apoptotic cells (green cells) and co-labeled with DAPI (blue cells). (A–B) Low power (10X) images of the utricle reveals few TUNEL-labeled cells scattered throughout the utricle of a (A) buffer-treated animal but more cells with TUNEL-labeling in the (B) gentamicin-treated animal. (C) Mean number of TUNEL-labeled cells (± SD) in the utricles of buffer- or gentamicin-injected zebrafish. *$p<0.05$ or ***$p<0.001$; n = 9–12; M = medial, R = rostral.

Discussion

Gentamicin-induced hair cell loss in the inner ear has been previously studied in several species of fish including oscar (*Astronotus ocellatus*) [47,48], goldfish (*Carassius auratus*) [51,52] and Atlantic Cod (*Gadus morhua*) [49,50]. Different species respond to aminoglycosides differently. For instance, gentamicin kills hair cells in the lagena and utricle but not the saccule of the oscar [47]. In fact, no damage was reported in the saccule following higher doses of gentamicin [47]. In contrast, hair cells in the saccule of the goldfish [51] and Atlantic cod [49,50], along with hair cells in both the utricle and saccule of the zebrafish, as reported here, are killed by systemic injection of gentamicin. We chose not to study the lagena since it is often damaged during excision of the saccule.

Hair cell uptake of GTTR in these vestibular organs (utricle and saccule) is variable, and this may underlie the susceptibility of some hair cells to undergo cytotoxicity and cell death compared to surviving hair cells in these organs. Modulation of gentamicin uptake by extracellular cations also modulates the susceptibility of lateral line neuromasts to cytotoxicity and cell death [15]. Variation in the uptake of aminoglycosides by inner ear hair cells in other fish species may also account for the observed variation in saccular and utricular hair cell death in differing species. Other experiments to measure aminoglycoside uptake in teleost inner ears are needed to determine this. In addition, the varied experimental paradigms also make comparison of their results more difficult to interpret. In three studies, repeated intramuscular injections of gentamicin to the oscar, goldfish, and Atlantic cod resulted in differing levels of damage. The Atlantic cod received multiple injections of gentamicin ranging from 5–80 mg/kg [49] whereas the oscars received multiple injections between 10–120 mg/kg. Unfortunately, further comparison between the goldfish study to the other two studies cannot be made as the dose given to goldfish was not reported. One major side effect of using repeated intramuscular injections are kidney problems as well as other health disorders in oscars [47,48], goldfish [53], and Atlantic cod [49].

Some studies used an intra-saccular injection of gentamicin, which caused hair cell death in Atlantic cod [49,50] and goldfish [54] since there are fewer side effects including less nephrotoxicity and death associated with this type of drug delivery. However, this procedure requires X-ray imaging in larger fish to determine if the needle is correctly positioned in the inner ear [49], and is not practical for smaller fish like zebrafish.

In this study, a single intraperitoneal injection of GTTR revealed trafficking of the conjugated drug into the inner ear, and that gentamicin caused significant saccular lesions and consequential auditory threshold shifts. GTTR was present in both hair cells and supporting cells in the both the saccule and utricle. The presence of GTTR in supporting cells is unsurprising and has also been observed in supporting cells (and hair cells) of frog, mouse, and guinea pig sensory epithelia [33,55,56].

While the dose of gentamicin in the current study was greater than in other teleost studies, these fish received only a single injection. Previous fish studies have given daily injections of gentamicin with varying onset of damage. For instance, the maximal amount of damage to the inner ear organs of the goldfish occurred 4 days after the beginning of gentamicin injections [51] versus the damage we observed 4 hours after a single injection. The onset of damage in the goldfish was not noted [51]. Gentamicin treatment can result in high mortality rates in zebrafish. Yet, a single dose was shown to be sufficient to produce a decrease in the number of hair cells. Four hours after injection of gentamicin, a noticeable increase in the number of apoptotic cells (as assessed by TUNEL labeling) and significant decrease of sensory hair cells in both saccules and utricles were observed. This is similar to lateral line neuromast hair cells. Within 4 hours of exposure to gentamicin or another aminoglycoside, neomycin,

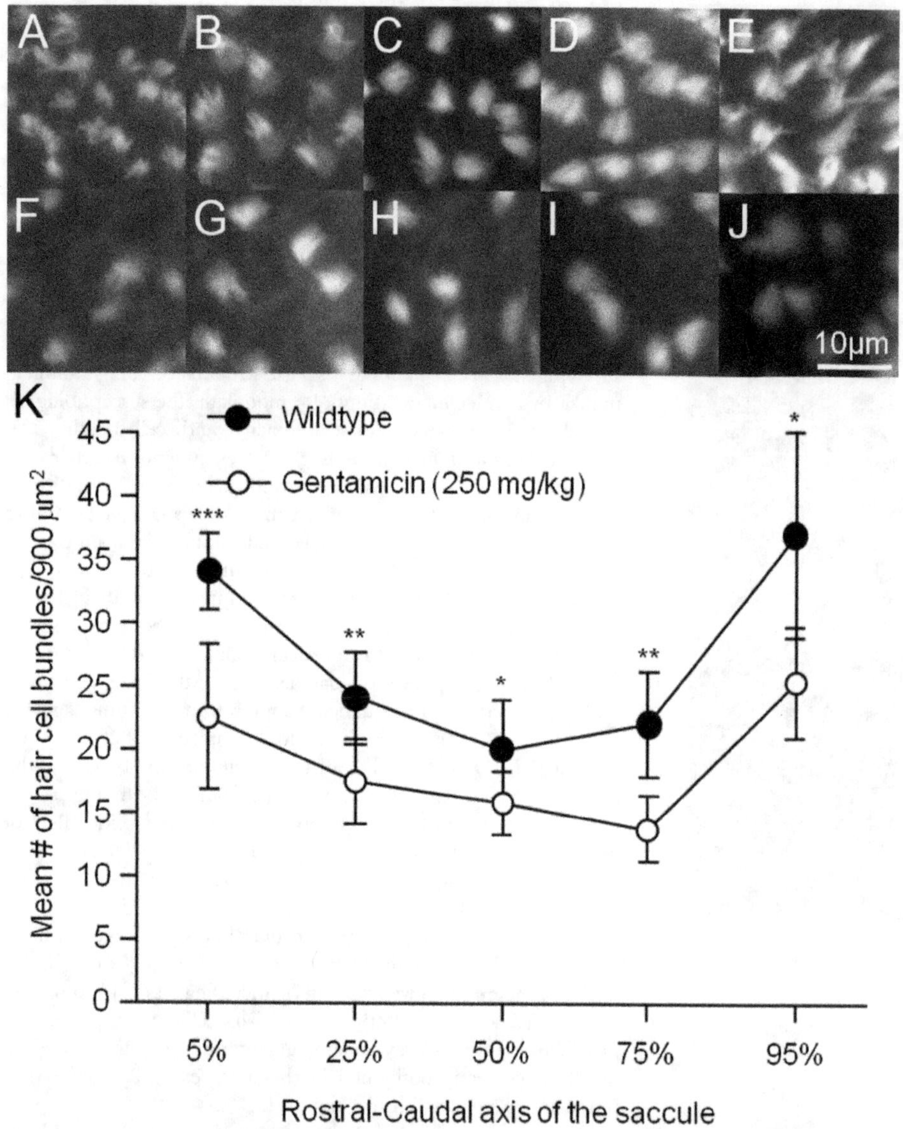

Figure 6. Gentamicin treatment resulted in fewer saccular hair bundles after 24 hours. Adult wildtype zebrafish received a single 250 mg/kg intraperitoneal injection of gentamicin and allowed to recover for 24 hours. Images of phalloidin-labeled cells were taken at (A, F) 5%, (B, G) 25%, (C, H) 50%, (D, I) 75%, and (E, J) 95% along the length of the saccule beginning at the rostral end in (A–E) untreated controls and (F–J) gentamicin-treated animals. (K) Mean (± SD) number of saccular hair cell bundles per 900 μm^2 of epithelia. Significantly fewer phalloidin-labeled hair bundles were counted at each area along the length of the saccule in gentamicin-treated animals compared to controls. *$p<0.05$ or **$p<0.01$; n = 6–13 saccules per area per condition.

there are significantly fewer neuromast hair cells in larval zebrafish [7,17]. Other studies of larval zebrafish show that functional mechanotransduction channels are required for GTTR to enter neuromast hair cells [56].

There have been studies in other species that compared a single injection versus multiple injections of gentamicin. In chickens, a single high dose of gentamicin (100 mg/kg) resulted in hair cell loss in the basal 20% of the cochlea and this occurred several days after injection [57]. Alternatively, multiple injections of gentamicin (50 mg/kg) for ten days resulted in the loss of the basal hair cells with a corresponding high-frequency hearing loss as measured by auditory brainstem responses [58,59]. Other studies have reported variation in susceptibility to systemic and audiological toxicity to different aminoglycosides among different mammals including guinea pigs, rats, humans, and different strains of mice [60,61]. Mechanisms of ototoxicity are not yet sufficiently understood to explain variation across species.

The speed with which gentamicin can induce zebrafish inner ear hair cell death and hearing loss has experimental advantages for studying hair cell regeneration. Most studies examining hair cell regeneration in the teleost inner ear have used an acoustic stimulus (either white noise or a low-frequency tone) that is played continuously for 40–48 hours to induce hair cell death and hearing loss [27,28,40]. Although minimal hearing loss (approximately 5 dB) is evident in goldfish within 10 minutes of white noise exposure, maximal threshold shifts occur approximately 24 hours later [38,39]. It has been assumed that it takes approximately one day for acoustically-damaged hair cells to become non-responsive, begin to undergo apoptosis, and begin to be ejected out of the sensory epithelia, although this has not been directly measured via hair cell counts or cell death assays at time points earlier than 40–48 hours post-sound exposure [27,28,40]. The gentamicin-injection protocol presented in this paper will be useful for future comparisons between acoustically- and ototoxic chemical-induced hair cell death and regeneration.

Previous studies using goldfish have shown that multiple intramuscular injections of gentamicin can cause auditory hair cell death and hearing loss [51,52]. In these studies, hearing loss was limited to frequencies between 300 and 600 Hz, whereas in this zebrafish study, hearing loss was evident at almost all frequencies between 100 and 4000 Hz. The extent of hearing loss (approximately 8–15 dB), though, was similar where threshold shifts were evident in both sets of studies. It is likely that differences in the two studies are a result of gentamicin dosage, rather than species differences since goldfish and zebrafish are closely-related cyprinids with similarly-shaped audiograms and inner ear structure [62]. Unfortunately, the gentamicin dosage cannot be directly compared between the two studies since the goldfish studies reported injected dosages as mg/ml without specifying the total volume injected per fish.

This study demonstrated the ototoxic effects of gentamicin on the saccule and utricle of adult zebrafish. Future studies will evaluate the effects of other aminoglycosides and the chemotherapeutic agent cisplatin on the inner ear hair cells of adult zebrafish. In addition, subsequent studies will evaluate the regeneration of inner ear sensory hair cells and auditory evoked potentials after gentamicin treatment and compare this recovery to studies that have investigated acoustically-induced damage in adult zebrafish [27,28,29].

Acknowledgments

The authors thank Bethany Coffey and Savannah Bell for collecting the auditory evoked potentials data.

Author Contributions

Conceived and designed the experiments: PMU HS KW CWC PSS MES JIM. Performed the experiments: PMU HS KW JDA CWC MES. Analyzed the data: PMU HS MES JIM. Contributed reagents/materials/analysis tools: QW PSS. Wrote the paper: PMU JDA PSS MES JIM.

References

1. Hudspeth AJ (1985) The cellular basis of hearing: the biophysics of hair cells. Science 230: 745–752.
2. Hudspeth AJ, Choe Y, Mehta AD, Martin P (2000) Putting ion channels to work: mechanoelectrical transduction, adaptation, and amplification by hair cells. Proc Natl Acad Sci USA 97: 11765–11772.
3. Gillespie PG, Muller U (2009) Mechanotransduction by hair cells: models, molecules, and mechanisms. Cell 139: 33–44.
4. Warchol ME (2010) Cellular mechanisms of aminoglycoside ototoxicity. Curr Opin Otolaryngol Head Neck Surg 18: 454–458.
5. Song J, Yan HY, Popper AN (1995) Damage and recovery of hair cells in fish canal (but not superficial) neuromasts after gentamicin exposure. Hear Res 91: 63–71.
6. Williams JA, Holder N (2000) Cell turnover in neuromasts of zebrafish larvae. Hear Res 143: 171–181.
7. Harris JA, Cheng AG, Cunningham LL, MacDonald G, Raible DW, et al. (2003) Neomycin-induced hair cell death and rapid regeneration in the lateral line of zebrafish (*Danio rerio*). J Assoc Res Otolaryngol 4: 219–234.
8. Murakami SL, Cunningham LL, Werner LA, Bauer E, Pujol R, et al. (2003) Developmental differences in susceptibility to neomycin-induced hair cell death in the lateral line neuromasts of zebrafish (*Danio rerio*). Hear Res 186: 47–56.
9. Santos F, MacDonald G, Rubel EW, Raible DW (2006) Lateral line hair cell maturation is a determinant of aminoglycoside susceptibility in zebrafish (*Danio rerio*). Hear Res 213: 25–33.
10. Chiu LL, Cunningham LL, Raible DW, Rubel EW, Ou HC (2008) Using the zebrafish lateral line to screen for ototoxicity. J Assoc Res Otolaryngol 9: 178–190.
11. Hernandez PP, Olivari FA, Sarrazin AF, Sandoval PC, Allende ML (2007) Regeneration in zebrafish lateral line neuromasts: expression of the neural progenitor cell marker sox2 and proliferation-dependent and-independent mechanisms of hair cell renewal. Dev Neurobiol 67: 637–654.
12. Ou HC, Raible DW, Rubel EW (2007) Cisplatin-induced hair cell loss in zebrafish (*Danio rerio*) lateral line. Hear Res 233: 46–53.
13. Ma EY, Rubel EW, Raible DW (2008) Notch signaling regulates the extent of hair cell regeneration in the zebrafish lateral line. J Neurosci 28: 2261–2273.
14. Owens KN, Santos F, Roberts B, Linbo T, Coffin AB, et al. (2008) Identification of genetic and chemical modulators of zebrafish mechanosensory hair cell death. PLoS Genet 4: e1000020.
15. Coffin AB, Reinhart KE, Owens KN, Raible DW, Rubel EW (2009) Extracellular divalent cations modulate aminoglycoside-induced hair cell death in the zebrafish lateral line. Hear Res 253: 42–51.
16. Ou HC, Cunningham LL, Francis SP, Brandon CS, Simon JA, et al. (2009) Identification of FDA-approved drugs and bioactives that protect hair cells in the zebrafish (*Danio rerio*) lateral line and mouse (*Mus musculus*) utricle. J Assoc Res Otolaryngol 10: 191–203.
17. Owens KN, Coffin AB, Hong LS, Bennett KO, Rubel EW, et al. (2009) Response of mechanosensory hair cells of the zebrafish lateral line to aminoglycosides reveals distinct cell death pathways. Hear Res 253: 32–41.
18. Coffin AB, Ou H, Owens KN, Santos F, Simon JA, et al. (2010) Chemical screening for hair cell loss and protection in the zebrafish lateral line. Zebrafish 7: 3–11.
19. Giari L, Dezfuli BS, Astolfi L, Martini A (2012) Ultrastructural effects of cisplatin on the inner ear and lateral line system of zebrafish (*Danio rerio*) larvae. J Appl Toxicol 32: 293–299.
20. Namdaran P, Reinhart KE, Owens KN, Raible DW, Rubel EW (2012) Identification of modulators of hair cell regeneration in the zebrafish lateral line. J Neurosci 32: 3516–3528.
21. Popper AN, Fay RR (1973) Sound detection and processing by teleost fishes: a critical review. J Acoust Soc Am 53: 1515–1529.
22. Popper AN, Fay RR (1999) The Auditory Periphery in Fishes. In: Fay RR, Popper AN, editors. Comparative Hearing: Fish and Amphibians: Springer. 43–100.
23. Higgs DM, Souza MJ, Wilkins HR, Presson JC, Popper AN (2002) Age- and size-related changes in the inner ear and hearing ability of the adult zebrafish (*Danio rerio*). J Assoc Res Otolaryngol 3: 174–184.
24. Higgs DM, Rollo AK, Souza MJ, Popper AN (2003) Development of form and function in peripheral auditory structures of the zebrafish (*Danio rerio*). J Acoust Soc Am 113: 1145–1154.
25. Raible DW, Kruse GJ (2000) Organization of the lateral line system in embryonic zebrafish. J Comp Neurol 421: 189–198.
26. Van Trump WJ, Coombs S, Duncan K, McHenry MJ (2010) Gentamicin is ototoxic to all hair cells in the fish lateral line system. Hear Res 261: 42–50.
27. Schuck JB, Smith ME (2009) Cell proliferation follows acoustically-induced hair cell bundle loss in the zebrafish saccule. Hear Res 253: 67–76.
28. Sun H, Lin CH, Smith ME (2011) Growth hormone promotes hair cell regeneration in the zebrafish (*Danio rerio*) inner ear following acoustic trauma. PLoS ONE 6: e28372.
29. Liang J, Wang D, Renaud G, Wolfsberg TG, Wilson AF, et al. (2012) The stat3/socs3a pathway is a key regulator of hair cell regeneration in zebrafish. J Neurosci 32: 10662–10673.
30. Xiao T, Roeser T, Staub W, Baier H (2005) A GFP-based genetic screen reveals mutations that disrupt the architecture of the zebrafish retinotectal projection. Development 132: 2955–2967.
31. Uribe PM, Mueller MA, Gleichman JS, Kramer MD, Wang Q, et al. (2013) Dimethyl sulfoxide (DMSO) exacerbates cisplatin-induced sensory hair cell death in zebrafish (*Danio rerio*). PLoS ONE 8: e55359.
32. Westerfield M (1994) The Zebrafish Book: A Guide for the Laboratory Use of Zebrafish. Eugene: Institute of Neuroscience, University of Oregon.
33. Dai CF, Mangiardi D, Cotanche DA, Steyger PS (2006) Uptake of fluorescent gentamicin by vertebrate sensory cells *in vivo*. Hear Res 213: 64–78.
34. Kinkel MD, Eames SC, Philipson LH, Prince VE (2010) Intraperitoneal injection into adult zebrafish. J Vis Exp 42: e2126.
35. Liang J, Burgess SM (2009) Gross and fine dissection of inner ear sensory epithelia in adult zebrafish (*Danio rerio*). J Vis Exp 27: e1211.
36. Corwin JT, Bullock TH, Schweitzer J (1982) The auditory brain stem response in five vertebrate classes. Electroencephalogr Clin Neurophysiol 54: 629–641.
37. Kenyon TN, Ladich F, Yan HY (1998) A comparative study of hearing ability in fishes: the auditory brainstem response approach. J Comp Physiol [A] 182: 307–318.
38. Smith ME, Kane AS, Popper AN (2004) Acoustical stress and hearing sensitivity in fishes: does the linear threshold shift hypothesis hold water? J Exp Biol 207: 3591–3602.
39. Smith ME, Kane AS, Popper AN (2004) Noise-induced stress response and hearing loss in goldfish (*Carassius auratus*). J Exp Biol 207: 427–435.
40. Smith ME, Coffin AB, Miller DL, Popper AN (2006) Anatomical and functional recovery of the goldfish (*Carassius auratus*) ear following noise exposure. J Exp Biol 209: 4193–4202.

41. Olivari FA, Hernandez PP, Allende ML (2008) Acute copper exposure induces oxidative stress and cell death in lateral line hair cells of zebrafish larvae. Brain Res 1244: 1–12.
42. Smith ME, Schuck JB, Gilley RR, Rogers BD (2011) Structural and functional effects of acoustic exposure in goldfish: evidence for tonotopy in the teleost saccule. BMC Neurosci 12: 19.
43. Corwin JT (1977) Morphology of the macula neglecta in sharks of the genus *Carcharhinus*. J Morphol 152: 341–362.
44. Corwin JT (1981) Postembryonic production and aging in inner ear hair cells in sharks. J Comp Neurol 201: 541–553.
45. Corwin JT (1983) Postembryonic growth of the macula neglecta auditory detector in the ray, *Raja clavata*: continual increases in hair cell number, neural convergence, and physiological sensitivity. J Comp Neurol 217: 345–356.
46. Corwin JT (1985) Perpetual production of hair cells and maturational changes in hair cell ultrastructure accompany postembryonic growth in an amphibian ear. Proc Natl Acad Sci USA 82: 3911–3915.
47. Yan HY, Saidel WM, Chang JS, Presson JC, Popper AN (1991) Sensory hair cells of a fish ear: evidence of multiple types based on ototoxicity sensitivity. Proc R Soc Lond B Biol Sci 245: 133–138.
48. Lombarte A, Yan HY, Popper AN, Chang JS, Platt C (1993) Damage and regeneration of hair cell ciliary bundles in a fish ear following treatment with gentamicin. Hear Res 64: 166–174.
49. Faucher K, Aas-Hansen O, Damsgard B, Stenklev NC (2008) Effects of systemic versus local gentamicin on the inner ear in the Atlantic cod, *Gadus morhua* (*L.*), relevance for fish hearing investigations. Hear Res 240: 12–21.
50. Faucher K, Aas-Hansen O, Damsgard B, Laukli E, Stenklev NC (2009) Damage and functional recovery of the Atlantic cod (*Gadus morhua*) inner ear hair cells following local injection of gentamicin. Int J Audiol 48: 456–464.
51. Ramcharitar JU, Brack CL (2010) Physiological dimensions of ototoxic responses in a model fish species. J Clin Neurosci 17: 103–106.
52. Ramcharitar J, Selckmann GM (2010) Differential ablation of sensory receptors underlies ototoxin-induced shifts in auditory thresholds of the goldfish (*Carassius auratus*). J Appl Toxicol 30: 536–541.
53. Liu M, Reimschuessel R, Hassel BA (2002) Molecular cloning of the fish interferon stimulated gene, 15 kDa (ISG15) orthologue: a ubiquitin-like gene induced by nephrotoxic damage. Gene 298: 129–139.
54. Matsuura S, Ikeda K, Furukawa T (1971) Effects of streptomycin, kanamycin, quinine, and other drugs on the microphonic potentials of goldfish sacculus. Jpn J Physiol 21: 579–590.
55. Steyger PS, Peters SL, Rehling J, Hordichok A, Dai CF (2003) Uptake of gentamicin by bullfrog saccular hair cells *in vitro*. J Assoc Res Otolaryngol 4: 565–578.
56. Wang Q, Steyger PS (2009) Trafficking of systemic fluorescent gentamicin into the cochlea and hair cells. J Assoc Res Otolaryngol 10: 205–219.
57. Janas JD, Cotanche DA, Rubel EW (1995) Avian cochlear hair cell regeneration: stereological analyses of damage and recovery from a single high dose of gentamicin. Hear Res 92: 17–29.
58. Tucci DL, Rubel EW (1990) Physiologic status of regenerated hair cells in the avian inner ear following aminoglycoside ototoxicity. J Otolaryng Head Neck Surg 103: 443–450.
59. Girod DA, Tucci DL, Rubel EW (1991) Anatomical correlates of functional recovery in the avian inner ear following aminoglycoside ototoxicity. Laryngoscope 101: 1139–1149.
60. Blakley BW, Hochman J, Wellman M, Gooi A, Hussain AE (2008) Differences in ototoxicity across species. J Otolaryngol Head Neck Surg 37: 700–703.
61. Wu WJ, Sha SH, McLaren JD, Kawamoto K, Raphael Y, et al. (2001) Aminoglycoside ototoxicity in adult CBA, C57BL and BALB mice and the Sprague-Dawley rat. Hear Res 158: 165–178.
62. Platt C (1993) Zebrafish inner ear sensory surfaces are similar to those in goldfish. Hear Res 65: 133–140.

23

KCNJ10 may not be a Contributor to Nonsyndromic Enlargement of Vestibular Aqueduct (NSEVA) in Chinese Subjects

Jiandong Zhao[1¶], Yongyi Yuan[1,2¶], Shasha Huang[1¶], Bangqing Huang[2¶], Jing Cheng[1], Dongyang Kang[1], Guojian Wang[1,2], Dongyi Han[1]*, Pu Dai[1,2]*

1 Department of Otolaryngology, PLA General Hospital, Beijing, People's Republic of China, **2** Department of Otolaryngology, Hainan Branch of PLA General Hospital, Sanya, People's Republic of China

Abstract

Background: Nonsyndromic enlargement of vestibular aqueduct (NSEVA) is an autosomal recessive hearing loss disorder that is associated with mutations in *SLC26A4*. However, not all patients with NSEVA carry biallelic mutations in *SLC26A4*. A recent study proposed that single mutations in both *SLC26A4* and *KCNJ10* lead to digenic NSEVA. We examined whether *KCNJ10* excert a role in the pathogenesis of NSEVA in Chinese patients.

Methods: *SLC26A4* was sequenced in 1056 Chinese patients with NSEVA. *KCNJ10* was screened in 131 patients who lacked mutations in either one or both alleles of *SLC26A4*. Additionally, *KCNJ10* was screened in 840 controls, including 563 patients diagnosed with NSEVA who carried biallelic *SLC26A4* mutations, 48 patients with nonsyndromic hearing loss due to inner ear malformations that did not involve enlargement of the vestibular aqueduct (EVA), 96 patients with conductive hearing loss due to various causes, and 133 normal-hearing individuals with no family history of hereditary hearing loss.

Results: 925 NSEVA patients were found carrying two-allele pathogenic *SLC26A4* mutations. The most frequently detected *KCNJ10* mutation was c.812G>A (p.R271H). Compared with the normal-hearing control subjects, the occurrence rate of c.812G>A in NSEVA patients with lacking mutations in one or both alleles of *SLC26A4* had no significant difference(1.53% vs. 5.30%, $\chi^2 = 2.798$, $p = 0.172$), which suggested that it is probably a nonpathogenic benign variant. *KCNJ10* c.1042C>T (p.R348C), the reported EVA-related mutation, was not found in patients with NSEVA who lacked mutations in either one or both alleles of *SLC26A4*. Furthermore, the normal-hearing parents of patients with NSEVA having two *SLC26A4* mutations carried the *KCNJ10* c.1042C>T or c.812G>A mutation and a *SLC26A4* pathogenic mutation.

Conclusion: *SLC26A4* is the major genetic cause in Chinese NSEVA patients, accounting for 87.59%. *KCNJ10* may not be a contributor to NSEVA in Chinese population. Other genetic or environmental factors are possibly play a role in the etiology of Chinese EVA patients with zero or monoallelic *SLC26A4* mutation.

Editor: Tao Cai, NIDCR/NIH, United States of America

Funding: This work was supported by funding from a grant from the Minister of Science and Technology (2012BAI09B02) and the 12th Five-Year National Key Technologies R & D program (No. 2012BAI12B01), Chinese National Nature Science Foundation Research Grants (30728030, 31071109, 81230020), and the State 863 High Technology R & D Key Project of China (SQ2010AA0221634001) to Dr. Pu Dai; the PLA General Hospital Culturing Foundation to Dr. Jiandong Zhao (12KMM32); a Chinese National Nature Science Foundation Research Grant (81070792) to Dr. Dongyi Han; and the Beijing Natural Science Foundation (7132177), Beijing Nova programme (2009B34) and Chinese National Nature Science Foundation (81371098) to Dr. Yongyi Yuan. The funders had no role in study design, data collection and analysis, decision to publish, or preparation of the manuscript.

Competing Interests: The authors have declared that no competing interests exist.

* Email: hdy301@263.net (DH); daipu301@vip.sina.com (PD)

¶ These authors contributed equally to this work.

Introduction

Nonsyndromic sensorineural hearing loss associated with an enlargement of the vestibular aqueduct (EVA) is a common form of inner ear malformation [1]. It occurs either congenitally or following some mild head injury and results in fluctuating and progressive hearing loss. Nonsyndromic enlargement of vestibular aqueduct (NSEVA) is an autosomal recessive hearing loss associated with mutations in the anion transporter *SLC26A4*, which encodes the anion transporter protein pendrin [2]. Located in the kidney, thyroid, and inner ear, pendrin is responsible for the transport of Cl^-, $HCO3^-$, OH^-, I^-, and formate [2,3]. In the inner ear, pendrin is expressed mainly in the external sulcus, endolym-phatic duct and sac, utricle, and saccule, and it maintains the endolymphatic balance by mediating Cl^-/HCO_3^- exchange [4–6]. Malfunction of the *SLC26A4* protein can cause NSEVA and Pendred syndrome (PS), a type of syndromic sensorineural hearing loss characterized by EVA, goiter, and in some cases Mondini malformation [7].

The underlying mechanisms for the etiology of NSEVA/PS remain elusive; however, studies that have screened for *SLC26A4* mutations in patients with NSEVA/PS and subsequent studies of these mutant proteins have been informative [2]. Some pendrin mutants fail to reach the cell surface and are retained in the endoplasmic reticulum, impairing anion transport and consequently the ionic balance of endolymph [8,9]. This imbalance causes endolymphatic dilatation, enlarges the membranous labyrinth, and disrupts the development of bone structures in the inner ear [9]. In addition, studies using *Slc26a4*$^{-/-}$ mouse models have demonstrated that the loss of pendrin expression decreases HCO_3^- secretion into the endolymph [10]. The resulting endolymphatic acidification inhibits Ca^{2+} reabsorption from endolymph, which further inhibits sensory transduction and promotes the degeneration of the sensory hair cells [10]. In China, NSEVA accounts for 20–25% of hereditary hearing loss cases, and biallelic mutations in *SLC26A4* represent nearly 90% of the genetic etiology of NSEVA [11]. However, the detection rate of *SLC26A4* biallelic mutations varies among different ethnicities (*e.g.*, 24% in Caucasians and 81% in Koreans) [12,13].

Although most previous studies in patients with NSEVA have focused on *SLC26A4*, not all patients with NSEVA carry biallelic mutations in *SLC26A4*. This discrepancy has led to the hypothesis that other genetic modifications or environmental factors may be involved. Yang et al. [14] proposed that single mutations in both *SLC26A4* and *KCNJ10* lead to digenic NSEVA. *KCNJ10* encodes a 42.5-kD member of the inward rectifier potassium channel family and is expressed mainly in the brain, kidney, and inner ear. The *KCNJ10* K^+ channel buffers the K^+ levels in brain glial cells, and mutations in this gene may lead to the so-called 'EAST/SeSAME syndrome,' which is manifested by seizures, sensorineural deafness, ataxia, mental retardation, and electrolyte imbalance [15,16]. In the inner ear, *KCNJ10* is expressed mainly in the intermediate cells of the stria vascularis. It maintains the K^+ concentration in the endolymph and generates endocochlear potential, which is the main driving force of sensory transduction that enables hearing [17,18]. In *Kcnj10*$^{-/-}$ mice, the endocochlear potential is abolished and hearing is greatly compromised [18].

Interestingly, studies using *Slc26a4*$^{-/-}$ mice have revealed an association between *SLC26A4* and *KCNJ10*. In these studies, the loss of pendrin reduced the protein expression of *KCNJ10*, which in turn eliminated endocochlear potential and impaired hearing [10,19]. Furthermore, Yang and colleagues have identified patients with NSEVA who carried single mutations in both *SLC26A4* and *KCNJ10* genes [14]. In one affected patient, Yang and colleagues identified the *KCNJ10* c.1042C>T (p.R348C) mutation as being in double heterozygosity with a *SLC26A4* mutation, whereas this was not observed in controls of European or Chinese descent with normal hearing [14]. In addition, they showed that haplo-insufficiency of *SLC26A4* in *Slc26a4*$^{+/-}$ mice reduced the *KCNJ10* levels. The *KCNJ10* mutants identified in their study displayed reduced K^+ conductance activity, a critical step in generating endocochlear potential [14]. Furthermore, the *KCNJ10* c.1042C>T mutation, which was suggested to be a potentially pathological mutation, was shown to reduce K^+ conductance activity [14]. Based on these findings, the authors postulated that single mutations in both *SLC26A4* and *KCNJ10* lead to digenic NSEVA.

In this study, we aimed to examine whether *KCNJ10* plays a role in the pathogenesis of NSEVA by screening *KCNJ10* mutations in Chinese patients with NSEVA who lacked mutations in one or both alleles of *SLC26A4*. This screening resulted in the identification of common *KCNJ10* mutations in the Chinese population. The conclusions from this study contribute important foundations for genetic diagnosis as well as prenatal diagnosis of deafness.

Subjects and Methods

Subjects

The subjects were recruited by the Department of Otolaryngology and Genetic Testing Center for Deafness, PLA General Hospital, BeiJing, China. Totally 1056 EVA patients were enrolled in the study. They were all screened the coding region of *SLC26A4* firstly. Then a cohort of 131 Chinese patients with NSEVA without mutation or with only one *SLC26A4* mutation was recruited for mutation screening for *KCNJ10*. In addition, we examined 840 controls, comprising the following four groups: 563 patients who were diagnosed with NSEVA and carried biallelic *SLC26A4* mutations, 48 patients with nonsyndromic hearing loss and inner ear malformation other than EVA, 96 patients with conductive hearing loss due to various causes (70 cases with chronic otitis media, 11 cases with secretory otitis media, 9 cases with conductive deafness due to unknown causes, three cases with otosclerosis, 2 cases with external auditory canal tumor, and 1 case with a jugular tumor sphere), and 133 normal-hearing individuals with no family history of hereditary hearing loss. Written informed consent was obtained from all subjects or guardians prior to blood sampling and genetic testing. The study protocol, including the consent procedure, was performed with the approval of the Ethics Committee of the Chinese PLA General Hospital.

Mutation screening of *KCNJ10*

Genomic DNA was isolated from whole blood through a modification of standard procedures [20]. Most DNA samples were collected by and stored at the Genetic Testing Center for Deafness. The only coding exon of *KCNJ10* was amplified in a 20-μl PCR reaction mixture containing 20 ng of genomic DNA template, 0.0625 units of Taq DNA polymerase (Biomed, Cat: Pc01, Lot: 211841XB), and 40 nM primers. The following three sets of PCR primers were used (5′→3′): forward, CGATAACCTCCATTATGCTG and reverse, AGGATGGTGGTGAGCACCAG; forward, TGGCTTCCGCTACATCAGTG and reverse, ACAACTTGGTCAAAAGGCTAA; forward, ACCCCTTACCTTCTATCATG and reverse, GTAGTATTCCTTACCAGGGC. To increase the specificity and sensitivity of PCR amplification, the technique of touchdown-PCR was employed: one cycle at 95°C for 1 min; 95°C for 30 s, 62°C for 30 s, and 72°C for 45 s, followed by 13 cycles at decreasing annealing temperatures in decrements of 0.5°C; 21 cycles of 95°C for 30 s, 56°C for 30 s, and 72°C for 45 s, with a final extension at 72°C for 7 min. The sizes of the PCR products were confirmed by 1% agarose gel electrophoresis. PCR products were sequenced using forward primers to screen for mutations in *KCNJ10* (Doobio Biotechnology Co., China). The detected mutations were confirmed by sequencing using reverse primers.

Statistics

SPSS 17.0 software was used in statistical analysis. Comparisons between groups were tested using the χ^2 or Fisher's exact tests. P value<0.05 was set for statistically significant difference.

Results

SLC26A4 analysis in NSEVA patients

Totally 925 NSEVA patients were found carrying two-allele pathogenic *SLC26A4* mutations, *SLC26A4* accounts for 87.59%

Table 1. Genotype of NSEVA patients with two-allele *SLC26A4* mutations.

Number	SLC26A4 Genotype		Number of patients
	Allele 1	Allele 2	
1	IVS7-2A>G	IVS7-2A>G	237
2	IVS7-2A>G	c.2168A>G(p.H723R)	103
3	IVS7-2A>G	c.1226G>A(p.R409H)	40
4	IVS7-2A>G	c.1975G>C(p.V659L)	35
5	IVS7-2A>G	c.1229C>T(p.T410M)	27
6	IVS7-2A>G	c.1174A>T(p.N392Y)	23
7	IVS7-2A>G	c.2027T>A(p.L676Q)	19
8	IVS7-2A>G	c.589G>A(p.G197R)	15
9	IVS7-2A>G	IVS15+5G>A	11
10	IVS7-2A>G	c.917insG	10
11	c.2168A>G(p.H723R)	c.2168A>G(p.H723R)	9
12	c.2168A>G(p.H723R)	c.1975G>C(p.V659L)	9
13	c.2168A>G(p.H723R)	c.1229C>T(p T410M)	8
14	IVS7-2A>G	c.281C>T(p.T94I)	6
15	IVS7-2A>G	c.1336C>T(p.Q446X)	6
16	IVS7-2A>G	c.1262A>C(p.Q421P)	5
17	IVS7-2A>G	IVS4+2T>C	5
18	c.1174A>T(p.N392Y)	c.1226G>A(p.R409H)	5
19	IVS7-2A>G	c.1225C>T(p.R409C)	5
20	IVS7-2A>G	c.1586T>G(p.I529S)	5
21	IVS7-2A>G	c.1687_1692insA	5
22	IVS7-2A>G	c.235C>T(p.R79X)	4
23	c.1229C>T(p.T410M)	c.1229C>T(p.T410M)	4
24	c.1975G>C(p.V659L)	c.2027T>A(p.L676Q)	4
25	IVS7-2A>G	c.1079C>T(p.A360V)	4
26	IVS7-2A>G	IVS13+9C>T	4
27	c.2168A>G(p.H723R)	c.2027T>A(p.L676Q)	4
28	c.2168A>G(p.H723R)	c.1226G>A(p.R409H)	4
29	IVS7-2A>G	c.1318A>T(p.K440X)	4
30	c.1540C>T(p.Q514X)	c.2168A>G(p.H723R)	3
31	c.2027T>A(p.L676Q)	c.589G>A(p.G197R)	3
32	IVS7-2A>G	c.1340delA	3
33	IVS7-2A>G	c.563T>C(p.I188T)	3
34	IVS7-2A>G	c.170C>A(p.S57X)	3
35	IVS7-2A>G	c.1594A>C(p.S532R)	3
36	IVS7-2A>G	c.946G>T(p.G316X)	3
37	IVS7-2A>G	c.1334T>G(p.L445W)	3
38	IVS7-2A>G	c.1343C>A(p.S448X)	3
39	c.1975G>C(p.V659L)	c.1229C>T(p.T410M)	3
40	IVS7-2A>G	c.2162C>T(p.T721M)	3
41	IVS7-2A>G	c.1540C>T(p.Q514X)	3
42	IVS7-2A>G	c.1693insA	3
43	IVS7-2A>G	c.1160C>T(p.A387V)	3
44	IVS7-2A>G	c.2167C>G(p.H723D)	3
45	IVS7-2A>G	c.1343C>A(p.S448X)	3
46	c.2168A>G(p.H723R)	c.563T>C(p.I188T)	3
47	IVS7-2A>G	c.1520delT	3
48	c.2168A>G(p.H723R)	c.589G>A(p.G197R)	3

Table 1. Cont.

Number	SLC26A4 Genotype		Number of patients
	Allele 1	**Allele 2**	
49	IVS7-2A>G	c.1173C>A(p.S391R)	3
50	c.1229C>T(p.T410M)	c.1174A>T(p.N392Y)	2
51	IVS7-2A>G	c.414delT	2
52	IVS7-2A>G	c.1548insC	2
53	c.1174A>T(p.N392Y)	IVS15+5G>A	2
54	IVS7-2A>G	IVS14-2A>G	2
55	c.235C>T(p.R79X)	c.2168A>G(p.H723R)	2
56	IVS7-2A>G	c.1699A>T(p.K567X)	2
57	IVS7-2A>G	c.1371C>A(p.N457K)	2
58	1240–1243GAGA>AAAG(p.E414K, p.S415G)	IVS14-6T>G	2
59	IVS7-2A>G	c.1670G>A(p.G557D)	2
60	IVS7-2A>G	c.665G>T(p.G222V)	2
61	IVS7-2A>G	c.1990G>A(p.A664T)	2
62	IVS7-2A>G	c.1238A>G(p.Q413R)	2
63	c.1079C>T(p.A360V)	c.2168A>G(p.H723R)	2
64	c.1229C>T(p.T410M)	c.1687_1692insA	2
65	IVS7-2A>G	c.1022delC	2
66	IVS7-2A>G	c.907G>C(p.E303Q)	2
67	IVS7-2A>G	c.2086C>T(p.Q696X)	2
68	c.2027T>A(p.L676Q)	c.2027T>A(p.L676Q)	2
69	IVS7-2A>G	c.269C>T(p.S90L)	2
70	c.1174A>T(p.N392Y)	c.2168A>G(p.H723R)	2
71	IVS7-2A>G	c.1363A>T(p.I455F)	2
72	c.1174A>T(p.N392Y)	c.2027T>A(p.L676Q)	2
73	c.1673A>T(p.N558I)	IVS14+1G>A	2
74	c.1318A>T(p.K440X)	c.1327G>C(p.E443Q)	2
75	IVS7-2A>G	c.1991C>T(p.A664V)	2
76	IVS7-2A>G	c.1595G>T(p.S532I)	2
77	c.1226G>A(p.R409H)	c.1226G>A(p.R409H)	2
78	c.946G>T(p.G316X)	c.2168A>G(p.H723R)	2
79	IVS7-2A>G	c.668T>C(p.F223S)	2
80	IVS7-2A>G	c.1970G>T(p.S657I)	2
81	c.1522A>G(p.T508A)	c.1522A>G(p.T508A)	1
82	c.1595G>T(p.S532I)	IVS4+7A>G	1
83	IVS7-2A>G	c.1720G>A(p.A574T)	1
84	c.1343C>A(p.S448X)	c.2167C>G(p.H723D)	1
85	c.1178delTCT	c.439A>G((p.M147V)	1
86	IVS7-2A>G	c.400A>G(p.R134G)	1
87	c.589G>A(p.G197R)	c.1105A>G(p.K369E)	1
88	IVS15+5G>A	c.1318A>T(p.K440X)	1
89	IVS7-2A>G	c.1367C>A(p.A456D)	1
90	IVS7-2A>G	c.249G>A(p.W83X)	1
91	c.1174A>T(p.N392Y)	c.1975G>C(p.V659L)	1
92	IVS7-2A>G	c.1964T>A(p.I655N)	1
93	IVS7-2A>G	c.2081delC	1
94	c.281C>T(p.T94I)	c.692T>A(p.V231E)	1
95	IVS7-2A>G	IVS9+1G>A	1
96	c.2168A>G(p.H723R)	c.439A>G((p.M147V)	1

Table 1. Cont.

Number	SLC26A4 Genotype		Number of patients
	Allele 1	Allele 2	
97	IVS7-2A>G	IVS10+1G>A	1
98	c.890delC	IVS7-2A>G	1
99	IVS7-2A>G	c.1829C>A(p.S610X)	1
100	IVS7-2A>G	c.218delA	1
101	c.1594A>C(p.S532R)	c.2168A>G(p.H723R)	1
102	c.1229C>T(p.T410M)	c.281C>T(p.T94I)	1
103	IVS7-2A>G	c.404A>G(p.H135R)	1
104	c.1022insC	c.1489G>A(p.G497S)	1
105	c.946G>T(p.G316X)	c.1343C>A(p.S448X)	1
106	IVS7-2A>G	c.230A>T(p.K77I)	1
107	IVS7-2A>G	c.1327G>C(p.E443Q)	1
108	c.1226G>A(p.R409H)	c.58T>C(p.Y20H)	1
109	c.2027T>A(p.L676Q)	IVS13+9C>T	1
110	c.249G>A(p.W83X)	c.2168A>G(p.H723R)	1
111	c.203T>C(p.L68P)	IVS4+2T>C	1
112	c.911T>A(p.V304E)	c.1238A>G(p.Q413R)	1
113	c.2027T>A(p.L676Q)	IVS15+5G>A	1
114	c.1343C>A(p.S448X)	c.1339delA	1
115	c.1976T>G(p.V659G)	c.2168A>G(p.H723R)	1
116	c.2027T>A(p.L676Q)	c.1520delT	1
117	IVS10+1G>A	IVS10+1G>A	1
118	c.1238A>G(p.Q413R)	c.1172G>A(p.S391N)	1
119	IVS7-2A>G	c.1634T>A(p.V545E)	1
120	IVS7-2A>G	c.2179C>T(p.L727F)	1
121	c.1343C>A(p.S448X)	c.1178delTCT	1
122	c.2086C>T(p.Q696X)	c.2168A>G(p.H723R)	1
123	c.754T>C(p.S252P)	c.86A>G(p.E29G)	1
124	c.2168A>G(p.H723R)	IVS4+2T>C	1
125	c.1229C>T(p.T410M)	c.1949T>A(p.V650D)	1
126	IVS7-2A>G	IVS5+2T>A	1
127	c.1229C>T(p.T410M)	c.1693insA	1
128	c.391G>A(p.G131R)	c.2168A>G(p.H723R)	1
129	IVS7-2A>G	c.2014G>A(p.G672R)	1
130	IVS7-2A>G	IVS12+1G>A	1
131	IVS7-2A>G	c.1373T>C(p.L458P)	1
132	c.754T>C(p.S252P)	c.2168A>G(p.H723R)	1
133	c.71G>A(p.R24Q)	c.2168A>G(p.H723R)	1
134	c.1174A>T(p.N392Y)	c.1829C>A(p.S610X)	1
135	c.439A>G((p.M147V)	c.1615A>G(p.I539V)	1
136	IVS7-2A>G	c.1615A>G(p.I539V)	1
137	c.1174A>T(p.N392Y)	c.1340delA	1
138	c.1975G>C(p.V659L)	c.1238A>G(p.Q413R)	1
139	c.589G>A(p.G197R)	c.589G>A(p.G197R)	1
140	c.1174A>T(p.N392Y)	c.249G>A(p.W83X)	1
141	c.1991C>T(p.A664V)	c.1336C>T(p.Q446X)	1
142	IVS7-2A>G	c.349delC	1
143	IVS7-2A>G	c.259G>T(p.D87Y)	1
144	IVS7-2A>G	c.1687_1692delA	1

Table 1. Cont.

Number	SLC26A4 Genotype		Number of patients
	Allele 1	Allele 2	
145	c.109G>T(p.E37X)	c.2168A>G(p.H723R)	1
146	c.917insG	c.2168A>G(p.H723R)	1
147	c.1226G>A(p.R409H)	IVS15+5G>A	1
148	IVS7+1G>A	c.2168A>G(p.H723R)	1
149	c.1334T>G(p.L445W)	c.1544T>C(p.F515S)	1
150	c.1489G>A(p.G497S)	c.414delT	1
151	IVS7-2A>G	c.1803G>C(p.K601N)	1
152	c.2168A>G(p.H723R)	c.279T>A(p.S93N)	1
153	c.235C>T(p.R79X)	c.589G>A(p.G197R)	1
154	IVS15+5G>A	c.2145G>T(p.K715N)	1
155	c.1229C>T(p.T410M)	c.1343C>A(p.S448X)	1
156	IVS7-2A>G	c.79T>A(p.Y27N)	1
157	c.1586T>G(p.I529S)	c.2168A>G(p.H723R)	1
158	IVS7-2A>G	c.2009T>C(p.V670A)	1
159	c.2027T>A(p.L676Q)	c.1586T>G(p.I529S)	1
160	c.1229C>T(p.T410M)	IVS19+2T>A	1
161	c.1264G>A(p.V422I)	c.2027T>A(p.L676Q)	1
162	IVS7-2A>G	c.1975G>C(p.V659L)	1
163	c.109G>T(p.E37X)	c.109G>T(p.E37X)	1
164	c.421T>C(p.F141L)	c.1343C>A(p.S448X)	1
165	IVS7-2A>G	c.227C>T(p.P76L)	1
166	c.1520delT	c.2168A>G(p.H723R)	1
167	c.249G>A(p.W83X)	c.1105A>G(p.K369E)	1
168	IVS7-2A>G	c.754T>C(p.S252P)	1
169	c.279T>A(p.S93N)	c.2183insT	1
170	c.1991C>T(p.A664V)	c.1173C>A(p.S391R)	1
171	c.1343C>A(p.S448X)	c.2168A>G(p.H723R)	1
172	c.249G>A(p.W83X)	c.1340delA	1
173	IVS7-2A>G	c.2168A>C(p.H723P)	1
174	c.1174A>T(p.N392Y)	c.1991C>T(p.A664V)	1
175	c.1975G>C(p.V659L)	c.2039delT	1
176	c.1975G>C(p.V659L)	c.281C>T(p.T94I)	1
177	IVS7-2A>G	c.1714T>G(p.F572V)	1
178	IVS7-2A>G	c.2000T>C(p.F667S)	1
179	c.574delC	c.2168A>G(p.H723R)	1
180	IVS7-2A>G	c.1835delA	1
181	c.1229C>T(p.T410M)	c.1079C>T(p.A360V)	1
182	c.1229C>T(p.T410M)	IVS1-2A>C	1
183	c.1334T>G(p.L445W)	c.2168A>G(p.H723R)	1
184	IVS7-2A>G	c.439A>G((p.M147V)	1
185	c.1318A>T(p.K440X)	c.2168A>G(p.H723R)	1
186	c.1229C>T(p.T410M)	c.1226G>A(p.R409H)	1
187	c.1517T>G(p.L506R)	c.2162C>T(p.T721M)	1
188	c.1174A>T(p.N392Y)	IVS13+9C>T	1
189	c.1174A>T(p.N392Y)	c.1334T>G(p.L445W)	1
190	c.917insG	c.281C>T(p.T94I)	1
191	c.1174A>T(p.N392Y)	c.668T>C(p.F223S)	1
192	c.1229C>T(p.T410M)	c.1594AG>T	1

Table 1. Cont.

Number	SLC26A4 Genotype		Number of patients
	Allele 1	Allele 2	
193	c.2027T>A(p.L676Q)	c.334C>T(p.P112S)	1
194	IVS15+5G>A	c.1520delT	1
195	c.387delC	c.2168A>G(p.H723R)	1
196	c.946G>T(p.G316X)	c.1522A>G(p.T508A)	1
197	IVS7-2A>G	c.587T>A(p.V196D)	1
198	IVS7-2A>G	c.1927G>T(p.E643X)	1
199	c.1687_1692insA	c.68C>A(p.S23X)	1
200	c.1829C>A(p.S610X)	c.2168A>G(p.H723R)	1
201	c.1343C>T(p.S448L)	c.2168A>G(p.H723R)	1
202	c.1174A>T(p.N392Y)	c.414delT	1
203	IVS7-2A>G	c.2118C>A(p.C706X)	1
204	c.2168A>G(p.H723R)	c.281C>T(p.T94I)	1
205	IVS7-2A>G	c.496delA	1
206	c.1540C>T(p.Q514X)	IVS13+9C>T	1
207	c.917insG	c.1229C>T(p.T410M)	1
208	c.2168A>G(p.H723R)	c.1548insC	1
209	IVS7-2A>G	c.1286C>A(p.A429E)	1
210	IVS15+5G>A	c.235C>T(p.R79X)	1
211	c.946G>T(p.G316X)	c.1226G>A(p.R409H)	1
212	c.1927G>T(p.E643X)	c.2168A>G(p.H723R)	1
213	c.2027T>A(p.L676Q)	c.1336C>T(p.Q446X)	1
214	c.1336C>T(p.Q446X)	c.1520delT	1
215	c.2T>C(p.M1T)	c.2168A>G(p.H723R)	1
216	c.1174A>T(p.N392Y)	c.1225C>T(p.R409C)	1
217	c.1174A>T(p.N392Y)	c.346G>A(p.G116S)	1
218	IVS7-2A>G	c.398C>T(p.S133L)	1
219	c.1226G>A(p.R409H)	c.281C>T(p.T94I)	1
220	c.917insG	c.2086C>T(p.Q696X)	1
221	IVS7-2A>G	c.1216G>A(p.A406T)	1
222	c.946G>T(p.G316X)	c.1586T>G(p.I529S)	1
223	c.1173C>A(p.S391R)	c.279T>A(p.S93N)	1
224	c.1985G>A(p.C662Y)	c.1687_1692insA	1
225	c.227C>T(p.P76L)	IVS4+2T>C	1
226	c.768delG	IVS15+5G>A	1
227	c.1174A>T(p.N392Y)	c.281C>T(p.T94I)	1
228	c.1225C>T(p.R409C)	c.1226G>A(p.R409H)	1
229	IVS9+1G>A	IVS18+3A>C	1
230	IVS7-2A>G	c.149T>C(p.L50P)	1
231	c.1174A>T(p.N392Y)	c.1594A>C(p.S532R)	1
232	IVS7-2A>G	c.1339delA	1
233	c.281C>T(p.T94I)	c.1318A>T(p.K440X)	1
234	c.1985G>A(p.C662Y)	IVS7-2A>G	1
235	c.1548insC	c.2086C>T(p.Q696X)	1
236	c.235C>T(p.R79X)	c.1022delC	1
237	c.1226G>A(p.R409H)	IVS5+2T>A	1
238	c.1229C>T(p.T410M)	c.279T>A(p.S93N)	1
239	IVS7-2A>G	c.1746delG	1
240	c.1226G>A(p.R409H)	c.589G>A(p.G197R)	1

Table 1. Cont.

Number	SLC26A4 Genotype		Number of patients
	Allele 1	Allele 2	
241	c.920C>A(p.T307K)	c.2174insCTAT	1
242	IVS7-2A>G	c.1264G>A(p.V422I)	1
243	c.1229C>T(p.T410M)	c.365delT	1
244	IVS7-2A>G	IVS7+2T>C	1
245	c.1229C>T(p.T410M)	c.235C>T(p.R79X)	1
246	c.1174A>T(p.N392Y)	c.1174A>T(p.N392Y)	1
247	c.754T>C(p.S252P)	c.349insC	1
248	IVS7-2A>G	c.387delC	1
249	c.2014G>A(p.G672R)	c.2168A>G(p.H723R)	1
250	c.249G>A(p.W83X)	c.281C>T(p.T94I)	1
251	c.1262A>C(p.Q421P)	c.2054G>T(p.R685I)	1
252	c.1687_1692insA	c.589G>A(p.G197R)	1
253	IVS7-2A>G	c.716T>A(p.V239D)	1
254	c.1229C>T(p.T410M)	c.1546C>T(p.P516S)	1
255	IVS7-3C>G	IVS15+5G>A	1
256	c.1975G>C(p.V659L)	c.2086C>T(p.Q696X)	1
257	c.1225C>T(p.R409C)	c.1225C>T(p.R409C)	1
258	c.2168A>G(p.H723R)	c.404A>G(p.H135R)	1
259	IVS7-2A>G	IVS3+84G>A	1
260	c.2006A>T(p.D669V)	c.439A>G((p.M147V)	1
261	IVS7-2A>G	c.403C>T(p.H135Y)	1
262	IVS7-2A>G	c.1673A>T(p.N558I)	1
263	c.1226G>A(p.R409H)	c.1340delA	1

(925/1056) of the genetic etiology in Chinese NSEVA patients. The *SLC26A4* mutation data were shown in Table 1 and Table 2.

Genetic analysis of *KCNJ10* among NSEVA patients lacking mutations in one or both alleles of *SLC26A4*

Among the 131 NSEVA patients lacking mutations in one or both alleles of *SLC26A4*, we identified the heterozygous missense mutation c.812G>A in *KCNJ10* in two cases (Fig. S1), with a mutation rate of 1.53% (2/131); the *KCNJ10* c.1042C>T mutation was not found. In the two cases with the *KCNJ10* c.812G>A mutation, Patient 195 carried no mutations in *SLC26A4* and Patient 1606 carried a heterozygous mutation in *SLC26A4* (c.225C>G). In addition, we screened *SLC26A4* and *KCNJ10* genes in the parents of Patient 195 (Table 3). Both Patient 195 and his father carried *KCNJ10* c.812G>A and wild-type *SLC26A4*; however, only Patient 195 developed NSEVA symptoms.

Genetic analysis of *KCNJ10* among NSEVA patients with two mutations in *SLC26A4*

As a control, we conducted *KCNJ10* mutation screening in 563 patients with NSEVA who carried two mutations in *SLC26A4*. We found 11 cases with a heterozygous *KCNJ10* c.812G>A mutation (1.95%, 11/563) and three cases with a heterozygous *KCNJ10* c.1042C>T mutation (0.53%, 3/563) (Fig. S1). We performed further testing for *KCNJ10* in one of the pedigrees containing 11 subjects with the *KCNJ10* c.812G>A mutation. Our result showed that Patient 2471 shared *SLC26A4* c.2027 T>A and *KCNJ10* c.812 G>A with his father, and *SLC26A4* IVS7-2 A>G with his mother. Patient 2471, with compound heterozygous mutations in *SLC26A4*, developed NSEVA, whereas his father, with double heterozygosity in both *SLC26A4* and *KCNJ10*, was not affected (Table 3).

We examined three patients with NSEVA in Pedigrees 4769 and 4814 who had biallelic *SLC26A4* mutations and the *KCNJ10* c.1042C>T mutation (Table 4). Hearing examinations showed that the hearing capabilities of the parents were normal, and high-resolution temporal bone computed tomography (CT) scans showed that EVA was not present in the parents. Because both parents in Pedigree 1134 were deceased, neither hearing examinations nor DNA sequencing could be done. However, the proband from Pedigree 3 reported to us that his parents had no hearing problems. We sequenced the *KCNJ10* and *SLC26A4* genes from the family members in Pedigrees 4769 and 4814. For Pedigree 4769, the proband's mother carried the *SLC26A4* c.2168A>G (p.H723R) and *KCNJ10* c.1042C>T (p.R348C) mutations. For Pedigree 4814, the proband's father carried the monoallelic *SLC26A4* IVS7-2A>G and *KCNJ10* c.1042C>T (p.R348C) mutations. IVS7-2A>G and c.2168A>G (p.H723R) are pathogenic mutations supported by both functional and molecular epidemiological studies [21–23]. They are also prevalent *SLC26A4* hotspot mutations in Chinese NSEVA. The finding that normal-hearing individuals carried both the *KCNJ10* c.1042C>T mutation and a *SLC26A4* pathogenic mutation

Table 2. Genotype of NSEVA patients with zero or one allele *SLC26A4* mutation.

Number	Genotype	Number of patients
1	IVS7-2A>G/wt	68
2	c.2168 A>G(p.H723R)/wt	11
3	c.2027T>A(p.L676Q)/wt	5
4	c.1174A>T(p.N392Y)/wt	5
5	IVS15+5G>A/wt	4
6	c.1229C>T(p.T410M)/wt	4
7	c.1226G>A(p.R409H)/wt	3
8	c.147C>G(p.S49R)/wt	2
9	c.235C>T(p.R79X)/wt	1
10	c.487G>C(p.R163L)/wt	1
11	c.471C>T(p.P157P)/wt	1
12	c.1339_1340delA/wt	1
13	c.1286C>A(p.A429E)/wt	1
14	c.1336C>T(p.Q446X)/wt	1
15	IVS18+1G>A/wt	1
16	c.1673A>T(p.N558I)/wt	1
17	c.917insG/wt	1
18	c.946G>T(p.G316X)/wt	1
19	c.1687_1692insA/wt	1
20	wt/wt	18

wt: wild-type.

suggests that *KCNJ10* c.1042C>T may not always act together with *SLC26A4* mutation in digenic inheritance related to the etiology of NSEVA in Chinese subjects.

Genetic analysis of *KCNJ10* among subjects with inner ear malformation

Among 48 patients with NSEVA and non-EVA inner ear malformations, we identified one case (1/48, 2.1%) with the missense mutation c.812G>A in *KCNJ10*.

Genetic analysis of *KCNJ10* among subjects with conductive hearing loss

Among the 96 inpatients with conductive hearing loss, we detected *KCNJ10* heterozygous c.812G>A in four cases (4/96, 4.2%), heterozygous c.811C>T in one case (1/96, 1.0%), and heterozygous c.1042C>T in one case (1/96, 1.0%).

Genetic analysis of *KCNJ10* among normal-hearing subjects

We completed *KCNJ10* mutation screening in 133 normal-hearing control subjects with no family history of hereditary hearing loss. Seven subjects carried a single heterozygous mutation of c.812G>A in *KCNJ10* (7/133, 5.3%), and one subject carried a single heterozygous mutation of c.1042C>T in *KCNJ10* (1/133, 0.8%). No other mutations in *KCNJ10* were detected. No statistical difference in the *KCNJ10* c.812G>A and c.1042C>T mutations was observed between the normal-hearing group and the NSEVA cases with zero, one, or two mutations in *SLC26A4*,

Table 3. The KCNJ10 c.812G>A mutation identified in Chinese patients with nonsyndromic enlargement of vestibular aqueduct (NSEVA).

Pedigree No.	Phenotype	*SLC26A4* mutation	*KCNJ10* mutation
195 proband	NSEVA	wt/wt	c.812G>A (p.R271H)/wt
P	Normal	wt/wt	c.812G>A (p.R271H)/wt
M	Normal	wt/wt	wt/wt
1606 proband	NSEVA	c.225C>G(p.L75L)/wt unknown	c.812G>A(p.R271H)/wt
P	Normal	Unknown	Unknown
M	Normal	Unknown	Unknown
2471 proband	NSEVA	IVS7-2 A>G/c.2027T>A(p.L676Q)	c.812G>A (p.R271H)wt
P	Normal	c.2027T>A(p.L676Q)/wt	c.812G>A (p.R271H)/wt
M	Normal	IVS7-2 A>G/wt	wt/wt

wt, wild-type; P, father of proband (paternal); M, mother of proband (maternal).

Table 4. Identification of the *KCNJ10* c.1042C>T mutation in three NSEVA pedigrees with biallelic mutations in *SLC26A4*.

Pedigree No.	Phenotype	*SLC26A4* mutation	*KCNJ10* mutation
4769 proband	NSEVA	IVS7-2 A>G/c.2168 A>G (p.H723R)	c.1042 C>T(p.R348C)/wt
P	Normal	IVS7-2 A>G/wt	wt/wt
M	Normal	c.2168 A>G (p.H723R)/wt	c.1042 C>T(p.R348C)/wt
4814 proband	NSEVA	IVS7-2 A>G/IVS7-2 A>G	c.1042 C>T(p.R348C)/wt
P	Normal	IVS7-2 A>G/wt	c.1042 C>T(p.R348C)/wt
M	Normal	IVS7-2 A>G/wt	wt/wt
S	NSEVA	IVS7-2 A>G/IVS7-2 A>G	c.1042 C>T(p.R348C)/wt
1134 proband	NSEVA	IVS7-2 A>G/c.249 G>A (p.W83X)	c.1042 C>T(p.R348C)/wt
P	Normal	Unknown	Unknown
M	Normal	Unknown	Unknown

wt, wild-type; P, father of proband (paternal); M, mother of proband (maternal); S, sibling of proband.

patients with inner ear malformation, or patients with conductive hearing loss ($\chi^2 = 6.287$, $P = 0.179$).

Discussion

NSEVA/PS is an autosomal recessive disorder that results in sensorineural hearing loss and is associated with mutations in the *SLC26A4* gene. The exact causal relationship between the *SLC26A4* genotype and pathological phenotypes remains controversial [24]. Some patients with NSEVA have biallelic mutations in *SLC26A4*, including homozygous mutations and compound heterozygous mutations, whereas others lack mutations in one or both alleles of *SLC26A4*. In addition, the ratios of *SLC26A4* biallelic and monoallelic mutations vary across different populations. For example, double and single mutation rates are 81% and 11% in South Korea [13], 77% and 13% in France [25], 47% and 13% in Japan [26], and 88% and 10% in China, respectively [27]. Several reasons may explain this seemingly confusing phenomenon. First, the efficiency and effectiveness of mutation screening are limited. Mutations in the promoter and intronic cryptic splicing regions could be missed [28]. Benign *SLC26A4* polymorphic variants could be misrecognized as pathogenic alleles [24]. Furthermore, the pathogenesis of NSEVA/PS, as for many complex multigenic disorders, may result from interactions among multiple genes and environmental factors. In patients with NSEVA/PS, mutations in *FOXI1*, a transcription factor of *SLC26A4*, have been identified either alone or in combination with mutations in *SLC26A4* [28]. Single mutations in both *SLC26A4* and *KCNJ10* have been suggested as another potential etiological mechanism [14].

Yang et al. [14] proposed that single mutations in both *SLC26A4* and *KCNJ10*, an inward rectifier potassium channel, lead to digenic NSEVA. *KCNJ10* c.1042C>T was shown to reduce K^+ conductance activity and was therefore considered a potential pathological mutation. *KCNJ10* c.1042C>T was not found in ESP 6500 and was regarded as a pathogenic SNV by 1000 Genomes. However, in our study, *KCNJ10* c.1042C>T was not found in patients with NSEVA with zero or one *SLC26A4* mutation (n = 131). But the facts that *KCNJ10* c.1042C>T was found in a normal-hearing control subject and that normal hearing parents of patients with NSEVA with two *SLC26A4* mutations carried both *KCNJ10* c.1042C>T and *SLC26A4* pathogenic mutations suggest that *KCNJ10* c.1042C>T might be a benign variant in the Chinese population.

The most frequently identified mutation of *KCNJ10* in this study was c.812G>A (p.R271H). *KCNJ10* c.812G>A was not found in ESP 6500 and was regarded as a benign SNV by 1000 Genomes. It was found in patients with NSEVA who carried no mutation, a monoallelic mutation, or two mutations in *SLC26A4*; in patients with inner ear malformation; in patients with conductive hearing loss; and in normal-hearing individuals. The occurrence rate of c.812G>A had no significantly difference among the above five group people, suggest that *KCNJ10* c.812G>A is a benign variant in the Chinese population. Interestingly, the hearing in the two individuals with the *SLC26A4* mutations and *KCNJ10* c.1042C>T (p.R348C) mutations was normal. It may be due to the likelihood of incomplete penetrance of the p.R348C mutation influenced by additional environmental factors, genetic modifiers or difference in genetic/ethnical background. Our observations also suggested another possibility that *KCNJ10* c.1042C>T (p.R348C) is a benign variant in the Chinese population.

Similar to our study, other genetic studies in patients with EVA/PS have failed to find convincing evidence that *KCNJ10* mutations contribute to these phenotypes. Jonard et al. [29] screened 25 patients with unilateral deafness and unilateral EVA, but found no mutations in *KCNJ10*. Mercer et al. [30] screened 51 patients with EVA and found no mutations in *KCNJ10*. Chen et al. [31] screened *SLC26A4* and *KCNJ10* in patients with bilateral deafness and inner ear malformations and found no mutations in *KCNJ10* in the 15 patients who had one or no *SLC26A4* mutations. Landa et al. screened *KCNJ10/FOXI1* in 68 EVA or Pendred syndrome patients with with monoallelic mutations of SLC26A4. They found no evidence for an association between mutations of *KCNJ10* or *FOXI1* with SLC26A4 mutations in the pathogenesis of EVA or Pendred syndrome [32].

To our knowledge, this report is the largest study to screen *KCNJ10* in patients with NSEVA with two, one, or no *SLC26A4* mutations. In addition, we screened *KCNJ10* in patients diagnosed with conductive hearing loss having non-EVA inner ear malformations. Interestingly, no statistical differences in *KCNJ10* mutation rates were detected among all of the above groups and the normal-hearing control group.

Conclusions

SLC26A4 is the major genetic cause in Chinese NSEVA patients, accounting for 87.59%. *KCNJ10* may not be a contributor to NSEVA. Other genetic or environmental factors are possibly playing a role in the etiology of Chinese NSEVA patients with zero or monoallelic *SLC26A4* mutation.

Supporting Information

Figure S1 The representative chromatograms of the Sanger sequencing data for wild, c.812G>A and c.1042C>T of KCNJ10. A: wild type of KCNJ10 in the 812 locus. B: sense strand of 812G>A mutation: wild type of KCNJ10 in the 1042 locus. D: sense strand of 1042C>T mutation. E: antisense strand of 1042C>T mutation.

Acknowledgments

We thank all the normal-hearing subjects who collaborated in this study. The English in this document has been checked by at least two professional editors, both native speakers of English. For a certificate, please see: http://www.textcheck.com/certificate/K8ZiA4.

Author Contributions

Conceived and designed the experiments: PD DH. Performed the experiments: JZ GW DK. Analyzed the data: JZ JC SH BH YY. Contributed reagents/materials/analysis tools: PD. Wrote the paper: JZ YY.

References

1. Mafee MF, Charletta D, Kumar A, Belmont H (1992) Large vestibular aqueduct and congenital sensorineural hearing loss. AJNR Am J Neuroradiol. 13: 805–819.
2. Dossena S, Rodighiero S, Vezzoli V, Nofziger C, Salvioni E, et al. (2009)Functional characterization of wild-type and mutated pendrin (SLC26A4), the anion transporter involved in Pendred syndrome. J Mol Endocrinol. 43: 93–103.
3. Mount DB, Romero MF (2004) The SLC26 gene family of multifunctional anion exchangers. Pflugers Arch. 447: 710–721.
4. Alper SL, Sharma AK (2013)The SLC26 gene family of anion transporters and channels. Mol Aspects Med. 34: 494–515.
5. Yoshino T, Sato E, Nakashima T, Nagashima W, Teranishi MA, et al (2004)The immunohistochemical analysis of pendrin in the mouse inner ear. Hear Res. 195: 9–16.
6. Shcheynikov N, Yang D, Wang Y, Zeng W, Karniski LP, et al. (2008)The Slc26a4 transporter functions as an electroneutral Cl-/I-/HCO3- exchanger: role of Slc26a4 and Slc26a6 in I- and HCO3- secretion and in regulation of CFTR in the parotid duct. J Physiol. 586: 3813–3824.
7. Maciaszczyk K, Lewinski A (2008) Phenotypes of SLC26A4 gene mutations: Pendred syndrome and hypoacusis with enlarged vestibular aqueduct. Neuro Endocrinol Lett. 29: 29–36.
8. Taylor JP, Metcalfe RA, Watson PF, Weetman AP, Trembath RC (2002) Mutations of the PDS gene, encoding pendrin, are associated with protein mislocalization and loss of iodide efflux: implications for thyroid dysfunction in Pendred syndrome. J Clin Endocrinol Metab. 87: 1778–1784.
9. Everett LA, Belyantseva IA, Noben-Trauth K, Cantos R, Chen A, et al. (2001) Targeted disruption of mouse Pds provides insight about the inner-ear defects encountered in Pendred syndrome. Hum Mol Genet. 10: 153–161.
10. Wangemann P, Nakaya K, Wu T, Maganti RJ, Itza EM, et al. (2007) Loss of cochlear HCO3- secretion causes deafness via endolymphatic acidification and inhibition of Ca2+ reabsorption in a Pendred syndrome mouse model. Am J Physiol Renal Physiol. 292: F1345–1353.
11. Wang QJ, Zhao YL, Rao SQ, Guo YF, Yuan H, et al. (2007) A distinct spectrum of SLC26A4 mutations in patients with enlarged vestibular aqueduct in China. Clin Genet. 72: 245–254.
12. Albert S, Blons H, Jonard L, Feldmann D, Chauvin P, et al. (2006) SLC26A4 gene is frequently involved in nonsyndromic hearing impairment with enlarged vestibular aqueduct in Caucasian populations. Eur J Hum Genet. 14: 773–779.
13. Park HJ, Lee SJ, Jin HS, Lee JO, Go SH, et al. (2005) Genetic basis of hearing loss associated with enlarged vestibular aqueducts in Koreans. Clin Genet. 67: 160–165.
14. Yang T, Gurrola JG, Wu H, Chiu SM, Wangemann P, et al. (2009) Mutations of KCNJ10 together with mutations of SLC26A4 cause digenic nonsyndromic hearing loss associated with enlarged vestibular aqueduct syndrome. Am J Hum Genet. 8: 651–57.
15. Reichold M, Zdebik AA, Lieberer E, Rapedius M, Schmidt K, et al. (2010) KCNJ10 gene mutations causing EAST syndrome (epilepsy, ataxia, sensorineural deafness, and tubulopathy) disrupt channel function. Proc Natl Acad Sci USA. 107: 14490–95.
16. Sala-Rabanal M, Kucheryavykh LY, Skatchkov SN, Eaton MJ, Nichols CG (2010) Molecular mechanisms of EAST/SeSAME syndrome mutations in Kir4.1 (KCNJ10). J Biol Chem. 28: 36040–8.
17. Jin Z, Ulfendahl M, Jarlebark L (2008) Spatiotemporal loss of K+ transport proteins in the developing cochlear lateral wall of guinea pigs with hereditary deafness. Eur J Neurosci, 27: 145–154.
18. Marcus DC, Wu T, Wangemann P, Kofuji P (2002)KCNJ10 (Kir4.1) potassium channel knockout abolishes endocochlear potential. Am J Physiol Cell Physiol. 282: C403–407.
19. Singh R, Wangemann P (2008) Free radical stress-mediated loss of Kcnj10 protein expression in stria vascularis contributes to deafness in Pendred syndrome mouse model. Am J Physiol Renal Physiol. 294: F139–148.
20. Grimberg J, Nawoschik S, Belluscio L, McKee R, Turck A, et al. (1989) A simple and efficient non-organic procedure for the isolation of genomic DNA from blood. Nucleic Acids Res. 17: 8390.
21. Yuan Y, Guo W, Tang J, Zhang G, Wang G, et al. (2012) Dai P. Molecular Epidemiology and Functional Assessment of Novel Allelic Variants of SLC26A4 in Non-Syndromic Hearing Loss Patients with Enlarged Vestibular Aqueduct in China. PLoS One 7(11): e49984.
22. Lu YC, Wu CC, Yang TH, Lin YH, Yu IS, et al. (2013) Differences in the pathogenicity of the p.H723R mutation of the common deafness-associated SLC26A4 gene in humans and mice. PLoS One. Jun 3; 8(6): e64906.
23. Lu YC, Wu CC, Shen WS, Yang TH, Yeh TH, et al. (2011) Establishment of a knock-in mouse model with the SLC26A4 c.919-2A>G mutation and characterization of its pathology. PLoS One. 6(7): e22150.
24. Choi BY, Stewart AK, Madeo AC, Pryor SP, Lenhard S, et al. (2009) Hypo-functional SLC26A4 variants associated with nonsyndromic hearing loss and enlargement of the vestibular aqueduct: genotype-phenotype correlation or coincidental polymorphisms? Hum Mutat. 30: 599–608.
25. Blons H, Feldmann D, Duval V, Messaz O, Denoyelle F, et al. (2004) Screening of SLC26A4 (PDS) gene in Pendred's syndrome: a large spectrum of mutations in France and phenotypic heterogeneity. Clin Genet. 66: 333–340.
26. Tsukamoto K, Suzuki H, Harada D, Namba A, Abe S, et al. (2003) Distribution and frequencies of PDS (SLC26A4) mutations in Pendred syndrome and nonsyndromic hearing loss associated with enlarged vestibular aqueduct: a unique spectrum of mutations in Japanese. Eur J Hum Genet. 11: 916–922.
27. Dai P, Stewart AK, Chebib F, Hsu A, Rozenfeld J, et al. (2009) Distinct and novel SLC26A4/Pendrin mutations in Chinese and U.S. patients with nonsyndromic hearing loss. Physiol Genomics. 38: 281–290.
28. Yang T, Vidarsson H, Rodrigo-Blomqvist S, Rosengren SS, Enerback S, et al. (2007) Transcriptional control of SLC26A4 is involved in Pendred syndrome and nonsyndromic enlargement of vestibular aqueduct (DFNB4). Am J Hum Genet. 80: 1055–1063.
29. Jonard L, Niasme-Grare M, Bonnet C, Feldmann D, Rouillon I, et al. (2010) Screening of SLC26A4, FOXI1 and KCNJ10 genes in unilateral hearing impairment with ipsilateral enlarged vestibular aqueduct. Int J Pediatr Otorhinolaryngol. Sep; 74(9): 1049–53.
30. Mercer S, Mutton P, Dahl HH (2011) Identification of SLC26A4 mutations in patients with hearing loss and enlarged vestibular aqueduct using high-resolution melting curve analysis. Genet Test Mol Biomarkers. May; 15(5): 365–8.
31. Chen K, Wang X, Sun L, Jiang H (2012) Screening of SLC26A4, FOXI1, KCNJ10, and GJB2 in bilateral deafness patients with inner ear malformation. Otolaryngol Head Neck Surg. Jun; 146(6): 972–978.
32. Landa P, Differ AM, Rajput K, Jenkins L, Bitner-Glindzicz M (2013) Lack of significant association between mutations of KCNJ10 or FOXI1 and SLC26A4 mutations in Pendred syndrome/enlarged vestibular aqueducts. BMC Med Genet. Aug 21; 14: 85.

Audiovisual Speech Perception at Various Presentation Levels in Mandarin-Speaking Adults with Cochlear Implants

Shu-Yu Liu[1,2,3¶], Grace Yu[4], Li-Ang Lee[5], Tien-Chen Liu[6], Yung-Ting Tsou[5], Te-Jen Lai[1,7*], Che-Ming Wu[5*¶]

1 Institute of Medicine, Chung Shan Medical University, Taichung, Taiwan, **2** School of Speech Language Pathology and Audiology, Chung Shan Medical University, Taichung, Taiwan, **3** Department of Otolaryngology, Chung Shan Medical University Hospital, Taichung, Taiwan, **4** Department of Otolaryngology - Head and Neck Surgery, National University Health System of Singapore, Singapore, Singapore, **5** Department of Otolaryngology, Chang-Gung Memorial Hospital, College of Medicine, Chang-Gung University, Linkou, Taiwan, **6** Department of Otolaryngology, National Taiwan University Hospital, Taipei, Taiwan, **7** Department of Psychiatry, Chung Shan Medical University Hospital, Taichung, Taiwan

Abstract

Objectives: (1) To evaluate the recognition of words, phonemes and lexical tones in audiovisual (AV) and auditory-only (AO) modes in Mandarin-speaking adults with cochlear implants (CIs); (2) to understand the effect of presentation levels on AV speech perception; (3) to learn the effect of hearing experience on AV speech perception.

Methods: Thirteen deaf adults (age = 29.1 ± 13.5 years; 8 male, 5 female) who had used CIs for >6 months and 10 normal-hearing (NH) adults participated in this study. Seven of them were prelingually deaf, and 6 postlingually deaf. The Mandarin Monosyllablic Word Recognition Test was used to assess recognition of words, phonemes and lexical tones in AV and AO conditions at 3 presentation levels: speech detection threshold (SDT), speech recognition threshold (SRT) and 10 dB SL (re:SRT).

Results: The prelingual group had better phoneme recognition in the AV mode than in the AO mode at SDT and SRT (both $p = 0.016$), and so did the NH group at SDT ($p = 0.004$). Mode difference was not noted in the postlingual group. None of the groups had significantly different tone recognition in the 2 modes. The prelingual and postlingual groups had significantly better phoneme and tone recognition than the NH one at SDT in the AO mode ($p = 0.016$ and $p = 0.002$ for phonemes; $p = 0.001$ and $p < 0.001$ for tones) but were outperformed by the NH group at 10 dB SL (re:SRT) in both modes (both $p < 0.001$ for phonemes; $p < 0.001$ and $p = 0.002$ for tones). The recognition scores had a significant correlation with group with age and sex controlled ($p < 0.001$).

Conclusions: Visual input may help prelingually deaf implantees to recognize phonemes but may not augment Mandarin tone recognition. The effect of presentation level seems minimal on CI users' AV perception. This indicates special considerations in developing audiological assessment protocols and rehabilitation strategies for implantees who speak tonal languages.

Editor: Christian Friedrich Altmann, Human Brain Research Center, Japan

Funding: This study was supported by research grants from the National Science Council of the Executive Yuan of Taiwan (NSC 100-2815-C-040-039-B). The funder had no role in study design, data collection and analysis, decision to publish, or preparation of the manuscript.

Competing Interests: The authors have declared that no competing interests exist.

* Email: tejenlai@hotmail.com (TJL); bobwu506@hotmail.com (CMW)

¶ SYL and CMW are co-first authors on this work.

Introduction

Verbal information transmitted to listeners via dual-modal (i.e., audiovisual, AV) stimulation is often thought to be more efficient than uni-modal (auditory-only, AO) stimulation [1–2]. Listeners, whether hearing-impaired or not, automatically watch talkers' facial, lip and jaw movements, especially when auditory information was degraded, distorted or noise-masked [3–5]. In fact, optical cues also provide useful information when auditory stimuli are clear [6]. For example, English listeners distinguish "threat" from "fret" better by observing the location of teeth and tongue of the talkers.

Cochlear implantation has been proven as an effective treatment to restore the hearing of patients with severe-to-profound sensorineural hearing loss [7]. It was reported that deaf patients with cochlear implants (CIs) made use of visual information to supplement the auditory stimulation they received from the CIs and in this way optimized their speech perception in daily communication (e.g., [8–10]). Their speech recognition was significantly better in the AV condition than in the AO condition

[10]. Higher AV gain was observed in the CI users than in the NH controls who were tested in the simulated or noise-masked conditions as a result of CI users' greater capability to integrate visual information with degraded auditory signals [11].

This AV integration ability in CI users was reported to correlate with the duration of the implant experience rather than the duration of deafness [12]. The neuroplasticity involving speech-related network in our brain seems to allow a more efficient AV integration of speech after cochlear implantation [13]. Yet, although visual speech perceptual skills that developed during periods of deafness could have positive implications for later perception of auditory speech signals [14], visual take-over found in the auditory cortex in some CI users may also lead to incomplete reversal of this deafness-induced cortical reorganization [15]. Due to the inconsistent results from the past studies, the effect of auditory experience on AV perception in CI patients is still in question.

However, although extensive research has been undertaken in non-tonal language users with CIs regarding AV speech processing, little information is available for the patients who speak tonal languages such as Mandarin Chinese. In Mandarin Chinese, each monosyllabic word comprises two lexical components: phoneme(s) and lexical tone. Words could be semantically different solely because of the lexical tone variations. Smith and Burnham [16] and Chen and Massaro [17] were the only ones we found who investigated the tone perception ability of Mandarin-speaking adults in the AV condition. They used normal-hearing participants and focused only on lexical tone discrimination. The authors found that visual information seemed less informative for Mandarin Chinese listeners than for non-tonal language users when discriminating Mandarin tones, meaning that native listeners of Mandarin Chinese depended more on auditory signals than visual ones to distinguish lexical tones.

The presentation levels of speech signals could also affect speech recognition performance in listeners with normal hearing [18] and with CIs [19–20]. In general, speech stimuli were more difficult to recognize at soft levels, and listeners often reported to take advantage of visual cues when auditory input was unreliable [3–5]. Thus, the degree of dependency on visual cues to distinguish speech stimuli increased with decreasing sensation levels in the normal-hearing listeners [21]. However, the loudness perception of speech stimuli in CI patients can be quite different from normal-hearing ones as they receive sounds through electrical hearing, making their dynamic range much narrower than normal-hearing listeners [20]. Firszt et al.'s study [19] indicated that the CI patients' recognition performances on monosyllabic words and sentences were strongly dependent on presentation levels as their scores decreased consistently when the stimulus level was reduced from 60 to 50 dB SPL. However, it is still unknown whether and how much the CI adults depend on visual information to better recognize the speech stimuli at various presentation levels. In this study, we intend to explore the effect of speech presentation level on visual benefits.

Therefore, the present study aimed (1) to evaluate the recognition performance at word-level, phoneme-level and tone-level in AV mode and in AO mode in Mandarin-speaking Chinese adults with CIs, (2) to understand the effect of presentation levels on their AV speech perception, and (3) to learn the possible effect of hearing experience on AV speech perception in CI listeners.

Materials and Methods

Participants

Thirteen (8 male and 5 female) deaf adults with CIs participated in this study (hereafter as the "CI group", Table 1). They had bilateral severe-to profound sensorineural hearing loss and received unilateral implantation. All of them were recruited from the CI center of Chang-Gung Memorial Hospital, Linkou, Taiwan. No neurological and psychological disorders were found in these subjects, and their verbal intelligence quotient was all higher than 70 (Wechsler Adult Intelligence Scale, 3rd edition) [22–23]. They aged between 18.1 years and 56.5 years (mean = 29.1±13.5; median =30.2; interquartile range, IQR =23.7) at the time this study took place and had been using the implants for more than 0.5 year (median =4.7; IQR =6.3). Seven of them were prelingually deafened (before the age of 5 years, the "prelingual group") and 6 were postlingually deafened (after the age of 5 years, the "postlingual group;" see Table 1). Ten (4 male and 6 female) healthy NH adults were recruited as controls (the "NH group"), aged between 19 years and 26 years (mean =21.6±2.9; median = 20.5; IQR =4.8). They did not have any middle ear anomalies or history of otological/neurological diseases. Their hearing thresholds at 500, 1000, 2000 and 4000 Hz were all below 25 dB HL. All of the CI subjects and NH controls were native Mandarin Chinese speakers and had normal or corrected-to-normal vision. The study protocol and written informed consent form was approved by the Institutional Review Board of the Chang Gung Memorial Hospital. All written informed consent forms signed by the participants involved in the present study were obtained before the test procedures took place.

Test materials

The Mandarin Monosyllablic Word Recognition Test (MMRT), developed by Tsai et al. [24], was used to assess the word recognition ability. A compact disc, offered by the authors of the test, was used as the test material in this study. The test contains standardized-recorded word stimuli, including 6 lists of phonemically balanced monosyllabic words, each with 25 items (i.e., 150 auditory stimuli in total). It has been reported with satisfactory reliability [25].

To measure AV perception of the participating listeners, a video film was recorded specifically by the authors of this study. A male talker produced the test items of MMRT and recorded using a video recording system. The speaking rate of each word was consistent with the auditory output of MMRT. The production of each word began and ended in a closed-mouth, that is, the neutral position. Then, the video film was edited with matched onsets and offsets of auditory stimuli and displayed simultaneously with the auditory signals.

Test procedures

The test protocol consisted of two sessions: an AO session (i.e., only auditory stimuli were presented to the participants) and an AV session (i.e., the auditory stimuli were presented together with corresponding visual stimuli shown on the displaying screen of a computer). Both sessions took place in a sound-treated booth where a 19-inch LCD monitor was positioned at the participant's eye level at a distance of 1 meter and one loudspeaker at ear level in front (0°) of the participants. The CI group took the test in the CI Center of Chang-Gung Memorial Hospital and the NH group in Chung Shan Medical University. The CI patients did the test with their implanted ear, while the non-implanted ear was not wearing a hearing aid. The NH control group was tested in one ear only. The ear for testing was randomly selected, and the other

Table 1. Demographical background of the prelingually deaf group, the postlingually deaf group and the normal-hearing (NH) group.

		Prelingual		Postlingual		NH	
		N	Median (IQR)	N	Median (IQR)	N	Median (IQR)
Gender (M/F)		3/4		5/1		4/6	
ImpSide (L/R)		4/3		5/1			
Age (y)			17.2 (0.8)		41.2 (6.4)		20.5 (4.8)
OnsetDeaf (y)			4.0 (4.1)		37.9 (9.1)		
DuraDeaf (y)			16.1 (4.4)		0.5 (0.5)		
AgeImp (y)			9.0 (5.1)		38.7 (8.4)		
DuraImp (y)			8.2 (1.7)		1.7 (1.4)		
SDT (dB HL)			25.0 (7.5)		20.0 (3.8)		−5.0 (10.0)
SRT (dB HL)			35.0 (7.5)		35.0 (11.3)		10.0 (0.0)
ImpPTA (dB HL)			30.0 (8.5)		33.5 (3.8)		
NonImpPTA (dB HL)			106.0 (7.5)		107.5 (3.3)		8.0 (6.5)
CI device	Nucleus CI24RE(CA)	5		3			
	Nucleus CI24R(CS)	2		2			
	Nucleus 24M	0		1			
VisionCon	Normal	3		1		2	
	Nearsighted	1		5		8	
	Presbyopic	2		0		0	
	Cataractous	1		0		0	

IQR: Interquartile range; ImpSide: Side of ear with a implant; OnsetDeaf: Onset of deafness; DuraDeaf: Duration of deafness; AgeImp: Age at implantation; DuraImp: Duration of implant use; SDT: Speech detection threshold; SRT: Speech recognition threshold; ImpPTA: Pure tone average of the implanted ear; NonImpPTA: Pure tone average of the non-implanted or normal-hearing ear; VisionCon: Vision condition.

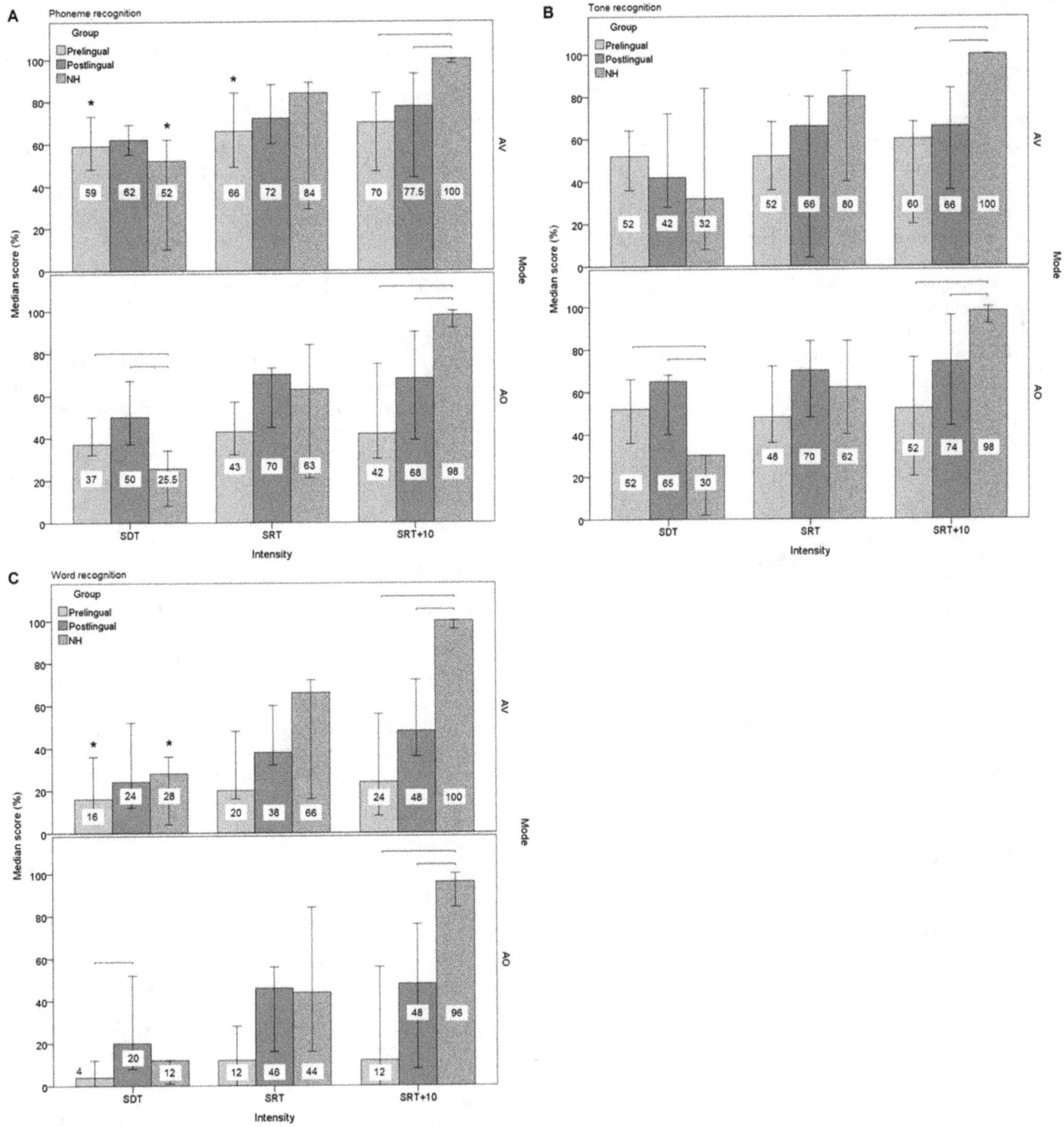

Figure 1. Median recognition scores obtained by the cochlear implanted groups and the normal-hearing group. Median recognition scores of (A) phonemes, (B) lexical tones and (C) words obtained by the prelingual group, the postlingual group and the normal-hearing (NH) group in audiovisual (AV) and auditory-only (AO) modes at the 3 presentation levels. The asterisk marks indicate significant difference between AV and AO modes. The horizontal bars indicate significant difference between groups. The vertical error bars represent 95% confidence interval.

ear was covered by a TDH-39 headphone set which introduced a masking noise to prevent possible cross-hearing.

The test started with measurements of warble-tone thresholds (at 500, 1000, 2000 and 4000 Hz), speech detection thresholds (SDT) and speech recognition thresholds (SRT) in sound field. Monosyllabic word recognition performances in AV and AO conditions were tested at their SDT, SRT and 10 dB SL above SRT (SRT+10), resulting in a total of 3 presentation levels in each test session. For example, if a participant's SDT was 30 dB HL and SRT 40 dB HL, his/her word recognition performance would be tested at 30, 40, 50 dB HL. We ensured that the subjects felt comfortable with each presentation level. The subjects wrote down each word they heard/saw after each test item was presented to them. The test procedures of the AV session were the same as those in the AO session except that the video stimuli were not presented in the latter condition. To avoid learning effects, the AO session took place one week after the AV session, and the word lists used to test each subject at each of the presentation levels were randomly selected without duplication in each session. Each word was scored based on the accuracy of the phonemes and the lexical tone. For example, if the test item was "ma3 (*horse*)," and the patient responded "ma4 (*scold*)", he/she would get 0 point for word recognition, 2 point for phoneme recognition, and 0 point for lexical tone recognition.

Statistical analysis

The descriptive statistics of these variables were presented as median and interquartile ranges because most of the distributions of the variables were not normal. The Kruskal-Wallis H test was implemented to compare the test results of the three groups, and the Mann-Whitney U test was conducted to compare two groups. The Wilcoxon signed-rank test and the Friedman test were used to make within-group comparisons of two or more than two conditions. Relationships between the recognition scores and scoring type (word, tone, phoneme), mode, intensity level and deafness- or implant-related variables – including onset of deafness, duration of deafness, age at implantation and duration of implant use – were assessed using Spearman correlation coefficient with adjustment (age and sex). Statistical analyses were conducted using SPSS software (version 17.0; SPSS; SPSS, Inc., Chicago, IL, USA). A value of $p<0.05$ was considered significant. The Bonferroni correction was used to adjust the p values of multiple comparisons; i.e., the differences between the three groups or intensity levels were significant when $p<\alpha/3=0.017$.

Results

Comparisons between AV and AO conditions at different presentation levels

The prelingual group, postlingual group and NH group all had a better phoneme recognition performance in the AV mode than in the AO mode (see Figure 1a). However, the significance was reached only in the prelingual group and NH group (both $p<0.001$). Using Wilcoxon signed-rank tests with correction for multiple comparisons, the difference between the two modes was significant at SDT and SRT in the prelingual group (both $p=0.016$), and at SDT in the NH group ($p=0.004$). Significance was not reached at SRT+10 in either group. For tone recognition, none of the three groups had significantly different performances in the two modes (see Figure 1b). Significantly better word recognition performance was noted in the AV mode than in the AO mode in the prelingual group ($p<0.001$) and the NH group ($p=0.005$; see Figure 1c). The significance was reached only at SDT in both groups ($p=0.016$ for the prelingual group; $p=0.010$ for the NH group).

Comparisons between groups with different hearing experiences

Using Kruskal-Wallis tests, we found significant differences in phoneme, tone and word recognition between the three groups at SDT and SRT+10 in the AO condition (at SDT, $p=0.001$, $p<0.001$, $p=0.029$ respectively for phoneme, tone, word recognition; at SRT+10, all $p<0.001$). In the AV mode, significance was only reached at SRT+10 (all $p<0.001$ for phoneme, tone and word recognition). No significant difference was noted at SRT.

Post hoc tests showed that, in the AO mode, the prelingual group and the postlingual group had significantly better phoneme recognition scores than the NH controls at SDT ($p=0.016$ and $p=0.002$ respectively), while the NH group outperformed the two CI groups at SRT +10 (both $p<0.001$; see Figure 1a). Similarly for tone recognition, the two CI groups obtained significantly higher scores than the NH group at SDT in the AO mode ($p=0.001$ and $p<0.001$ respectively), and were outperformed by the NH controls at SRT+10 ($p<0.001$ and $p=0.002$ respectively; see Figure 1b). For word recognition, the prelingual group performed worse than the postlingual group at SDT in the AO mode ($p=0.013$), and the two CI groups both obtained lower scores than the NH group at SRT+10 (both $p<0.001$; see Figure 1c). When the test was given in the AV mode, no significant difference was found between the three groups at SDT and SRT. However, at SRT+10, the NH group obtained significantly higher phoneme, tone and word recognition scores than the two CI groups did (all $p<0.001$; see Figure 1a-c).

Correlation analysis

The recognition scores had a significant correlation with group when age and sex were controlled (rho $=0.276$, $p<0.001$). The prelingual group's recognition scores were significantly correlated with scoring type (word, tone or phoneme), mode (AV or AO) and duration of deafness (see Table 2). The postlingual group's recognition scores had significant correlation with scoring type. The recognition scores of the NH group were significantly correlated only with mode and intensity level.

Discussion

Researchers have undertaken many studies on audiovisual speech perception in CI users who speak non-tonal languages; however, the performance of the Mandarin-speaking patient group is seldom discussed. Our results indicate that the visual cues from talker's lip and face are informative for phoneme recognition in our prelingually deaf patients with CIs. Yet, vision do not augment Mandarin tone recognition in our CI and NH adults. The presentation level does not affect recognition performance in the CI listeners as much as it does in the NH ones whether in AO or AV mode. The CI users who were deaf at early childhood show poorer speech recognition performance in AV and AO modes and depend more on vision to distinguish phonemes than those patients who were postlingually deafened.

The present study indicates that auditory signals seem to play a major role in identifying lexical tones in Mandarin monosyllabic words for both NH and CI listeners. In other words, visual cues are not found to benefit tone perception at the three intensity levels tested in this study. This finding is similar to Smith and Burnham's study [16] which uses normal-hearing adults and reports that the Mandarin Chinese listeners have worse Mandarin tone recognition scores than the non-tonal Australian English listeners in a visual-only condition. As we know, the pitch variations produced from vocal folds are accessible primarily from audition rather than from vision. However, the signal processing strategies of current CI devices do not transform fundamental frequency of speech stimuli which is important for accurate perception of lexical tones.

On the contrary, visual cues do help phoneme recognition in the prelingual group and the NH group, yet only at threshold levels (i.e., SDT and SRT). It suggests that visual information is required for the NH subjects and the prelingually deaf ones with CIs to recognize phonemes when the auditory information is insufficient. However, the postlingual group performs in a different manner that their phoneme recognition score does not significantly decrease in the absence of visual cues even when the speech intensity is lower than their SRT level. This trend is also found in word recognition that visual cues help the prelingual group and the NH group to better recognize words at SDT, while no

Table 2. Spearman correlation coefficients between deafness-related parameters, test conditions and recognition scores.

	Prelingual		Postlingual		NH	
Correlated item	**Coefficient***	***p* value**	**Coefficient***	***p* value**	**Coefficient***	***p* value**
Scoring type[1]	0.657	<0.001	0.542	<0.001	n/s	
Mode[2]	0.237	0.008	n/s		0.152	0.044
Intensity	n/a		n/s		0.840	<0.001
OnsetDeaf	n/a		n/s		n/a	
DuraDeaf	−0.439	<0.001	n/s		n/a	
AgeImp	n/s		n/s		n/a	
DuraImp	n/s		n/s		n/a	

OnsetDeaf: Onset of deafness; DuraDeaf: Duration of deafness; AgeImp: Age at implantation; DuraImp: Duration of implant use; n/s: Not significant; n/a: Not applicable.
*Spearman's correlation coefficients adjusted by sex and age.
[1]Scoring type coded as word = 1, tone = 2, phoneme = 3.
[2]Mode coded as auditory-only = 1, audiovisual = 2.
Only significant correlations are shown.

significant visual benefit is noted in the postlingual group at any of the intensity levels. The finding that the postlingual group is less dependent on visual information may have some association with their pre-implant language experiences and the automatic gain control provided by the CI. These two factors may allow the postlingual group to show lower dependency on visual information than the prelingual group (who does not have pre-implant hearing experiences) and the NH group (whose acoustic hearing does not adjust loudness input when the intensity level is too low). Because the speech signals experienced by CI patients is transformed by electrical stimulation and the electrical dynamic range of the recipient differs in threshold (T) and comfort (C) levels, microphone sensitivity and volume control, their loudness perception can be quite different from the acoustic hearing perceived by normal listeners. The two CI groups could thus have louder perception at threshold levels than the NH controls. Yet, it also needs to be noted that the median SDT of the NH group is minus 5 dB HL, which does not commonly occur in everyday activities. This may also account for NH controls' lower performance at SDT.

The automatic gain control offered by CI and the narrower dynamic range could make the implantees less sensitive to the changes in the input intensity level as the NH controls are. Unlike the NH subjects whose word recognition performance improves markedly with the increasing sensation levels (scores increased by 72 percentage points from SDT to SRT+10), the CI subjects do not necessarily perform better at higher levels (scores increased by only 8 percentage points in the prelingual group, and by 24 percentage points in the postlingual group; see Figure 1c).

Their lack of sensitivity to the intensity levels in the current study could also be a result that the presentation level at 10 dB SL (re: SRT) is not high enough for them to correctly recognize the word stimuli given the fact that the median presented level at SRT+10 is only 45 dB HL. Therefore, even though the postlingual group manages to score higher than the prelingual group – thanks to their pre-implant hearing experiences – the former still demonstrates worse speech recognition than the NH group. For further studies, degraded sound stimuli (e.g., by using a noise-band vocoder) could be used as the test material for NH controls in order to avoid the ceiling effect observed in our NH subjects and allow a better comparability between CI users and NH listeners. Also, special training on AV integration may be helpful to the CI patients with postlingual deafness as they do not seem to take advantage of the visual information and rely primarily on auditory input even when the acoustic speech signals are barely audible. Yet, further validation using larger sample or data from other institutions is required to test the generalizability of these results.

Furthermore, given that visual information does not help Mandarin tone recognition in our subjects, auditory training programs with a focus on tonal perceptual skills may be helpful for CI users who speak tonal language because lexical tones carry semantic importance and correct lexical tone recognition depends primarily on auditory input. This implies special considerations in developing audiological evaluation protocols and rehabilitation strategies for CI listeners who speak tonal languages.

Some previous studies claim that visual-only lipreading ability deteriorates with age [26–27]. Older people may thus gain limited benefit from visual information [28]. However, the result of Cienkowski and Carney [27] study shows that older adults and younger adults actually have similar AV integration ability at syllable level. The poorer visual-only lipreading ability of the older adults does not have a significant influence on successful integration of bisensory information. In the present study, the recognition scores are significantly correlated with group with age and sex controlled, which also implies that age difference is not the cause of the significant between-group difference found in our study. For further studies, visual-only condition is suggested to be taken into consideration to validate the current findings.

Lastly, it should be noted that this study uses monosyllabic words as test materials and that visual cues have different effects on the CI groups' recognition of words, tones and phonemes. It implies that detail analysis of the components of speech signals may help us differentiate the perceptual benefits the implanted devices may provide. Further investigations are required to show the effect of visual information on the CI users when they deal with different forms of speech signals, such as multisyllabic words or sentences.

Conclusions

Our preliminary results show that vision may help prelingually deaf CI patients to recognize phonemes at threshold presentation levels (i.e., SDT and SRT). However, visual cues may not augment Mandarin tone recognition, at least in our CI and NH subjects. It suggests that auditory training programs with a focus on tonal perceptual skills could be helpful for Mandarin-speaking CI adults to enhance their speech recognition performance as correct perception of tones depends mainly on audition. Moreover, the recognition performance of the CI subjects, whether prelingually or postlingually deafened, does not seem to be significantly affected by the presentation levels regardless of the accessibility of visual cues. These findings indicate special considerations in developing audiological assessment protocols and rehabilitation strategies for CI listeners who speak tonal languages. Further validation is required to test the generalizability of these results, including data from other institutions and other tonal languages.

Author Contributions

Conceived and designed the experiments: SYL GY TJL CMW. Performed the experiments: GY. Analyzed the data: SYL GY LAL YTT. Contributed reagents/materials/analysis tools: LAL TCL CMW. Contributed to the writing of the manuscript: SYL YTT. Critically reviewed and revised the manuscript: TCL TJL CMW.

References

1. Grant KW, Walden BE, Seitz PF (1998) Auditory-visual speech recognition by hearing-impaired subjects: consonant recognition, sentence recognition, and auditory-visual integration. J Acoust Soc Am 103: 2677–2690.
2. Arnold P, Hill F (2001) Bisensory augmentation: A speechreading advantage when speech is clearly audible and intact. Br J Psychol 92: 339–355.
3. Sumby W, Pollack I (1954) Visual contribution to speech intelligibility in noise. J Acoust Soc Am 26: 212–215.
4. Sanders DA, Goodrich SJ (1971) The relative contribution of visual and auditory components of speech to speech intelligibility as a function of three conditions of frequency distortion. J Speech Hear Res 14: 154–159.
5. Massaro DW, Cohen MM (1995) Perceiving talking faces. Current Directions in Psychological Science 4: 104–109.
6. Campbell R (2008) The processing of audio-visual speech: empirical and neural bases. Philos Trans R Soc Lond B Biol Sci 363: 1001–1010.
7. Waltzman SB (2006) Cochlear implants: current status. Expert Rev Med Devices 3: 647–655.
8. Moody-Antonio S, Takayanagi S, Masuda A, Auer ET Jr, Fisher L, et al. (2005) Improved speech perception in adult congenitally deafened cochlear implant recipients. Otol Neurotol 26: 649–654.
9. Kirk KI, Hay-McCutcheon MJ, Holt RF, Gao S, Qi R, et al. (2007) Audiovisual Spoken Word Recognition by Children with Cochlear Implants. Audiol Med 5: 250–261.
10. Tyler RS, Fryauf-Bertschy H, Kelsay DM, Gantz BJ, Woodworth GP, et al. (1997) Speech perception by prelingually deaf children using cochlear implants. Otolaryngol Head Neck Surg 117: 180–187.
11. Rouger J, Fraysse B, Deguine O, Barone P (2008) McGurk effects in cochlear-implanted deaf subjects. Brain Res 1188: 87–99.
12. Desai S, Stickney G, Zeng FG (2008) Auditory-visual speech perception in normal-hearing and cochlear-implant listeners. J Acoust Soc Am 123: 428–440.
13. Rouger J, Lagleyre S, Démonet JF, Fraysse B, Deguine O, et al. (2012) Evolution of crossmodal reorganization of the voice area in cochlear-implanted deaf patients. Hum Brain Mapp 33: 1929–1940.
14. Mitchell TV, Maslin MT (2007) How vision matters for individuals with hearing loss. Int J Audiol 46: 500–511.
15. Sandmann P, Dillier N, Eichele T, Meyer M, Kegel A, et al. (2012) Visual activation of auditory cortex reflects maladaptive plasticity in cochlear implant users. Brain 135: 555–568.
16. Smith D, Burnham D (2012) Faciliation of Mandarin tone perception by visual speech in clear and degraded audio: implications for cochlear implants. J Acoust Soc Am 131: 1480–1489.
17. Chen TH, Massaro DW (2008) Seeing pitch: visual information for lexical tones of Mandarin-Chinese. J Acoust Soc Am 123: 2356–2366.
18. Beattie RC, Raffin MJ (1985) Reliability of threshold, slope, and PB max for monosyllabic words. J Speech Hear Disord 50: 166–178.
19. Firszt JB, Holden LK, Skinner MW, Tobey EA, Peterson A, et al. (2004) Recognition of speech presented at soft to loud levels by adult cochlear implant recipients of three cochlear implant systems. Ear Hear 25: 375–387.
20. Donaldson GS, Allen SL (2003) Effects of presentation level on phoneme and sentence recognition in quiet by cochlear implant listeners. Ear Hear 24: 392–405.
21. Binnie CA (1973) Bi-sensory articulation functions for normal hearing and sensorineural hearing loss patients. Journal of Academic Rehabilitation in Audiology 6: 43–53.
22. Wechsler D (1997) Wechsler Adult Intelligence Scale-Third Edition. San Antonio, TX: The Psychological Corporation.
23. Chen Y, Chen H (2002) Wechsler Adult Intelligence Scale-Third Edition (Mandarin Version). Taipei: Chinese Behavioral Science Corporations.
24. Tsai KS, Tseng LH, Wu CJ, Young ST (2009) Development of a mandarin monosyllable recognition test. Ear Hear 30: 90–99.
25. Wu CJ (2009) Reliability of the Mandarin Monosyllable Recognition Test in Hearing-Impaired Listeners. MA Thesis, National Taipei University of Nursing and Health Sciences, Taipei, Taiwan.
26. Shoop C, Binnie C (1979) The effects of age on the visual perception of speech. Scandinavian Audiology 8: 3–8.
27. Cienkowski KM, Carney AE (2002) Auditory-visual speech perception and aging. Ear Hear 23: 439–449.
28. Sommers MS, Tye-Murray N, Spehar B (2005) Auditory-visual speech perception and auditory-visual enhancement in normal-hearing younger and older adults. Ear Hear 26: 263–275.

25

Mandarin Speech Perception in Combined Electric and Acoustic Stimulation

Yongxin Li[1], Guoping Zhang[1], John J. Galvin III[2], Qian-Jie Fu[2]*

1 Department of Otolaryngology, Head and Neck Surgery, Beijing TongRen Hospital, Capital Medical University, Beijing, 100730, P. R. China, **2** Department of Head and Neck Surgery, David Geffen School of Medicine, University of California Los Angeles, Los Angeles, California, United States of America

Abstract

For deaf individuals with residual low-frequency acoustic hearing, combined use of a cochlear implant (CI) and hearing aid (HA) typically provides better speech understanding than with either device alone. Because of coarse spectral resolution, CIs do not provide fundamental frequency (F0) information that contributes to understanding of tonal languages such as Mandarin Chinese. The HA can provide good representation of F0 and, depending on the range of aided acoustic hearing, first and second formant (F1 and F2) information. In this study, Mandarin tone, vowel, and consonant recognition in quiet and noise was measured in 12 adult Mandarin-speaking bimodal listeners with the CI-only and with the CI+HA. Tone recognition was significantly better with the CI+HA in noise, but not in quiet. Vowel recognition was significantly better with the CI+HA in quiet, but not in noise. There was no significant difference in consonant recognition between the CI-only and the CI+HA in quiet or in noise. There was a wide range in bimodal benefit, with improvements often greater than 20 percentage points in some tests and conditions. The bimodal benefit was compared to CI subjects' HA-aided pure-tone average (PTA) thresholds between 250 and 2000 Hz; subjects were divided into two groups: "better" PTA (<50 dB HL) or "poorer" PTA (>50 dB HL). The bimodal benefit differed significantly between groups only for consonant recognition. The bimodal benefit for tone recognition in quiet was significantly correlated with CI experience, suggesting that bimodal CI users learn to better combine low-frequency spectro-temporal information from acoustic hearing with temporal envelope information from electric hearing. Given the small number of subjects in this study (n = 12), further research with Chinese bimodal listeners may provide more information regarding the contribution of acoustic and electric hearing to tonal language perception.

Editor: Manuel S. Malmierca, University of Salamanca- Institute for Neuroscience of Castille and Leon and Medical School, Spain

Funding: QF and JG were supported by the National Institute of Health, grants R01-DC004792 and R01-DC004993. The funders had no role in study design, data collection and analysis, decision to publish, or preparation of the manuscript.

Competing Interests: The authors have declared that no competing interests exist.

* Email: qfu@mednet.ucla.edu

Introduction

For cochlear implant (CI) users with residual acoustic hearing in the contralateral ear, speech understanding may be greatly improved when the CI is combined with a hearing aid (HA). Many studies with English-speaking CI users have shown better sentence recognition in noise for combined use of CI+HA ("bimodal" listening) than with either device alone [1–11]. The HA provides fundamental frequency (F0) information that is not well-represented by the CI. Acoustic F0 information is especially beneficial for CI users when listening to speech in dynamic noise or competing talkers [5,12–13].

Significant bimodal benefits (defined here as the difference in performance between the CI+HA and the CI alone) have been observed for monosyllabic words and phonemes [6,9,14–16]. Depending on the upper limit of aided acoustic hearing, the HA may provide useful first and second formant (F1 and F2) information for vowels and voicing information for consonants. Yoon et al. [9] found a significant bimodal benefit for perception of F1 and F2 information in vowel recognition and voicing information in consonant recognition with the CI+HA versus the CI alone, but mostly for CI subjects with "good" aided acoustic hearing (pure-tone average, or PTA <55 dB HL). Sheffield and Zeng [15] also found significantly better perception of F1 and F2 information in vowel recognition and voicing information in consonant recognition with the CI+HA compared with the CI alone. These results suggest that the bimodal benefit may be due to phonemic features besides F0 transmitted by the HA.

The amount of residual hearing has been associated with bimodal benefit in many studies. In studies where the bandwidth of available acoustic information was systematically varied, the bimodal benefit increased as the bandwidth was increased [11,17–18]. Bimodal benefit has also been correlated with hearing function of the non-implanted ear. Yoon et al. [9] found that aided acoustic low-frequency pure-tone average (PTA) thresholds, calculated between 250 and 1000 Hz, were significantly correlated with the bimodal benefit for vowel recognition at low signal-to-noise ratios (SNRs). Sheffield and Zeng [15] found that vowel recognition was significantly correlated with the slope of unaided audiometric threshold functions. Zhang et al. [16] found a significant correlation between HA-aided audiometric thresholds and bimodal benefit for speech performance and quiet and in noise, as well as a significant correlation between bimodal benefit and the spectral resolution of the non-implanted ear. These studies suggest that the HA may provide useful acoustic information beyond F0, depending on audibility.

While bimodal benefits have been shown for English-speaking CI users, very few studies have examined bimodal benefits for tonal languages such as Mandarin Chinese. For tonal languages, the perception of lexical tones depends strongly on fundamental frequency (F0) cues [19]. However, the functional spectral resolution of the CI is not sufficient to support complex pitch perception needed for difficult listening tasks such as music perception, talker identification, and speech understanding in noise [20]. Efforts to improve CI users' pitch by modifying the signal processing have shown relatively little benefit [21–24]. Previous studies with Mandarin-speaking CI users have shown moderately good tone recognition performance, ranging between approximately 50–80% correct [25–32], most likely due to access to amplitude contour and duration cues that co-vary with F0 in naturally uttered Chinese tones [29,32]. When Mandarin-speaking CI users must rely exclusively on F0 information, tone recognition is generally poorer [30,34–35].

For patients with some residual acoustic hearing, combining a HA with the CI may represent the best opportunity to improve CI users' Chinese tone recognition. Luo and Fu [36] investigated the contribution of low frequency acoustic information to Chinese speech perception in Mandarin-speaking normal-hearing (NH) subjects listening to an acoustic simulation of bimodal listening (i.e., low frequency acoustic information presented to one ear and a CI simulation presented to the other ear). Results showed that acoustic information below 500 Hz contributed strongly to tone recognition, while acoustic information above 500 Hz contributed strongly to phoneme recognition; Chinese sentence recognition in noise improved as the bandwidth of acoustic information was increased. These results suggest that, for CI patients with residual acoustic hearing, preserving low-frequency acoustic information can improve Chinese speech recognition in noise.

While combined acoustic-electric hearing is not unusual in adult English-speaking CI patients, there are relatively few Mandarin-speaking adults who regularly use both the CI and HA. Because most of cochlear implantees in China have been children, adult CI users are less common, though those numbers will increase as the children grow older and implant criteria change. Currently, the recommended criteria for cochlear implantation for adults in China include severe-to-profound bilateral deafness, with unaided audiometric threshold PTAs (0.5–4 kHz) >80 dB HL [37]. These criteria for adults are more restrictive than in the United States, where moderate-to-severe bilateral sensorineural hearing loss is indicated. As such, it is somewhat unusual to find native adult Chinese CI users with substantial acoustic hearing in the non-implanted ear. Such patients would provide great insight into the contribution of aided acoustic hearing to Chinese CI users' speech perception. In this study, Chinese tone, vowel, and consonant recognition in quiet and in noise were evaluated in adult Mandarin-speaking subjects who regularly used a CI and HA. Subjects were tested while listening with the CI-only, or with the CI+HA. Due to the better F0 information provided by the HA, we hypothesized that lexical tone recognition would greatly benefit from the addition of the HA to the CI. We also hypothesized that vowel recognition would be better for subjects with greater acoustic hearing range, as the HA may provide useful formant information. Finally, we hypothesized that the bimodal benefit would be greater in noise than in quiet, consistent with previous studies [3–4,6–7,38].

Methods

Subjects

Twelve Mandarin-speaking bimodal CI patients (6 male and 6 female) participated in this study. Subjects were native speakers of Mandarin Chinese and were between the ages of 16 to 24 years old. All CI subjects had more than six months of experience with their device at the time of testing. Subjects were recruited from the Department of Otolaryngology, Head and Neck Surgery of Beijing TongRen Hospital (which specifically approved this study), with no particular consideration of age at implantation, duration of profound deafness, period for bimodal experience, etiology, CI or HA type, configuration, or processor strategy. Subject demographics are shown in Table 1.

Ethics statement

All subjects provided written informed consent prior to participating in the study, in compliance with the Institutional Review Board protocol of Beijing TongRen Hospital, Capital Medical University, China, which specifically approved this study. In terms of the minors/children enrolled in the study, the written informed consent was obtained from the next of kin, caretakers, or guardians on behalf of the minors/children enrolled in the study.

Stimuli

Stimuli for tone, consonant, and vowel recognition tests were drawn from the Chinese Standard Database [39]. For Chinese tone recognition, two male and two female speakers each produced four tones for the four Mandarin Chinese monosyllabic words "ba", "bi", "bu", "bo", resulting in a total of 64 tone tokens. For Chinese vowel recognition, two male and two female speakers each produced sixteen Mandarin Chinese monosyllabic words in a/d/-vowel context with tone 1 (/a/,/i/,/u/,/ai/,/ao/,/ou/,/iao/,/iu/,/uo/,/ui/,/ang/,/eng/,/ong/,/ing/,/uan/, and/un/), resulting in a total of 64 vowel tokens. Key acoustic features of vowel stimuli are shown in Table 2. For Chinese consonant recognition, two male and two female speakers each produced tone 1 for/a/in a consonant-/a/context, for the 20 Mandarin Chinese initial consonants (/b/,/p/,/m/,/f/,/d/,/t/,/l/,/g/,/k/,/h/,/j/,/q/,/x/,/zh/,/ch/,/sh/,/z/,/c/,/s/and/w/), resulting in a total of 80 consonant tokens.

Procedure

Closed-set identification tasks were used to measure Chinese tone recognition (4-alternative, forced choice, or 4AFC), vowel recognition (16AFC), and consonant recognition (20AFC). For each trial within a given test, a stimulus was randomly selected from the token list without repetition and presented to the subject, who responded by clicking on one of the response choices shown on screen. For tone recognition, the 4 response choices were labeled "Tone 1", "Tone 2", "Tone 3", and "Tone 4". For vowel recognition, each of the 16 response choices was labeled in a d/V/ context using Pinyin symbol and the corresponding Chinese character. For the consonant recognition, each of the 20 response choices was labeled in a C/a/using Pinyin symbol and the corresponding Chinese character. Responses were collected by the experimental software (Mandarin i-CAST software developed by Qian-Jie Fu and freely available at http://icast.emilyfufoundation.org) and scored in terms of percent correct. No trial-by-trial feedback or training was provided. Because of time constraints (data were collected following a routine clinical appointment) and the number of conditions and tests [2 listening (CI, CI+HA)×2 noise (quiet, noise)×3 tests (tone, vowel, consonant) = 12], only one

Table 1. Bimodal CI subject demographics.

Subject	Gender	Age	Ethology	CI exp (yrs)	Dur Deaf (yrs)
S1	F	22	LVAS	3.4	14.0
S2	F	21	Unknown	0.6	5.0
S3	F	20	Unknown	0.5	8.0
S4	M	24	LVAS	4.9	10.0
S5	M	23	Ototoxicity	3.8	12.0
S6	M	16	Unknown	2.5	5.0
S7	F	22	Unknown	6.0	16.0
S8	F	21	LVAS	0.5	21.0
S9	F	20	Unknown	2.8	17.0
S10	M	23	Unknown	4.4	19.0
S11	M	16	Unknown	2.0	14.0
S12	M	16	LVAS	1.0	13.0

CI exp = cochlear implant experience; Dur deaf = duration of deafness; F = female; M = male; LVAS = large vestibular aqueduct syndrome.

run was collected for each test and listening condition. The total amount of time required to complete all tests was 2–3 hours.

Chinese tone, vowel, and consonant recognition were measured in quiet and in noise under two listening conditions: CI alone and combined CI+HA. Because of time constraints and subject availability, the HA alone condition was not tested. For the CI alone condition, the HA was removed but the HA ear was not plugged. The two listening conditions were evaluated in random order for each subject. For testing in noise, speech-weighed steady noise (1000-Hz cutoff frequency, −12 dB/octave) was used. The SNR was fixed at +5 dB, and was calculated in terms of the long-term root-mean square (RMS) of the speech signal and noise. The onset and offset of the noise was 500 ms before the target speech token. Speech and noise were mixed at the target SNR of +5 dB, and the combined signal and noise was then scaled to the output (65 dBA). Testing was conducted in a sound-treated booth. Subjects were seated directly facing a single loudspeaker 1 m away. CI subjects were tested with their clinical CI and HA settings; these settings were not changed during testing.

Results

Figure 1 shows CI subjects' unaided (white symbols) and HA-aided (black symbols) audiometric thresholds at 0.25, 0.5, 1, 2, and 4 kHz. Audiometry was conducted in sound field using warble tones. Unaided pure-tone average (PTA) thresholds between 0.25 and 2 kHz ranged from 54 to 101 dB HL; with the exception of subject S11, unaided thresholds were above the range of conversational speech levels (gray shaded areas in each panel). HA-aided PTA thresholds ranged from 38 to 75 dB HL; in many cases, the HA amplification boosted thresholds within the range of conversational speech levels. With the CI-only, PTA thresholds ranged from 24 to 48 dB HL. With the CI+HA, PTA thresholds ranged from 23 to 41 dB HL. With the CI-only or with the CI+HA, thresholds were well within the range of conversational speech levels. Note that no "real-ear" measurements were conducted to confirm sound pressure levels in the HA ear.

Figure 2 shows boxplots of tone, vowel, and consonant recognition in quiet and in noise, with the CI only or with the CI+HA. All scores were corrected for chance level performance (25% for tones, 6.25% for vowels, and 5% for consonants).

Relative to the CI-only, mean tone recognition with the CI+HA improved from 66.8% to 74.1% correct in quiet (+7.3 points), and from 31.1% to 44.5% correct in noise (+13.4 points). A two-way repeated measures of variance (RM ANOVA), with listening condition (CI-only, CI+HA) and SNR (quiet, 5 dB) as factors, showed that tone recognition was significantly affected by listening condition [$F(1,11) = 16.3$, $p = 0.002$] and SNR [$F(1,11) = 40.0$, $p < 0.001$]; there were no significant interactions. Post-hoc Bonferroni pairwise comparisons showed that performance was significantly better in quiet than in noise for both the CI-only and CI+HA listening conditions ($p < 0.05$ in both cases). Post-hoc Bonferroni pairwise comparisons also showed that tone recognition was significantly better with the CI+HA in noise ($p < 0.05$), but not in quiet ($p > 0.05$).

Relative to the CI-only, mean vowel recognition with the CI+HA improved from 58.9% to 71.0% correct in quiet (+12.1 points), and from 37.9% to 47.8% correct in noise (+9.9 points). A two-way RM ANOVA, with listening condition and SNR as factors, showed that vowel recognition was significantly affected by listening condition [$F(1,11) = 10.9$, $p = 0.007$] and SNR [$F(1,11) = 42.5$, $p < 0.001$]; there were no significant interactions. Post-hoc Bonferroni pairwise comparisons showed that performance was significantly better in quiet than in noise for both the CI-only and CI+HA listening conditions ($p < 0.05$ in both cases). Different from tone recognition, post-hoc Bonferroni pairwise comparisons showed that vowel recognition was significantly better with the CI+HA in quiet ($p < 0.05$), but not in noise ($p > 0.05$).

Relative to the CI-only, mean consonant recognition with the CI+HA improved from 45.8% to 53.6% correct in quiet (+7.8 points), and from 21.9% to 25.84% correct in noise (+3.5 points). Note that subject S12 was unable to complete the consonant recognition tests. A two-way RM ANOVA, with listening condition and SNR as factors, showed that consonant recognition was significantly affected by listening condition [$F(1,10) = 6.15$, $p = 0.033$] and SNR [$F(1,10) = 88.6$, $p < 0.001$]; there were no significant interactions. Post-hoc Bonferroni pairwise comparisons showed that performance was significantly better in quiet than in noise for both the CI-only and CI+HA listening conditions ($p < 0.05$ in both cases). However, post-hoc Bonferroni pairwise comparisons showed no significant difference in consonant

Table 2. Production-based acoustic features for vowel stimuli.

Talker	F0 (Hz) Mean	F0 Min	F0 Max	F1 (Hz) Mean	F1 Min	F1 Max	F2 (Hz) Mean	F2 Min	F2 Max
f1	285	267	297	582	299	979	1707	867	2827
f2	278	268	291	600	295	1116	1636	767	2932
f AVE	282	268	294	591	297	1048	1672	817	2880
m1	165	135	187	566	309	857	1670	906	2427
m2	177	163	188	589	303	897	1777	949	2454
m AVE	171	149	188	578	306	877	1724	928	2441
AVE	228	212	241	587	301	967	1711	878	2663

f = female; m = male; F0 = fundamental frequency; F1 = first formant; F2 = second formant.

recognition between the CI-only and CI+HA listening conditions in quiet or in noise ($p > 0.05$ in both cases).

Paired to t-tests showed no significant difference in bimodal benefit (CI+HA–CI-only) between quiet and noise for tones ($p = 0.201$), vowels ($p = 0.332$), or consonants ($p = 0.107$). Figure 3 shows boxplots of the bimodal benefit for tones, vowels, and consonants in quiet and in noise; data are grouped according to CI subjects with "better" (<50 dB HL; n = 5) or "poorer" (>50 dB HL; n = 7) HA-aided PTA thresholds averaged across 0.25, 0.5, 1, and 2 kHz. The frequency range for PTAs was similar as used by Wang et al. [35] when measuring residual acoustic hearing. The bimodal benefit was calculated using the scores corrected for chance level.

For tone recognition, the mean bimodal benefit in quiet was 9.1 percentage points (range: −2.1–20.9) for the poorer group and 5.1 points (range: −8.3–14.5) for the better group. In noise, the mean bimodal benefit in quiet was 11.0 points (range: 2.1–27.1) for the poorer group and 16.7 points (range: 5.1–45.1) for the better group. A split-plot RM ANOVA, with SNR (quiet, 5 dB) as the within subject factor and HA-aided threshold (poorer, better) as the between subject factor, showed no significant effects for SNR [$F(1,10) = 1.14$, $p = 0.311$, observed power = 0.17] or HA-aided threshold [$F(1,10) = 0.03$, $p = 0.874$, observed power = 0.16].

For vowel recognition, the mean bimodal benefit in quiet was 7.6 points (range: 3.4–11.7) for the poorer group and 18.3 points (range: 5.0–43.3) for the better group. In noise, the mean bimodal benefit in quiet was 6.3 points (range: 3.3–15.0) for the poorer group and 15.0 points (range: −6.6–45.0) for the better group. A split-plot RM ANOVA, with SNR as the within-subject factor and HA-aided threshold as the between-subject factor, showed no significant effects for SNR [[$F(1,10) = 0.2$, $p = 0.665$, observed power = 0.07] or HA-aided threshold [$F(1,10) = 2.29$, $p = 0.161$, observed power = 0.28].

For consonant recognition, the mean bimodal benefit in quiet was 3.6 points (range: −1.3–10.5) for the poorer group and 13.7 points (range: 9.2–17.2) for the better group. In noise, the mean bimodal benefit in quiet was −0.4 points (range: −11.8–17.1) for the poorer group and 10.2 points (range: 2.6–14.5) for the better group. A split-plot RM ANOVA, with SNR as the within-subject factor and HA-aided threshold as the between-subject factor, showed no significant effect for SNR [$F(1,9) = 0.02$, $p = 0.994$, observed power = 0.05], but a significant effect for HA-aided threshold [$F(1,9) = 10.7$, $p = 0.010$, observed power = 0.82].

Key demographic variables were compared to CI-only performance, CI+HA performance, and bimodal benefit; scores were corrected for chance level performance. As all subjects were implanted at 16 yrs or later, only duration of deafness and CI listening experience were used as demographic variables. The significance level was adjusted to correct for family-wise error (Bonferroni-adjusted $p < 0.003$). A significant was found only between CI experience and bimodal benefit for tone recognition in quiet ($r = 0.79$; $p = 0.003$). There were no significant correlations between CI experience and CI-only or CI+HA performance for any of the speech tests in quiet or in noise, and there were no significant correlations between CI experience and bimodal benefit for vowel or consonant recognition in quiet or in noise, or for tone recognition in noise. There were no significant correlations between duration of deafness and CI-only performance, CI+HA performance, or bimodal benefit for any of the speech tests.

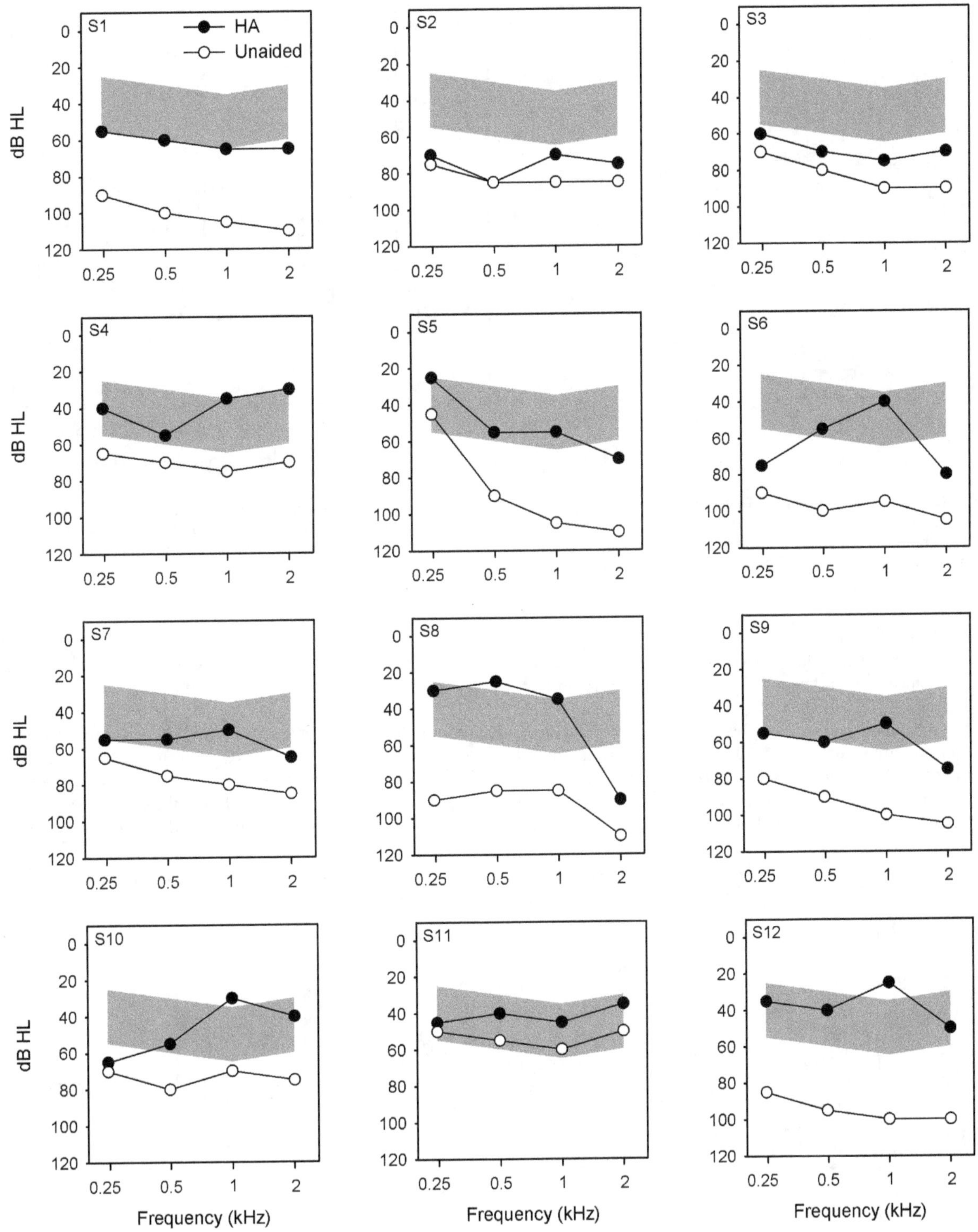

Figure 1. Aided and unaided thresholds for bimodal subjects. The x-axis shows audiometric frequency and the y-axis shows threshold in dB HL. The open circles show unaided threshold and the filled circles show HA-aided thresholds. The shaded area shows the range of hearing levels for conversational speech levels (i.e., the "speech banana"). HA = hearing aid.

Discussion

The present results showed a clear bimodal benefit for tone, consonant, and vowel recognition in quiet, and for tone and vowel recognition in noise. The bimodal benefit appeared to be greater for CI subjects with better HA-aided PTA thresholds, especially for consonant recognition. Greater CI experience was associated with greater bimodal benefit for tone recognition in quiet. Below, we discuss the results in greater detail.

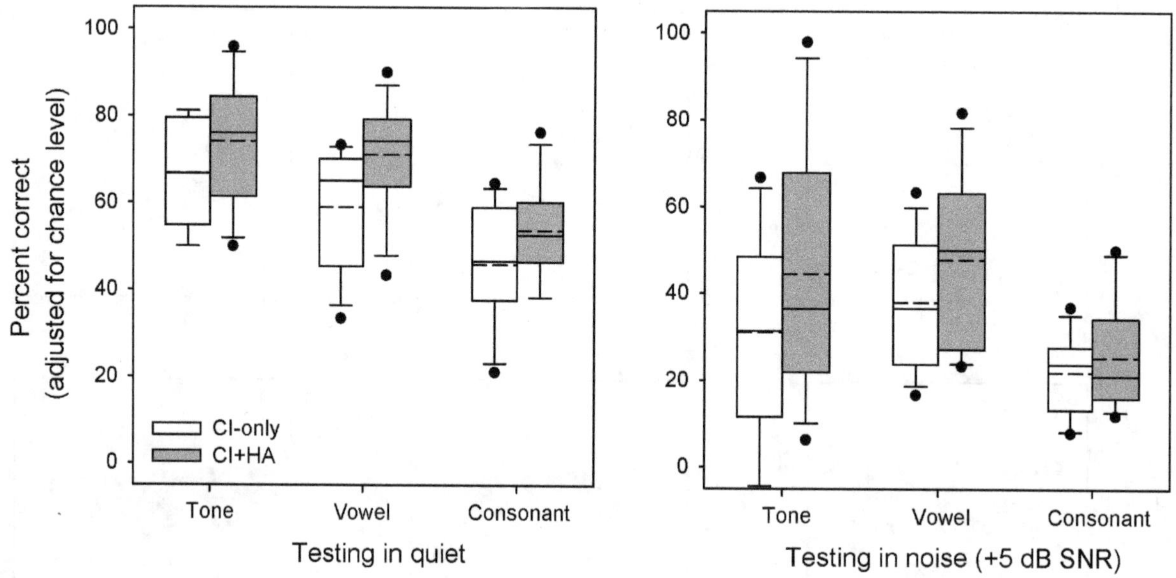

Figure 2. Boxplots for speech performance with CI-only or with CI+HA. The left panel shows performance measured in quiet and the right panel shows performance measured in noise. The white boxes show CI-only performance and the gray boxes show CI+HA performance. The boxes show the 25th and 75th percentiles, the short dashed lines show median value, the solid lines show mean value, the error bars show the 10th and 90th percentiles, and the circles show outliers. CI = cochlear implant; HA = hearing aid.

Bimodal benefit in quiet

Given the dependence on F0 cues for tone recognition, one might have expected that the greatest bimodal benefit would have been for tones, as the addition of the HA would have provided low-frequency pitch cues. For the present tone stimuli, amplitude contour and duration cues were available, as stimuli were natural productions of Chinese tones. These cues are known to co-vary with F0 [19,33,40–41]. It is possible that the availability of amplitude and duration cues may have weakened the dependence on F0 cues and therefore, the bimodal benefit relative to vowels and consonants. Note that for some subjects, the bimodal benefit for tones was substantial (18.7 and 20.9 points, after correcting for chance level, for subjects S5 and S7, respectively). With the CI alone, only 33.3% of subjects scored 75% percent correct or better (after correcting for chance level performance); with the CI+HA, 50% of subjects scored 75% percent correct or better. This suggests that the addition of the HA to the CI was key to good tone recognition performance for many of the present CI subjects.

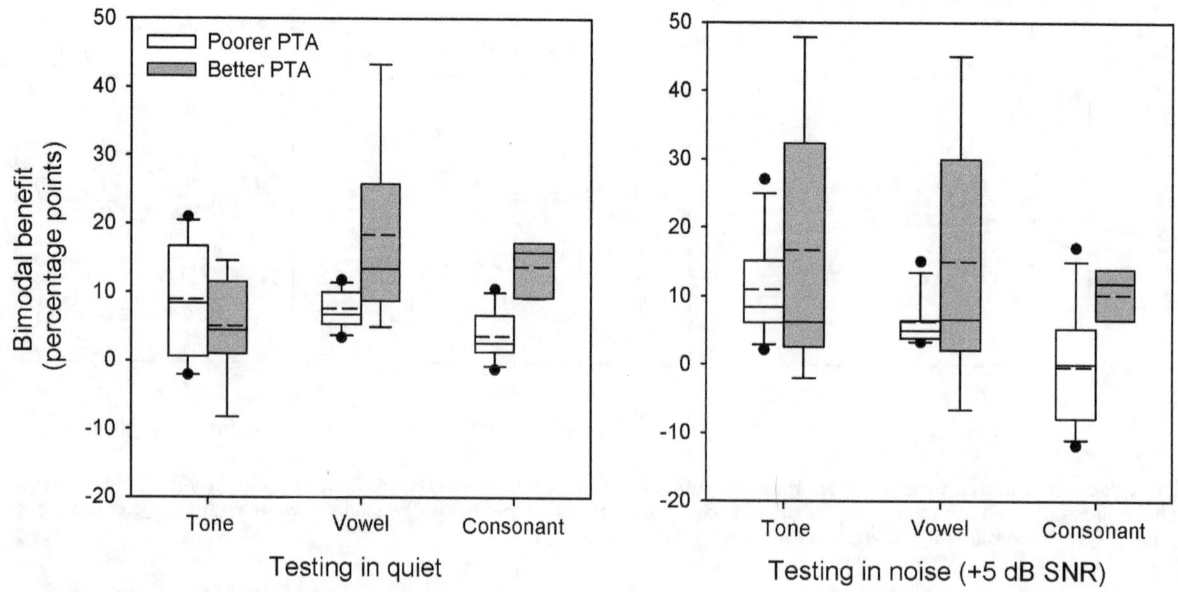

Figure 3. Boxplots for bimodal benefit. The left panel shows performance measured in quiet and the right panel shows performance measured in noise. The white boxes show performance for the CI group with poorer HA-aided PTA thresholds (>50 dB HL for audiometric frequencies between 0.25 and 2 kHz) for the CI group with better HA-aided PTA thresholds (<50 dB HL) The boxes show the 25th and 75th percentiles, the short dashed lines show median value, the solid lines show mean value, the error bars show the 10th and 90th percentiles, and the circles show outliers. CI = cochlear implant; HA = hearing aid; PTA = pure-tone average.

Similarly, one might expect that the bimodal benefit would have been weakest for consonants, as high-frequency information would have been largely represented by the CI. However, the mean bimodal benefit was similar for tones and consonants. Again, some subjects experienced substantial bimodal benefit (15.8, 17.2, and 17.2 points for subjects S4, S8, and S11, respectively, after correcting for chance level performance). The addition of the HA may have strengthened voice cues and may have provided better coding of aperiodic consonant information.

The greatest bimodal benefit in quiet was observed for vowels. Again, some subjects experienced substantial bimodal benefit (20.0 and 43.1 points for subjects S8 and S4, respectively, after correcting for chance level performance). While F0 information is not required for vowel recognition, the HA may have provided better representation of F1 (which ranged from 301 to 967 Hz for the present stimuli) and even F2 information (which ranged from 878 to 2663 Hz), depending on the audibility of aided acoustic hearing.

Bimodal benefit in noise

Mean speech performance was significantly poorer in noise than that in quiet for all speech measures and listening conditions. Interestingly, a significant bimodal benefit was observed for tone recognition in noise, but not in quiet. The bimodal benefit for tone recognition in noise was substantial for some subjects (27.1, 27.1, and 47.9 points, after correcting for chance level performance, for subjects S6, S8, and S4, respectively). The bimodal advantage for tone recognition in noise is consistent with previous studies that show a bimodal advantage for sentence recognition in noise [5,12–13]. However, some subjects experienced nearly no benefit or even a deficit with the CI+HA, relative to the CI alone (2.1 and −2.0 points, after correcting for chance level performance, for subjects S3 and S11, respectively). Different from testing in quiet, there was no significant bimodal benefit for vowel recognition in noise. Again, the bimodal benefit for vowel recognition in noise was substantial for some subjects (15.0, 25.0, and 45.0 points, after correcting for chance level performance, for subjects S7, S8, and S4, respectively).

The lack of bimodal benefit for consonants in noise may have been due to the relatively low SNR (+5 dB), which was calculated according to the long-term RMS of the noise and the speech token. For consonants, most of the energy in the speech token was for the vowel portion of the C/a stimuli which would have contributed strongly to the estimate of the long-term RMS. As such, the consonant portion may have been masked by the noise. Even so, some subjects received a substantial bimodal benefit (13.2, 14.5, and 17.1 points, after correcting for chance level performance, for subjects S4, S10, and S7, respectively). However, some subjects also received a substantial bimodal deficit (−7.8 and −11.8 points, after correcting for chance level performance, for subjects S1 and S7, respectively). It is unclear whether such large bimodal deficits are due to sub-optimal HA settings or to other factors.

Previous sentence recognition studies with English-speaking CI users have shown that the bimodal benefit was generally greater in noise than in quiet [3–4,6–7]. Previous phoneme recognition studies with English-speaking bimodal CI users have also shown that the bimodal benefit was generally small in quiet and greater in noise. Kong and Braida [14] found no significant difference in vowel or consonant recognition in quiet between the CI-only and CI+HA. Sheffield and Zeng [15] found no significant difference in overall vowel recognition in quiet between the CI-only and CI+HA; however, overall vowel recognition in noise and information transfer of F1 and F2 information was significantly better with the CI+HA than with the CI alone. In this study, a significant bimodal benefit for vowel recognition was observed in quiet, but not in noise. In Sheffield and Zeng [15], consonant recognition was significantly better with the CI+HA than with the CI alone in quiet, but not in noise. In this study, there was no significant bimodal benefit for consonant recognition in quiet or in noise. Differences in speech materials, testing methods, and subject groups may explain some of the inconsistencies between the present and previous studies.

Improved perception of F0 information with the HA may allow bimodal CI users to better segregate speech from noise, typically measured using sentence materials. In this study, the bimodal benefit was assessed for lexical tones, vowels and consonants. It is possible that the lack of contextual cues focused listeners' attention to other cues afforded by the HA besides F0, such as F1 and F2 information, depending on the amount of residual aided acoustic hearing. Averaged across all talkers and vowel stimuli, the mean range of F1 was 301–967 Hz and the mean range of F2 was 878–2663 Hz. F1 and F2 cues may have been in the audible range with the HA for some subjects (see Fig. 1). As such, the HA provides important acoustic features for phoneme recognition that is beneficial in both quiet and noise.

Dependence of bimodal benefit on aided acoustic hearing

The bimodal benefit for consonant recognition appeared to depend on the audibility of acoustic information provided by the HA, coarsely divided in this study according to whether PTA thresholds were above or below 50 dB HL (see Fig. 3). This result is consistent with previous speech recognition studies that have shown that the bimodal benefit depends on the amount of residual acoustic hearing [9,15–16,42]. For example, Yoon et al. [9] found that the CI subjects with "better" HA-aided PTA thresholds (< 55 dB HL across audiometric frequencies 0.25, 0.5, 0.75, and 1 kHz) exhibited a clear bimodal benefit for vowel and sentence recognition in noise, while CI subjects with "poorer" PTA thresholds (>55 dB) received little bimodal benefit across speech tests and SNRs. In this study, PTA thresholds were averaged across 0.25, 0.5, 1, and 2 kHz, and the breakpoint between "better" and "poorer" HA-aided thresholds was 50 dB HL.

For tone and vowel recognition, there was no significant relationship between HA-aided thresholds and bimodal benefit. Note that statistical power was quite low for these analyses, given the limited number of subjects. With the exception of tone recognition in quiet, the mean bimodal benefit was greater for subjects with better HA-aided thresholds for nearly all tests in quiet and in noise. Besides the limited number of subjects, the lack of statistical significance may be due to adequate audibility for tone and vowel cues even when HA-aided thresholds were greater than 50 dB HL.

It is important to note that PTA thresholds reported and analyzed in this study provide only partial information regarding the audibility of signals with aided acoustic hearing. In this study, the effects of HA compression and signal processing were unknown, and there was no verification of sound pressure level at the ear canal, as is common in clinical practice. HA prescription has been also shown to greatly affect CI users' bimodal benefit [43]. The present subjects were all tested using their clinically assigned HAs and CIs, presumably set for conversational speech; these settings were not changed during testing. Further testing with a greater number of Chinese bimodal CI users, as well as greater control of HA variables (e.g., threshold, compression, etc.) may provide greater insight into the role of aided acoustic hearing levels on bimodal benefit. Such information is needed to optimize HAs for optimal use with contralateral CIs.

Demographic factors

Only the bimodal benefit for tone recognition in quiet was correlated with CI experience; no other demographic variables were correlated with CI-only performance, CI+HA performance, or bimodal benefit for any of the remaining speech measures in quiet or in noise. Subjects in the present study were all adults, late-implanted with long-term experience of acoustic hearing, whether aided or unaided. As such, the relatively late onset of auditory deprivation may not be comparable to that of pre-lingually deafened CI users. In studies with pediatric Mandarin-speaking CI users, age at implantation has been negatively correlated with speech performance [28,44–45] In these studies, the duration of deafness was generally calculated between birth and age at implantation, and speech development worsens as the auditory deprivation increases. With the present adults, the auditory deprivation may have occurred after sufficient development of speech patterns via acoustic hearing.

Unfortunately, little information was available regarding the extent of acoustic hearing (aided or unaided) or unaided for the present subjects. As such, the correlation with duration of deafness may not reflect age-accurate diagnoses of onset of sever-to-profound deafness. Although CI experience was not significantly correlated with speech scores in quiet or in noise, it was significantly correlated with the bimodal benefit for tone recognition in quiet. This suggests that CI users must learn to combine acoustic and electric stimulation for tone recognition after implantation. As mentioned earlier, the perception of lexical tones depends strongly F0 cues [19] in acoustic hearing. While CIs do not provide strong F0 cues due to coarse spectral resolution, CI users are able to perceive some tonal information by using temporal cues such as periodicity-related amplitude fluctuations and similarities between the fundamental F0 contour and the amplitude envelope [23,33]. The correlation between CI experience and bimodal benefit for lexical tones suggests that CI patients are able to learn to combine fine structure cues via acoustic hearing with temporal envelope cues via electric hearing. Combining these acoustic and electric cues may require longer bimodal listening experience or even explicit training.

Implications for Mandarin-speaking CI users

Because of the current restrictive criteria (severe-to-profound bilateral deafness) for cochlear implantation in adult Chinese individuals, it is difficult to find large numbers of adult, post-lingually deafened bimodal listeners in China. This difficulty contributed to the small sample size (n = 12) of the present study. However, the present data suggest that residual acoustic hearing in the non-implanted ear can improve many aspects of Mandarin speech perception by CI users. As such, less restrictive criteria for adults, as found in the United States (moderate-to severe bilateral deafness), may allow for some contribution of aided acoustic hearing to electric hearing, thereby providing a better overall benefit for cochlear implantation. As the number of Chinese bimodal listeners increases, further research with more patients may provide additional information regarding the benefit of combined acoustic and electric hearing for tonal language perception.

There was a clear benefit for combined use of a CI and HA for most speech measures. If possible, residual acoustic hearing should be combined with electric hearing to maximize the benefit of cochlear implantation. The correlation between bimodal benefit and CI experience for tone recognition suggests that bimodal CI users should wear both devices as much as possible to learn to combine acoustic and electric hearing. Alternatively, bimodal training may accelerate this learning process. With English-speaking CI users, Zhang et al. [16] found significant improvements in bimodal speech performance after bimodal training on home computers, although the benefit was largely due to improved CI-only performance.

Combined with findings from previous studies showing that increased bandwidth for acoustic hearing is associated with better bimodal performance [11,17–18], efforts should be made to implant patients with substantial aided acoustic hearing. Alternatively, HA signal processing may be modified ("frequency transposition") to better preserve formant frequency cues as well as F0. It is unclear if how frequency transposition in acoustic hearing may interact with the apical frequency mismatch associated with electric hearing. If HA signal processing is optimized for use with a CI, bimodal listening experience and/or training may help Mandarin-speaking CI users to better combine speech cues from acoustic and electric hearing.

Conclusions

Chinese tone, vowel and consonant recognition was measured in 12 adult Mandarin-speaking subjects who regularly used a HA with their CI; speech performance was measured with the CI-only and with the CI+HA. Major findings include:

1. Performance was significantly better with the CI+HA than with the CI alone for tone recognition in noise and vowel recognition in quiet. There was no significant difference in consonant recognition between the CI+HA and the CI alone in quiet or in noise.
2. There was no significant difference in bimodal benefit (CI+HA–CI alone) between quiet and noise for tones, vowels, or consonants. In quiet, the bimodal benefit was greatest for vowels, suggesting that the HA provided important formant information beyond F0. In noise, the bimodal benefit was similar for tones and vowels, with no benefit for consonants.
3. When CI subjects were group according to "better" (<50 dB HL) and "poorer" (>50 dB HL) HA-aided PTA thresholds, the mean bimodal benefit was generally greater for subjects with better HA-aided thresholds. However, a significant difference between these two groups was only observed in consonant recognition, possibly because of improved audibility of voicing cues.
4. Among demographic factors, only CI experience was significantly correlated with the bimodal benefit for tone recognition in quiet, suggesting that bimodal CI users must learn to combine fine structure cues from acoustic hearing with temporal envelope cues from electric stimulation.

Acknowledgments

We thank all the CI subjects who participated in this study. We are grateful to Dr. Li Xu and anonymous reviewer for useful suggestions on an earlier draft of this paper.

Author Contributions

Conceived and designed the experiments: YL QF. Performed the experiments: GZ YL. Analyzed the data: YL GZ JG QF. Contributed reagents/materials/analysis tools: QF. Contributed to the writing of the manuscript: JG QF.

References

1. Ching TY, Incerti P, Hill M (2004) Binaural benefits for adults who use hearing aids and cochlear implants in opposite ears. Ear Hear 25: 9–21.
2. Hamzavi J, Pok SM, Gstoettner W, Baumgartner W (2004) Speech perception with a cochlear implant used in conjunction with a hearing aid in the opposite ear. Int J of Aud 43: 61–65.
3. Mok M, Grayden D, Dowell RC, Lawrence D (2006) Speech perception for adults who use hearing aids in conjunction with cochlear implants in opposite ears. J Speech Hear Res 49: 338–351.
4. Kiefer J, Pok M, Adunka O, Stürzebeche RE, Baumgartner W, et al. (2005) Combined electric and acoustic stimulation of the auditory system: results of a clinical study. Aud Neurotol 10: 134–144.
5. Kong YY, Stickney GS, Zeng FG (2005) Speech and melody recognition in binaurally combined acoustic and electric hearing. J Acoust Soc Am 117: 1351–1361.
6. Gifford RH, Dorman MF, McKarns SA, Spahr AJ (2007) Combined electric and contralateral acoustic hearing: word and sentence recognition with bimodal hearing. J Speech Hear Res 50: 835–843.
7. Dorman MF, Gifford RH, Spahr AJ, McKarns SA (2008) The benefits of combining acoustic and electric stimulation for the recognition of speech, voice and melodies. Aud Neurotol 13: 105–112.
8. Morera C, Cavalle L, Manrique M, Huarte A, Angel R, et al. (2012) Contralateral hearing aid use in cochlear implanted patients: multicenter study of bimodal benefit. Acta Otolaryngol 132: 1084–1094.
9. Yoon YS, Li Y, Fu QJ (2012) Speech recognition and acoustic features in combined electric and acoustic stimulation. J Speech Lang Hear Res 55: 105–124.
10. Zhang T, Dorman MF, Fu QJ, Spahr AJ (2012) Auditory training in patients with unilateral cochlear implant and contralateral acoustic stimulation. Ear Hear 33: e70–79.
11. Neuman AC, Svirsky MA (2013) Effect of hearing aid bandwidth on speech recognition performance of listeners using a cochlear implant and contralateral hearing aid (bimodal hearing). Ear Hear 34: 553–561.
12. Turner CW, Gantz BJ, Vidal C, Behrens A, Henry BA (2004) Speech recognition in noise for cochlear implant listeners: benefits of residual acoustic hearing. J Acoust Soc Am 115: 1729–1735.
13. Brown CA, Bacon SP (2009) Achieving electric-acoustic benefit with a modulated tone. Ear Hear 30: 489–493.
14. Kong YY, Braida LD (2011) Cross-frequency integration for consonant and vowel identification in bimodal hearing. J Speech Lang Hear Res 54: 959–980.
15. Sheffield BM, Zeng FG (2012) The relative phonetic contributions of a cochlear implant and residual acoustic hearing to bimodal speech perception. J Acoust Soc Am 131: 518–530.
16. Zhang T, Spahr AJ, Dorman MF, Saoji A (2013) Relationship between auditory function of nonimplanted ears and bimodal benefit. Ear Hear 34: 133–141.
17. Zhang T, Dorman MF, Spahr AJ (2010) Information from the voice fundamental frequency (F0) region accounts for the majority of the benefit when acoustic stimulation is added to electric stimulation. Ear Hear 31: 63–69.
18. Sheffield SW, Gifford RH (2014) The Benefits of Bimodal Hearing: Effect of Frequency Region and Acoustic Bandwidth. Audiol Neurootol 19: 151–163.
19. Lin MC (1988) The acoustic characteristics and perceptual cues of tones in Standard Chinese. Chinese Yuwen 204: 182–193.
20. Shannon RV, Fu QJ, Galvin JJ 3rd (2004) The number of spectral channels required for speech recognition depends on the difficulty of the listening situation. Acta Otolaryngol Suppl 552: 50–54.
21. Geurts L, Wouters J (2001) Coding of the fundamental frequency in continuous interleaved sampling processors for cochlear implants. J Acoust Soc Am 109: 713–726.
22. Geurts L, Wouters J (2004) Better place-coding of the fundamental frequency in cochlear implants. J Acoust Soc Am 115: 844–852.
23. Luo X, Fu QJ (2004) Enhancing Chinese tone recognition by manipulating amplitude envelope: implications for cochlear implants. J Acoust Soc Am 116: 3659–3667.
24. Green T, Faulkner A, Rosen S, Macherey O (2005) Enhancement of temporal periodicity cues in cochlear implants: effects on prosodic perception and vowel identification. J Acoust Soc Am. 118: 375–385.
25. Huang TS, Wang NM, Liu SY (1995) Tone perception of Mandarin-speaking postlingually deaf implantees using the Nucleus 22-Channel Cochlear Mini System. Ann Otol Rhinol Laryngol Suppl 166: 294–298.
26. Wei WI, Wong R, Hui Y, Au DK, Wong BY, et al. (2000) Chinese tonal language rehabilitation following cochlear implantation in children. Acta Otolaryngol 120: 218–221.
27. Lee KY, van Hasselt CA, Chiu SN, Cheung DM (2002) Cantonese tone perception ability of cochlear implant children in comparison with normal-hearing children. Int J Pediatr Otorhinolaryngol 63: 137–147.
28. Wu JL, Yang HM (2003) Speech perception of Mandarin Chinese speaking young children after cochlear implant use: effect of age at implantation. Int J Pediatr Otorhinolaryngol 67: 247–253.
29. Fu QJ, Hsu CJ, Horng MJ (2004) Effects of speech processing strategy on Chinese tone recognition by nucleus-24 cochlear implant users. Ear Hear 25: 501–508.
30. Luo X, Fu QJ, Wei CG, Cao KL (2008) Speech recognition and temporal amplitude modulation processing by Mandarin-speaking cochlear implant users. Ear Hear 29: 957–970.
31. Tao D, Deng R, Jiang Y, Galvin JJ 3rd, Fu QJ, et al. (2014) Melodic pitch perception and lexical tone perception in Mandarin-speaking cochlear implant users. Ear Hear. 2014 Aug 5.
32. Zhou N, Huang J, Chen X, Xu L (2013) Relationship between tone perception and production in prelingually deafened children with cochlear implants. Otol Neurotol. 34: 499–506.
33. Fu QJ, Zeng FG, Shannon RV, Soli SD (1998) Importance of tonal envelope cues in Chinese speech recognition. J Acoust Soc Am 104: 505–510.
34. Luo X, Fu QJ, Wu HP, Hsu HJ (2009) Concurrent-vowel and tone recognition by Mandarin-speaking cochlear implant users. Hear Res 256: 75–84.
35. Wang W, Zhou N, Xu L (2011) Musical pitch and lexical tone perception with cochlear implants. Int J Audiol 50: 270–278.
36. Luo X, Fu QJ (2006) Contribution of low-frequency acoustic information to Chinese speech recognition in cochlear implant simulations. J Acoust Soc Am 120: 2260–2266.
37. Chen Z, Yu D, Wu Y, Zhou H, Shi H, et al. (2009) Indications and common surgical approaches for cochlear implantation in China. ORL J Otorhinolaryngol Relat Spec. 71: 187–191.
38. Gstoettner W, Kiefer J, Baumgartner WD, Pok S, Peters S, et al. (2004) Hearing preservation in cochlear implantation for electric acoustic stimulation. Acta Otolaryngolol 124: 3 48–352.
39. Wang RH (1993) The standard Chinese database. University of Science and Technology of China, internal materials.
40. Whalen DH, Xu Y (1992) Information for Mandarin Tones in the amplitude contour and in brief segments. Phonetica 49: 25–47.
41. Fu QJ, Zeng FG (2000) Effects of envelope cues on Mandarin Chinese tone recognition. Asia-Pacific J Speech Lang Hear 5: 45–57.
42. Jang JH, Lee JH, Chang SO, Oh SH (2014) Effect of Aided Hearing in the Nonimplanted Ear on Bimodal Hearing. Otol Neurotol. [Epub ahead of print].
43. Dillon MT, Buss E, Pillsbury HC, Adunka OF, Buchman CA, et al. (2014) Effects of hearing aid settings for electric-acoustic stimulation. J Am Acad Audiol. 25: 133–40.
44. Wu JL, Lin CY, Yang HM, Lin YH (2006) Effect of age at cochlear implantation on open-set word recognition in Mandarin speaking deaf children. Int J Pediatr Otorhinolaryngol. 70: 207–211.
45. Li B, Soli SD, Zheng Y, Li G, Meng Z (2014) Development of Mandarin spoken language after pediatric cochlear implantation. Int J Pediatr Otorhinolaryngol. 78: 1000–1009.

Targeted Exome Sequencing Identified Novel *USH2A* Mutations in Usher Syndrome Families

Xiu-Feng Huang[1,2]⁹, Ping Xiang[1,2]⁹, Jie Chen[3], Dong-Jun Xing[1,2], Na Huang[1,2], Qingjie Min[4], Feng Gu[2], Yi Tong[5], Chi-Pui Pang[6], Jia Qu[2], Zi-Bing Jin[1,2,3]*

1 Division of Ophthalmic Genetics, Laboratory for Stem Cell & Retinal Regeneration, The Eye Hospital of Wenzhou Medical College, Wenzhou, China, **2** The State Key Laboratory Cultivation Base and Key Laboratory of Vision Science, Ministry of Health P. R. China, Wenzhou, China, **3** Center for Excellence in Low Vision and Visual Rehabilitation, The Eye Hospital of Wenzhou Medical College, Wenzhou, China, **4** The Institute of Genomic Medicine, Wenzhou Medical College, Wenzhou, China, **5** Fuzhou Southeastern Eye Hospital, Fuzhou, China, **6** Department of Ophthalmology and Visual Sciences, The Chinese University of Hong Kong, Hong Kong, China

Abstract

Usher syndrome (USH) is a leading cause of deaf-blindness in autosomal recessive trait. Phenotypic and genetic heterogeneities in USH make molecular diagnosis much difficult. This is a pilot study aiming to develop an approach based on next-generation sequencing to determine the genetic defects in patients with USH or allied diseases precisely and effectively. Eight affected patients and twelve unaffected relatives from five unrelated Chinese USH families, including 2 pseudo-dominant ones, were recruited. A total of 144 known genes of inherited retinal diseases were selected for deep exome resequencing. Through systematic data analysis using established bioinformatics pipeline and segregation analysis, a number of genetic variants were released. Eleven mutations, eight of them were novel, in the *USH2A* gene were identified. Biparental mutations in *USH2A* were revealed in 2 families with pseudo-dominant inheritance. A proband was found to have triple mutations, two of them were supposed to locate in the same chromosome. In conclusion, this study revealed the genetic defects in the *USH2A* gene and demonstrated the robustness of targeted exome sequencing to precisely and rapidly determine genetic defects. The methodology provides a reliable strategy for routine gene diagnosis of USH.

Editor: Andreas R. Janecke, Innsbruck Medical University, Austria

Funding: This study was supported by the National Natural Science Foundation of China (H1208/81170879), the National Key Basic Research Program (2013CB967502), and the MOST Major Projects (2012YQ12008004). The funders had no role in study design, data collection and analysis, decision to publish, or preparation of the manuscript.

Competing Interests: The authors have declared that no competing interests exist.

* E-mail: jinzb@mail.eye.ac.cn

⁹ These authors contributed equally to this work.

Introduction

Usher syndrome (USH) is an autosomal recessive disorder characterized by visual loss due to retinitis pigmentosa (RP), sensorineural hearing impairment and variable vestibular dysfunction, with remarkable clinical and genetic heterogeneity [1]. According to the disease severity and progression, three subtypes of USH have been descrobed. Type I (USH1) is the most severe form characterized by prepubertal onset of RP, profound hearing loss, and vestibular dysfunction. Type II (USH2) is characterized by postpuberal onset RP and moderate deafness without vestibular dysfunction. Type III (USH3) is featured as postlingual deafness, teenage-onset RP and varying degree of vestibular dysfunction. To date, at least 12 loci have been mapped for the three types of USH in human chromosomes and 10 genes have been identified [2]. These genes totally comprise 321 coding exons spanning a length of 59,430-nt (Table S1). Reported mutations of USH widely spread over the coding regions of these causative genes. Genetic screening through traditional approaches, such as direct sequencing is therefore difficult. A high-throughout and cost-effective method to detect the genetic defects is needed. Targeted or whole exome sequencing has been proved to be a powerful tool to discover novel disease-related genes or genetic mutations in large genomic regions [3]. With the progresses on next-generation sequencing (NGS) and bioinformatics, it has been demonstrated to have higher efficiency but lower cost comparing with previous methods [4]. In this study, we utilized targeted exome sequencing (TES) to study genetic defects in five USH families and attempted to establish a strategy useful for genetic diagnosis of USH patients.

Materials and Methods

Patient Recruitment

This study adhered to the tenets of the Declaration of Helsinki. The protocol was approved by the ethics committee of The Eye Hospital of Wenzhou Medical College and written informed consent has been obtained from all study subjects. Comprehensive ophthalmic examination, including routine eye tests, perimetry, electroretinography (ERG), and optical coherence tomography (OCT), were carried out in each patient. Detailed family history was obtained through personal interviews with patients and their relatives (Figure 1). Peripheral blood samples were collected from both the affected patients and unaffected kinships.

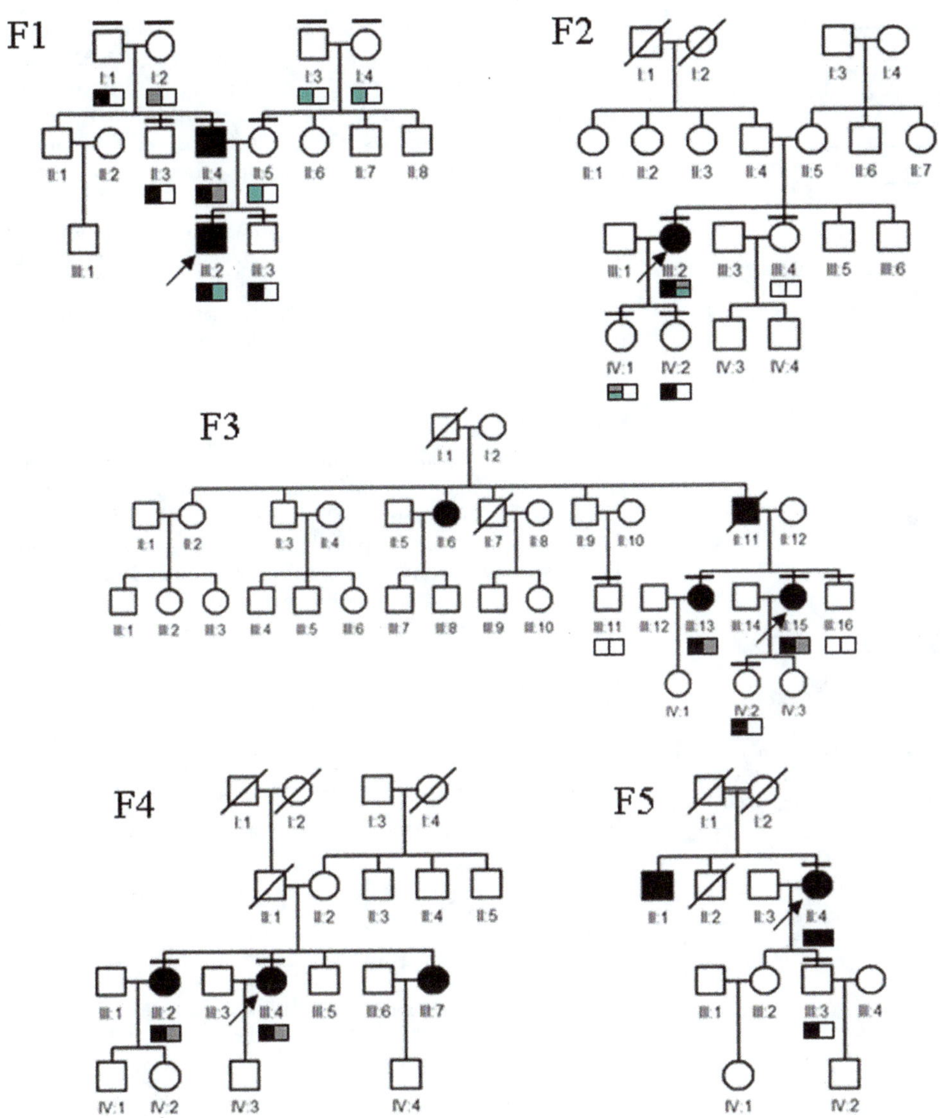

Figure 1. Families with Usher syndrome. Pedigrees of the Usher syndrome in this study. Closed symbol represents affected patient and open symbol indicates unaffected subject. The bar over the symbol indicates examined subjects in this study. Arrow indicates proband. Slash represents deceased person. The box labeled with different color indicates different mutation in each pedigree.

Illumina Library Preparation

Genomic DNA was extracted from whole blood using a DNA Extraction kit (TIANGEN, Beijing) using the manufacturer's instructions. The DNA was quantified with Nanodrop 2000 (Thermal Fisher Scientific, DE). A minimum of 3 μg DNA was used for the indexed Illumina libraries according to manufacturer's protocol. The final library size 350 bp–450 bp including adapter sequences was selected.

Disease Genes Enrichment and Sequencing

A total of 144 disease genes (Table S2) were selected by a gene capture strategy, using GenCap custom enrichment kit (MyGenostics, Beijing) based on previously described technologies [5,6]. The biotinylated single-strand capture probes were designed to tile along the exonic non-repeated regions of the genes (Table S3). The capture experiment was conducted according to manufacturer's protocol. In brief, 1 μg DNA library was mixed with Buffer BL and GenCap probe (MyGenostics, Beijing), heated at 95°C for 7 min and 65°C for 2 min on a PCR machine; 23 μl of the 65°C prewarmed Buffer HY (MyGenostics, Beijing) was then added to the mix, and the mixture was hold at 65°C with PCR lid heat on for 22 hours for hybridization. 50 μl MyOne beads (Life Technology) was washed in 500 μL 1Xbinding buffer for 3 times and resuspended in 80 μl 1Xbinding buffer. Sixty-four μl 2Xbinding buffer was added to the hybrid mix, and transferred to the tube with 80 μl MyOne beads. The mix was rotated for 1 hour on a rotator. The beads were then washed with WB1 buffer at room temperature for 15 minutes once and WB3 buffer at 65°C for 15 minutes three times. The bound DNA was then eluted with Buffer Elute. The eluted DNA was finally amplified for 15 cycles using the following program: 98°C for 30 s (1 cycle); 98°C for 25 s, 65°C for 30 s, 72°C for 30 s (15 cycles) and 72°C for 5 min (1 cycle). The PCR product was purified using SPRI beads (Beckman Coulter) according to manufacturer's protocol. The enrichment libraries were sequenced on Illumina Solexa HiSeq 2000 sequencer for paired read 100bp.

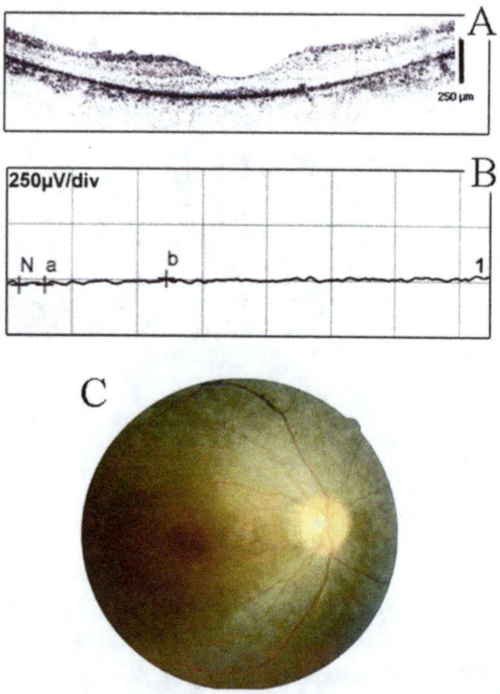

Figure 2. Clinical examination. A. OCT examination demonstrated thinned retina in the proband patient with Usher syndrome (F3-III-15); B. ERG testing showed extinguished rod response; C. representative fundography of the patient.

Bioinformatics Analysis

After Solexa HiSeq 2000 sequencing, high-quality reads were retrieved from raw reads by filtering out the low quality reads and adaptor sequences using the Solexa QA package [7] and the cutadapt program (http://code.google.com/p/cutadapt/), respectively. SOAPaligner program [8] was then used to align the clean reads to the reference human genome (hg19). After the PCR duplicates were removed by the Picard software, [9] the SNPs was firstly identified using the SOAPsnp program, [8] Subsequently, we realigned the reads to the reference genome using BWA [10] and identified the insertions or deletions (InDels) using the GATK program [11], The identified SNPs and InDels were annotated using the Exome-assistant program (http://122.228.158.106/exomeassistant). MagicViewer [12] was used to view the short read alignment and validate the candidate SNPs and InDels. Nonsynonymous variants were evaluated by four algorithms, PolyPhen, SIFT, PANTHER and Pmut as described previously, to determine pathogenicity [13]. Sequencing data were deposited in NIH Short Read Archive (PRJNA189497).

Expanded Validation

DNA samples of all the family members (Figure 1) were taken for the same targeted exome sequencing and filtering strategy. Furthermore, coding regions of the mutations identified as described above were amplified by polymerase chain reaction (PCR) for conventional direct sequencing. Purified PSR products were cycle-sequenced on an ABI 3500 Genetic Analyzer (Applied Biosystems, CA). Sanger sequencing results were analyzed by

Table 1. Clinical manifestations of the proband patients.

Proband	M/F	Age	Onset	NB	Deaf	Vertigo	BCVA (R/L)
F1-III-2	M	29	5	+	+	–	0.7/0.8
F2-III-2	F	33	<5	+	+	–	0.3/0.3
F3-III-15	F	31	10	+	+	+	0.15/0.15
F4-III-4	F	40	<5	+	+	–	0.2/0.3
F5-II-4	F	65	<5	+	+	+	FC/0.1*

M, male; F, female; NB, night blindness; BCVA, best corrected visual acuity; R, right eye, L, left eye. Asterisk indicates BCVA after cataract surgery in the left eye.

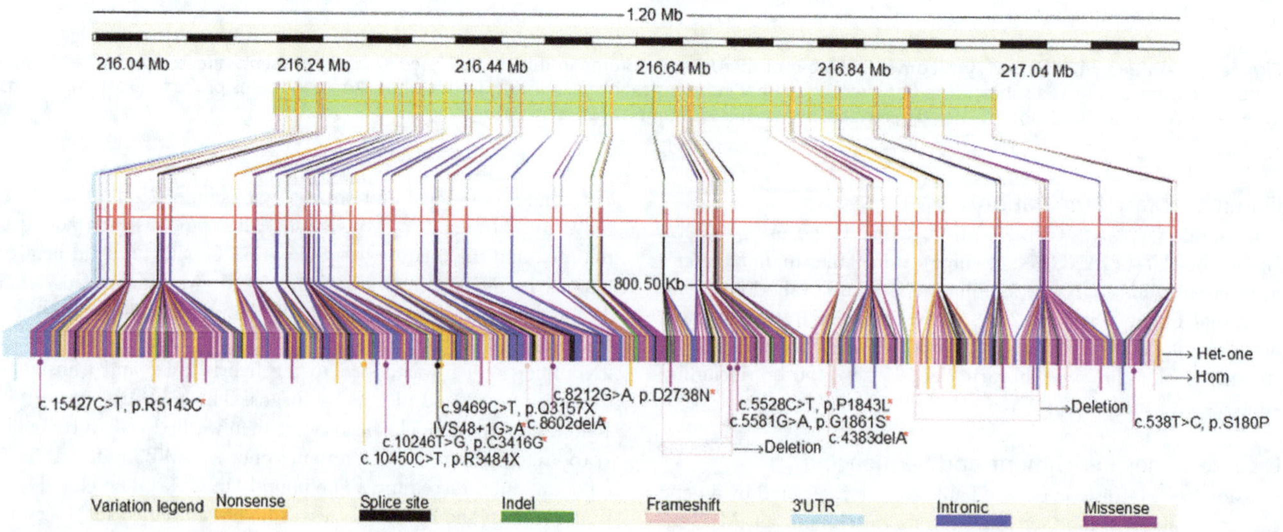

Figure 3. Mutation spectrum in the *USH2A* gene. Gene level overview of the summarized *USH2A* mutations. The gene is comprised of 71 exons which harbored 1000 distinct mutations so far have been reported. The new identified mutations are marked as arrows in the schema. Each color of the box in the figure represents a mutation type: orange, nonsense mutation; black, splice site mutation; green, indel; pink, frameshift mutation; sky blue, mutation in 3'UTR; blue, intronic mutation; purple, missense mutation. Red asterisk indicates novel mutation discovered in this study. Het-one, single heterozygous mutation; homo, homozygous mutation.

Table 2. Identified mutations in *USH2A* gene.

Family	Proband	Phenotype	Mutation	Type	Amino acid	Reported
F1	III-2	+	c.10450C>T	hetero	R3484X	Reported
			c.9469C>T	hetero	Q3157X	Reported
F2	III-2	+	c.5581G>A	hetero	G1861S	Novel
			c.15427C>T	hetero	R5143C	Novel
			c.8602delA	hetero	frameshift	Novel
F3	III-15	+	c.538T>T	hetero	S180P	Reported
			IVS48+1G>A	hetero	Splice site	Novel
F4	III-4	+	c.8212G>A	hetero	D2738N	Novel
			c.5528C>T	hetero	P1843L	Novel
F5	II-4	+	c.4383delT	homo	frameshift	Novel

Mutation Surveyor (Softgenetics, PA) and reconfirmed by the same procedure.

Results

Phenotypic Determination

Typical RP signs in the fundi, including bone-spicule hyperpigmentation and attenuated arteries, were observed in all patients. ERG showed extinguished response of the rods and OCT clearly displayed thinner retinal thickness and disorganized inner or outer segment structure (Figure 2). Three proband patients complained progressive night blindness and mild deafness, indicating a diagnosis of type II Usher syndrome. However, another two probands clearly showed a vertigo symptom, supporting a type III diagnosis (Table 1). Among these patients, more severe visual dysfunction was present in the elders. These clinical evidences suggested diagnosis of Usher syndrome type II or III.

Targeted Exome Sequencing Identified Candidate Mutations

We performed targeted exome resequencing of 144 genes implicated in inherited retinal degeneration. For the samples subjected to TES, the average sequencing depths on the targeted regions were yielded from 104.38 to 140.13 (Table S4). Each sample had more than 98.0% targeted regions covered. Meanwhile, coverage of targeted exons for >10 reads were ranged from 90.7% to 92.3% and >20 reads from 81.6% to 85.0%. By using the SOAPsnp program [8], an average of 474 to 650 variants was identified for each sample. Among them, non-synonymous variants were ranged from146 to 178 including missense, nonsense and splicing variants. The amounts were further narrowed down to 15–27 respectively through excluding the variants reported in the HapMap 28 and the SNP release of the 1000 Genome Project with a MAF>0.05. In case of the missense variants, computational prediction by four algorithms (PolyPhen, SIFT, PANTHER and Pmut) and consistency of genetic transmission mode further confined the number of candidate mutations to less than 8. For the 6–27 coding InDels initially identified in the samples using the GATK program [11], we totally identified 2 variants based on the sample filtering strategy. By the stepwise approach as described, candidate mutations in all patients were successfully identified.

Expanded Familial Validation and Sanger Sequencing Confirmation

Among the 5 USH families, pedigrees F1 and F3 (Figure 1) showed a pseudo-dominant transmission, which is definitely different with previous reports [2]. In family F1, both the proband (F1-III-2) and his father (F1-II-4) were diagnosed as typical USH based on their clinical features. Since the F1-I-1 and F1-I-2 were completely normal, it is thus conceivable that F1-II-4 carried a *de novo* dominant mutation, which was afterward transmitted to F1-III-2. Family F3 also showed a genetic continuity which was considered as a dominant pedigree. However, the TES results of the two probands were probably indicated to be the *USH2A* gene defects. To validate the TES results from proband, we extended the same procedure to the parents and a sibling in the F1 pedigree. Interestingly, expanded familial validation successfully revealed two compound heterozygous *USH2A* mutations (C3416G and R3484X) in the affected father (F1-II-4), a heterozygous *USH2A* mutation (Q3157X) in the unaffected mother (F1-II-5) and a heterozygous *USH2A* mutation (R3484X) in the unaffected sibling (F1-III-3), while the proband (F1-III-2) harbored two compound heterozygous *USH2A* mutations (Q3157X and R3484X) (Figure 1). Sanger sequencing of the coding region further confirmed that the mutation (R3484X) was transmitted from the paternal grandfather (F1-I-1) and the mutation (C3416G) was inherited from F1-I-2. The mutation (Q3157X) in the unaffected F1-II-5 was derived from maternal grandfather (F1-I-3). These results suggested the occurrence of compound heterozygosity in *USH2A* for USH. Taken together, the two causatives mutations in the proband (F1-III-2) were inherited from the paternal grandfather and maternal grandfather respectively. Furthermore, the affected father (F1-II-4) harbored another mutation in *USH2A* leading to the disease. Co-segregation analysis was performed to confirm the extracted mutations in the other 4 pedigrees. As a result, all mutations were confirmed to co-segregate well with the disease in these families. In the pseudo-dominant family F3, both the proband (F3-III-15) and the affected sister (F3-III-13) were revealed to have two compound heterozygous mutations, c.538T>C (p.S180P) and IVS48+1G>A. The splice site mutation was transmitted from proband to her unaffected son (F3-IV-2). It was suspected that the deceased affected mother (F3-II-6) carried another unknown mutation in the *USH2A* gene. In family F2, the proband (F2-III-2) was found to carry three mutations. This rare condition was further confirmed by intra-familial validation. Two heterozygous mutations, c.15427C>T (p.R5143C) and c.5581G>T (p.G1861S), were confirmed in the elder daughter (F2-IV-1) who was unaffected, which indicates the bi-mutation (c.5581G>A and c.15427C>T) in the maternal allele; while another frameshift mutation, c.8602delA, was identified in the unaffected younger daughter (F2-IV-2). In the pedigree F4, two affected siblings (F4-III-2 and F4-III-4) were revealed with the same heterozygous mutations, c.8212G>A (p.D2738N) and c.5528C>T (p.P1843L). In the last pedigree F5, a novel homozygous frameshift mutation (c.4383delT) was identified in the proband (F5-II-4). The unaffected son (F5-III-3) was proved to be a carrier. Taken together, causative mutations (Tables 2, S5 and Figure S1) were successfully finalized in all USH families via expanded TES, Sanger sequencing, and co-segregation analysis.

In this study a total of 11 identified mutations were presumed to be pathological. Both the nonsense and frameshift mutations were predicted to create a premature stop codon, strongly indicating the protein dysfunction. The splicing site mutation, IVS48+1G>A, is predicted to be damaging in silico. In addition, all missense mutations were located in highly conserved (Figure S2) and functional domains as reported previously [14]. Taken together, these results strongly indicated disease-causing mutations in the *USH2A* gene.

Mutation Spectrum in the *USH2A* Gene

The mutation distribution had been summarized in previously reported *USH2A* mutations [15–17] and novel mutations identified in this study (Table 2). It is observed that the mutations spread over the whole region of the gene. Mutations identified in the present study, including the new ones, did not show specific distribution, suggesting that it may be absence of mutation hot spot in the *USH2A* in the population (Figure 3).

Discussion

Usher syndrome is a severe disease with significant vision and hearing impairments. The prevalence worldwide ranged from 1/12,500 to 1/29,000 as previous studies have been shown [1]. Based on the phenotypic characterization, the disease has been classified into three subtypes. Seven loci (USH1B-H) have been mapped and five genes have been identified for type 1, four loci (USH2A-D) have been mapped and three genes have been identified for type 2, and two genes (USH3A, USH3B) have been identified for type 3. However, a number of studies have demonstrated phenotypic variation and crossover of the phenotype-genotype subtyping [18]. Together with the fact that a large number of coding exons exist in these genes, traditional screening of each region is infeasible for clinical application. In this study, we thus attempted to target on a group of genes responsible for inherited retinal degeneration, including RP and USH. As a result, we have proved deep exome sequencing of target 144 known causative genes of inherited retinal degeneration can serve as a fast and efficient way to perform the diagnosis. The cost was much lower compared with direct sequencing in a conservative estimation, while the amount of work is saved even more. Notably, only a single sample from the proband in each family is sufficient to identify causative mutation and intra-familiar mutation validation and co-segregation analysis can enhance the finalization.

In our USH families, mutations in the *USH2A* gene predispose the disease, suggesting the high prevalence of the *USH2A* mutation in Chinese USH population. Meantime, unaffected individuals, such as F1-II-5 from a completely normal family, were eventually found to carry a heterozygous mutation. It is worthwhile to be underlined that eight mutations have not yet been reported so far among the 11 mutations identified in this study. As there are few reports of molecular diagnosis on Chinese USH families [19], our results indicate a distinctive mutation spectrum in the population, which may require further investigation in more cohorts.

It is notable that in our strategy revealed genetic mutations in several extraordinary cases in this study. USH is well known as an autosomal recessive disease, however, among our families, pedigree F1 showed a successive transmission in a pseudo-dominant trait. This unusual case raised a question whether the patient F1-II-4 carried a *de novo* dominant mutation. Our results well addressed an autosomal recessive trait based on the discovery of a heterozygous mutation which is easily ignored in the proband's mother (F1-II-5). In family F2, we identified three distinct *USH2A* mutations in the proband (F2-III-1). In these cases, targeted exome sequencing allows excavating complete information of genetic defects which may be undetectable by traditional methods.

In the present study, we have successfully performed genetic diagnosis of Usher syndrome by utilization of NGS and have proved that it can serve as a rapid, high-throughput and efficient screening strategy. In brief, targeted exome sequencing of the 144 known genes is sufficient and clinically utilizable to comprehensively reveal genetic defects in patients with genetic retinal disease.

Supporting Information

Figure S1 Identified mutations confirmed by Sanger sequencing. Corresponding chromatograms showing mutant and wild-type alleles are as indicated.

Figure S2 Conserved amino acid sequence. Conservation of amino acid residue across species is highlighted.

Table S1 Known causative genes responsible for Usher syndrome.

Table S2 List of the genes captured in the present study.

Table S3 List of all probes used to enrich for the target genes.

Table S4 Data summary of the targeted exome resequencing. Asterisk indicates proband patient.

Table S5 Expanded familial validation.

Acknowledgments

We thank all patients and family members for their participation in this study.

Author Contributions

Conceived and designed the experiments: JQ ZBJ. Performed the experiments: XFH PX JC DJX NH QM. Analyzed the data: XFH PX QM FG CPP ZBJ. Contributed reagents/materials/analysis tools: JQ ZBJ CPP YT. Wrote the paper: XFH ZBJ.

References

1. Wleber RG, Gregory-Evans K (2006) Retinitis Pigmentosa and Allied Disorders. In: Ryan SJ, ed. Retina, Fourth ed: Elsevier-Mosby, p395–498.
2. Bonnet C, El-Amraoui A (2012) Usher syndrome (sensorineural deafness and retinitis pigmentosa): pathogenesis, molecular diagnosis and therapeutic approaches. Curr Opin Neurol 25: 42–49.
3. Bras J, Guerreiro R, Hardy J (2012) Use of next-generation sequencing and other whole-genome strategies to dissect neurological disease. Nat Rev Neurosci 13: 453–464.
4. Bowne SJ, Sullivan LS, Koboldt DC, Ding L, Fulton R, et al. (2011) Identification of disease-causing mutations in autosomal dominant retinitis pigmentosa (adRP) using next-generation DNA sequencing. Invest Ophthalmol Vis Sci 52: 494–503.
5. He J, Wu J, Jiao Y, Wagner-Johnston N, Ambinder RF, et al. (2011) IgH gene rearrangements as plasma biomarkers in Non- Hodgkin's lymphoma patients. Oncotarget 2: 178–185.
6. Wu J, Matthaei H, Maitra A, Dal Molin M, Wood LD, et al. (2011) Recurrent GNAS mutations define an unexpected pathway for pancreatic cyst development. Sci Transl Med 3: 92ra66.
7. Cox MP, Peterson DA, Biggs PJ (2010) SolexaQA: At-a-glance quality assessment of Illumina second-generation sequencing data. BMC Bioinformatics 11: 485.
8. Li R, Yu C, Li Y, Lam TW, Yiu SM, et al. (2009) SOAP2: an improved ultrafast tool for short read alignment. Bioinformatics 25: 1966–1967.
9. Li H, Handsaker B, Wysoker A, Fennell T, Ruan J, et al. (2009) The Sequence Alignment/Map format and SAMtools. Bioinformatics 25: 2078–2079.

10. Li H, Durbin R (2009) Fast and accurate short read alignment with Burrows-Wheeler transform. Bioinformatics 25: 1754–1760.
11. DePristo MA, Banks E, Poplin R, Garimella KV, Maguire JR, et al. (2011) A framework for variation discovery and genotyping using next-generation DNA sequencing data. Nat Genet 43: 491–498.
12. Hou H, Zhao F, Zhou L, Zhu E, Teng H, et al. (2010) MagicViewer: integrated solution for next-generation sequencing data visualization and genetic variation detection and annotation. Nucleic Acids Res 38: W732–736.
13. Jin ZB, Mandai M, Yokota T, Higuchi K, Ohmori K, et al. (2008) Identifying pathogenic genetic background of simplex or multiplex retinitis pigmentosa patients: a large scale mutation screening study. J Med Genet 45: 465–472.
14. van Wijk E, Pennings RJ, te Brinke H, Claassen A, Yntema HG, et al. (2004) Identification of 51 novel exons of the Usher syndrome type 2A (USH2A) gene that encode multiple conserved functional domains and that are mutated in patients with Usher syndrome type II. Am J Hum Genet 74: 738–744.
15. Dreyer B, Brox V, Tranebjaerg L, Rosenberg T, Sadeghi AM, et al. (2008) Spectrum of USH2A mutations in Scandinavian patients with Usher syndrome type II. Hum Mutat 29: 451.
16. Nakanishi H, Ohtsubo M, Iwasaki S, Hotta Y, Usami S, et al. (2011) Novel USH2A mutations in Japanese Usher syndrome type 2 patients: marked differences in the mutation spectrum between the Japanese and other populations. J Hum Genet 56: 484–490.
17. Nakanishi H, Ohtsubo M, Iwasaki S, Hotta Y, Mizuta K, et al. (2009) Identification of 11 novel mutations in USH2A among Japanese patients with Usher syndrome type 2. Clin Genet 76: 383–391.
18. Besnard T, Vache C, Baux D, Larrieu L, Abadie C, et al. (2012) Non-USH2A mutations in USH2 patients. Hum Mutat 33: 504–510.
19. Xu W, Dai H, Lu T, Zhang X, Dong B, et al. (2011) Seven novel mutations in the long isoform of the USH2A gene in Chinese families with nonsyndromic retinitis pigmentosa and Usher syndrome Type II. Mol Vis 17: 1537–1552.

Mcph1-Deficient Mice Reveal a Role for MCPH1 in Otitis Media

Jing Chen[1¤], Neil Ingham[1¤], Simon Clare[1], Claire Raisen[1], Valerie E. Vancollie[1], Ozama Ismail[1], Rebecca E. McIntyre[1], Stephen H. Tsang[2], Vinit B. Mahajan[3], Gordon Dougan[1], David J. Adams[1], Jacqueline K. White[1], Karen P. Steel[1*¤]

1 Wellcome Trust Sanger Institute, Hinxton, Cambridgeshire, United Kingdom, **2** Edward S. Harkness Eye Institute, Columbia University, New York, New York, United States of America, **3** Omics Laboratory, Department of Ophthalmology and Visual Sciences, University of Iowa, Iowa City, Iowa, United States of America

Abstract

Otitis media is a common reason for hearing loss, especially in children. Otitis media is a multifactorial disease and environmental factors, anatomic dysmorphology and genetic predisposition can all contribute to its pathogenesis. However, the reasons for the variable susceptibility to otitis media are elusive. *MCPH1* mutations cause primary microcephaly in humans. So far, no hearing impairment has been reported either in the *MCPH1* patients or mouse models with *Mcph1* deficiency. In this study, *Mcph1*-deficient ($Mcph1^{tm1a/tm1a}$) mice were produced using embryonic stem cells with a targeted mutation by the Sanger Institute's Mouse Genetics Project. Auditory brainstem response measurements revealed that $Mcph1^{tm1a/tm1a}$ mice had mild to moderate hearing impairment with around 70% penetrance. We found otitis media with effusion in the hearing-impaired $Mcph1^{tm1a/tm1a}$ mice by anatomic and histological examinations. Expression of Mcph1 in the epithelial cells of middle ear cavities supported its involvement in the development of otitis media. Other defects of $Mcph1^{tm1a/tm1a}$ mice included small skull sizes, increased micronuclei in red blood cells, increased B cells and ocular abnormalities. These findings not only recapitulated the defects found in other *Mcph1*-deficient mice or *MCPH1* patients, but also revealed an unexpected phenotype, otitis media with hearing impairment, which suggests *Mcph1* is a new gene underlying genetic predisposition to otitis media.

Editor: Patrick Callaerts, VIB & Katholieke Universiteit Leuven, Belgium

Funding: This work was supported by the Wellcome Trust (grant number 098051) www.wellcome.ac.uk, Medical Research Council (grant number G0300212) http://www.mrc.ac.uk, European Commission (EUMODIC contract no. LSHG-CT-2006-037188) www.eumodic.org and Cancer Research UK (grant number C20510/A13031) http://www.cancerresearchuk.org. The funders had no role in study design, data collection and analysis, decision to publish, or preparation of the manuscript.

Competing Interests: The authors have declared that no competing interests exist.

* E-mail: karen.steel@kcl.ac.uk

¤ Current address: Wolfson Centre for Age-Related Diseases, King's College London, London, United Kingdom

Introduction

Otitis media (OM), inflammation of the middle ear, is the most common cause of hearing impairment in children. As a multifactorial disease, the pathogenesis of OM is complicated. Based on previous research, many factors are thought to contribute to the development and persistence of OM including: environmental factors such as smoking and type of child care; anatomical dysmorphology; Eustachian-tube function; adaptive and innate immune system function; viral and bacterial load; and genetic predisposition. However, the mechanisms underlying OM are still elusive. Heritability estimated from twin studies [1,2] and linkage analysis [3] indicates a strong genetic component is involved in OM. Outcomes vary in different patients with similar symptoms after standardised treatment, also suggesting differences in their underlying pathophysiology that may have a genetic component. Clinical studies of OM are limited by the wide range of environmental elements involved. Mice, however, can be bred in a controlled environment, minimising the variation arising from the environment, making it a useful model for building an understanding of the genetic pathways and mechanisms underlying OM. Due to our very limited knowledge of the genetic etiology of OM in humans, it is hard to anticipate which genes may contribute to this disorder. As summarised in a recent review [4], mouse models involving disruption of genes functioning as transcription factors, and genes involved in apoptosis, the immune system, ciliary function and in mucopolysaccharidoses revealed that many pathways and processes can contribute to the development of OM.

In the present study, microcephalin 1 (*Mcph1*)-deficient ($Mcph1^{tm1a/tm1a}$) mice were found to exhibit hearing impairment as a part of the Sanger Institute's Mouse Genetics Project (MGP). The MGP uses the Knockout Mouse Project and the European Conditional Mouse Mutagenesis Program (KOMP/EUCOMM) resource of over 17,000 genes targeted in ES cells [5] and aims to generate and screen the phenotype of mutants for 160 genes per year. The hearing screening uses the Auditory Brainstem Response (ABR) test at 14 weeks of age and is part of the standardised battery of primary phenotypic tests.

MCPH1 mutations cause primary microcephaly in humans characterized by a markedly reduced brain size and mental retardation [6,7]. The *MCPH1* gene (also known as *BRIT1*,

BRCT-repeat inhibitor of hTERT expression) encodes MCPH1, which contained three BRCT domains: one in its N terminus and two in its C terminus. BRCT domains have been found predominantly in proteins involved in cell cycle checkpoint functions and in proteins involved in the DNA damage response [8,9]. Because the MCPH1 protein contains three BRCT domains, previous studies focused on and implicated MCPH1 in DNA damage response [8], DNA damage regulation in the ATM/ATR pathways [10], co-ordination of the regulation of Cdc25A and Cdk1–cyclin B1 activity and thus, in regulation of mitotic entry [11], and homologous recombination repair through the Condensin II complex [12]. MCPH1 also has a role in coupling the centrosome cycle with mitosis, which is required for precise mitotic spindle orientation and regulation of progenitor cell division to maintain brain size. Neuroepithelial cells have apical-basal polarity, and the switch from proliferative, symmetric to neurogenic, asymmetric division is controlled by the orientation of the spindle pole during mitotic division. Primary microcephaly is caused by mutations of centrosomal proteins and is thought to arise from an increase in asymmetric divisions that reduces the size of the neural progenitor pool available for future brain growth [13]. Finally, MCPH1 has been proposed to function as a tumor suppressor gene that contributes to both cancer initiation and cancer progression in a variety of cancer lineages [10].

The broad phenotypic screening of the MGP revealed that $Mcph1^{tm1a/tm1a}$ mouse mutants not only had some expected features such as small skull size and increased micronuclei reflecting genome instability, but also showed some unexpected phenotypes including susceptibility to OM implicating MCPH1 in genetic predisposition to OM. This finding implicates a new molecule in the pathogenesis of OM that is relevant to understanding the underlying mechanisms irrespective of the initial trigger for OM.

Materials and Methods

All mouse breeding and investigation was carried out with authorization of the UK Home Office. Mice were killed by cervical dislocation and decapitation. All efforts were made to minimize suffering.

Production of $Mcph1^{tm1a/tm1a}$ mice

Mcph1-deficient ($Mcph1^{tm1a(EUCOMM)Wtsi}$, abbreviated to $Mcph1^{tm1a}$ in this report) mice carry a knockout-first allele [5], in which a promoterless cassette including *LacZ* and *neo* genes were inserted in intron 3–4 of the *Mcph1* gene (Figure 1A). In the knockout-first allele design, the knockout is obtained by introduction of a splice acceptor/reporter cassette with a strong polyA site into an endogenous intron upstream of a critical exon. By computer analysis based on defined criteria (http://www.knockoutmouse.org/kb/entry/102/), exon 4 of *Mcph1* was chosen as the critical exon. The vectors containing the *Mcph1* knockout-first allele were electroporated into embryonic stem cells (JM8F6) derived from C57BL/6N mice. Targeted embryonic stem cell lines were selected using neomycin and screened by long range PCR after homologous recombination. The presence of the *LoxP* site was confirmed by sequencing. Correct integration of the 5′ arm and 3′ arm was confirmed by long range PCR using a universal primer and two genome-specific primers, and the subsequent PCR amplicon was verified by sequencing. The positive stem cells were injected into host mouse blastocysts and were used to generate chimeras containing the targeted allele. Male chimeras with 80–90% of targeted cells were bred with C57BL/6Brd-Tyr^{c-Brd} females and germ line transmission of the *Mcph1* knockout-first allele was confirmed by a series of genotyping PCR analyses (http://www.knockoutmouse.org/kb/25/) using the mouse tissue DNA as template. These heterozygous mice were inter-crossed to expand the colony. The mice were maintained in individually-ventilated cages at a standard temperature and humidity and in specific pathogen-free conditions on the mixed C57BL/6N and C57BL/6Brd-Tyr^{c-Brd} genetic background. To genotype animals (Figure 1B), DNA was extracted from the tissue of ear-clips and used as the template for short range PCR using the forward primer for the wild type allele: TGGAGTTTGGAGGGTGCTTC, and the reverse primer: CTTGGGGAATGAGGAAGGTG. The mutant allele shares the same forward primer with wild type, and the reverse primer: TCGTGGTATCGTTATGCGCC.

Reverse transcription PCR and real-time quantitative PCR

RNA was isolated from the tissues of middle ear, inner ear and forebrain. Littermates were used (wild type mice, n = 3; heterozygous mice, n = 3; homozygous mice, n = 3, at postnatal day 3). Total RNA was isolated with QIAshredder columns (QIAgen, cat. no. 79654) and RNAeasy mini kit (QIAgen, cat. no. 74104). cDNA was synthesized with normalization of the same original amount of RNA using oligo dT and SuperScrip II (Invitrogen). Primers were designed to amplify part of exon 9–13 (forward primer: AGAAGAAAAGCCAACGAGAACATT, reverse primer: CTGAGGGGCTGGGCTGACTTG) and exon 14 (3′ UTR, forward primer: CGTGCCATCATCAGGTCAATCA, reverse primer: GGGGCGAGGAGCAAGTCTGTA). Real-time PCR was performed in quadruplicate for each sample using the probe (Applied Biosystem, Mm00557495_m1, covering exon 3–4 boundary) in an ABI Prism 7000 (Applied Biosystem). Hypoxanthine-guanine phosphoribosyltransferase (Hprt) was amplified simultaneously (Applied Biosystem, Mm01318747_g1) as the internal reference. The relative quantity of *Mcph1* RNA was calculated using $2^{-\Delta\Delta Ct}$ method [14].

Auditory Brainstem Response

Mice were anaesthetised by ketamine hydrochloride (100 mg/Kg, Ketaset®, Fort Dodge Animal Health) and xylazine hydrochloride (10 mg/Kg, Rompun®, Bayer Animal Health) and subcutaneous needle electrodes were inserted on the vertex (active), and over the left (reference) and right (ground) bullae. A calibrated sound system was used to deliver free-field click (0.01 ms duration) and tone pip (various frequencies from 6–30 or 6–42 kHz of 5 ms duration, 1 ms rise/fall time) stimuli at a range of intensity levels in 3 or 5 dB steps. Averaged responses to 256 stimuli, presented at 42.2 per second, were analysed and thresholds established as the lowest sound intensity giving a visually detectable ABR response. The peak-peak amplitude of wave 1 of click-evoked ABRs (P1-N1 amplitude) was measured and plotted as a function of sound level above threshold to produce input-output functions (IOFs). The IOF slope from 0–35 dB above threshold was calculated since 0–35 dB above threshold covered the more linear range before the function begins to flatten towards a plateau and also to ensure that a similar dB SL (sensation level) range was covered in both wild type and $Mcph1^{tm1a/tm1a}$ mice. In more severely impaired mutants, it was not possible to record in the higher ranges of dB SL. A *t*-test was used to compare the slopes.

Anatomy and histology of temporal bone

Mice used for recurrent ABR measurements were sacrificed after the last measurement and the anatomy of their middle ears was examined. Briefly, the external ear canals, tympanic membranes, ossicles and middle ear cavities were carefully dissected, examined and imaged. The inner ears were dissected

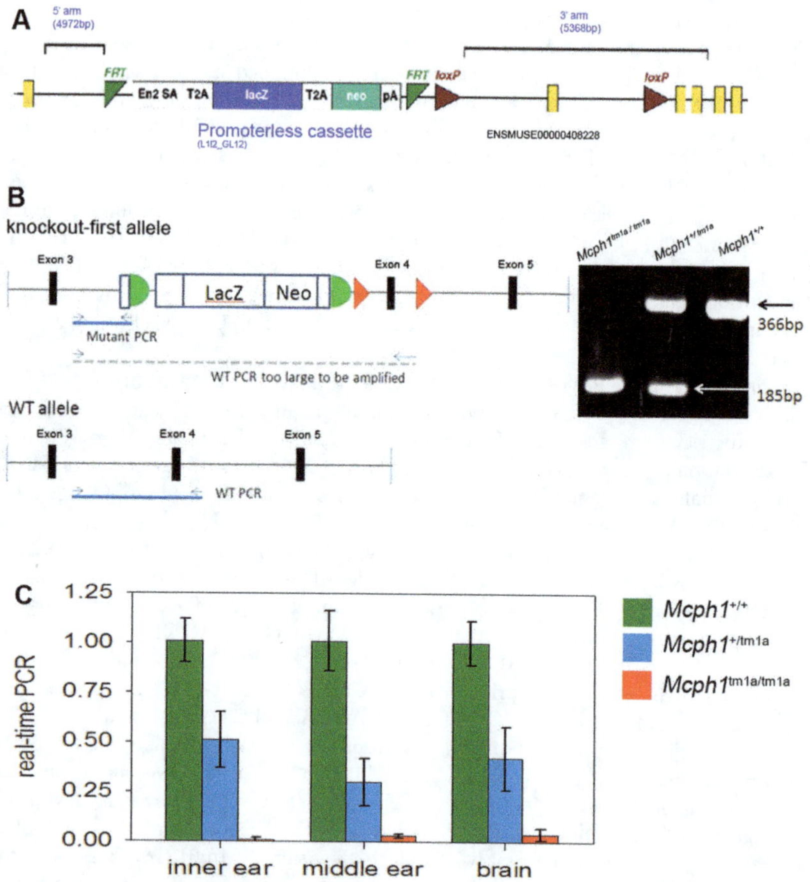

Figure 1. Production of *Mcph1*-deficient (*Mcph1*$^{tm1a/tm1a}$) mice. (A) Schematic of knockout strategy for *Mcph1* gene based on knockout-first design. A promoterless cassette including *LacZ* and *neo* genes was inserted in the third intron of *Mcph1* gene flanked by FRT sites. *LoxP* sites flank the critical exon (exon4 of *Mcph1* gene in knockout-first design). See http://www.knockoutmouse.org/martsearch/project/41705 for more details. (B) Short range PCR for genotyping. Wild type allele produces one band of 366bp. Due to the insertion of the cassette, primers designed for the wild type allele do not have product for the mutant allele using the short range PCR (illustrated as the left panel, schematic illustration is not in scale). The homozygous allele produces only one band of 185 bp. The heterozygotes produce two bands of 185 bp and 366 bp. (C) Quantitative real-time PCR showed largely reduced transcript of *Mcph1* in *Mcph1*$^{tm1a/tm1a}$ (n = 3) mice compared to wild type mice (n = 3) and the residual levels vary in different organs.

out, fixed in 4% paraformaldehyde and examined following inner ear clearing in glycerol [15]. Skulls from 17 mice (wild type mice, n = 4 at 4–5 weeks old; heterozygous mice, n = 2 at 5 weeks old, n = 1 at 60 weeks old; homozygous mice, n = 7 at 4–6 weeks old, n = 3 at 59–61 weeks old) were collected after the ABR measurement and fixed in 10% buffered formalin, decalcified in 10% EDTA until the tissues were soft, dehydrated and embedded in paraffin. Eight-micrometer-thick sagittal sections were obtained before hematoxylin-eosin staining.

Scanning Electron Microscopy

Inner ears of six mice at postnatal day 4 (three mice each of homozygote and wild type) were fixed by 2.5% glutaraldehyde in 0.1 M sodium cacodylate buffer with 3 mM $CaCl_2$ at room temperature for 3 hours. Cochleae were finely dissected in PBS. This was followed by further processing by an osmium-thiocarbohydrazide-osmium (OTOTO) method [16]. The samples were dehydrated in increasing concentration of ethanol, critical-point dried, mounted and examined under a HITACHI S-4800 scanning electron microscope.

Immunohistochemistry

Immunohistochemistry staining was performed using the Ventana Discovery machine (Roche) and reagents according to the manufacturer's instructions. Paraffin sections from wild type mice at postnatal day 7 (n = 3) and 4 weeks old (n = 5) were obtained as described above. The expression of Mcph1 was detected by using Mcph1 antibody (Abcam: ab2612, 1:3000).

X-ray assay and brain weight measurement

Digital X-ray images are acquired using a Faxitron system MX20 (Faxitron X-ray corporation) in 14-week old mice (wild type mice, n = 7M & 7F; homozygous mice, n = 6M & 7F). Mice were anaesthetised and up to five standard images were taken for each mouse. The entire skeleton morphology was assessed using a standardised protocol capturing 41 parameters. To extract the brains, a vertical incision was made through the scalp and both sides were peeled back. Then a vertical cut was made through the midline of the skull using a pair of scissors and the skull was peeled off with a pair of fine forceps. Brains were then removed using a fine spatula and weighed on a Sartorius TE212, accurate to two decimal places.

Micronucleus assay

The prevalence of micronucleated normochromatic erythrocytes (MN-NCE) was determined using a flow cytometric assay of micronucleus formation [17]. Flow cytometry analysis was performed as described previously [17].

Pathogen challenge experiment

Salmonella enterica serovar Typhimurium M525 [18] and Citrobacter rodentium [19] were grown at 37°C as stationary overnight cultures in Luria-Bertani (LB) broth (Difco) containing ampicillin (100 µg/mL Sigma) or naladixic acid (100 µg/mL Sigma) respectively. For oral inoculation, overnight cultures were centrifuged at 15,000× g for 10 min and resuspended in the original volume in phosphate-buffered saline (PBS). Bacteria were administered with a blunt-tipped gavage needle. For intravenous inoculation, overnight cultures were diluted in PBS and injected into the lateral tail vein. Inocula were cultured retrospectively on LB agar to determine the administered dose. At regular time points post-infection, faecal samples from individual mice were collected in separate sterile tubes. Faecal samples were weighed and for every 0.01 g of faeces 100 µL of sterile PBS was added. Faecal samples were homogenised on a vortex and serially diluted. The number of viable bacteria was determined by viable count on LB agar containing naladixic acid (100 µg/mL Sigma). At selected time points post-infection, mice were killed by cervical dislocation and surface-sterilized with 70% ethanol. Livers and spleens were removed aseptically into bags and weighed. Organs were homogenised in 5 mL of sterile double distilled water using a Seward Stomacher 80 (Seward, London UK) for 2 minutes at high speed. The number of viable bacteria in organ homogenates was determined by serial dilution and viable count on LB agar supplemented with an appropriate antibiotic.

Peripheral Blood Lymphocyte profile

Flow analysis was performed on heparinised blood collected from 16-week old mice (wild type mice, n = 35F & 29M; homozygous mice, n = 7F & 7M). The following parameters were analysed: percentages of total T cells, CD4+ and CD8+ T cells, NKT cells, NK cells, B cells, Granulocytes and Monocytes are presented relative to the total CD45+ WBC population. Percentages of memory CD4 and CD4+CD25+ Treg cells are presented relative to the total CD4+ T cell population. Percentages of memory CD8 and mature IgD+ B cells are presented relative to the total CD8+ T cell and B cell populations respectively. All samples are analysed on a BD LSR II.

Antibody level assay

Recipient mice (wild type mice, n = 2F & 4M; homozygous mice, n = 2F & 4M) were immunized by intranasal inhalation of 30 µl PBS containing 10 mg TetC (gift from Omar Qazi, Imperial College London) combined with 1 mg heat-labile toxin of *Escherichia coli* (gift of Rino Rappuoli, Chiron) adjuvant. Mice were boosted on days 7 and 21. Serum samples were collected on days 28. Detection of TetC-specific antibodies from sera was performed by ELISA. For the measurements of antibody levels, mouse blood was collected by cardiac puncture, and serum was prepared and stored at −20°C. For antigen specific antibody measurements in mouse serum, Nunc MaxiSorp plates were coated overnight at 4°C with 2 mg/ml tetanus toxin fragment C recombinant protein (TetC) in 0.1 M Na2HPO4 (pH 9.0), blocked with 3% (w/v) BSA in PBS for 1 h, and incubated with 5-fold serial dilutions of mouse serum in PBS with 1% BSA for 1 h. The plates were developed with anti-mouse Ig HRP-conjugated Abs (Dako), followed by o-phenylenediamine substrate tablets (Sigma-Aldrich) dissolved in water. Absorbance was read at 490 nm and optical densities represented as titres.

Ocular assessment and histological examination

Mice underwent ophthalmic screening at 15 weeks of age. They were assessed for gross morphological changes to the eye using a slit lamp (Zeiss SL130) and ophthalmoscope (Heine Omega 500). The eye was examined both undilated and dilated (tropicamide). Images using the slit lamp were collected using a Leica DFC420 camera. The mice were culled under terminal anaesthesia followed by cervical dislocation and six eyes from 3 male homozygous mutants and 3 wild type mice were removed and fixed. Pupil-optic nerve sections were processed with hematoxylin and eosin, and standard images were captured under light microscopy for review [20].

Haematology of peripheral blood

Blood was collected at 16 weeks of age into ETDA microvette tubes (Startedt) and analyzed on an analyzer (SciIVet Animal Blood Counter) with ten parameters tested.

Clinical chemistry

16-week-old mice were terminally anaesthetized and blood was collected from the retro-orbital sinus into lithium-heparin tubes. The plasma was immediately analyzed on an Olympus AU400 Analyzer with 28 parameters tested.

Glucose tolerance

We assessed glucose tolerance in mice fed on a high-fat diet (Western RD, 829100, Special Diets Services) from 4 weeks of age until 13 weeks of age. At 13 weeks, mice were fasted overnight before a blood sample was taken and glucose was measured using an Accu-Chek Aviva (Roche). A bolus of glucose (2 mg/g) was administered intraperitoneally and blood glucose concentration from the tail tip was measured using Accu-Chek Aviva (Roche) after 15, 30, 60 and 120 min.

Results

Production of *Mcph1*-deficient mice

Targeted ES cells from the EUCOMM resource were used by the MGP to generate the *Mcph1* mutant on a C57BL/6 genetic background. The mutant allele is designated *Mcph1*$^{tm1a(EUCOMM)Wtsi}$, and abbreviated to *Mcph1*^{tm1a} in this study. The design of the *Mcph1*^{tm1a} allele and genotyping protocol are illustrated in Figure 1A and 1B. The homozygous mutants are viable, but the frequency of homozygous mutant offspring from heterozygous intercross matings is 14%, which is below the expected Mendelian ratio (χ^2 test, $p<0.001$). Both male and female homozygous mutants are infertile, similar to other *Mcph1* mutants reported previously [9,13]. There was no evidence of retarded growth in *Mcph1*$^{tm1a/tm1a}$ mice (data not shown). Reverse transcription PCR was performed to test the effect of the mutation of *Mcph1* on transcription. The homozygous mutants, heterozygous and wild type mice produced bands of expected size and sequencing of the PCR products validated the results. This indicated that there was residual *Mcph1* transcript in *Mcph1*$^{tm1a/tm1a}$ mice. Quantitative real-time PCR revealed the residual transcript of *Mcph1* in the homozygous mice is only 1–4% of the level compared to the wild type mice and the residual levels vary in different organs (Figure 1C).

Mcph1-deficient mice have mild to moderate hearing impairment

Hearing impairment was discovered by ABR measurement in 14 week old *Mcph1*$^{tm1a/tm1a}$ mice as part of the standard MGP phenotypic screen (phenotyping overview is available from http://www.sanger.ac.uk/mouseportal/). *Mcph1*$^{tm1a/tm1a}$ mice showed mild to moderate hearing impairment with increases of 10–50 decibels (dB) compared to the normal thresholds for both click and pure tone stimuli (6–30 kHz) (Figure 2A). To further characterise the hearing ability of *Mcph1*$^{tm1a/tm1a}$ mice and to ask whether the hearing impairment is progressive with age, recurrent ABR measurements were performed in *Mcph1*$^{tm1a/tm1a}$, *Mcph1*$^{+/tm1a}$ and *Mcph1*$^{+/+}$ littermates from 3 weeks to 24 weeks at 3-week intervals. *Mcph1*$^{+/tm1a}$ (n = 17) and *Mcph1*$^{+/+}$ (n = 13) mice showed normal ABR thresholds, whereas elevated thresholds can be detected in *Mcph1*$^{tm1a/tm1a}$ mice as early as 3 weeks of age (n = 13). Thresholds were generally stable over time, although there was progressive or fluctuating hearing impairment over time in some mice (Figure 3A). Heterozygous mice were found to have normal hearing, in accordance with the recessive model of inheritance for patients with *MCPH1* mutations (Figure 3A). *Mcph1*$^{tm1a/tm1a}$ mice behaved normally suggesting normal vestibular function. We defined three out of six stimuli tested (click and pure tone stimuli) above the normal hearing reference range as affected in this study, and the penetrance of hearing impairment in *Mcph1*$^{tm1a/tm1a}$ mice is around 70% based on this criterion.

Input-output function analysis showed that growth of amplitude of wave 1 of the click-evoked ABR with increasing sound level above threshold appeared similar in wild type and *Mcph1*$^{tm1a/tm1a}$ mice (Figure 2B). ABR waveforms were comparable in shape in mutants compared with controls (Figure 4).

Anatomical and histological analysis indicates otitis media

To assess the causes of hearing impairment in the *Mcph1*$^{tm1a/tm1a}$ mice, anatomical analysis of the middle ear was performed after the completion of the recurrent ABR measurements. All the *Mcph1*$^{+/tm1a}$ (n = 17) and *Mcph1*$^{+/+}$ (n = 13) mice showed a transparent tympanic membrane, air-filled middle ear cavity, and normal morphology of ossicles (apart from one heterozygous mouse that had some white secretion in the hypotympanum in the right middle ear cavity). Dissection of *Mcph1*$^{tm1a/tm1a}$ mice (n = 13) that had elevated ABR thresholds revealed a range of defects in the middle ear including thickened and white bone forming the bulla instead of the normal thin and transparent bone, retracted tympanic membrane, bubbles present underneath the tympanic membrane, or middle ear cavities filled with clear or cloudy fluid. In addition, two *Mcph1*$^{tm1a/tm1a}$ mice had an amorphous tissue mass in the middle ear cavity (Figure 3D). The ossicles displayed normal gross morphology, but the mice that had pus-like effusions or amorphous material in the middle ear had a rough surface of the ossicles. However, we did not see bony outgrowths, otorrhea or perforation of the tympanic membrane, which is different from some reported OM mouse models [21]. The correlation between the middle ear effusion and recurrent ABR measurement results is noticeable (Figure 3C–F). Watery secretion with bubbles in the middle ear cavity was seen in the mice that displayed fluctuating ABR thresholds. One mouse that had a pus-like secretion within the middle ear demonstrated relatively stable raised ABR thresholds through all the recurrent ABR measurements. Progressive hearing loss was observed in the mice that had amorphous material in the middle ear cavity, in which we found that the auditory ossicular chain was severely impeded (Figure 3B).

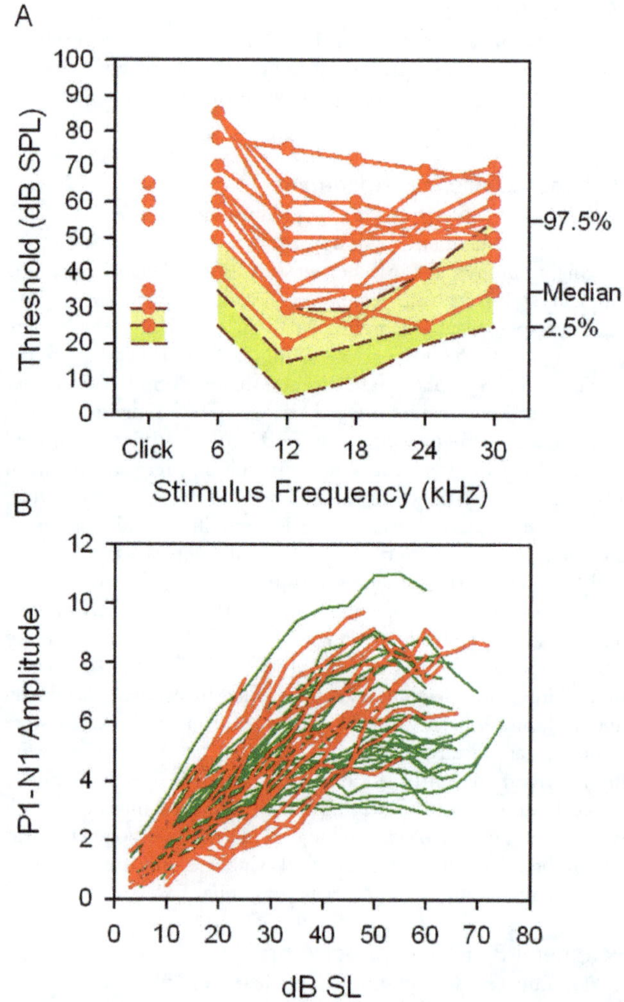

Figure 2. *Mcph1*-deficient mice have mild to moderate hearing impairment characterized with conductive hearing impairment. (A) ABR measurement results of 14 week old *Mcph1*$^{tm1a/tm1a}$ mice (n = 11) in MGP showed mild to moderate hearing impairment, or normal hearing compared to control mice. The green baseline area shows a reference range for the control wild type mice with the same genetic background, plotting the median and 2.5 to 97.5 percentile of the population (n = 440). (B) Input-output function (IOF) analysis. The peak-peak amplitude of wave 1 (P1-N1 amplitude) of click-evoked ABRs is plotted as a function of dB SL (Sensation Level, dB above threshold) for wild type (green) and *Mcph1*$^{tm1a/tm1a}$ (red) mice. There was no significant difference of IOF slopes of *Mcph1*$^{tm1a/tm1a}$ (n = 24, slope = 0.144+/−0.066; mean +/− SD) and wild type mice (n = 36, slope = 0.133+/−0.048) (t-test, $p = 0.444$).

Histological examination was performed to investigate the pathological change (Figure 5). Hearing was evaluated by ABR measurement before sectioning the temporal bone. The middle ear cavities of *Mcph1*$^{+/tm1a}$ and *Mcph1*$^{+/+}$ mice were clear and lined with thin mucoperiosteum. The middle ear cavities of the hearing-impaired *Mcph1*$^{tm1a/tm1a}$ mice were filled with exudate and lined with a thickened mucoperiosteum, and occasionally formation of fibrous polyps of mucoperiosteum stroma, indicative of otitis media. The middle ear effusions included a variable amount of inflammatory cells in different mice (mainly granulocytes and scattered foamy macrophages according to the morphology in the haematoxylin/eosin-stained slides). The effusion was confined within the middle ear cavity and did not appear to extend through

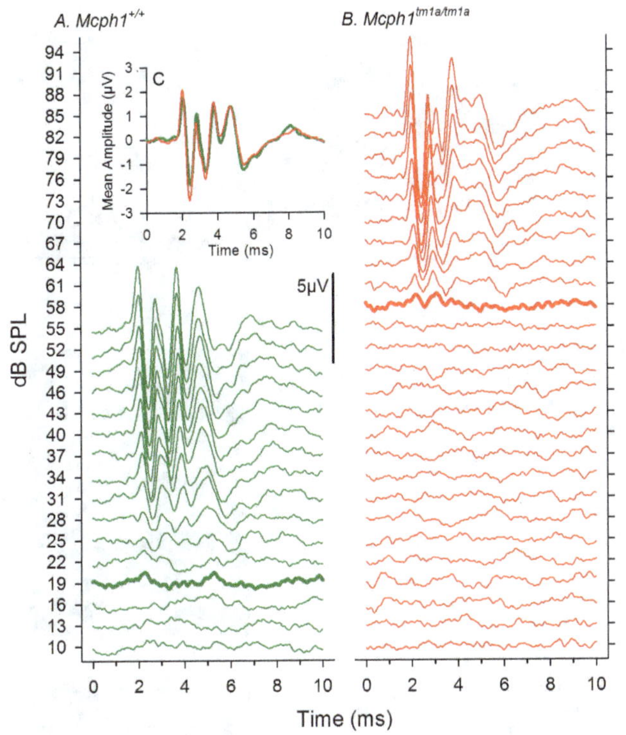

Figure 3. Recurrent ABR measurement indicated the relation between the hearing profile and middle ear defects. (A) Results of recurrent ABR measurement (click thresholds) with age. Hearing impairment can be detected as early as 3 weeks old in *Mcph1^tm1a/tm1a^* mice (n = 13). Hearing profile of the *Mcph1^tm1a/tm1a^* mice showed either a stable, progressive, or fluctuating pattern with age (three of them marked dark). All the wild type (n = 13) and heterozygous (n = 17) mice displayed normal click thresholds with age. (B) Auditory chain (incus-stapes joint) and oval window sound transduction was severely impeded. Normal incus-stapes joint of auditory chain in a *Mcph1^+/+^* mouse, and a clear oval window is necessary for sound vibration conduction. After removing some of the amorphous material in the middle ear cavity of a *Mcph1^tm1a/tm1a^* mouse, the incus-stapes joint (arrow head) and the oval window (arrow) is present but embedded in the amorphous material. Scale bar, 1 mm. (C–F) Correlation between middle ear defects and hearing sensitivity change with time. (C) Normal ABR thresholds and middle ear structure in a wild type mouse: normal middle ear cavity is full of air, tympanic membrane is transparent and normal morphology of ossicles. (D) Progressively elevated ABR thresholds with age in a *Mcph1^tm1a/tm1a^* mouse. Amorphous mass filled the middle ear cavity and outgrew into external ear canal. Ossicles were embedded in the amorphous mass and appeared to have thinner bony structure. (E) Fluctuating ABR thresholds in a *Mcph1^tm1a/tm1a^* mouse. Watery effusion with bubbles was seen in the middle ear cavity and normal gross morphology of ossicles. (F) Stable and moderate hearing impairment in a *Mcph1^tm1a/tm1a^* mouse. The middle cavity was filled with pus-like secretion. Normal gross morphology of ossicles but with rough surface. Scale bar, 1 mm.

the round window. In two out of three 60-week old *Mcph1^tm1a/tm1a^* mice, we saw only a few inflammatory cells scattered in the middle ear cavity, but the thickened mucoperiosteum was still present (data not shown). The Eustachian tube had a similar appearance in mutant (n = 4) and control (n = 2 heterozygotes, 2 wild types) mice in serial sections through the tube as it exits the middle ear (data not shown).

We collected tissue from the nasopharynx, middle ears and external ear canal of *Mcph1^tm1a/tm1a^* and wild type mice. DNA was extracted from these and the 16S rRNA gene was amplified via PCR with universal bacterial primers (7f and 1510r). From this, 16S rRNA clone libraries were created for a *Mcph1^tm1a/tm1a^* and wild type mouse for each tissue sampled. The predominant phylotype found to be present in the nasopharynx of both mutant and wild type mice was matched through BLAST analysis to a previously-uncultured *Streptococcus* sequence (ERD01G accession number GQ456229.1) [22]; however, it was also present in the middle ear of the mutant *Mcph1^tm1a/tm1a^* mouse. We were then able to culture this bacterium from the mutant middle ear by plating it onto a variety of media under micro-aerophilic conditions, thus confirming its presence within the tissue. The identity of this isolate as *Streptococcus* bacterium (Strep ERD01G) was confirmed by 16S rRNA PCR (Derek Pickard, Trevor Lawley and Mark Stares, personal communication).

Normal inner ear structure

To learn whether *Mcph1^tm1a/tm1a^* mice have inner ear defects, scanning electron microscopy (SEM) and temporal bone sections were used to examine cochleae in young pups and adult mice respectively. At postnatal day 4, *Mcph1^tm1a/tm1a^* mice showed normal morphology of the upper surface of the organ of Corti by SEM (Figure 6A). Adult *Mcph1^tm1a/tm1a^* mice showed a normal gross anatomy of the inner ear (data not shown) and there was no evidence of any abnormality of the cochlea in *Mcph1^tm1a/tm1a^* mice (4–5 week old, Figure 6B).

Expression of Mcph1 in the middle ear

Expression of Mcph1 in epithelial cells of the middle ear cavity (Figure 7) was revealed by immunohistochemistry. Before maturation of the middle ear (postnatal day 7), Mcph1 was expressed in the epithelial cells of the middle ear cavity and appeared stronger in the ciliated cells than the non-ciliated cells. The expression was seen in some cells of the middle ear mesenchyme as well at P7. In adult mice (4–5 weeks old), the expression appeared stronger than that of P7 mice and was present and appeared similar in both ciliated and non-ciliated cells.

Smaller skull size with normal skull structure

We examined the skeleton of the *Mcph1^tm1a/tm1a^* mice by X-ray at 1eeks of age. *Mcph1^tm1a/tm1a^* mice showed a similar skull structure compared with the wild type mice (Figure 8A). However, skull width and length of female *Mcph1^tm1a/tm1a^* mice were significantly smaller than those of wild type mice (Figure 8B). The weight of the brain was measured at 16 weeks old, and both male and female *Mcph1^tm1a/tm1a^* mice had lighter brain weight than wild type mice.

Increased prevalence of micronucleated normochromatic erythrocytes

There was an increased prevalence of micronucleated normochromatic erythrocytes (MN-NCE) in *Mcph1^tm1a/tm1a^* mice compared to the control mice (Figure 9) indicating increased genomic instability.

Normal control of *Salmonella* Typhimurium and *Citrobacter rodentium* challenge

Following a systemic *Salmonella* Typhimurium challenge, *Mcph1^tm1a/tm1a^* mice had a similar change of body weight compared to control mice over a 21 day period following the infection (Figure 10A). Counts of bacteria in the livers and spleens at day 21 were no different in *Mcph1^tm1a/tm1a^* mice compared to control mice and the mice cleared the bacteria from the system (Figure 10B). When challenged with the gastric pathogen *Citrobacter rodentium,*

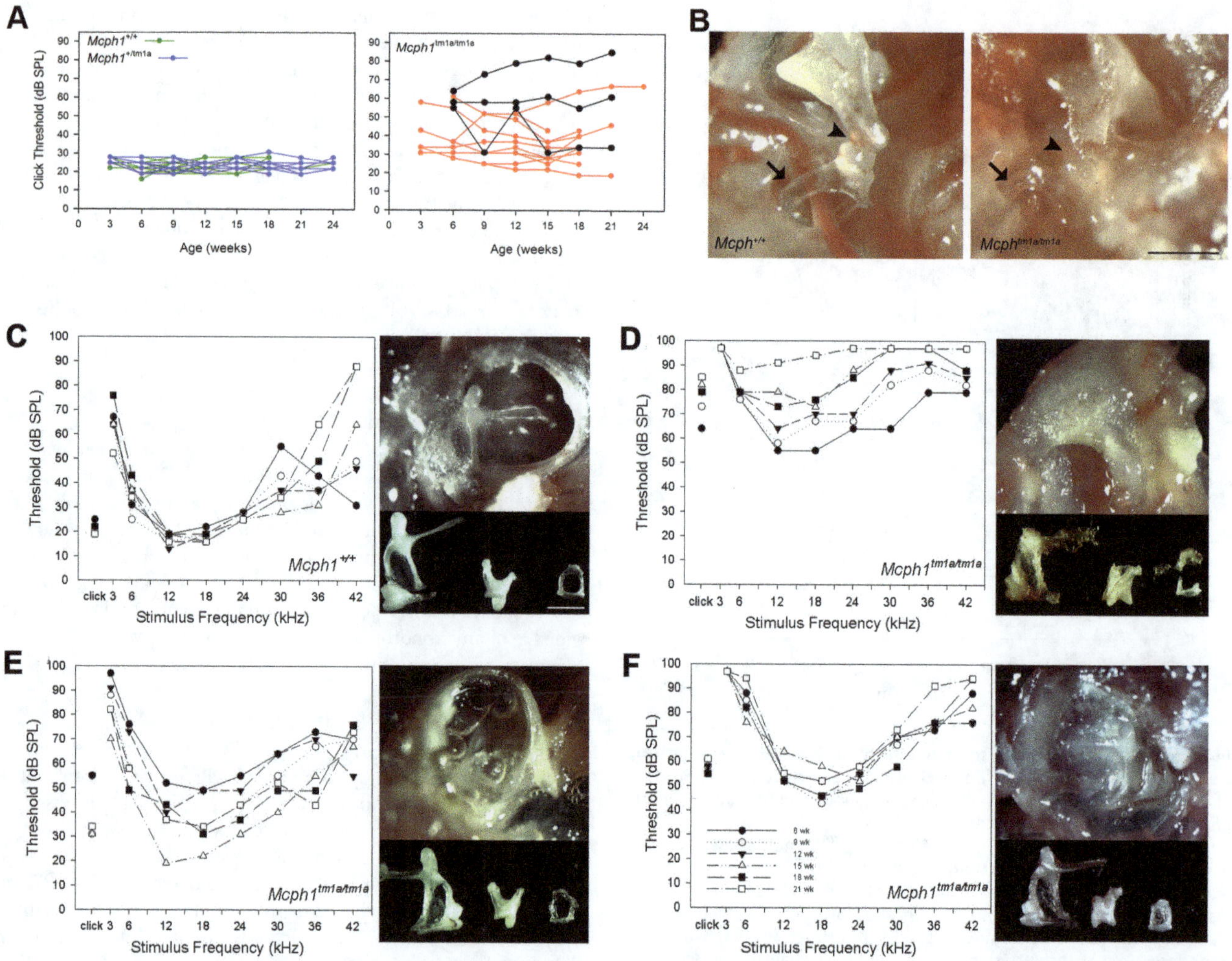

Figure 4. Similar ABR waveforms in $Mcph1^{tm1a/tm1a}$ and wild type mice at 9 weeks old. A & B illustrate click-evoked ABR waveforms recorded in a wildtype (green) and a$Mcph1^{tm1a/tm1a}$ (red) mouse, respectively. The dB SPL of the click stimulus for each response is indicated on the abscissa. The scale bar indicates 5 μV amplitude of response. The heavy lines indicate the click-ABR threshold allocated to each mouse. C. (inset) Mean click-evoked ABR waveforms recorded at 21 dB sensation level for wildtype (n = 8, green) and $Mcph1^{tm1a/tm1a}$ (n = 8, red).

there was no difference between *Mcph1*$^{tm1a/tm1a}$ and control mice in colonisation and bacterial shedding in the stool of infected mice (Figure 10C).

Increased B cells but normal antibody production

There was no evidence of any immune defects or activation after analysis of the peripheral blood leukocytes by flow cytometry (data not shown). The only significant difference was an increase in the circulating B cell frequency in female *Mcph1*$^{tm1a/tm1a}$ mice, however there was no difference in the maturity of these B cells as determined by cell surface IgD expression (data not shown). To test if this alteration to the B cell frequency resulted in any changes in antibody production, we performed a prime boost immunisation with Fragment C of tetanus toxin. However, in agreement with the normal response to infection there was no significant change in antibody level in the *Mcph1*$^{tm1a/tm1a}$ mice (Figure 11).

Ocular abnormalities

A significant proportion of *Mcph1*$^{tm1a/tm1a}$ mice displayed ocular abnormalities including corneal opacity and vascularisation (Figure 12A). Abnormal histopathology of *Mcph1*$^{tm1a/tm1a}$ mice was revealed by sections in the pupil-optic nerve plane including collapsed anterior and posterior chambers, cataracts of lens, and disorganized and degenerated retinal layers (Figure 12B).

Other screening tests

Mcph1$^{tm1a/tm1a}$ mice did not show any abnormalities in other screening tests such as haematology of peripheral blood, clinical chemistry or intraperitoneal glucose tolerance tests (for more details refer to http://www.sanger.ac.uk/mouseportal/).

Discussion

We report here a new mouse with a targeted mutation of *Mcph1* (*Mcph1*$^{tm1a(EUCOMM)Wtsi}$, knockout-first design [5]) resulting in a severe reduction in transcript level of *Mcph1* in the homozygous mutant mice to less than 4% of the wild type level. During the standardised phenotypic screen of these mutants, we found an unexpected phenotype: mild to moderate hearing impairment. ABR thresholds were raised uniformly across all frequencies tested and the growth of amplitude of the waveform with increasing sound stimulation above threshold was similar in mutants and controls, both features consistent with a conductive hearing

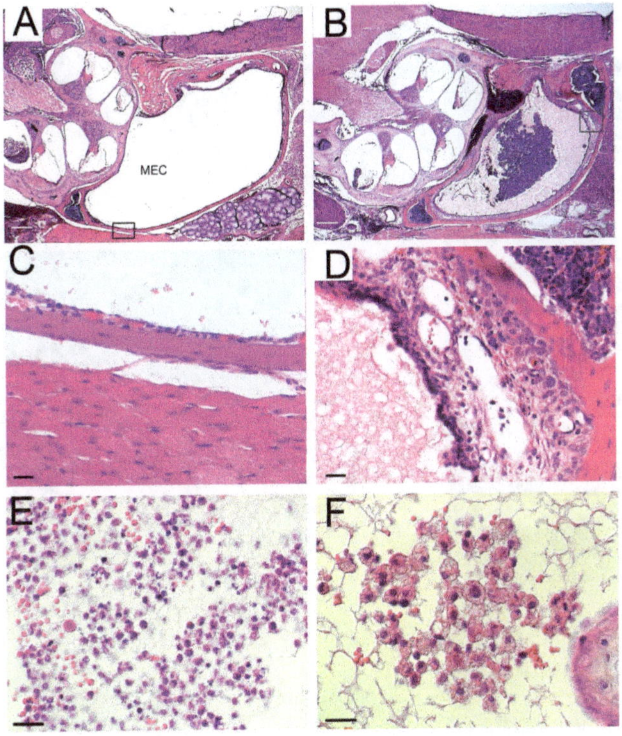

Figure 5. Hematoxylin and eosin staining of the middle ear in adult mice indicated otitis media. Clear middle ear cavity (MEC) and thin mucoperiosteum in wild type mice (A,C). MECs of *Mcph1*$^{tm1a/tm1a}$ mice (B,D) were filled with exudate and lined with thickened mucoperiosteum. High magnification for mucoperiosteum of MEC framed in A and B (C,D). Inflammatory cells (E,F) in MECs. Scale bar, 200 μm (A,B), 20 μm (C–F).

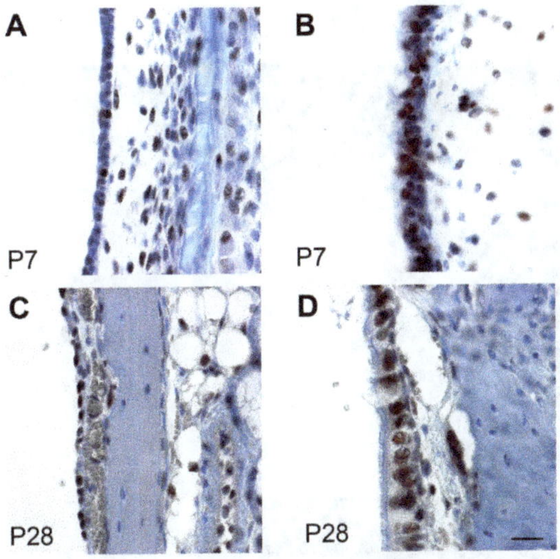

Figure 7. Mcph1 is expressed in the middle ear. Immunochemistry using an antibody shows that Mcph1 (brown labelling) is expressed in epithelial cells of the middle ear cavity at P7 (A,B) and P28 (C,D) wild type mice. Mcph1 is expressed in both ciliated (B,D) cells close to orifice of Eustachian tube and non-ciliated cells (A,C). Scale bar, 20 μm.

impairment. Subsequent ABR measurement, dissection of the middle ear and histopathology indicated otitis media with effusion was present to varying degrees in the mutant middle ears. We found expression of Mcph1 in the epithelia lining the middle ear consistent with its involvement in otitis media. These findings suggest that *Mcph1*$^{tm1a/tm1a}$ mice are a model for one form of heritable otitis media and reveal a new molecule involved in the pathogenic pathways underlying otitis media that can be used to

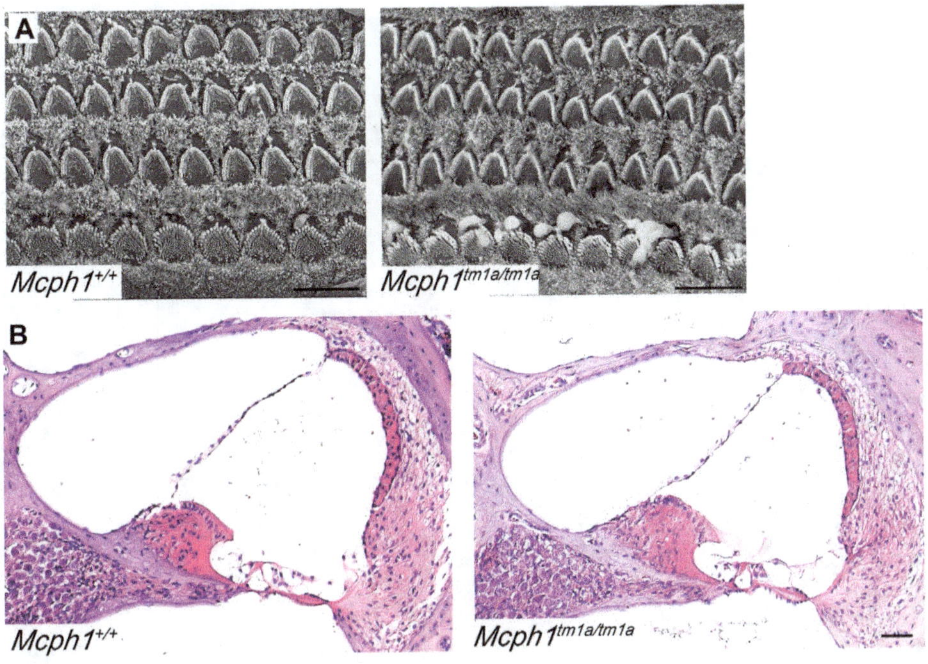

Figure 6. Normal inner ear structure in *Mcph1*$^{tm1a/tm1a}$ mice. (A) Scanning electron microscope (SEM) showed normal development of hair cells at P4 in *Mcph1*$^{tm1a/tm1a}$ mice (*Mcph1*$^{+/+}$, n = 3; *Mcph1*$^{tm1a/tm1a}$, n = 3. scale bar, 10 μm). (B) HE slides displayed comparable structure of inner ears (basal turn) in *Mcph1*$^{+/+}$ and *Mcph1*$^{tm1a/tm1a}$ mice at 4–5 weeks old (*Mcph1*$^{+/+}$, n = 3; *Mcph1*$^{tm1a/tm1a}$, n = 3. scale bar, 50 μm).

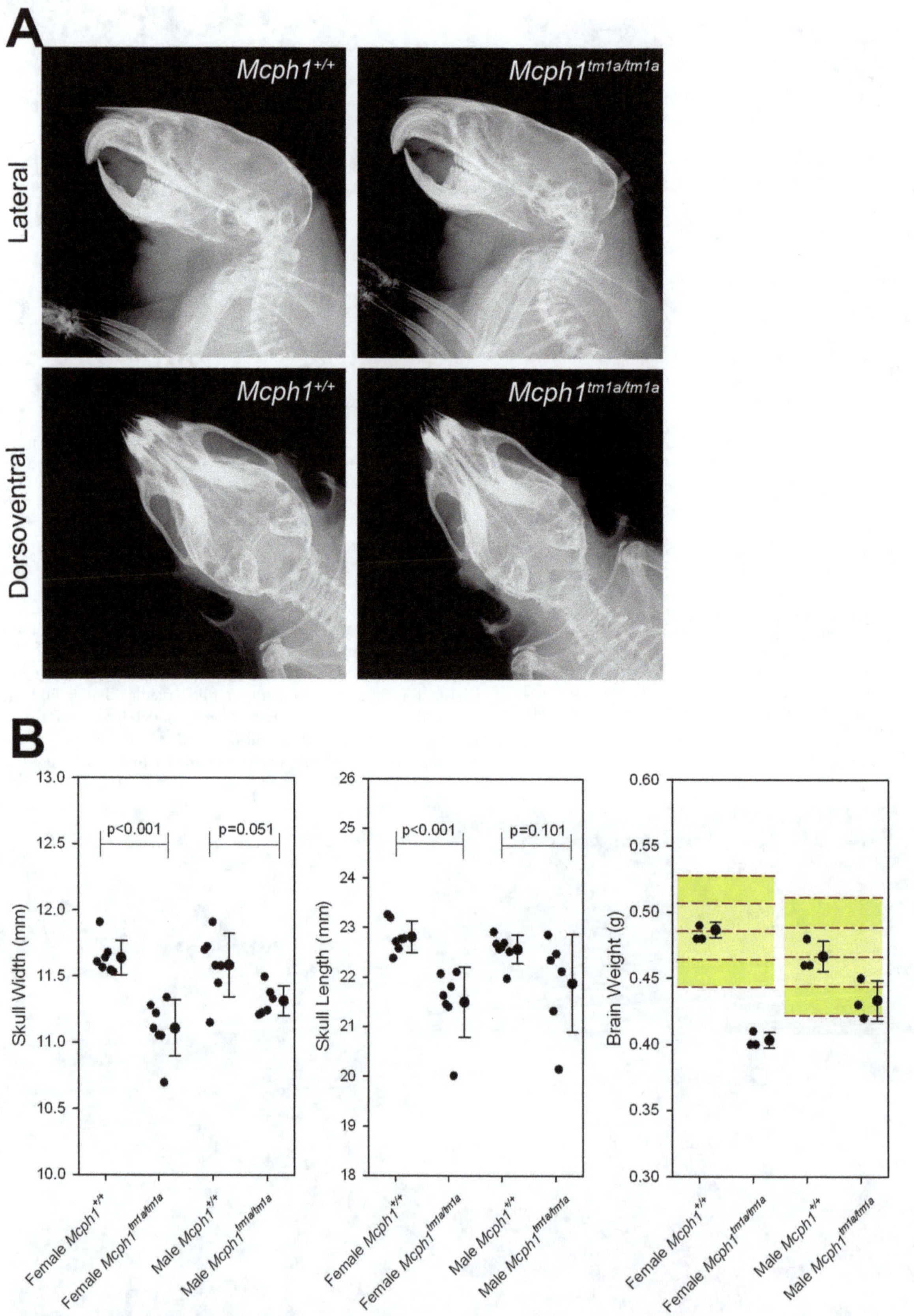

Figure 8. ***Mcph1*$^{tm1a/tm1a}$ mice have normal skull structure but smaller skull size.** (A) X-ray assay showed comparable structure of craniofacial skeleton between wild type and *Mcph1*$^{tm1a/tm1a}$ mice at 14 weeks old. (B) Measurement showed that skull width and length in female *Mcph1*$^{tm1a/tm1a}$ mice (n = 6) are significantly smaller than those of wild type mice (n = 7) (Rank Sum test). The weight of the brain was measured at 16 weeks of age showed that female and male *Mcph1*$^{tm1a/tm1a}$ mice (n = 3, each sex) had lighter brain than the local control mice (n = 3, each sex) and MGP wild type mouse baseline (female, n = 10; male n = 187).

unravel the underlying mechanisms irrespective of the initial trigger.

ABR has been used extensively for assessment of mouse auditory function and can detect moderately-raised thresholds due to middle ear inflammation among many other mechanisms underlying hearing impairment [23]. Compared to using the clickbox, which produces an intense auditory stimulus and can only be used to search for deaf or severely hearing-impaired mice by lack of a Preyer reflex (ear flick), ABR measurement has the advantage of detecting mild to moderate hearing loss [24], which is the expected threshold elevation in conductive hearing impairment. ABR is efficient for detecting mild alteration of hearing function, although some mice with OM assessed by histology may have normal ABR thresholds if the effusion accumulated in the middle ear is not enough to interfere with normal sound transmission. All the mice in this study were bred in a specific pathogen-free animal facility and had a penetrance of hearing impairment around 70%, but there may be a higher penetrance if the mice are bred in a conventional environment.

Previous studies showed that the inner ear might be involved in long-term hearing threshold elevations in OM [25,26] and the round window was proposed as the most likely site of entry of inflammatory mediators and noxious substances [27–30]. However, we did not observe obvious degeneration of the spiral ganglion, hair cells or lateral wall, or serous labyrithitis in sections of hearing-impaired *Mcph1*$^{tm1a/tm1a}$ mice. Furthermore, round windows appeared intact and the exudate was confined within the middle ear cavity. Most *Mcph1*$^{tm1a/tm1a}$ mice showed ABR threshold elevations no higher than 40 dB, which is what is expected in conductive hearing impairment and all tested frequencies were affected which is another characteristic of conductive hearing impairment. Furthermore, input-output function analysis suggested that there is no evidence for a recruitment-type effect in the hearing-impaired *Mcph1*$^{tm1a/tm1a}$ mice, where a steeper slope would be seen and be indicative of recruitment of additional auditory nerve fibers into the ABR wave 1 component with increasing sound levels as a result of sensorineural hearing loss. Thus, the features of hearing impairment seen in the *Mcph1*$^{tm1a/tm1a}$ mice are consistent with conductive impairment. We noticed a few *Mcph1*$^{tm1a/tm1a}$ mice had ABR threshold elevation higher than 40 dB (Figure 4D), so there may be some sensorineural component involved, in which case, the noxious substances may permeate through an intact round window membrane [31].

The Eustachian tube is a tube that links the nasopharynx to the middle ear and plays a critical role in the development of OM due to its functions in pressure equalization and mucus drainage and it is thought to be the main route of infection into the middle ear. Eustachian tube dysfunction can be caused by developmental anatomical anomalies [32,33], adenoid [34] or tumor [35] blockage in the nasopharynx, or cilial defects in the Eustachian

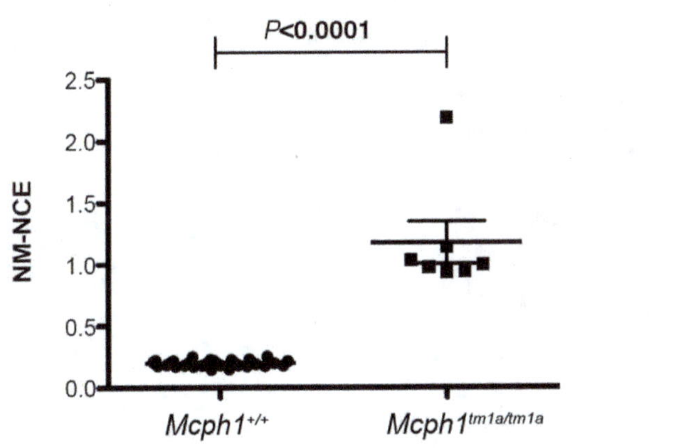

Figure 9. *Mcph1*$^{tm1a/tm1a}$ mice show evidence of genomic instability. Adult *Mcph1*$^{tm1a/tm1a}$ (n = 7) mice showed increased genomic instability when compared to wild type mice (n = 34) as determined by an increased prevalence of micronucleated normochromatic erythrocytes (MN-NCE). Data is presented as the Mean ± SEM.

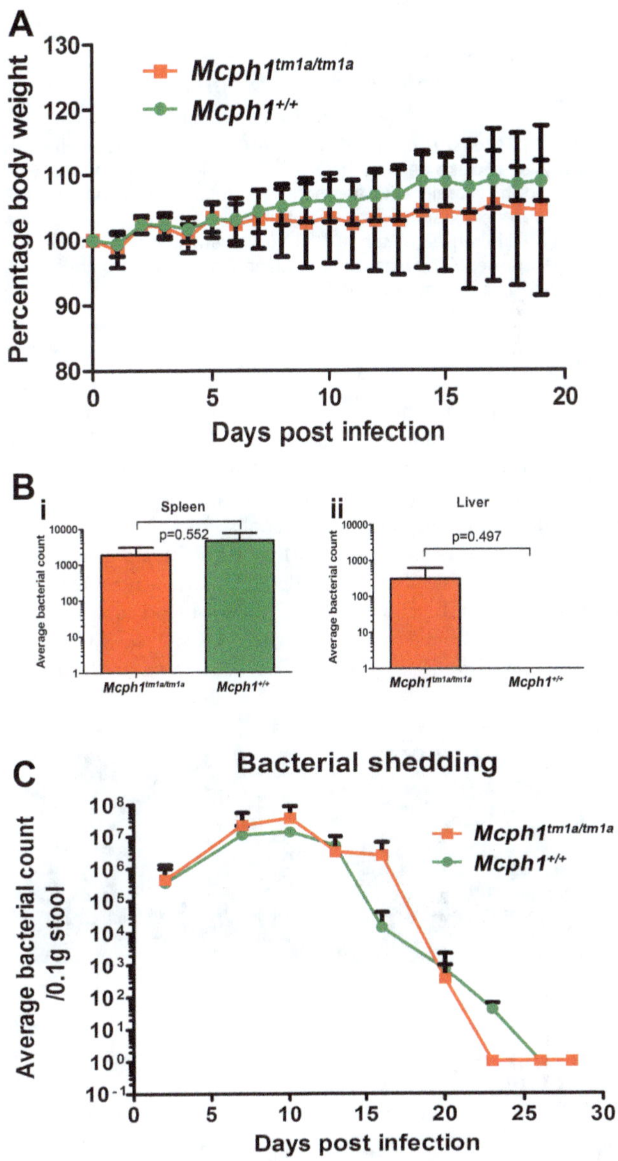

Figure 10. *Mcph1*$^{tm1a/tm1a}$ mice had normal control of *Salmonella* Typhimurium and *Citrobacter rodentium* challenge. (A) No difference of weight change (Mean ± SEM) between *Mcph1*$^{tm1a/tm1a}$ (n = 4) and *Mchp1*$^{+/+}$ (n = 8) mice infected by *Salmonella* Typhimurium and monitored by weight loss for 21 days. (B) Viable bacterial counts from the spleen (i) and the liver (ii) from the same mice infected by *Salmonella* Typhimurium at 21 days post infection. There was only one *Mcph1*$^{tm1a/tm1a}$ mouse out of 4 tested with any bacteria present in the liver. Mann Whitney U tests were used, p (two-tailed) is indicated in the figure. (C) Viable bacterial counts (Mean ± SEM) being shed in the stool from *Mcph1*$^{tm1a/tm1a}$ (n = 5) and *Mchp1*$^{+/+}$ (n = 5) mice were similar over a 28 day infection of *Citrobacter rodentium*.

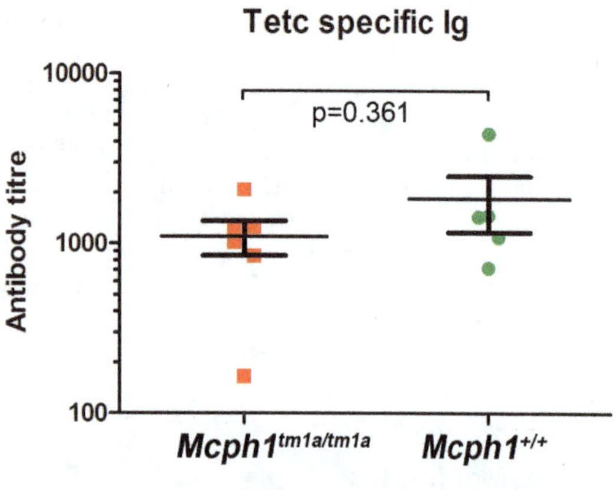

Figure 11. Measurement of anti-TetC specific antibodies in immunised mouse serum. *Mcph1*$^{tm1a/tm1a}$ and *Mchp1*$^{+/+}$ mice were immunised intranasally with fragment C of tetanus toxin on day 0, 7 and 21. Presence of antigen-specific Ig in serum isolated at day 28 was showed no difference in *Mcph1*$^{tm1a/tm1a}$ (n = 6) and *Mchp1*$^{+/+}$ (n = 5). The solid bar represents the Mean ± SEM. Mann Whitney U tests were used, p (two-tailed) is indicated in the figure.

tube [36,37]. We observed that some *Mcph1*$^{tm1a/tm1a}$ mice had fluctuating ABR thresholds, and one possible explanation for this may be that the accumulated effusion in middle ear cavities can be drained through the Eustachian tube, through which hearing can be restored partially. However, we saw no obvious abnormality in the Eustachian tube of mutants in serial sections.

The clinical classification of OM remains a topic of disagreement [38]. One classification divides cases into acute OM, OM with effusion (OME), chronic suppurative OM, and adhesive OM. In this study, we did not see typical signs of acute OM (red eardrum) or chronic suppurative OM (perforated eardrum and discharge/otorrhoea). OME is the most common cause of hearing impairment in children in the developed world [39] and a prospective twin study suggested that genetics played a large role in OME [1]. In our study of *Mcph1*^{tm1a} mutants, dissection of the middle ears revealed effusion or amorphous mass which appeared more like the signs of OM with effusion or adhesive OM. So we suggest that *Mcph1*$^{tm1a/tm1a}$ mouse is a suitable mouse model for research into human OME and adhesive OM. There are no signs of multi-systemic inflammation or any indications of immunodeficiency in *Mcph1*$^{tm1a/tm1a}$ mice indicating normal overt immune function. The only difference was the increased B cell percentage in the blood of female mutants. This observation in naïve animals is further supported by the ability of these mice to control their response to *Salmonella* and *Citrobacter*, which are pathogens that challenge the immune system both systemically and at a mucosal surface. Furthermore, antibody production after immunisation was the same in *Mcph1*$^{tm1a/tm1a}$ and control mice. Overall these findings suggest that *Mcph1*$^{tm1a/tm1a}$ are not immunocomprised and do not display any indications of autoimmunity or inflammation.

MCPH1 protein is ubiquitously expressed [40]. When we examined the expression of Mcph1 in the middle ear, we found Mcph1 was expressed in middle ear mucosal cells and was especially marked in 4–5 week old adults. Four-five weeks old is within the time of occurrence of OM. The major part of the middle ear is lined with simple, non-keratinizing squamous cells with or without microvilli. Ciliated and secretory cells are concentrated around the Eustachian tube orifice [41]. Non-ciliated secretory cells including goblet cells, completely filled with secretory granules, that produce the mucin [42] and ciliated cells are important for the clearance of the mucus. The expression of *Mcph1* in both non-ciliated and ciliated cells is consistent with a role for Mcph1 in the production and clearance of middle ear mucus.

Mcph1 localises to centrosomes [13,43] suggesting that it may affect the primary cilium. OM in *Mcph1*$^{tm1a/tm1a}$ mice may be due

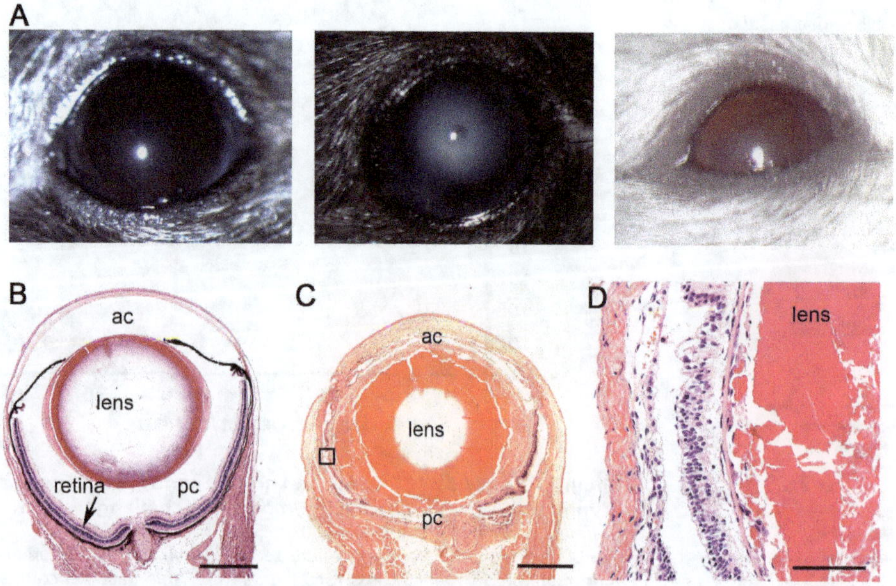

Figure 12. *Mcph1*$^{tm1a/tm1a}$ mice have ocular abnormalities. (A) Slit lamp images (12× magnification) revealed corneal (center) opacity and vascularisation (right) in *Mcph1*$^{tm1a/tm1a}$ mice. The difference of ocular abnormality portion is significant between wild type (n = 23) and *Mcph1*$^{tm1/tm1a}$ (n = 14) mice (Fischer's exact test: p = 0.002). (B) Wild type eye shows normal lens and retina. The anterior and posterior chamber spaces are well defined. ac = anterior chamber; pc = posterior chamber. (C) *Mcph1*$^{tm1a/tm1a}$ eye shows cataractous lens and thin retina. The anterior and posterior chambers are collapsed. Scale bar, 500 μm (B,C). (D) Inset from (C) with solid line shows cataractous lens and loss of retinal cell layers. Scale bar, 100 μm.

to a cilium dysfunction causing reduced clearance leading to accumulation of mucin. Disorganized and degenerated retinal layers in eyes, where photoreceptors have an integral cilium, and male infertility also may be explained by any cilium defects. These hypotheses need future investigation. However, *Mcph1*$^{tm1a/tm1a}$ mice did not display phenotypes normally associated with ciliopathies, such as situs inversus or renal cystic disease, suggesting that sufficient amounts of Mcph1 are available in the mutant for functional cilia formation in the majority of cells.

Very recently, three different *Mcph1*-deficient mouse models have been reported [9,13,44]. *Mcph1*$^{tm1a/tm1a}$ mice in our study had some similarities with the reported mouse models such as reduced birth rate and infertility in both sexes. Increased genomic instability is another common phenotype shared by all the *Mcph1*-deficient mouse models. One of these three mutants clearly exhibited small brains, mimicking microcephaly in humans [13]. The lack of microcephaly in one mouse model was associated with a hypomorphic mutation generated by inserting a gene-trap cassette into intron 12 [44]. We found that female *Mcph1*$^{tm1a/tm1a}$ mice had smaller skull sizes, as observed in *MCPH1* patients. There is a small amount of residual transcript revealed by real-time PCR in *Mcph1*$^{tm1a/tm1a}$ mice, suggesting that the lack of a microcephaly phenotype cannot be explained simply by the presence of residual Mcph1 mRNA or protein. Lymphoblastoid cell lines carrying a *MCPH1* patient mutation C74G (S25X) also suggest a more complex explanation, as these cells expressed residual MCPH1 protein but were derived from a patient with microcephaly [11].

OM or hearing impairment has not been reported in human patients or mouse models with *MCPH1* mutations previously. One possible explanation for this is that hearing impairment can easily be missed in the mouse. Also, owing to practical difficulties [40], OM occurrence in microcephaly patients may be overlooked. As OM has been detected frequently in these mouse mutants, it may be worth looking specifically for OM in patients with microcephaly, as OM can cause long-term problems if untreated.

Besides OM, hearing impairment and smaller brain and skull sizes, we observed other defects in *Mcph1*$^{tm1a/tm1a}$ mice. Similar to studies of other *Mcph1* mutants, we found that *Mcph1*-deficient mice have defects in DNA damage repair revealed by the increased prevalence of micronucleated normochromatic erythrocytes. Eye abnormalities revealed by gross morphology and histopathology present to varying degrees in the mutants implicating *Mcph1* function in vision, but have not previously been reported in *MCPH1* patients or mouse models.

Mcph1 was proposed as a potential tumour suppressor because decreased levels of Mcph1 were detected in several types of human cancer including breast and ovarian cancers [10]. The high level of micronuclei in erythrocytes of *Mcph1*$^{tm1a/tm1a}$ mutants suggests genomic instability so is consistent with a role in cancer. However, the four available *Mcph1* mutant mouse lines have not been reported to show any excess of tumours, although none have been systematically aged and examined appropriately to detect tumours. Furthermore, there is anecdotal evidence that the incidence of cancer in *MCPH1* patients is low [40]. The inconsistency between the reduced *MCPH1* expression in human cancer cells and increased micronuclei in the mice reported here on the one hand and the lack of reported tumour development in mouse *Mcph1* mutants and *MCPH1* patients on the other hand may reflect the small numbers of individuals studied appropriately.

The knockout-first allele which *Mcph1*$^{tm1a/tm1a}$ mice carry can produce reporter knockouts, conditional knockouts, and null alleles following exposure to site-specific recombinases Flp and Cre [5], so the *Mcph1*$^{tm1a/tm1a}$ mouse could provide useful tools for further research to unravel the underlying mechanism of OM. The discovery of a role for *Mcph1* in predisposition to OM expands our knowledge of genetic factors underlying OM. Rapid advances in sequencing technologies have already proved valuable in finding novel OM genes [45]. Undoubtedly, combining mouse models with methods for analysing human populations such as genome wide association studies and massively parallel sequencing will contribute to the long-term goal of the development of preventative and therapeutic approaches for OM.

Acknowledgments

We thank Selina Pearson for assistance with ABR measurements and Johanna Pass, Zahra Hance and Michelle Trudeau Fleming for assistance with genotyping, Anneliese Speak for immunology analysis, MaryAnn Mahajan for ocular histopathology analysis, and the staff of the Sanger Institute's Mouse Genetics Project for generating the mutant mice for screening.

Author Contributions

Conceived and designed the experiments: JC KPS GD. Performed the experiments: JC NI SC CR VEV OI REM SHT. Analyzed the data: JC NI SC CR VEM OI REM VBM DJA JKW KPS. Wrote the paper: JC KPS.

References

1. Casselbrant ML, Mandel EM, Fall PA, Rockette HE, Kurs-Lasky M, et al. (1999) The heritability of otitis media: a twin and triplet study. JAMA 282: 2125–2130.
2. Kvaerner KJ, Tambs K, Harris JR, Magnus P (1997) Distribution and heritability of recurrent ear infections. Ann Otol Rhinol Laryngol 106: 624–632.
3. Daly KA, Brown WM, Segade F, Bowden DW, Keats BJ, et al. (2004) Chronic and recurrent otitis media: a genome scan for susceptibility loci. Am J Hum Genet 75: 988–997.
4. Rye MS, Bhutta MF, Cheeseman MT, Burgner D, Blackwell JM, et al. (2011) Unraveling the genetics of otitis media: from mouse to human and back again. Mamm Genome 22: 66–82.
5. Skarnes WC, Rosen B, West AP, Koutsourakis M, Bushell W, et al. (2011) A conditional knockout resource for the genome-wide study of mouse gene function. Nature 474: 337–342.
6. Jackson AP, McHale DP, Campbell DA, Jafri H, Rashid Y, et al. (1998) Primary autosomal recessive microcephaly (MCPH1) maps to chromosome 8p22-pter. Am J Hum Genet 63: 541–546.
7. Woods C, Bond J, Enard W (2005) Autosomal Recessive Primary Microcephaly (MCPH): A Review of Clinical, Molecular, and Evolutionary Findings. The American Journal of Human Genetics 76: 717–728.
8. Lin SY, Rai R, Li K, Xu ZX, Elledge SJ (2005) BRIT1/MCPH1 is a DNA damage responsive protein that regulates the Brca1–Chk1 pathway, implicating checkpoint dysfunction in microcephaly. Proc Natl Acad Sci U S A 102: 15105–15109.
9. Liang Y, Gao H, Lin SY, Peng G, Huang X, et al. (2010) BRIT1/MCPH1 is essential for mitotic and meiotic recombination DNA repair and maintaining genomic stability in mice. PLoS Genet 6: e1000826.
10. Rai R, Dai H, Multani AS, Li K, Chin K, et al. (2006) BRIT1 regulates early DNA damage response, chromosomal integrity, and cancer. Cancer Cell 10: 145–157.
11. Alderton GK, Galbiati L, Griffith E, Surinya KH, Neitzel H, et al. (2006) Regulation of mitotic entry by microcephalin and its overlap with ATR signalling. Nat Cell Biol 8: 725–733.
12. Wood JL, Liang Y, Li K, Chen J (2008) Microcephalin/MCPH1 associates with the Condensin II complex to function in homologous recombination repair. J Biol Chem 283: 29586–29592.
13. Gruber R, Zhou Z, Sukchev M, Joerss T, Frappart PO, et al. (2011) MCI regulates the neuroprogenitor division mode by coupling the centrosomal cycle with mitotic entry through the Chk1-Cdc25 pathway. Nat Cell Biol 13: 1325–1334.
14. Livak KJ, Schmittgen TD (2001) Analysis of relative gene expression data using real-time quantitative PCR and the 2(-Delta Delta C(T)) Method. Methods 25: 402–408.

15. Steel KP, Smith RJ (1992) Normal hearing in Splotch (Sp/+), the mouse homologue of Waardenburg syndrome type 1. Nat Genet 2: 75–79.
16. Hunter-Duvar IM (1978) A technique for preparation of cochlear specimens for assessment with the scanning electron microscope. Acta Otolaryngol Suppl 351: 3–23.
17. Shima N, Hartford SA, Duffy T, Wilson LA, Schimenti KJ, et al. (2003) Phenotype-based identification of mouse chromosome instability mutants. Genetics 163: 1031–1040.
18. Izhar M, DeSilva L, Joysey HS, Hormaeche CE (1990) Moderate immunodeficiency does not increase susceptibility to Salmonella typhimurium aroA live vaccines in mice. Infect Immun 58: 2258–2261.
19. Wiles S, Clare S, Harker J, Huett A, Young D, et al. (2004) Organ specificity, colonization and clearance dynamics in vivo following oral challenges with the murine pathogen Citrobacter rodentium. Cell Microbiol 6: 963–972.
20. Mahajan VB, Skeie JM, Assefnia AH, Mahajan M, Tsang SH (2011) Mouse eye enucleation for remote high-throughput phenotyping. J Vis Exp.
21. Parkinson N, Hardisty-Hughes RE, Tateossian H, Tsai HT, Brooker D, et al. (2006) Mutation at the Evi1 locus in Junbo mice causes susceptibility to otitis media. PLoS Genet 2: e149.
22. Scharschmidt TC, List K, Grice EA, Szabo R, Renaud G, et al. (2009) Matriptase-deficient mice exhibit ichthyotic skin with a selective shift in skin microbiota. J Invest Dermatol 129: 2435–2442.
23. MacArthur CJ, Hefeneider SH, Kempton JB, Parrish SK, McCoy SL, et al. (2006) Evaluation of the mouse model for acute otitis media. Hear Res 219: 12–23.
24. Jero J, Coling DE, Lalwani AK (2001) The use of Preyer's reflex in evaluation of hearing in mice. Acta Otolaryngol 121: 585–589.
25. Ryding M, Konradsson K, Kalm O, Prellner K (2002) Auditory consequences of recurrent acute purulent otitis media. Ann Otol Rhinol Laryngol 111: 261–266.
26. Sorri M, Maki-Torkko E, Alho OP (1995) Otitis media and long-term follow-up of hearing. Acta Otolaryngol 115: 193–195.
27. Kawauchi H, DeMaria TF, Lim DJ (1989) Endotoxin permeability through the round window. Acta Otolaryngol Suppl 457: 100–115.
28. Suzuki M, Kawauchi H, Fujiyoshi T, Mogi G (1989) Round window membrane and perilymph in experimental otitis media with effusion. Ann Otol Rhinol Laryngol 98: 980–987.
29. Gloddek B, Lamm K, Haslov K (1992) Influence of middle ear immune response on the immunological state and function of the inner ear. Laryngoscope 102: 177–181.
30. Juhn SK, Jung TT, Lin J, Rhee CK (1997) Effects of inflammatory mediators on middle ear pathology and on inner ear function. Ann N Y Acad Sci 830: 130–142.
31. Yoshida K, Ichimiya I, Suzuki M, Mogi G (1999) Effect of proinflammatory cytokines on cultured spiral ligament fibrocytes. Hear Res 137: 155–159.
32. Depreux FF, Darrow K, Conner DA, Eavey RD, Liberman MC, et al. (2008) Eya4-deficient mice are a model for heritable otitis media. J Clin Invest 118: 651–658.
33. Miura M, Sando I, Hirsch BE, Orita Y (2002) Anomaly of the eustachian tube and its associated structures in patients with multiple congenital malformation: a histopathological and morphometric study. Int J Pediatr Otorhinolaryngol 64: 207–216.
34. Marseglia GL, Caimmi D, Pagella F, Matti E, Labo E, et al. (2011) Adenoids during childhood: the facts. Int J Immunopathol Pharmacol 24: 1–5.
35. Lukens A, Dimartino E, Gunther RW, Krombach GA (2012) Functional MR imaging of the eustachian tube in patients with clinically proven dysfunction: correlation with lesions detected on MR images. Eur Radiol 22: 533–538.
36. Voronina VA, Takemaru K, Treuting P, Love D, Grubb BR, et al. (2009) Inactivation of Chibby affects function of motile airway cilia. J Cell Biol 185: 225–233.
37. Ibanez-Tallon I, Gorokhova S, Heintz N (2002) Loss of function of axonemal dynein Mdnah5 causes primary ciliary dyskinesia and hydrocephalus. Hum Mol Genet 11: 715–721.
38. Harkness P, Topham J (1998) Classification of otitis media. Laryngoscope 108: 1539–1543.
39. Kubba H, Pearson JP, Birchall JP (2000) The aetiology of otitis media with effusion: a review. Clin Otolaryngol Allied Sci 25: 181–194.
40. Thornton GK, Woods CG (2009) Primary microcephaly: do all roads lead to Rome? Trends Genet 25: 501–510.
41. Chole RA, Chiu M (1985) Ultrastructure of middle ear mucosa in the Mongolian gerbil, Meriones unguiculatus. Acta Otolaryngol 100: 273–288.
42. Hentzer E (1984) Ultrastructure of the middle ear mucosa. Acta Otolaryngol Suppl 414: 19–27.
43. Jeffers LJ, Coull BJ, Stack SJ, Morrison CG (2008) Distinct BRCT domains in Mcph1/Brit1 mediate ionizing radiation-induced focus formation and centrosomal localization. Oncogene 27: 139–144.
44. Trimborn M, Ghani M, Walther DJ, Dopatka M, Dutrannoy V, et al. (2010) Establishment of a mouse model with misregulated chromosome condensation due to defective Mcph1 function. PLoS ONE 5: e9242.
45. Hilton JM, Lewis MA, Grati M, Ingham N, Pearson S, et al. (2011) Exome sequencing identifies a missense mutation in Isl1 associated with low penetrance otitis media in dearisch mice. Genome Biol 12: R90.

Permissions

All chapters in this book were first published in PLOS ONE, by The Public Library of Science; hereby published with permission under the Creative Commons Attribution License or equivalent. Every chapter published in this book has been scrutinized by our experts. Their significance has been extensively debated. The topics covered herein carry significant findings which will fuel the growth of the discipline. They may even be implemented as practical applications or may be referred to as a beginning point for another development.

The contributors of this book come from diverse backgrounds, making this book a truly international effort. This book will bring forth new frontiers with its revolutionizing research information and detailed analysis of the nascent developments around the world.

We would like to thank all the contributing authors for lending their expertise to make the book truly unique. They have played a crucial role in the development of this book. Without their invaluable contributions this book wouldn't have been possible. They have made vital efforts to compile up to date information on the varied aspects of this subject to make this book a valuable addition to the collection of many professionals and students.

This book was conceptualized with the vision of imparting up-to-date information and advanced data in this field. To ensure the same, a matchless editorial board was set up. Every individual on the board went through rigorous rounds of assessment to prove their worth. After which they invested a large part of their time researching and compiling the most relevant data for our readers.

The editorial board has been involved in producing this book since its inception. They have spent rigorous hours researching and exploring the diverse topics which have resulted in the successful publishing of this book. They have passed on their knowledge of decades through this book. To expedite this challenging task, the publisher supported the team at every step. A small team of assistant editors was also appointed to further simplify the editing procedure and attain best results for the readers.

Apart from the editorial board, the designing team has also invested a significant amount of their time in understanding the subject and creating the most relevant covers. They scrutinized every image to scout for the most suitable representation of the subject and create an appropriate cover for the book.

The publishing team has been an ardent support to the editorial, designing and production team. Their endless efforts to recruit the best for this project, has resulted in the accomplishment of this book. They are a veteran in the field of academics and their pool of knowledge is as vast as their experience in printing. Their expertise and guidance has proved useful at every step. Their uncompromising quality standards have made this book an exceptional effort. Their encouragement from time to time has been an inspiration for everyone.

The publisher and the editorial board hope that this book will prove to be a valuable piece of knowledge for researchers, students, practitioners and scholars across the globe.

List of Contributors

Yoshifumi Matsumoto, Kei-ichi Katayama, Noriko Takashima and Jun Aruga
Laboratory for Behavioral and Developmental Disorders, RIKEN Brain Science Institute (BSI), Wakoshi, Japan

Takehito Okamoto and Soichi Nagao
Laboratory for Motor Learning Control, RIKEN Brain Science Institute (BSI), Wako-shi, Japan

Kazuyuki Yamada
Support Unit for Animal Experiments, RIKEN Brain Science Institute (BSI), Wako-shi, Japan

Diane S. Lazard
Bionics Institute, Melbourne, Australia

Christophe Vincent
Service d'otologie et d'otoneurologie, Hôpital R.-Salengro, CHRU de Lille, Lille, France

Frédéric Venail
CHU Gui de Chauliac, Service d'ORL et Chirurgie Cervico-Faciale, Montpellier, France

Henryk Skarzynski
Institute of Physiology and Pathology of Hearing, Warsaw, Poland,

Karen Schauwers
The Eargroup, Antwerp, Belgium

Norbert Dillier
Department of Otorhinolaryngology, University Hospital of Zurich, Zurich, Switzerland

Simon Landry
Centre de Recherche en Neuropsychologie et Cognition (CERNEC), Montréal, Québec, Canada

Benoit A. Bacon
Centre de Recherche en Neuropsychologie et Cognition (CERNEC), Montréal, Québec, Canada
Department of Psychology, Bishop's University, Sherbrooke, Québec, Canada

François Champoux
Centre de Recherche en Neuropsychologie et Cognition (CERNEC), Montréal, Québec, Canada
Centre de recherche interdisciplinaire en réadaptation du Montréal métropolitain, Institut Raymond-Dewar École d'orthophonie et d'audiologie, Université de Montréal, Montréal, Québec, Canada

Jacqueline Leybaert
Université libre de Bruxelles, Bruxelles, Belgique

Jean-Pierre Gagné
Centre de recherche interdisciplinaire en réadaptation du Montréal métropolitain, Institut Raymond-Dewar École d'orthophonie et d'audiologie, Université de Montréal, Montréal, Québec, Canada

Alexander U. Brandt, Hanna Zimmermann and Falko Kaufhold
Neuro Cure Clinical Research Center, Charité – Universitätsmedizin Berlin, Berlin, Germany

Jan Dörr
Neuro Cure Clinical Research Center, Charité – Universitätsmedizin Berlin, Berlin, Germany Clinical and Experimental Research Center for Multiple Sclerosis, Department of Neurology, Charité – Universitätsmedizin Berlin, Berlin, Germany

Friedemann Paul
Neuro Cure Clinical Research Center, Charité – Universitätsmedizin Berlin, Berlin, Germany Clinical and Experimental Research Center for Multiple Sclerosis, Department of Neurology, Charité – Universitätsmedizin Berlin, Berlin, Germany
Experimental and Clinical Research Center, Max Delbrück Center for Molecular Medicine and Charité – Universitätsmedizin Berlin, Berlin, Germany

Julia Promesberger
Department of Ophthalmology, University of Münster, Münster, Germany

Sven Schippling
Institute for Neuroimmunology and Clinical Multiple Sclerosis Research (inims), University Medical Center Hamburg Eppendorf, Hamburg, Germany

David Finis
Department of Ophthalmology, University Medical Center, Heinrich-Heine-University, Düsseldorf, Germany

Orhan Aktas, Marius Ringelstein and Hans-Peter Hartung
Department of Neurology, University Medical Center, Heinrich-Heine- University, Düsseldorf, Germany

Christian Geis
Department of Neurology, University of Würzburg, Würzburg, Germany

E. Bernd Ringelstein and Ilka Kleffner
Department of Neurology, University of Münster, Münster, Germany

Viviane Baral, Asma Chaoui, Yuli Watanabe and Nadege Bondurand
INSERM, U955, equipe11, Créteil, France
Universite´ Paris Est, Faculté de Médecine, Créteil, France

Michel Goossens and Veronique Pingault
INSERM, U955, equipe11, Créteil, France
Université Paris Est, Faculté de Médecine, Créteil, France
AP-HP, Hôpital H.Mondor-A. Chenevier, Service de biochimie et génétique, Créteil, France

Tania Attie-Bitach
INSERM U781, Université Paris Descartes, Hôpital Necker-Enfants Malades, Paris, France

Sandrine Marlin
Service de Génétique, Centre deréférence "Surdités génétiques", INSERM U587, Hôpital Armand Trousseau, APHP, Paris, France

Fatima T. Husain
Department of Speech and Hearing Science, University of Illinois at Urbana-Champaign, Champaign, Illinois, United States of America
Brain Imaging and Modeling Section, National Institute on Deafness and Other Communication Disorders, National Institutes of Health, Bethesda, Maryland, United States of America

Nathan M. Pajor, Jason F. Smith and Barry Horwitz
Brain Imaging and Modeling Section, National Institute on Deafness and Other Communication Disorders, National Institutes of Health, Bethesda, Maryland, United States of America

H. Jeff Kim, Susan Rudy, Christopher Zalewski and Carmen Brewer
Otolaryngology Branch, National Institute on Deafness and Other Communication Disorders, National Institutes of Health, Bethesda, Maryland, United States of America

Yu Sun, Yu-Juan Hu, Yang Yang, Ling-Li Yao, Xing-Xing Zhou, Hao Wang and Rui Zhang
Department of Otorhinolaryngology, Union Hospital, Tongji Medical College, Huazhong University of Science and Technology, Wuhan, People's Republic of China

Lisa Wu
Department of Otorhinolaryngology, Union Hospital, Tongji Medical College, Huazhong University of Science and Technology, Wuhan, People's Republic of China
Department of Otolaryngology-Head and Neck Surgery, Xiangya Hospital, Central South University, Changsha, People's Republic of China

Wei-Jia Kong
Department of Otorhinolaryngology, Union Hospital, Tongji Medical College, Huazhong University of Science and Technology, Wuhan, People's Republic of China
Institute of Otorhinolaryngology, Union Hospital, Tongji Medical College, Huazhong University of Science and Technology, Wuhan, People's Republic of China
Key laboratory of Neurological Disease, Ministry of Education, Wuhan, People's Republic of China

Xiang Huang
Institute of Otorhinolaryngology, Union Hospital, Tongji Medical College, Huazhong University of Science and Technology, Wuhan, People's Republic of China

Alma Janeth Moreno-Aguirre, Efraín Santiago-Rodríguez, Thalía Harmony and Antonio Fernández-Bouzas
Unidad de Investigación en Neurodesarrollo "Dr. Augusto Fernández Guardiola", Instituto de Neurobiología, Universidad Nacional Auto´noma de Me´xico (UNAM), Campus Juriquilla, Queré taro, México

Huiqun Zhou, Zhengnong Chen, Haibo Shi, Yaqin Wu and Shankai Yin
Department of Otolaryngology, Affiliated Sixth People's Hospital to Shanghai Jiao Tong University, Shanghai, China
Otolaryngology Institute, Shanghai Jiao Tong University, Shanghai, China

Ye Zheng and James E. Arnold
Department of Otolaryngology-Head and Neck Surgery, University Hospitals of Cleveland, Case Western Reserve University School of Medicine, Cleveland, Ohio, United States of America

Qing Yin Zheng
Department of Otolaryngology-Head and Neck Surgery, University Hospitals of Cleveland, Case Western Reserve University School of Medicine, Cleveland, Ohio, United States of America
Department of Genetics and Genome Sciences, Case Western Reserve University School of Medicine, Cleveland, Ohio, United States of America
Case Comprehensive Cancer Center, Cleveland, Ohio, United States of America
The Transformative Otology and Neuroscience Center, Binzhou Medical University, Yantai, Shandong Province, China

Cong Tian
Department of Otolaryngology-Head and Neck Surgery, University Hospitals of Cleveland, Case Western Reserve University School of Medicine, Cleveland, Ohio, United States of America
Department of Genetics and Genome Sciences, Case Western Reserve University School of Medicine, Cleveland, Ohio, United States of America
The Transformative Otology and Neuroscience Center, Binzhou Medical University, Yantai, Shandong Province, China

Heping Yu and Fengchan Han
Department of Otolaryngology-Head and Neck Surgery, University Hospitals of Cleveland, Case Western Reserve University School of Medicine, Cleveland, Ohio, United States of America
The Transformative Otology and Neuroscience Center, Binzhou Medical University, Yantai, Shandong Province, China

Cynthia F. Bartels, Deborah Schelling and Peter C. Scacheri
Department of Genetics and Genome Sciences, Case Western Reserve University School of Medicine, Cleveland, Ohio, United States of America

Bin Yang
The Transformative Otology and Neuroscience Center, Binzhou Medical University, Yantai, Shandong Province, China

Jau-Min Wong
Institute of Biomedical Engineering, National Taiwan University, Taipei, Taiwan

Ying-Chang Lu
Institute of Biomedical Engineering, National Taiwan University, Taipei, Taiwan
Department of Otolaryngology, National Taiwan University Hospital, Taipei, Taiwan

Wen-Sheng Shen, Ting-Hua Yang and Te-Huei Yeh
Department of Otolaryngology, National Taiwan University Hospital, Taipei, Taiwan

Chen-Chi Wu
Department of Otolaryngology, National Taiwan University Hospital, Taipei, Taiwan
Graduate Institute of Clinical Medicine, College of Medicine, National Taiwan University, Taipei, Taiwan
Department of Medical Genetics, National Taiwan University Hospital, Taipei, Taiwan

Chuan-Jen Hsu
Department of Otolaryngology, National Taiwan University Hospital, Taipei, Taiwan
Department of Otolaryngology, College of Medicine, National Taiwan University, Taipei, Taiwan

Pei-Jer Chen
Graduate Institute of Clinical Medicine, College of Medicine, National Taiwan University, Taipei, Taiwan

I-Shing Yu and Shu-Wha Lin
Transgenic Mouse Models Core (TMMC), Division of Genomic Medicine, Research Center for Medical Excellence, National Taiwan University, Taipei, Taiwan

Qing Chang and Xi Lin
Department of Otolaryngology, Emory University School of Medicine, Atlanta, Georgia, United States of America

Georgios Mantokoudis, Claudia Dähler, Patrick Dubach, Martin Kompis, Marco D. Caversaccio and Pascal Senn
University Department of Otorhinolaryngology, Head & Neck Surgery, Inselspital, Bern, Switzerland

Lorenzo Monasta, Luca Ronfani, Marcella Montico and Chiara Barbiero
Epidemiology and Biostatistics Unit, Institute for Maternal and Child Health - IRCCS "Burlo Garofolo", Trieste, Italy

Federico Marchetti
Department of Paediatrics, Institute for Maternal and Child Health - IRCCS "Burlo Garofolo", Trieste, Italy

Liza Vecchi Brumatti and Giorgio Tamburlini
Research Direction, Institute for Maternal and Child Health - IRCCS "Burlo Garofolo", Trieste, Italy,

Alessandro Bavcar
Unit for Health Services Research and International Health, Institute for Maternal and Child Health - IRCCS "Burlo Garofolo", Trieste, Italy

Domenico Grasso
Ear, Nose and Throat Unit, Department of Paediatric Surgery, Institute for Maternal and Child Health - IRCCS "Burlo Garofolo", Trieste, Italy

Concetta Aloi, Alessandro Salina, Katia Perri, Chiara Russo, Ramona Tallone, Renata Lorini and Giuseppe d'Annunzio
Pediatric Clinic, University of Genoa, IRCCS G. Gaslini Institute, Genoa, Italy

Lorenzo Pasquali
Pediatric Clinic, University of Genoa, IRCCS G. Gaslini Institute, Genoa, Italy
Centro de Investigacion Biomedica en Red (CIBER) de Diabetes y Enfermedades Metabolicas Asociadas (CIBERDEM), Barcelona, Spain

Francesca Lugani
Pediatric Clinic, University of Genoa, IRCCS G. Gaslini Institute, Genoa, Italy
Division of Nephrology, Department of Medicine, Columbia University, New York, New York, United States of America
Laboratory on Pathophysiology of Uremia and Department of Nephrology, IRCCS G. Gaslini Institute, Genoa, Italy

Gian Marco Ghiggeri
Laboratory on Pathophysiology of Uremia and Department of Nephrology, IRCCS G. Gaslini Institute, Genoa, Italy

Shi-Ming Yang, Wei-Wei Guo, Jian-He Sun and Wie-Yen Young
Department of Otolaryngology—Head and Neck Surgery, Institute of Otolaryngology, Chinese PLA General Hospital, Beijing, China

Wei Chen
Department of Otolaryngology— Head and Neck Surgery, PLA Air Force General Hospital, Beijing, China

Shuping Jia, Hui-Zhan Liu and David Z. Z. He
Department of Biomedical Sciences, Creighton University School of Medicine, Omaha, Nebraska, United States of America

Emilie Friberg, Catarina Jansson, Ellenor Mittendorfer-Rutz and Kristina Alexanderson
Division of Insurance Medicine, Department of Clinical Neuroscience, Karolinska Institutet, Stockholm, Sweden

Ulf Rosenhall
Department of Clinical Neuroscience, Center for Hearing and Communication Research, Karolinska Institutet, Stockholm, Sweden
Department of Audiology, Karolinska University Hospital, Stockholm, Sweden

Bamini Gopinath, George Burlutsky and Paul Mitchell
Centre for Vision Research, Department of Ophthalmology and Westmead Millennium Institute, University of Sydney, New South Wales, Australia

Julie Schneider and Stephen R. Leeder
Menzies Centre for Health Policy, University of Sydney, Sydney, New South Wales, Australia

Catherine M. McMahon
HEARing Co-operative Research Centre, University of Melbourne, Melbourne, Victoria, Australia
Centre for Language Sciences, Linguistics Department, Macquarie University, Sydney, New South Wales, Australia

Xueqing Chen, Bo Liu, Sha Liu, Ying Kong, Jun Zheng, Yongxin Li, Shusheng Gong, Demin Han and Luo Zhang
Department of Otolaryngology, Head and Neck Surgery, Beijing Tongren Hospital and Beijing Institute of Otolaryngology, Capital Medical University, Beijing, China

Fei Yan
Department of Radiology, Beijing Tongren Hospital, Capital Medical University, Beijing, China

Juen-Haur Hwang
Graduate Institute of Clinical Medicine, College of Medicine, National Taiwan University, Taipei, Taiwan
Department of Otolaryngology, Buddhist Dalin Tzu-Chi General Hospital, Chiayi, Taiwan
School of Medicine, Tzu Chi University, Hualien, Taiwan

Wei-Shiung Yang
Graduate Institute of Clinical Medicine, College of Medicine, National Taiwan University, Taipei, Taiwan
Department of Internal Medicine, National Taiwan University, Hospital, Taipei, Taiwan
Research Center for Developmental Biology and Regenerative Medicine, National Taiwan University, Taipei, Taiwan

Chuan-Jen Hsu and Tien-Chen Liu
Department of Otolaryngology, National Taiwan University, Hospital, Taipei, Taiwan

Wei-Hsuan Yu
Institute of Biochemistry and Molecular Biology, College of Medicine, National Taiwan University, Taipei, Taiwan

Jau-Min Wong
Institute of Biomedical Engineering, National Taiwan University, Taipei, Taiwan

Ying-Chang Lu
Institute of Biomedical Engineering, National Taiwan University, Taipei, Taiwan
Department of Otolaryngology, National Taiwan University Hospital, Taipei, Taiwan

Ting-Hua Yang and Yin-Hung Lin
Department of Otolaryngology, National Taiwan University Hospital, Taipei, Taiwan

Chen-Chi Wu
Department of Otolaryngology, National Taiwan University Hospital, Taipei, Taiwan
Department of Medical Genetics, National Taiwan University Hospital, Taipei, Taiwan

Chuan-Jen Hsu
Department of Otolaryngology, National Taiwan University Hospital, Taipei, Taiwan
Department of Otolaryngology, College of Medicine, National Taiwan University, Taipei, Taiwan

I-Shing Yu and Shu-Wha Lin
Transgenic Mouse Models Core (TMMC), Division of Genomic Medicine, Research Center For Medical Excellence, National Taiwan University, Taipei, Taiwan

Qing Chang and Xi Lin
Department of Otolaryngology, Emory University School of Medicine, Atlanta, Georgia, United States of America

Ramesh Reddy and Rima Slim
Departments of Human Genetics and Obstetrics-Gynecology, McGill University Health Centre, Montreal, Canada

Somayyeh Fahiminiya and Jacek Majewski
McGill University and Genome Quebec Innovation Centre and Department of Human Genetics, Montreal, Canada

Elie El Zir
Department of Otorhinolaryngology, Ho^ pital Sacre´-Coeur, Baabda, Lebanon

Ahmad Mansour
Department of Ophthalmology, American University of Beirut, Beirut, Lebanon

Andre Megarbane
Unité de génétique médicale, Faculté de médecine, Université Saint Joseph, Beirut, Lebanon

Phillip M. Uribe, Kevin Wang, James D. Asuncion, Chien-Wei Chen and Jonathan I. Matsui
Department of Neuroscience, Pomona College, Claremont, California, United States of America

Huifang Sun and Michael E. Smith
Department of Biology and Biotechnology Center, Western Kentucky University, Bowling Green, Kentucky, United States of America

Qi Wang and Peter S. Steyger
Oregon Hearing Research Center, Department of Otolaryngology, Oregon Health & Science University, Portland, Oregon, United States of America

Jiandong Zhao, Shasha Huang, Jing Cheng, Dongyang Kang and Dongyi Han
Department of Otolaryngology, PLA General Hospital, Beijing, People's Republic of China

Yongyi Yuan, Guojian Wang and Pu Dai
Department of Otolaryngology, PLA General Hospital, Beijing, People's Republic of China
Department of Otolaryngology, Hainan Branch of PLA General Hospital, Sanya, People's Republic of China

Bangqing Huang
Department of Otolaryngology, Hainan Branch of PLA General Hospital, Sanya, People's Republic of China

Shu-Yu Liu
Institute of Medicine, Chung Shan Medical University, Taichung, Taiwan
School of Speech Language Pathology and Audiology, Chung Shan Medical University, Taichung, Taiwan
Department of Otolaryngology, Chung Shan Medical University Hospital, Taichung, Taiwan

Te-Jen Lai
Institute of Medicine, Chung Shan Medical University, Taichung, Taiwan
Department of Psychiatry, Chung Shan Medical University Hospital, Taichung, Taiwan

Grace Yu
Department of Otolaryngology - Head and Neck Surgery, National University Health System of Singapore, Singapore, Singapore

Li-Ang Lee, Yung-Ting Tsou and Che-Ming Wu
Department of Otolaryngology, Chang-Gung Memorial Hospital, College of Medicine, Chang-Gung University, Linkou, Taiwan

Tien-Chen Liu
Department of Otolaryngology, National Taiwan University Hospital, Taipei, Taiwan

Yongxin Li and Guoping Zhang
Department of Otolaryngology, Head and Neck Surgery, Beijing TongRen Hospital, Capital Medical University, Beijing, 100730, P. R. China

John J. Galvin III and Qian-Jie Fu
Department of Head and Neck Surgery, David Geffen School of Medicine, University of California Los Angeles, Los Angeles, California, United States of America

Xiu-Feng Huang, Ping Xiang, Dong-Jun Xing and Na Huang
Division of Ophthalmic Genetics, Laboratory for Stem Cell & Retinal Regeneration, The Eye Hospital of Wenzhou Medical College, Wenzhou, China
The State Key Laboratory Cultivation Base and Key Laboratory of Vision Science, Ministry of Health P. R. China, Wenzhou, China

Zi-Bing Jin
Division of Ophthalmic Genetics, Laboratory for Stem Cell & Retinal Regeneration, The Eye Hospital of Wenzhou Medical College, Wenzhou, China
The State Key Laboratory Cultivation Base and Key Laboratory of Vision Science, Ministry of Health P. R. China, Wenzhou, China
Center for Excellence in Low Vision and Visual Rehabilitation, The Eye Hospital of Wenzhou Medical College, Wenzhou, China

Feng Gu and Jia Qu
The State Key Laboratory Cultivation Base and Key Laboratory of Vision Science, Ministry of Health P. R. China, Wenzhou, China

Jie Chen
Center for Excellence in Low Vision and Visual Rehabilitation, The Eye Hospital of Wenzhou Medical College, Wenzhou, China

Qingjie Min
The Institute of Genomic Medicine, Wenzhou Medical College, Wenzhou, China

Yi Tong
Fuzhou Southeastern Eye Hospital, Fuzhou, China

Chi-Pui Pang
Department of Ophthalmology and Visual Sciences, The Chinese University of Hong Kong, Hong Kong, China

Jing Chen, Neil Ingham, Simon Clare, Claire Raisen, Valerie E. Vancollie, Ozama Ismail, Rebecca E. McIntyre, Gordon Dougan, David J. Adams, Jacqueline K. White and Karen P. Steel
Wellcome Trust Sanger Institute, Hinxton, Cambridgeshire, United Kingdom

Stephen H. Tsang
Edward S. Harkness Eye Institute, Columbia University, New York, New York, United States of America

Vinit B. Mahajan
Omics Laboratory, Department of Ophthalmology and Visual Sciences, University of Iowa, Iowa City, Iowa, United States of America

Index

www.ingramcontent.com/pod-product-compliance
Lightning Source LLC
LaVergne TN
LVHW081025210926
848485LV00004B/947